PRACTICE MADE PERFECT

A Complete Guide to Veterinary Practice Management

2ND EDITION

Marsha L. Heinke, DVM, EA, CPA, CVPM

With contributions by John B. McCarthy, DVM, MBA

AAHA
press

American Animal Hospital Association Press
12575 West Bayaud Avenue
Lakewood, Colorado 80228

Find the companion website to this book at aaha.org/PMP and enter passcode XPW213 to download free forms and templates.

ISBN 978-1-58326-172-9

Library of Congress Cataloging-in-Publication Data

Heinke, Marsha L., 1955-
    Practice made perfect : a complete guide to veterinary practice management / Marsha L. Heinke ; with contributions by John B. McCarthy. — 2nd ed.
        p. ; cm.
    Includes bibliographical references and index.
    ISBN 978-1-58326-172-9 (pbk. : alk. paper)
    1. Veterinary medicine—Practice. I. McCarthy, John B. II. American Animal Hospital Association. III. Title.
    [DNLM: 1. Practice Management—organization & administration. 2. Veterinary Medicine—organization & administration. 3. Hospitals, Animal—organization & administration. SF 756.4]
    SF756.4.H45 2012
    636.089'068—dc23
                            2012007075

Aquisitions Editor: Bess Maher
Developmental Editor: Katherine H. Streckfus
Cover design: Robin Baker
Interior design: Erin Farrell / Factor E Creative

Printed in the United States of America

12 13 14 / 10 9 8 7 6 5 4 3 2 1

Contents

Acknowledgments

Thanks to the reviewers of this second edition: Lisa B. Bell; Robin Brogdon, MA; Amanda L. Donnelly, DVM, MBA; Michelle Guercio-Winter, CVT, CVPM; Charlotte Lacroix, DVM, JD; John L. Meyer, PhD; Carolyn C. Shadle, PhD; and Gary Truman Esq. Their comments and additions greatly enhanced this publication. Thanks also to the first edition's editorial board: Laurel Collins, DVM, ABVP; Richard Goebel, DVM; Charles Hickey, DVM; Clayton McKinnon, DVM; and Hal Taylor, DVM.

List of Figures

* Go to www.aaha.org/PMP and enter passcode XPW213 to download free forms and templates.

Recommended Reading

AAHA Press offers high-quality, easy-to-use practice management resources for practice owners and managers. Order online at press.aaha.org or call 800-883-6301.

FINANCE AND MANAGEMENT

101 Inventory Questions Answered
James E. Guenther, DVM, MBA, MHA, CVPM

Inventory doesn't manage itself. This hands-on reference contains expert answers to your inventory questions—from how to compete with online retailers and big box stores to keeping overhead low.

101 Veterinary Practice Management Questions Answered
Amanda L. Donnelly, DVM, MBA

Managers like you pose their most pressing questions, and experts answer them. This handy reference is filled with smart, practical ideas and suggestions.

Compensation and Benefits

Widely regarded as the most trusted and comprehensive resource for veterinary professionals, *Compensation and Benefits* will help you offer competitive packages that attract and retain motivated, long-term employees.

Financial and Productivity Pulsepoints

This perennial bestseller offers sound advice—backed by solid data collected from hundreds of hospitals across the country. *Pulsepoints* delivers the measurements, insights, and tools you need to take the competitive edge and run your business brilliantly. The companion website includes benchmarking tools, simulators, a five-episode podcast series on key performance indicators, and more.

Financial Management of the Veterinary Practice
Justin Chamblee, CPA, MAcc, and Max Reiboldt, CPA

Easy to understand and full of examples, *Financial Management of the Veterinary Practice* will help you establish sound operational processes, make informed decisions, and obtain financial stability.

The Veterinary Fee Reference

The most complete and reliable fee resource available, this reference will help you price your services and products correctly and competitively for your market. You'll want the newest edition for information on how often fees should be reviewed and updated, how to price preventive health visits and wellness plans, and more.

HUMAN RESOURCES AND STAFF TRAINING

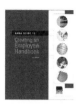

AAHA Guide to Creating an Employee Handbook, Third Edition
Edited by Amanda L. Donnelly, DVM, MBA

Establishing ground rules and expectations up front strengthens your hospital's team. A fully customizable electronic version of the handbook accompanies this guide, where you can access every section of the handbook, choose the wording you like best, and tailor it to your needs. Then simply print out your new policies or forms to create a handbook or expand your existing handbook.

AAHA Veterinary Safety Training
Philip J. Seibert, Jr., CVT

Your team's safety is critical to your practice's success. Get your team on board with hospital safety protocols, meet OSHA requirements, and control the risk of a work-related accident or illness with this two-part award-winning program. Veterinary-specific videos to train every member of the team come on a durable flashdrive, and workbooks for each participant complete this interactive program.

Be a Champion: 80 Tips to Work Smarter, Save Money, and Show the Love to Clients and Pets

Gathered from AAHA-accredited practices, these little tips can make a big difference in your hospital, inspiring your team to work smarter, not harder, to increase profitability, improve patient care and client service, and make the experience at your hospital a cut above the rest.

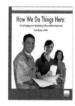

How We Do Things Here: Developing and Teaching Office-Wide Protocols
Nan Boss, DVM

Competent, capable, well-trained team members are the most important contributing factor to a practice's success. Avoid generic training materials and start using this interactive training program that can be customized with all of your practice's procedures and protocols. The materials have been specifically designed for all new employees—regardless of their job position—and they also serve as a quick reference for experienced team members and doctors alike.

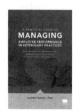

A Practical Guide to Managing Employee Performance in Veterinary Practices
Karen Parker, DVM

Start effecting positive change with your performance reviews. This guide outlines how to provide outstanding reviews that improve communication, motivation, job satisfaction, growth, productivity, and ultimately, profitability. Complete with customizable review templates for every member of the practice team and practical advice for feedback and disciplinary action, this book is your key to managing performance every day.

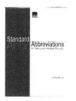

Standard Abbreviations for Veterinary Medical Records, Third Edition

Every member of your team must be able to quickly and easily understand a patient's record. Ensure that communication within your practice and with other hospitals is consistent by using this quick and concise record of universally accepted abbreviations, compiled with input from practicing veterinarians and technicians as well as veterinary education experts.

INTRODUCTION TO MANAGEMENT

What You Need to Know About Management

Financially successful and professionally rewarding veterinary practices result from good management. Good management doesn't happen by accident. It originates in a strong professional and career vision and in thoughtful planning and decision making. Although management may be intuitive in some respects, managers of superior veterinary practices purposefully plan, design, and implement management systems and protocols.

Once a burgeoning field drawing from general business resources, veterinary hospital management has evolved into a specialized and essential component of successful veterinary practices. It is founded in well-educated and skilled personnel. Acquiring comprehensive knowledge and a full array of management skills may require formal education in business and management. Nevertheless, basic practice management information can be helpful to a wide variety of veterinary professionals, including practice owners, associate veterinarians, veterinary students, office managers, bookkeepers, any employee with supervisory responsibilities, and other stakeholders in the veterinary profession.

Why Veterinary Practice Management?

Traditionally, veterinary practice managers have learned about managing hospital operations through trial and error, through supplementary coursework, or simply by trusting in fate to ensure adequate profit. The prime tenet has been "Practice good medicine and all else will follow."

However, practicing good medicine isn't something most clients can see. The tangible effects of good management increase client satisfaction and consequently client retention. Keeping a practice well managed is a little like training a thoroughbred. Simply owning a good horse doesn't produce a Triple Crown winner. Success requires a wise trainer who knows her team and uses her available resources. A systematic conditioning program, superb nutrition and health care, an expert blacksmith, and an experienced jockey are all needed, in addition to the racehorse's veterinarian, to create a consistent winner.

Similarly, a manager must have a broad range of skills and knowledge to run a veterinary hospital well. Financial management, facility development and maintenance, personnel training and oversight, and regulatory compliance are just a few areas of management import. Today's challenge is to become a competent manager in all of these areas while keeping the practice team fully attentive to client communication and patient care.

Good managers are stewards of the veterinary practice. They think proactively, bring creative ideas to the table, follow through and execute directives, acknowledge their own limitations, constantly seek self-improvement, and exhibit passion for and belief in the veterinary profession.

In *The Practice of Management*, renowned management guru Peter F. Drucker wrote, "In a competitive economy, above all, the quality and performance of the managers determine the success of a business; indeed, they determine its survival" (Drucker 1954 [1993], 1). Best-selling author Jim Collins has spent years researching companies, managers, and their teams to discern what makes for sustainable success, or what Collins calls greatness. In his 2001 book, *Good to Great: Why Some Companies Make the Leap . . . And Others Don't*, Collins concludes that business greatness results primarily from conscious choice and discipline rather than from lucky circumstances. One important key to practice success and survival is manager discipline to unfailingly adhere to core principles.

This handbook of veterinary practice management provides information and resources that will support your development of the skills, fortitude, and attitude needed to effectively manage. Your disciplined performance as a manager may well determine the sustained success, survival, and even greatness of the animal hospital you are managing.

Why You Need Management Information

Veterinary practices are no different from other small service-based businesses. Even in a competitive, high-tech, consumer-driven market, great opportunities and potential financial and professional success beckon. The entrepreneurial spirit nurtures a strong competitive drive. Every passionate practice manager envisions a thriving veterinary practice that accomplishes better animal care, more effective employee teamwork, and higher economic return than does any other practice.

Indeed, personal energy and burning excitement support your determination to meet the many challenges of building a practice: establishing a business plan, obtaining financing, acquiring real estate, buying equipment, hiring employees, attracting clients, and actively working in an admired profession. However, all this furious activity can blind a manager to the difficulties that may ensue as a successful veterinary practice grows. You cannot afford to ignore the potential adversities that exist, especially for practices that grow quickly without a solid plan or governance.

All businesspeople encounter challenges that can undermine their dreams. Even the most successful business owner can recount serious errors of judgment or other shortcomings that hindered his own business in some way. Eventual success can spring from the ashes of failure, but surely it is better to sidestep the errors that others have made by being a good student. And, without doubt, too many management mistakes can bankrupt a veterinary practice as easily as they can any other small business.

The U.S. Small Business Administration, citing statistics from 2000 compiled by the U.S. Department of Commerce and the U.S. Department of Labor, Bureau of Labor Statistics, stated that 69 percent of new businesses survive for at least two years, but only half survive for at least five years. There can be many different reasons for business failure or inability to thrive, and common management mistakes are among them. Significant factors that threaten business success have been identified by both the Small Business Administration and Dun & Bradstreet Credibility Corporation (see References). They include the following:

Inadequate Experience. Lack of business and management experience can be an obstacle to success in many professions, including veterinary practice. Most practice owners are doctors of veterinary medicine. Doctors may have years of veterinary medical experience, but formal training in any aspect of business management is the exception and not the norm.

Lack of a Business Plan. The formality of planning forces a business owner to engage in careful and strategic thought about business threats while analyzing service offerings, marketing, fees, financing, competition, demographics, equipment and inventory needs, and more.

Poor Capital Structure. New business owners often take on too much debt. This can be a very real problem in today's tech-heavy veterinary practice environment, which is replete with extensive computer networks, tablet computers, lasers, digital imaging, laboratory equipment linked with electronic record systems, and much more as computerization of medical, surgical, and management functions increases.

A corollary problem is *excessive capital investment in fixed assets*. Veterinary hospitals that emphasize diagnostics, surgery, dentistry, and emergency care often must purchase and maintain high-value equipment. These practices must ensure good utilization of equipment through adequate caseloads in order to justify the investment made. While it is nice to have a wide array of veterinary equipment, a manager has to ascertain all costs of ownership and plan pricing levels, case volume, and break-even requirements on fixed-asset investments accordingly.

Inadequate Reserve Funds. The possibility of encountering inadequate reserves worries many managers and especially threatens practices during volatile economic times. Even when markets are stable, a practice needs a money cushion to self-insure against foreseen and unforeseen events, such as vendor price increases, equipment breakage, and natural disasters. Increased operational costs may result from seasonal fluctuations or from unexpected causes.

Excessive and Premature Profit-Taking by Owners. Excessive profit-taking saps a business's ability to meet emergencies and support investments already made in a workforce. Client service and repeat business are supported by practice reinvestment. For example, owners must be sure to invest continually in employee training and education. These areas may become truncated when cash is diverted instead to profit distributions.

Unplanned Expansion and Overexpansion. Overexpansion can result in overspending, that is, spending that exceeds practice activity and outstrips the operating revenue a practice can realistically achieve within an adequate period of time for client acquisition.

Unsuitable Location. A poor location for practice operations is a common problem. It may be related to inadequate population density for the number of competing practices in an area, poor visibility and road access, and similar factors.

Mismanaged Inventory. An oft-cited cause of business failure, mismanaged inventory can be a significant problem for veterinary practices. Issues can include poor purchasing procedures, theft, waste, and pricing considerations.

Poor Internal Controls and Execution. This issue relates to much more than inventory problems. Management failure in accounting controls, client service consistency, and overall employee cross-training is a common challenge for keeping a veterinary practice healthy.

Lax Credit-Granting Practices. Extending credit to clients who are slow to pay or don't pay at all contributes to poor cash flow. Loose credit policies can result in a community reputation that makes it increasingly difficult to collect and may cause friction in client relations, as well as with employees who expect comparable financing for animal care.

Ineffective Marketing and Self-Promotion. Poorly executed marketing plans can hurt practices in at least two ways. First, it's easy to blow the entire marketing budget on initiatives that do little either to gain new clients who establish permanent relationships with the practice or to expand services to existing clients. Second, in service-based businesses like veterinary practices, both managers and veterinarians often underestimate the importance of personal relationships and word-of-mouth referral, even in virtual communities on the Internet.

Underestimating the Competition. Not realizing that veterinary services operate in a competitive market can lead to apathetic attitudes about clients and slack, irregular service. Clients have a lot of choices, and the Internet has exponentially expanded opportunities for buying products and finding information, even if it is incorrect. Veterinary practices must maintain an edge with expert and consistent information that leads to the highest level of client loyalty and compliance with care recommendations.

Failure to Change. Businesses sometimes fail simply through failure to change with the times when change is rapid and inevitable. Flexibility and adaptation in moving fluidly into new areas of expertise are key characteristics of businesses that survive even in the toughest of economic times.

As this list of mistakes suggests, the most common reasons for business failure are poor management and insufficient planning. If the veterinary business you manage is to be successful, you will have to be on a constant mission of learning and continually use management information and skills to think, plan, and direct your team strategically.

The Definition of Management

The verb *manage* derives from the Italian word *maneggiare*, which originally referred to handling a horse or certain objects, such as tools. This word in turn came from the Latin word for hand, *manus*. The meaning developed further in the seventeenth and eighteenth centuries, when the word *mesnagement* developed in Middle French. It referred to management of the household economy, and later, treatment of other people.

Modern definitions of management usually encompass human relationships as well as the functions of accomplishing business goals. The industrial revolution spawned many leaders in scientific management theory and application, such as Frederick Winslow Taylor (1856–1915), Henri Fayol (1841–1925), and others. The definition of management as "the art of getting things done through people" is commonly attributed to Mary Parker Follet (1868–1933).

Since then, many other writers have incorporated art and science, relationship, functional, and goal-setting concepts into definitions of management. Paul Hersey and Kenneth Blanchard define management simply as "working with and through individuals and groups to accomplish organizational goals" (Hersey and Blanchard 1982, 3).

In all business activities and organizations, including veterinary practices, management means getting people to work together to accomplish the organization's goals and objectives (mission) by using available resources efficiently and effectively. Key to successful management is the idea of working through and with other people. People are your largest, most expensive resource and become a valuable asset in a service business like veterinary practice.

Veterinary hospital managers commonly err by trying to do everything themselves rather than realizing they can accomplish mission objectives through a teamwork approach with others. Chapter 3 explores the topic of strategic planning, including how to define the mission of your veterinary practice and set goals. Effectively working through others may be one of the more important personal-skill goals you set for yourself as a manager, knowing that you have to be somewhat knowledgeable about what is being delegated to effectively oversee methods and outcomes.

Doctors of veterinary medicine are especially prone to the "do-it-yourself" management style. Rather than relying on other knowledgeable and skilled individuals, they may try to become "jacks-of-all-trades." In fact, by insisting on handling the bulk of management tasks, managing veterinarians may give less attention to the important duty for which they are best suited—practicing veterinary medicine. As a result, the management tasks may not be completed as quickly or as adeptly as they would have been if other individuals had been consulted, and the veterinary work may also suffer.

Clearly, to be a competent manager, you must learn to delegate. Doing everything yourself is not "managing." A successful manager knows what needs to be done and, while not abdicating responsibility for the results, enlists others to accomplish the necessary tasks.

The Management Process

Working with others to obtain the best possible results requires an insightful manager who is active throughout the management process. This process has four basic steps. These activities are all equal in importance, and each is present in all managing situations. Ignore one, and even close attention to the others becomes inconsequential (see Figure 1.1).

1. *Planning.* Determining the goals of the business and developing the strategy and tactics to accomplish these goals
2. *Organizing.* Communicating the plan to those who will carry it out and developing the team framework and resources required to successfully implement the plan
3. *Directing.* Using personnel management skills to motivate people to accomplish various steps of the plan through appropriate allocation of resources
4. *Evaluating.* Measuring and analyzing the success of the management process and providing the information required to adapt and modify management decisions

We cannot always make a clear distinction between these steps. They are part of an ongoing workflow process, and so they tend to overlap and do not always occur in a strict numerical order. Goals and activities will have to be modified throughout the process as you listen to employees, interact with clients, and observe how operations within the practice respond to your decisions and direction. A good manager will not be frustrated by such changes but will face them with flexibility, creativity, and optimism.

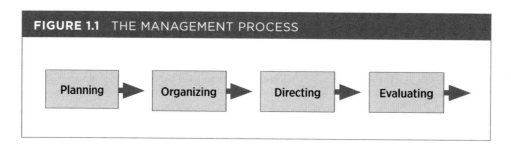

FIGURE 1.1 THE MANAGEMENT PROCESS

Although all four steps are equally important, not all managers are involved equally in all parts of the management process for every practice goal or activity. You may provide little input into the planning function on a specific project. For example, if the practice brochure has to be updated by a particular time, you may be responsible only for the strategic overview and for organizing and directing the project so that it is accomplished on schedule. Understanding your role within the practice will help you to clarify your responsibilities in any particular situation. See "Management Roles" in Chapter 2 for a discussion on different types of managers. We use one term, "manager," because hospitals divide managerial roles up differently, but these definitions will help you to determine the scope of your position within the practice. In addition to different types of managers, practices also may have team members who take on certain managerial roles, such as inventory management.

If you are a manager who is not an owner, understanding your role is especially important. Practice owners must execute and communicate long- and short-range practice planning. If they do not, the practice manager may have a very difficult time carrying out other management functions and processes effectively. Many times, practice owners identify goals but do not communicate them well. Or they may expect the manager to achieve goals using only certain resources and a particular method. If the manager simply tries to guess owner expectations without clarifying them, she will likely fail in her role.

THE PLANNING STAGE

Planning in small businesses sometimes is ignored altogether or is confused with procedure implementation. Practice procedures and systems should be the direct result of planning and not the result of random attempts at management. Successful businesses are goal oriented rather than procedure oriented.

Because planning is such an important aspect of your success as a manager, it is covered in more depth in Chapter 3, as mentioned earlier. You will learn useful planning techniques and goal-setting strategies. For now, we will explore some basic practice-planning concepts that are a foundation for all that follows.

First, you must know how to distinguish between goal-oriented and procedure-oriented work efforts. To understand the difference, consider medical records. Every veterinary clinic has a set of procedures for how these are prepared, formatted, and stored. In a procedure-oriented practice, record-handling may be based on little more than how things happened to evolve. Such methods are unplanned and may depend on individual doctors' personal preference. Styles of notation and treatment instructions do not further specific practice goals, and the system may be inefficient, incomplete, or insufficient for the type of patient care the practice aims to provide. In a goal-oriented practice, records are prepared and stored according to a well-thought-out plan that is based on practice goals related to agreed parameters of patient care, fee capture, and client communications. The difference between procedure- and goal-oriented approaches is compounded when other areas of practice management are added to the equation (e.g., when not only records management but also medical protocols, billing procedures, and inventory management are affected by a particular approach).

Three general types of planning occur in business, depending on the level and duration of the plan:

1. *Strategic planning:* Long-range planning (five to ten years into the future). Even though it is sometimes hard to envision the future in the face of rapid changes taking place all around us, practice owners and managers must attempt to predict and plan how the practice will be positioned down the road in relation to other practices and the marketplace. Strategic planning envisions practice size and location, type and number of clients, level of veterinary service demand, and philosophy and style of animal-care delivery.

2. *Tactical planning:* Planning for the near future (one to three years ahead). Tactical plans specify the steps, or tactics, required to attain the overall long-range strategy. They might include facility expansion, employee acquisition and training, identification of service specialization, budgeting, and the like.

3. *Operational planning:* Short-range planning (for the days and weeks immediately ahead). Operational planning evolves from tactical planning. An operational plan identifies specific steps, indicates who will accomplish them, and ensures that resources are budgeted to achieve the various tactics. Once the operational plan is designed and implemented, a manager must monitor the results and adapt the plan as needed to keep the practice in line with the longer-range tactical and strategic plans.

Whether strategic, tactical, or operational, plans should be realistic and have attainable goals. Usually strategic and tactical goals represent a significant challenge because, if they are to succeed, they must represent the philosophy of the practice owners. Simply parroting another veterinary hospital's goals without considering the owners' philosophy and beliefs is a recipe for discouragement, if not failure.

The following strategic goals are examples of possible practice owner aspirations:

- Produce the best possible medical care and service for patients and clients.
- Provide reasonable financial return for the owners, which will enable the owners to provide reasonable compensation and benefits for employees.
- Provide time for the owners to pursue special professional interests, time to devote to organized veterinary medicine and community activities, and time for personal and family enjoyment.

These examples might not be appropriate for every animal hospital, as owners may place greater weight on other goals to be articulated. Every owner and practice manager must think about how to state goals that truly reflect the values, philosophy, and beliefs that are important to the practice stakeholders.

Tactical goals designed to achieve the strategic vision should include target dates whenever possible. For example, one tactical goal might be to increase the number of patients seen by 25 percent in the next six months. Another might be to increase the gross income of the hospital by 15 percent in the next twelve months. A third tactical goal might be to allow each owner to take a one-month vacation in the next year.

Operational goals designed to achieve the tactical goal of increasing the number of patients might include (1) to arrange three speaking engagements within the next six months with local schools, civic organizations, youth groups, or pet clubs; (2) to send direct mailings to new families in the practice area; and (3) to develop new interactive client communication via social-media venues.

ORGANIZING

The second management duty, organizing, is founded in how well you, as practice manager (or hands-on owner), manage your team. Effective communication skills are a large part of successfully empowering others to carry out various plan initiatives. How well you manage employee behavior and emotions, as well as your own behavior and emotions, often dictates success in both organizing and the next step of management, directing others.

Chapter 2 about manager characteristics and Chapter 4 about personnel management specifics delve into aspects of communication and human resource management to expand your knowledge about organizing and directing the practice team.

DIRECTING

The third step of the management process, directing, calls upon your personnel management skills as you motivate your practice team to accomplish various stages of the plan. Efficient and effective directing requires you to be aware of employee skills, knowledge, and aptitude.

Although it may sound silly, it must be said: Practice managers can lose track of specific employee capabilities. Practice workforces normally evolve gradually. People are interviewed and hired for certain open job positions at one point in time. Résumés, however, may reveal that some employees have knowledge and skills that overlap with other job positions and functions.

Often, managers lose sight of the employees' strengths and potential areas of expertise, and they assign work based on perceived rather than actual capabilities. Team members may end up with assignments that are better suited to another employee, and they may not be given opportunities to grow and develop in areas in which they show promise. As a result, employees may not be as satisfied with their work as they could be.

A good technique for finding a better fit between employees and duties involves regular résumé updates by employees and management reading of those résumés. Assign all employees to revise their *curricula vitae* annually, adding any continuing education classes, special training, and other activities, such as community service, in which they have participated. Take time to read these updates and review your employees' educational histories. You'll be surprised at what you have forgotten about them and how they are adding skills annually. You could possibly increase their job satisfaction, and their longevity at the practice, too, if you use these reviews to refresh their job descriptions in ways that benefit both them and the practice. When employees know you do this on a regular basis, it encourages them to pursue educational opportunities and other interests applicable to their job.

EVALUATING

In the fourth step of management, evaluating, managers determine how to measure the results of their efforts. Although different managers use different methods of quantifying results, there are some concepts that are standard. These four attributes are cornerstones for marking the progress of a business's success strategy:

1. The financial success of the business (financial success metric)
2. The ability of the staff to work as a team (efficiency of internal processes metric)
3. The level of motivation and contentment among employees (employee development metric)
4. The level of client satisfaction as measured by new client referrals (client retention and loyalty metric)

The veterinary practice manager completes the four steps of the management process—planning, organizing, directing, and evaluating—in four distinct areas of activity. Some managers develop deeper strengths in one area or another, often because of personal preference. Truly effective, diversely talented managers are aware of their weakest skills. They continuously seek to expand and improve so that they can be competent administrators in each of the four areas.

Areas of Management in a Veterinary Practice

Following are the four basic management activities:

1. *Personnel and human resources:* Human resource management (HR or HRM) is the management of an organization's employees and includes hiring, training, firing, supervising employee activities, coordinating work of the professional and support staff, and fulfilling legal and regulatory requirements of employee management.
2. *Operations and maintenance:* Operations management designs and oversees the efficient use of practice resources in effectively meeting client demand for veterinary services and

products. Responsibilities include client reception and front-desk management, inventory management, insurance and workplace safety control, and care of buildings and equipment, including computer system management.

3. *Finance and economics:* Business finance deals with monetary decisions and the tools and analysis a manager uses to make those decisions. Knowledge of general and industry economic (*macroeconomic*) forces, as well as local economy and veterinary competitive (*microeconomic*) forces, is an important factor affecting a manager's financial decisions. This area includes revenue enhancement, accounting, bookkeeping, purchasing, debt collection, budgeting, capital acquisitions and financing, data management, record-control and risk-management systems, and compliance with legal requirements for tax reporting and remittance.

4. *Marketing and client relations:* Marketing management is the practical application of techniques and practice resources that efficiently and effectively influence positive client acquisition and retention, while respecting and aligning patient care outcomes in accord with practice guidelines. This area includes developing marketing techniques for finding and keeping clients, increasing public awareness of the need for veterinary services, advertising products available through the hospital, and enhancing the image and reputation of the practice in the community.

We will discuss these basic areas of management in more detail throughout the remainder of this book. You will explore how to apply the best practices in management to a host of areas in your day-to-day operations and long-range plans in order to make your practice thrive.

What Does It Take to Be a Manager?

When you accept the title of manager, you accept responsibility for organizing, directing, and evaluating the behavior of others. A manager leads and guides others while managing the tension between cost and care as well as between innovation and routine. If the idea of taking on these responsibilities seems exciting and challenging to you, you are likely ready to take that step. If they seem overwhelming, you may not be ready to manage.

As you read, ask yourself whether you are truly ready to become a manager. And if so, ask the following: "How will I, as a manager, evolve beyond a routine, bureaucratic mindset to one that is more creative and anticipatory? How will I embrace and advance the wonderful possibilities of veterinary practice without ignoring the day-to-day tasks that are a necessary part of the practice?"

You may be sharing managerial duties with others, or you may be responsible for all aspects of administration. You may be a top-level or a mid-level manager. Know your role. Be clear about the function you perform within the organization. Be self-aware. Understand enough about yourself to discern whether you can fulfill the real expectations of your role, not simply the defined job description.

Shouldering Responsibility

Taking on a management role means assuming the heady responsibility of ensuring business success through the decisions you make. The decision-making process can be a heavy burden on anyone managing a veterinary practice. Managers can be caught between the desire to help an animal to the fullest extent possible and the need to accept the economic constraints that might prohibit the client from paying for those same services.

The veterinary profession is highly regarded as caring and compassionate. Medical, technological, and research advancements result in ever-increasing resources for superb preventive care and disease treatment of animal patients. These marvelous advancements are embraced by doctors and expected by clients. Yet these medical services may be costly to provide, a fact many clients don't consider because of their own health insurance or other subsidized health care. Staying "in the black" can be a tough balancing act, and it is the practice management team that sees the numbers and must ensure profitability.

Veterinary hospital staff and doctors, who often do not have an implicit understanding of practice economics, may unwittingly put pressure on the practice manager to make exceptions to the rules. Trying to live up to the profession's compassionate, caring reputation, these employees may be tempted to bypass practice management systems, possibly because they do not fully understand the adverse financial outcomes that can result from making these allowances too often. Flexibility is often necessary, but as a practice manager, you may also frequently have to become the "bad guy": the one who must enforce attentiveness to management procedures such as collection policies, appropriate fee structures, accurate pre-service estimates, and signed client consent forms. Finding the right balance is an imperative. Otherwise, the practice will not thrive.

No matter how much wonderful, modern medical care the practice team offers clients for their animals' well-being, a veterinary practice will be challenged to survive if it has poor or absent management. As a practice manager, you will make daily decisions that affect the health of your veterinary hospital operation, despite whatever pressures exist. Be thoughtful and purposeful to ensure that your actions result in good outcomes supporting the longevity of the practice. Success will be measured through increasing profitability, leading to reinvestment in well-trained people, advanced technology, and new equipment.

Only if your practice sustains reasonable cash flow through profit can it continue to serve its clients and animals with excellent care, a high level of compassion, and state-of-the-art protocols. As a practice manager, you owe it to the practice, the employees, the clients, and the animals to ensure the success of your hospital by applying good management skills and knowledge.

Embracing Change

As with any professional body of knowledge, management knowledge is not static. A manager learns with experience and assimilates skills over time. Each practical application brings new understanding. Pay attention to areas in which you need to improve your knowledge base, and try to develop your skills with the interest of your practice in mind.

Managing a successful, growing practice requires ongoing attentiveness to both internal and external forces. Change is constant and should be expected. Employee ability and expertise, client expectations and demands, and animal-care technology, pharmacology, treatment modalities, and diagnostic protocols continuously evolve.

In addition, as suggested earlier, management does require significant flexibility. This requirement can present a bit of a dilemma. Veterinary practices must have defined protocols and prescribed ways of doing things that employees can follow so that necessary tasks are done correctly and efficiently. By its very definition, management creates and enforces rules and protocols to keep the practice running on track. Sometimes when there are rules surrounding how work is accomplished, however, people can become inflexible, which causes resistance to new ways of thinking and a failure to respond appropriately to new situations or in the face of change. To be a good manager, you have to lead your team in following procedure, yet be flexible enough to make sure the practice can adapt to change. (For more information on helping employees adjust to necessary changes to a business model and protocols to promote growth and health, see the section "Managing Change" in Chapter 5.)

No magic "shots" exist for any management dilemma or opportunity. Often no clear answer is apparent. Experience and knowledge are good friends to a manager, as is common sense. Any good manager knows her limitations and when necessary will seek competent assistance from others. Informed, intelligent advice helps a manager advance a practical action plan while continuing to remain open to alternative solutions. Be flexible as situations change and more information becomes available.

Management Roles

Veterinary practices continue to evolve in complexity and size. According to the American Veterinary Medical Association (AVMA) Biennial Economic Survey, the average number of full-time-equivalent veterinarians per private practice increased from 2.08 in 1999 to 2.44 in 2009. For practices concentrating on companion animals, solo practices are now less common than practices with more than three veterinarians (Burns 2011).

The practice size by number of full-time veterinarians and gross revenues relates directly to management needs and level of specialization within the management team. Yet even in larger practices, management authority and power can be limited by owner dictate. Job titles may not always synchronize with the duties expected, and the autonomy to execute them fully.

The veterinary profession recognizes three basic job titles, each relating to the level of practice management entailed: office manager, practice manager, and hospital administrator. An office manager has the lowest level of authority; the hospital administrator the highest level.

An office manager has specific, routine tasks to complete and is given authority to execute these low-risk assignments. Office management is generally one of repetitive organization with a "check-the-box" methodology. A person with an office manager title must give little anticipatory thought to management duties outside of the routine tasks of the position. An office manager follows detailed instructions to complete specific assignments given by someone with higher authority, such as an owner or a practice manager or administrator. She will likely be responsible for training and supervising front-office staff, ensuring that front-office protocols are followed, managing the client/patient database, processing payments, and handling customer relations.

At the highest level is the hospital (or practice) administrator, who bears a high degree of authority for planning and executing decisions with substantial risks to the financial stability and success of the practice. For this reason, practice administrators often have ownership stakes in their practices. Few practice owners may be willing to relinquish significant authority to others, which might put their own financial well-being at risk. A hospital administrator, if not an owner, reports to the practice's board of directors and is usually not a practicing veterinarian. He oversees human resources, finance, marketing, and all operations and long-term planning.

The job title of "practice manager" generally refers to someone performing duties that fall in between those of the administrator and the office manager. A practice manager is expected to anticipate and plan as well as identify issues that should be addressed and managed. Yet, performing the duties of the classic practice manager requires common sense and good judgment. The practice manager makes most of the day-to-day management decisions, including financial, budgeting, inventory, marketing, personnel, and facility-management decisions.

However, the practice manager must be able to recognize which projects she can resolve without extensive direction or permission from the owner or administrator and which ones must be submitted for decision making by these higher authorities. Often, the manager will need not only to identify the issues requiring further research, but also to investigate these issues and outline possible solutions, and then to present them to a higher authority for input and specific direction.

If You Are a Manager, but Not an Owner

A nonowner practice manager may have a challenging role as the "middle child" in the hospital family. To the employee, you are the experienced, mediating sibling who leads and directs, yet does not quite possess the ultimate authority of the owner—the oldest, autocratic, and pioneering child. To the practice owner, you are the negotiator, communicator, and pragmatist. You hold the younger children in check through skills that fluctuate between those of a parent and those of a friend.

Another useful way of understanding these relationships is offered by John Sheridan and Owen McCafferty (1993, 4), who describe three key character styles in the business arena: the entrepreneur, the professional, and the manager. In the veterinary practice, there will be interplay among these three personality types. Potentially conflicting forces are in place among the people playing these roles, but the dynamic that evolves may also be positive and productive.

The entrepreneur tends to be an energizing, dream-painting visionary. He impassions himself and the veterinary team with plans of the perfect practice. The entrepreneur can see, touch, taste, and describe the future as if it were here today, and this vision spurs energy, action, and risk-taking. Details of how the future vision will be attained may be blurry or downright lacking. In fact, the day-to-day details of practice operations may simply irk the entrepreneur (ibid.).

The professionals in a veterinary practice are the veterinarian, the veterinary technician, and the ward or other animal caretaker assistants. With a penchant for medical and technical proficiency, the task-oriented and conscientious professional delivers efficient and exacting veterinary care. If an animal needs diagnosis or treatment, the professional will make sure the tests are run, the medications are administered, and the surgical procedures completed. As individualists with intense ego strength, professionals may resist disciplined management systems that get in the way of their art of practice.

The third force radiates from the careful and methodical mind of the manager. As the conductor of planning, organization, and order, the manager acts as a buffer between the entrepreneur and the veterinary professional. The manager pragmatically identifies practice weaknesses, carries out the realistically obtainable ideas of the entrepreneur, and establishes practical approaches to problem solution and goal attainment. The manager develops systems of control that result in a predictable course of events.

Herein lies a potential dilemma for a nonowner practice manager. Sheridan and McCafferty observed how conflicts can arise: "To the manager, the veterinarian becomes a problem to be controlled. To the veterinarian, the manager becomes a bureaucratic meddler to be avoided. To the [visionary practice owner and] entrepreneur, the manager and the veterinarian are precious resources who are recruited to deal with the chore of working for today to accommodate tomorrow" (Sheridan and McCafferty 1993; see also Gerber 1995).

A growing, thriving veterinary practice keeps a good balance of all three forces, even though the resulting triangle can cause conflict. Entrepreneurial spirit identifies opportunities and drives the change that allows veterinary practices to evolve and adapt successfully to the fluidity of client demand and the economy. Professional competency and technical know-how help assure optimal patient outcomes. Managerial proficiency drives successful systems for supporting client service and the professional team, guiding the practice through the chaos of change, which often, in turn, is invoked by entrepreneurism. If any one of the three is missing or lacking, or too forceful, the practice will suffer. But if the balance among the forces is right, then the friction leads to forward movement.

Special Skills of Managers

Chapter 1 identified four steps in the management process: planning, organizing, directing, and evaluating. To balance the needs of each step, progressing from creative entrepreneurial vision to follow-through on details, you will need a variety of skills. Three general skill sets described by Hersey and Blanchard (1982, 5) will help you balance the complexities of veterinary practice and accomplish business directives and management responsibilities:

1. *People skills:* The ability to understand the people with whom you work and what motivates them, given their past behaviors, attitudes, and work styles, and to predict and direct future behavior through effective leadership.
2. *Technical skills:* The ability to apply management knowledge; familiarity with equipment, supplies, and hospital systems; and creativity to execute actions, projects, and plans.
3. *Conceptual skills:* The ability to sense how well your role, training, and leadership style fits into overall hospital operations and how the hospital is affected by and affects its external environment.

The foundation of the first skill is positive leadership, effective communication, and behavioral competence. The rest of this chapter will focus on these qualities.

BECOMING A HUMAN RELATIONS EXPERT

Novices in veterinary medicine are surprised to learn that, first and foremost, it is a people business. Like any service-based industry, veterinary medicine depends on satisfied clients who make decisions about spending money on a discretionary commodity. Client satisfaction depends on trained, customer-focused employees. Insightful veterinary staffers learn to work effectively with people so that the animal receives compassionate care.

The first skill to add to your bag of management tricks is the ability to work with and for other people. Not all people relate well to other people. For some, shyness, lack of assertiveness, submissiveness, and poor communication skills make it difficult to relate to others. At the opposite extreme are highly domineering, egocentric, and irritable individuals whose people skills are equally poor, if not worse.

Any combination of the above characteristics could preclude a person from becoming an effective manager. This is not to say that very shy or very bossy people cannot be managers. In fact, some of the most famous CEOs have been geniuses who were notoriously hard to work with. Nevertheless, in most cases effective managers who are well tolerated by clients, employees, and practice owners are the ones who are able to work well with people. If this did not come naturally, they have been willing to work at it and learn.

If you identify traits in yourself that impair healthy interpersonal relationships as a manager and a coworker, remember that this behavior can be modified if you have enough motivation. Knowledge, training, self-monitoring, and continual practice will support your efforts and your success in the workplace, regardless of the extent of a management role you take.

Know yourself well. Moving into a managerial role will not in and of itself change your behavior and attitude over the long run. In fact, taking on management responsibilities can accentuate the deficiencies you have and highlight them to others. You may have superb technical skills and excel in your current work position, yet without adequate interpersonal skills, a promotion to a management position where you are called upon to lead others may result in failure.

If you have ascended from the ranks, don't expect other staff to automatically recognize your authority. The title of "manager" won't cure the coworker communication breakdowns you may already have experienced. You have to earn respect.

How does one earn respect? What characteristics are important in working with people? Whether you are shy, domineering, or perfectly suited to the management role, you will want to consider two key elements of people skills: leadership and communication.

UNDERSTANDING LEADERSHIP

Leadership occurs anytime you attempt to influence the behavior of an individual or group. No manager can survive without the ability to lead, but not all leaders are successful managers (Hersey and Blanchard 1982, 3). In management, leadership must be directed toward accomplishing the goals of the business.

Effective hospital management clearly requires leadership abilities. Your positive leadership is a consistently exhibited behavior and attitude that encourages others in the veterinary practice to uphold the values, mission, and goals of the practice. Expect to be judged as a manager by your ability to effectively lead others to efficiently carry out tasks and duties that advance the practice philosophy and goals.

Take care not to harm or destroy your leadership options. Veterinary hospital teams tend to be close-knit groups. Friendships form easily as people work intensely with one another in sometimes stressful situations. These friendships often extend beyond the workplace, so that personal life and work life blend.

If you have management responsibilities and also maintain friendships or relationships with coworkers, you may discover that it can be hard to find a balance between friendship and leadership. Some employees will think that you are showing favoritism toward others because you are friends with them. Work disruption and friction between various staff members may result.

If team members view you as a friend and equal, you may have less authority. Employees may have a hard time envisioning a close friend as a leader. They may not consistently follow your directives as practice manager. Your management requests for follow-through on specific tasks may be politely deferred or outright ignored. You may find it difficult, if not impossible, to reprimand a coworker who is a friend.

Guard your leadership authority through a discreet and cordial segregation of friendship from duty, but take care that your management efforts are not destroyed through too much authoritarian behavior or an elitist attitude. A truly effective manager is able to balance healthy leadership behavior and duty execution with true respect for and belief in the other people on the veterinary practice team. (See Chapter 3 for a more in-depth examination of leadership skills and work behavior.)

COMMUNICATION IS CRITICAL

The most important skill for executing management directives is the ability to communicate clearly, succinctly, and pleasantly. Your ability to communicate will have an effect on every directive made and every action taken. Effective communication occurs in six primary ways: thinking clearly, acting appropriately, talking sparingly, listening carefully, writing concisely, and reading copiously (Stockner 1983).

Thinking Clearly. Thinking things through is the first step in good communication. Don't jump to conclusions or react before you understand all of the important issues. Take time to let events unfold. You must have the facts and interpret what they mean before you can act rationally, justly, and with dignity.

Just because you are a manager doesn't mean you have to immediately solve each and every problem as soon as it arises. Don't pressure yourself into making a rash decision. Use good judgment; collect the facts while keeping your own counsel. Know whom you can trust to give factual evidence rather than hearsay or rumor. In some cases, you may not need to do anything more than this. Successful managers quickly learn to let time work on their side to resolve problems, without direct intervention, where possible.

Actions Speak Louder Than Words. The best way to communicate with others is through good manners. Practice simple courtesy, gracious behavior, and nonthreatening body language to gain trust and respect. Employers, staff, and clients judge you not only by how you treat them personally, but by what they observe in your demeanor and attitude toward others.

You can also communicate through the example of your own work ethic. You might arrive before anyone else and be available throughout the day. You might be available on weekends. Or you might make it clear that at certain times you are not available. Whatever you do, you communicate an expectation that others will follow your example. Define what you expect of your staff and team members and behave accordingly yourself. Showing people what you expect by doing it yourself is far more effective than simply telling them what to do.

Talking. Speech is the most commonly used means of communication, and it may seem like the easiest, but in fact it is the most dangerous. Talking too much is as much of a problem as not talking enough.

Important information can be lost in a flood of verbal minutiae. Overwhelmed with auditory inputs, we may remember little of the speaker's intended message. As your hospital grows and the number of employees becomes larger, you will see that you cannot communicate solely by talking.

Think carefully about the information you wish to convey. How important is it? How detailed is it? Is speech the best way to convey it? Or would it be better to put it in writing?

If your communication style relies too much on speech, employers, especially task-oriented doctors, may perceive much of what you say as a waste of valuable staff time and payroll dollars. Employees may perceive it as sermonizing and tune out all spoken information, including critical facts. If you use speech to communicate everything, people may come to resent it as incessant babble. The person at the other end of your management sermon may be thinking, "Get to the point. I don't have time for this" (Crossen 1997).

Effective talking can be learned, with practice. Listen to your tone. Do you speak with enthusiasm, or do you have a monotone delivery? You might need to practice using shorter, more succinct sentences. Make sure you're not speaking too slowly. The human brain can process more than 500 words every minute, while the average speech rate is 120 to 150 words per minute. If your speech slows, your listener's attention may move elsewhere (ibid.). Finally, think about what you are going to say before you say it. Be cognizant of your own body language. A pleasant expression on your face and good eye contact support effective message delivery.

Listening. Perhaps the most overlooked, underutilized tool of communication, listening has become something of a lost art. In modern society, people often feel that it is more fun to talk than to listen. We consider talking to be active and dominant, while listening seems more passive and deferential. We are living the old joke, "The opposite of talking isn't listening; it's waiting to talk" (ibid.).

Yet listening effectively is the key to success in managing staff and client service. Listening encompasses much more than hearing. Listening is the ability to receive, attend to, interpret, and respond to verbal messages and other cues, such as body language (Carlson Learning Company n.d.).

Attentive, careful listening encourages information flow. Putting good listening skills to work increases trust, enhances individual and team performance, and breaks down communication barriers. When you listen, you learn a great deal about people and their fears, needs, and goals. Remember, you have two ears, two eyes, and only one mouth. There is a very good reason for this. Listen up!

In a medically based practice, the art of listening becomes especially important. Like poor talking skills, poor listening skills can cause people to tune out information, which can result in serious medical mistakes. Malpractice suits can result from communication breakdown among clients and doctors, or among team members (Crossen 1997).

Although communication breakdown might result in a major medical catastrophe, more typically it produces relatively small, time-wasting mistakes. Take the example of the receptionist who scheduled an appointment for the doctor to make a farm call to treat a horse. She believed the horse owner to be a longtime client. The doctor drove to the farm and then waited and waited at the appointed time for the no-show client. He finally treated the horse with the help of a neighboring horse owner. On the way back to the office, he found out that the appointment was really for a new client with the same last name at a barn on the other side of town. This client had been waiting all day for the doctor to arrive.

This is a true story. It happened because the receptionist wasn't listening carefully. She failed to solicit key information from a new client because she jumped to the conclusion that she was speaking with an established client.

Writing. E-mail has become a primary method of communicating with colleagues, coworkers, and clients. Wireless Internet connections are available almost everywhere, and the widespread use of smartphones enables nearly instantaneous text communication.

Paper memorandums, meeting minutes, and mail might be lost in the ever-mounding pile on the desk. E-mail is usually read promptly, but, as for any mode of communication, e-mail can lose its effectiveness and impact if overused. Cry wolf too often and deaf ears result. (For more information, see textbox on "E-mail Etiquette.")

Text messaging is rapidly growing in popularity for use by both businesses and individuals. Veterinary practices are no exception to this trend. Texting as a means of communicating with clients and coworkers has some clear advantages over e-mail. Text messages can be read anywhere, whereas not everyone has cell-phone e-mail capability. Additionally, 97 percent of all marketing text messages are opened, with more than 80 percent being read within one hour of receipt (Cohen 2009).

There are a number of ways in which a veterinary practice can employ text messaging. Most practices send out postcards or letters to remind clients that their pet is due for a visit. Why not send a text message, as well? Text messaging can also be a great way to share important information with clients that they might not otherwise hear. For instance, pet-food and animal-product recalls can easily be relayed to your clients through this medium.

Another consideration with text messaging is creation and use of templates. To appear professional and help prevent misspellings, grammatical errors, and a lack of clarity, create specific templates for most (or all) of the routine text messages sent. Templates help ensure that messages meet practice quality-control standards for communications of all kinds. Humans are prone to error, and even something as simple as an appointment-reminder text message can be done incorrectly without a template. In a hurry, an employee can leave out a crucial piece of information, or even word the text message in an unclear manner. Taking the time up front to create templates will help save time in the long run.

E-MAIL ETIQUETTE

Here are some rules for e-mail use, many of which are equally applicable to paper office mail, memos, and reports (Heinke 1999).

- *Consider the purpose of the message:* Is e-mail the right approach? E-mail and other informal forms of communication are usually not appropriate for performance reviews, discharges, or disciplinary action.

- *Research your response before writing it:* If you need some time to do this, respond with something like, "Let me check, and I will get back to you." This assures the sender that you received his message. Then, e-mail a full answer later.

- *Know when to stop:* Ask yourself whether a response to an e-mail message is really necessary. It may be best to let the other person have the last word. For instance, if you receive an e-mail saying, "Thank you," don't feel you have to respond to say, "You're welcome."

- *Think about legal ramifications:* Spoken words evaporate into the air, but written words do not. Like any other form of written communication, e-mail documents what was said. Most e-mail systems save even deleted messages. Be careful what you say or promise.

- *Protect confidentiality:* When you send e-mail, you do not necessarily know where it will end up. What was intended for only one person's eyes may be cut and pasted and sent around the world. A devious person could even alter your words with a few choice additions or subtractions. Any sensitive e-mail attachments should be encrypted or protected with a password.

- *Protect your reputation:* Don't forget that when you send e-mail, it still contains your address in its history even after it has been forwarded ten or twenty times. Think twice about what you want your name to be associated with.

- *Keep it short:* If you send e-mail to people who receive a lot of e-mail from different sources, you want to ensure that your e-mails are read. When e-mail is opened, the most important part of the message should be viewable on one screen, without requiring the reader to scroll down. Keep paragraphs short and succinct and keep the language simple. Avoid run-on sentences.

- *Keep it simple:* Colored fonts and clip art may provide attractive adjuncts, but it takes time to cut, paste, and append these styles and images. If you send artsy e-mail, others may wonder whether you have too much free time on your hands. If you feel you must experiment with artwork, save it for the e-mails you send as marketing pieces to clients.

CONTINUES >

- *Create multiple versions:* Some individuals in your organization will need a long, detailed version of a message. Others will only need the first few lines. Create versions that are appropriate for your recipient list, and offer everyone the most detailed version upon request.

- *Read between the lines:* Might the recipient take offense or be hurt by what you have typed? Because it lacks the nuance that tone and body language give to speech, the written word can easily be misinterpreted. Even in a simple e-mail, you might unintentionally convey emotions or attitudes that anger the recipient. Be careful. Also, try to be forgiving of messages you receive that appear to "cop an attitude." It probably wasn't intended.

- *Use concise subject headers:* The e-mail subject line should announce the purpose of the message in ten words or less (preferably five or less). An e-mail should never be sent with the subject line left blank. This line helps the recipient determine whether the message can wait or should be addressed immediately.

- *Consider the recipient(s):* Who gets what? Decide who really needs to receive a group e-mail. Sending the message to people who don't really need to know the information only negates the impact of e-mails that are truly important for them. It also wastes a lot of time. Use discretion.

- *Check the address:* Few things are more embarrassing than sending a sensitive e-mail to the wrong party. The classic electronic Freudian slip is sending unfavorable comments about an employee to that employee, when you intended the message for the practice administrator. Even with nonsensitive e-mail, sending a message to the wrong address may convey a lack of thoroughness and carefulness to the recipient.

- *Be cautious with forwards:* Sometimes long threads of e-mails develop as a message is forwarded back and forth. Before sending an accumulated group of messages like this on to someone, make sure you really want to send the entire thread.

- *Stop and think before clicking <send>:* Rush to answer an e-mail and you may regret your words later. If the issue is touchy or if you feel annoyed, write the message now but save it as a draft. Review it later. You will probably choose to revise it or not to send it at all because (1) it reveals too much emotion, (2) it doesn't make sense, (3) it contains misspellings or other errors, (4) it is too wordy, or (5) you forgot to consider key points.

- *Ensure that all attachments are attached:* It is a common mistake to click <send> prior to adding necessary attachments, which requires you to resend the e-mail, cluttering

CONTINUES >

> E-MAIL ETIQUETTE, CONT.

up the recipient's inbox with unnecessary information and wasting your own precious time.

- *Obtain your own e-mail account for personal use:* Using company e-mail to send jokes, snide comments about coworkers, or personal letters carries a slight but very real risk that someone else will read your e-mail and get you into trouble. (Even in a personal account, however, snide comments about coworkers are inappropriate. Let's face it: All e-mail you write becomes a history of who you are.)

- *Write important personal notes by hand:* Consider the power of a signature and a few kind, handwritten words. The veterinary profession abounds with cute, animal-oriented note cards. Lay in a stock of these and use them for personal thank-you notes to team members, employers, and special clients. E-mail will never replace the thoughtfulness of handwritten notes when a particularly special message is needed.

Possibly one of the most important text-messaging rules to follow is to keep mass text messages to a minimum. If you send more than two text messages per month to your clients, your practice is in danger of being considered an annoying source of spam. Overwhelming clients with too much information increases the possibility that they will begin to ignore all text messages from your practice. (See also textbox entitled "Electronic Text Primer.")

Reading. Reading is an exceptionally valuable method of improving your own communication, leadership, and administrative skills. Astute managers are avid students who read constantly and widely. Read to stay abreast of what is going on in the community and in the larger business world in addition to keeping up with more specialized veterinary publications. In generalized business material that is applicable to any small business, you can find fresh ideas that you can apply to your practice. The veterinary literature keeps you abreast of key veterinary medical issues, both local and national, that your clients will be hearing about. Reading helps you to anticipate their questions and to recognize new opportunities for expanded services and client education.

Don't expect the members of your practice team to have the time to read much of this material on their own, but do express appreciation to those who bring interesting articles to your attention. Another way to encourage reading is to share what you read. For example, you might distill a pertinent item, paraphrasing it into a short "news flash" that keeps the reader's attention and succinctly imparts key information, or you might photocopy interesting articles for distribution, highlighting pertinent paragraphs.

Electronic Text Primer

All of the recommendations already stated for e-mail use pertain to text messaging. In addition, consider these pointers:

- *Keep text messages short:* Text messages are a means of conveying a very succinct communication (for example, "Fluffy's surgery went well. She is in recovery. Please call xxx-xxx-xxxx for more information").
- *Only send text messages with client permission:* Ask for the preferred means of communication: phone call, text or e-mail. Do not assume that just because a client has a cell phone, she sends or receives text messages.
- *Ask clients if they want to receive text messages:* If a client is scheduling an appointment over the phone, for example, you can ask, "Would you like a text-message reminder sent to your phone the day before your appointment?" If a pet is receiving inpatient treatment, ask, "Would you like to receive a text message, phone call, or both when Fluffy is ready for discharge?"
- *Do not abbreviate:* Do not use text-message slang. Using "2" instead of "to," or abbreviations such as "4u" and "gr8" may come off as unprofessional or pandering (Cohen 2009).
- *Pay attention to spelling and grammar:* You wouldn't want to send an e-mail with "there" being used in place of "their," or "too" instead of "two," so make sure you take the time to prevent those mistakes in text messages.

CONTINUES >

Look for dual-purpose uses for articles (for example, items that can be used in client e-newsletter broadcasts as well as for employee education and training). A third purpose might be citation in practice social-media venues such as Facebook.

Employees should be familiar with information in the hospital procedure and guideline manuals. However, don't rely on extensive training manuals, written instruction guides, and lengthy reports to explain desired hospital protocol or to replace training. It is unlikely that your average employees will read everything you assign them unless you give them some incentive to do so. To share information that is especially important, such as safety rules or new hospital procedures, some practice managers distribute reading material in addition to providing one-on-one training or group training and administering brief tests on the key points of required knowledge.

However, understand that written documentation outlining information such as job descriptions or hospital procedures is a valid part of establishing consistent management systems

> ELECTRONIC TEXT PRIMER, CONT.

- *Do not text-message negative information:* If there was a complication in surgery or a prescription is not going to be filled on time, the client needs to receive a phone call. Texting negative information will likely come across as inconsiderate and impersonal and could lead to lost business.
- *Brainstorm with your team:* Discuss exactly how you want to use text messaging and put strict protocols in place.
- *Keep text messaging to a minimum:* For example, limit the number of employees using text messaging with clients. The more employees who are texting, the greater the chances that protocols will not be followed and that miscommunication will occur. Some clients might receive the same text message more than once, while other clients might not receive a text message that they are expecting.
- *Automate:* Various marketing services provide text messaging solutions for businesses that can assist in setting up automatic text messaging for notices and discounts. Some services even work in conjunction with practice management software to automatically text appointment reminders. The benefits of such services may very well outweigh the cost savings achieved by minimizing employee time requirements.

and organization. This kind of documentation helps to ensure that important information is communicated without being lost, forgotten, or overlooked. Remember that to be effective, you need a well-organized and convenient means of distributing documentation, such as a bulletin board that employees know to check on a regular basis, a practice intranet, an internal newsletter, or employee mailboxes. (See also textbox entitled "Practice Procedure Examples.")

Don't depend on memory (whether yours or someone else's). Document all pertinent facts as well as the reasoning and conclusions that have led to an important course of action. Keep a personal diary of your own business life in which you explore ideas for improvement, goals, discussions, future projects, and present accomplishments. Diaries are an excellent way to keep your personal career development on track and parallel with your practice's progress.

Delegating Duties and Assigning Responsibilities. Knowing when and how to delegate responsibilities to other employees is the hallmark of a good manager. Not only do you have to know each person's abilities and work attitudes, but you also have to know how much oversight and guidance to provide. Some employees will require very little guidance, but abdicating total responsibility to any employee, providing no oversight at all, can result not only in disappointment, but also in serious problems.

Practice Procedure Examples

Examples of effective documentation include:

- Well-constructed and legible medical records
- Comprehensive and well-organized personnel policy manual and office and hospital policy manual
- Clear and concise employee performance evaluations
- Relevant and easy-to-understand employee and client satisfaction surveys
- Well-organized staff meeting minutes
- Error-free computer-generated letters and messages
- Simple notes to employees, management, or clients

Delegation of responsibility implies empowerment. When you empower people to make decisions, you also empower them to make mistakes. No one can succeed unless they sometimes fail, but failures can be costly unless you can control the level of failure. If you control the level of failure too much, however, you restrict the ability of the person to perform.

Delegating management duties to a nonmanagement employee can liberate you for other tasks, but the expense can be high. You need to understand the intense level of responsibility you have as a manager of other people in the practice.

Too much willingness to empower without the appropriate level of oversight can result in bankruptcy. This is especially true if you empower the wrong people. Oversight is managed consistently through systems of internal control. Internal control is the responsibility of owners and managers and cannot be delegated. You might assign nonmanagerial employees, for example, the responsibility for tasks such as drug and supply ordering or reconciling the daily receipts; but you should always have the override and keep an eye on the results. Without oversight, serious problems can occur.

For example, say a nonmanagerial employee is given the authority to make purchases, but because of a friendship with a particular vendor, he makes purchasing decisions that are based on affinity toward that salesperson rather than on cold, hard logic about cost. Perhaps Joseph, the office assistant, has the authority to purchase office supplies. This task is not supervised. Susceptible to romantic overtures from the sales rep, Joseph tends to order the most expensive, brand-name toner cartridges from the sales rep. Over time, this costs the practice quite a bit of money. Or imagine a case where an employee is responsible for making sure that reminders are sent to clients on a scheduled basis, but he fails to complete the task. The manager thought it was being handled, so she did not follow up. The problem may not be discovered until so many clients are missing appointments that someone begins to investigate.

Working closely with different individuals over time, you will come to know whom you can rely on to follow through on work assignments with a minimum of oversight. Competent, self-motivated employees will chafe under too much oversight, which they may perceive as micromanagement or distrust. Achieving the correct balance is an ongoing management challenge that requires good people skills and intuition.

Empowerment tends to become a reflection of economic well-being. The busier a practice, the more willing the owner is to empower the manager, and in turn, the more willing the manager is to empower other personnel. The less busy the practice, the less willingness there is to empower.

When you do assign tasks or projects, give adequate information to the employee and detail the resources available. Sketch out exactly what you want accomplished. The assigned personnel should fully understand:

- Why the activity is needed
- What the goal or desired outcome is
- Who is responsible for each task
- What resources are available
- When to ask for permission to change the procedure or request additional resources
- When and how to report progress or results to you (set specific dates)
- How much time is allotted for the assigned task or project
- What the deadlines are

Keep a tickler system to remind you which tasks have been delegated, to whom, and when to check up on them. As a practice manager, you will need to monitor your own responsibilities and accountability as well.

Behavioral Competency and Professionalism. Leadership and communication skills are outward manifestations of a manager's professionalism. The sum total of a person's demeanor, body language, communication style, interpersonal relationship skills, and other work-life behaviors can be a predictor of success in a management role.

A high level of behavioral aptitude is required of managers. You will need to hone skills related to your awareness of other people's emotions as well as your own and your ability to manage them and relate to people in positive ways. Many authors who write about a manager's skill in this area call it emotional intelligence, referring to a conceptual framework for identifying, assessing, and managing these emotions. "EQ" is as important as "IQ" when it comes to managing your practice team.

Certified Veterinary Practice Manager (CVPM) Recommendation Form

1. Ability to command respect
    a. Captures the respect and trust of others.
    b. Group members look to him for guidance.
    c. Is a source of motivation for others.
2. Supervisory skills
    a. Sets clear performance standards for people he supervises.
    b. Provides guidance and direction to subordinates.
    c. Delegates work tasks effectively to competent employees.
3. Ability to follow through on projects
    a. Finds the necessary resources to complete tasks.
    b. Completes tasks quickly and effectively.
    c. Does what is necessary to get the job done well.
4. Ability to be self-motivated
    a. Meets predetermined targets and deadlines.
    b. Effectively organizes and prioritizes work tasks.
    c. Keeps pushing to succeed in the face of obstacles.
    d. Takes initiative on projects.
5. Communication skills
    a. Presents messages clearly and forcefully when speaking to others.
    b. Speaks in clear and articulate manner.
    c. Gives full attention to what others are saying.
6. Ability to control emotions
    a. Keeps his emotions in check.
    b. Hides his anger and frustration in front of others.
    c. Accepts criticism from others in a calm manner.

Behavioral competency is such an important aspect of a manager's* job description that to be certified as a veterinary practice manager, candidates must be able to establish baseline proficiency in six key behavioral areas. The first five areas are the behavioral abilities to com-

* Veterinary managers can beecome certified by the Veterinary Hospital Managers Association (VHMA), a process, according to the VHMA, born out of "the increasing need among veterinarians and practice managers for a program that would qualify the knowledge and experience necessary to successfully manage veterinarian practices."

mand respect, to delegate, to follow through on projects, to be self-motivated, and to control personal emotions. Communication skills round out the essential competencies. (See textbox, "Certified Veterinary Practice Manager (CVPM) Recommendation Form.")

We will look in more detail at behavioral styles in management in Chapter 4.

Acquiring Skills and Information

Whether you need resources for training others or for enhancing your own skills, there are many tools at your disposal. We will outline a few of them here (see also "Additional Resources" at the end of this book).

EXPERIENCE

The most effective way to develop management skills is through experience. Experiential knowledge gained by working with or for an experienced manager will offer more than all of the books and magazine articles ever written on the subject. Experience on its own, however, is not an effective teacher. An old saying criticizes the person who has worked for twenty years but has only reexperienced the first year twenty times over. You learn from experience only if it allows you to make tentative generalizations as a guide, which you then test against every new experience.

Another good way to acquire management skills is to observe the mistakes of others and learn from them (Gaedeke and Tootelian 1985, 32). When you see others using strategies that are not working, try to understand why they are not working. The Veterinary Hospital Managers Association (VHMA) recognizes the value of both experience and observation. Many of the VHMA-sponsored management meetings feature roundtable discussions in which practice managers discuss problems they have experienced and mistakes they have made and find insights in the group's broad experience.

Any manager, experienced or not, must always be on the lookout for new ways to accomplish goals. Sometimes, old ideas can be applied to new problems; other times, new ideas can be applied to old problems. Always stay open to new ideas, but be sensible about implementation. Weigh every new idea against its cost, against its potential effectiveness in improving the standard of patient care, and against client willingness to pay. Remember, your practice is not a democracy. You are not obligated to implement every new idea suggested by employees or touted in the press.

TRAINING

Variety is the key to a manager's quest for new skills. If you just studied books on management, but did not attend any classes or seminars, your training would be lacking. Likewise, if you only attended classes and seminars, or watched videos, but refused to read books on management by the best in the field, your training would also be lacking. You may even become bored with your training because of the repetition. Vary your learning modalities, and you will continue to make gains in knowledge.

In addition to books, CDs, videos, and Internet materials, watch for lectures, conferences, and workshops that are geared to your areas of management weakness. Attend lectures and seminars that focus on topics specific to animal hospitals, where you will meet and network with other managers who share similar problems. Meet with your colleagues at management conferences to brainstorm for solutions to common practice issues.

Reassess your management skills and weaknesses on a regular basis. Keep pushing yourself to advance. If you are a practice manager and have not done so already, for example, consider applying for examination as a certified veterinary practice manager (CVPM). Applying for examination requires you to have experience in a wide variety of general practice responsibilities. The application process itself is a valuable learning experience and will help you take stock of your skills.

Local community colleges provide an economical method of enhancing your formal education. Courses in several disciplines will help you gain management skills, even though they are not specifically tailored to veterinary hospital management. (See textbox, "Courses on Management.")

Focus on education that enhances your value to the practice and the profession. Veterinary practice management can be a lifelong career. The demand has never been higher for qualified individuals with the right attitude and vision. You owe it to yourself to keep expanding your talents beyond what your current employment situation demands. You never know when you might be moving on to a new exciting opportunity.

OTHER RESOURCES

There are many tools to help you stay aware of laws and regulations affecting veterinary practice, especially those pertaining to personnel. However, it is also important to develop strong relationships with a competent accounting firm and a law firm with special interest in small, closely held businesses. The practice CPA and attorney should be trusted advisers with whom you can consult on a regular basis. (See Chapter 11 for more information on choosing an accountant.)

A well-versed, successful manager will be familiar with several management-oriented periodicals. Maintain membership in groups that share solutions for management headaches. The VHMA and the American Animal Hospital Association (AAHA) are excellent choices.

To find veterinary practice management books and aids to add to your library, start with the AAHA Press. Lifelearn, Veterinary Economics, Wiley-Blackwell, and Elsevier also publish books on veterinary practice management. Internet newsletters from Advanstar (dvm360.com)

Courses on Management

Taking courses can introduce you to valuable knowledge and give you new ideas for solving management problems and inspiring your team. Consider the following pertinent disciplines and courses:

- **Accounting**
  - » Introduction to Accounting
  - » Principles of Accounting
  - » Financial Statement Analysis
  - » Management Accounting
  - » Business Income Taxation
  - » Intermediate Accounting
  - » Advanced Accounting
  - » Statistics
- **Economics/Finance**
  - » Basic Economics
  - » Introduction to Finance
  - » Principles of Finance
  - » Financial Decisions
  - » Investments
  - » Business Finance
  - » Banking
- **Computer Science**
  - » Introduction to Computers
  - » Computer Programming
  - » Data Processing
  - » Systems Analysis
- **Marketing**
  - » Introduction to Marketing
  - » Marketing Principles
  - » Market Research
  - » Methods of Marketing
  - » Consumer Behavior
  - » Advertising
  - » Marketing Policy

CONTINUES >

> COURSES ON MANAGEMENT, CONT.

- **Management**
  - » Introduction to Management
  - » Business Ethics
  - » Strategic Planning
  - » Entrepreneurship
  - » Communication
- **Labor Relations and Human Resources**
  - » English
  - » Speech
  - » Personnel Administration
  - » Labor Relations
  - » Behavioral Problem Solving
  - » Human Resource Management
  - » Introduction to Psychology
  - » Psychology of Personnel Management
  - » Managerial Leadership
  - » Personnel Training
  - » Performance Appraisals
- **Law/Taxation**
  - » Business Law
  - » Introduction to Taxation
  - » Business Taxation
  - » Tax Principles
  - » Federal Income Taxation

contain good information, as do the newsletters from the North American Veterinary Conference (see My Exceptional Veterinary Team at http://myevt.com/). But don't stop with veterinary management books. Cross over into the general business realm to explore your options. The list of additional resources at the end of this book suggests books, periodicals, videotape s, training programs, practice aid resources, websites, and other relevant resources. This list, though by no means comprehensive, will help you to identify opportunities for education and continuing education in management. Delve into these resources as much as possible, and you will find yourself growing in your management skills and in your career.

As you grow as a manager, you will find that there is always more to learn. As you seek to be the best manager you can be, you will hone your interpersonal skills. Your problem-solving skills will increase. You will learn how to plan and set goals in many different areas, and you will learn how to reach these goals while motivating others to do the same. It's a career that has great potential for personal and professional fulfillment.

3

Strategic Planning

The management process, as discussed in Chapter 1, involves planning, organizing, directing, and evaluating. These are the four fundamentals of management, and each is necessary to a successful practice. This chapter zeroes in on the planning stage, with an emphasis on strategic planning. The success of the organizing, directing, and evaluating stages depends on how well you plan. The models and frameworks described in this chapter will help you to develop strategy, tactics, and operational management objectives, right down to making goals and evaluating progress.

Business management understanding has evolved over the past one hundred years in ways that apply to the conduct of veterinary medicine in a practice setting. Using these models from the outset in the planning stage will help you to be a more effective manager. Strategic planning frameworks help you design roadmaps to follow for the entire management process.

In fact, it can be helpful to think of the management of a veterinary practice as a journey. As in a journey, in veterinary practice you must have an overall destination; otherwise you are only engaging in aimless wandering. And, as in a journey, in veterinary practice you will reach the destination step by step. We will use this analogy throughout the chapter (see textbox, "Management As a Journey"). Before getting started on your practice management journey, you will need to pack some good planning concepts and tools.

Thinking Strategically

Veterinary consultants and practice owners have long recognized several weaknesses in veterinary practice management. These areas continue to present challenges, despite the attention and recognition they have received. Two of these areas are strategic planning and evaluation of progress.

In fact, strategic planning is often missing entirely in practice management. However, it is possible to apply ideas from outside the veterinary profession to repair this shortcoming. To use the journey analogy, the strategic plan is a roadmap showing the steps you will take on

Management As a Journey

Management models often correlate well with the concept of a journey. Here are some examples of how the analogy works:

Journey: A three-part process with a beginning; day-by-day, week-by-week, and year-by-year progress, reached by means of a strategy and tactical goals; and an ultimate destination.

Ultimate destination: The vision you have of veterinary medicine and your practice. It involves not only vision but also strategy and mission.

Daily destination: On-time delivery of client value (value chain model).

Roadmaps: The strategic plan, tactical plan, and operational plan, which must be flexible to meet the ever-changing variables you encounter.

Rules of the road: The laws and regulations affecting your management decisions.

Weather: The economic conditions (requiring the manager to forecast and plan for worst and best possible scenarios).

Mode of transportation: Species mix and service offerings.

Vehicle: Practice plant and equipment accessories.

Drivers: Practice leader(s) (drivers may rotate in and out, depending on the circumstances).

Passengers: Employees, clients, and patients. It is important to have the right ones to make the journey fun and rewarding.

Cargo: Client value (value chain model).

Routine maintenance: Planned continuing education, performance reviews, financial analysis, and meetings, for example.

Dashboard gauges: Key performance indicators (for example, a speedometer (revenues); fuel gauge (expenses); temperature (client satisfaction, patient outcomes); tachometer (operating efficiency); odometer (patient numbers, profits).

Brakes: Common sense applied with knowledge and wisdom.

your journey. Without it, you will not know how to reach the destination. In a more formal sense, an effective business strategy consists of the methods and tactics you will use to achieve the goals, purpose, and vision of the practice.

Most practice owners have some sort of strategic plan in mind, but often it is not written down or even articulated. Like hospital policies and procedures, however, a plan is not a plan until it is written down. Even when it is written down, the failure rate for plan execution is high. Many sources state that well under 50 percent of American business strategic plans actually get implemented. In reality, probably no more than 30 percent are implemented; the figure may even be as low as 10 percent (Raps 2004). There could be many reasons for the failure to implement strategic plans. For example, the strategic plans may not be realistic, or the follow-through in organizing, directing, and evaluating may not be optimal.

Strategic planning is a formal design of the practice's future activities. It is based on the answers of key stakeholders in the business to three fundamental questions:

1. What do we do?
2. For whom do we do it?
3. How do we excel?

The typical overall strategic planning process follows the diagram shown in Figure 3.1. It involves taking many smaller steps. For a breakdown of these steps, see the textbox "Step by Step." In this chapter, we will look at these steps in more detail. The entire process begins with the formulation of a *vision statement* and a *mission statement*. These inspirational statements provide dual guiding lights for the practice stakeholders, articulating core values and behavior expectations that energize people to obtain defined goals.

As you begin to plan strategically, re-

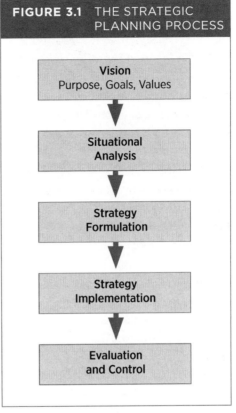

FIGURE 3.1 THE STRATEGIC PLANNING PROCESS

Adapted from Quick MBA, www.quickmba.com/strategy/strategic-planning/

member that strategic planning is not so much about the destination itself as it is about the journey. To be sustainable, the path your team takes as it follows the strategic plan must be enjoyable, inspiring all concerned to do their best. If it is not, the practice may end up with a plan that it cannot follow.

Defining the Practice's Vision and Mission

Vision and mission statements are closely related but also distinct, with each serving a different purpose. Both are based on the practice's core values. Thus, if you are just starting out, or due for a major rethinking of overall practice goals and strategy, it will be essential for the practice principals to define the underlying human values that serve to guide how the practice team behaves to accomplish day-to-day objectives as well as long-range goals. These core values will

Step by Step

To conduct strategic planning in veterinary practice, follow the steps outlined below.

- **Memorialize practice vision and mission in separate statements**
  - » Describe steadfast, irrevocable core values that cement expectations of behavior
  - » Describe an inspiring common vision of the practice's future
  - » Identify the practice's core purpose and primary objectives
  - » Create, critique, and update the practice's vision statement and mission statement
- **Conduct situational analysis**
  - » Analyze external practice forces
  - » Analyze internal practice organization and processes
  - » Determine critical success factors
- **Formulate strategy**
  - » Establish concrete goals to achieve defined success factors
  - » Decide on critical measures to evaluate progress over time
  - » Prioritize goals
- **Implement strategy**
  - » Communicate with key personnel, delegate and establish accountability and reporting requirements
  - » Establish budgets to allocate resources
  - » Educate and train team
- **Evaluate and control**
  - » Measure results against critical measures of success
  - » Analyze success and failure
  - » Give feedback
  - » Coach and support team
  - » Adapt goals and communicate

be the values that all practice leaders agree are foundational. They will serve as the basis for all other decisions to be made for the practice. In addition to identifying core values, the members of the practice leadership team must explore their visionary goals for the practice, identify the practice's core purpose, and take account of any legal or ethical principles that might affect these foundational elements of the practice. Each of these steps is described below.

When these steps are completed, the practice leaders will be ready to write a vision statement. This is a concise, inspirational statement that articulates how the practice will contribute to the community. It seeks to energize the practice team on its journey toward the purposes envisioned for the practice. When shared publicly, a vision statement also helps to shape how clients view the practice and why they want to use the practice's services.

The mission statement is also guided by the core values and core purpose but is more specifically focused on identifying the goals and objectives of the practice. In strategic planning, you will build an enduring practice mission by breaking these goals and objectives into achievable stages and documenting them each step of the way. Whereas the vision statement gives an inspirational, public-facing perspective of the practice's vision and commonly held values, the mission statement presents an internally facing and motivational definition of key measures of the practice's success in accomplishing its purpose and objectives. The mission statement, along with the core values, will guide practice leadership decisions. It often includes financial objectives supporting long-term practice success and value.

Both the vision statement and the mission statement describe what you would like the organization's life path to look and feel like. The practice vision statement describes the meaningful work the practice team does and aspires to do, while the mission statement describes key goals and measures of success.

DESCRIBE VISIONARY GOALS

The best place to start a strategic plan is by simply fantasizing. That's right, daydreaming. But this is not an open-ended, vague exercise. Practice stakeholders will take a specific amount of time, such as an hour, to envision and memorialize the kind of veterinary practice they wish to work toward. Try having the leadership team follow these steps. All participants should write down their answers as they reflect:

- Revisit the time of your life when you first decided you wanted to be a doctor of veterinary medicine and/or manage a veterinary practice. How did you think your life would look?
- If you are a veterinarian, revisit your years in veterinary school. When did you decide you wanted to be a veterinary practice owner? How did you envision your career then?
- Next, think about where you are now. Going forward from this very minute, imagine how you want your career and life to look. Write your vision of how the practice will look and feel.

Following this exercise, share and discuss your responses. How are they similar? How are they different? What are the visionary goals that should guide the practice vision and mission statements?

DESCRIBE CORE VALUES

The practice vision and culture should reflect the core values of its leaders, owners, and other vested stakeholders. Core values are the ultimate standards, those which the owners consider to be inviolate. They steer the veterinary practice as guiding principles of practice conduct, and they are the basis for the rules by which the principals and the rest of the practice team live and make daily decisions (Nyland and Heinke 2006).

Usually, core values come down to four or five deeply held principles that are independent of the current business environment and management fads (Collins and Porras 1996). Core values do not change over time. With different circumstances, they are still supported. In a different industry, core values would still resonate and be considered assets to the business.

Here are some ideas for exploring your core values. Again, all practice principals should participate in identifying these:

- *Tap your youth:* What values do you hold, and where did they come from? What prompted you to enter the veterinary profession? Did you learn important life lessons in a youth organization, such as 4-H, Future Farmers of America, or Girl Scouts or Boy Scouts? (Nyland and Heinke 2006).
- *Revisit books on core values:* One of these might be Robert Fulghum's *All I Really Need to Know I Learned in Kindergarten* (1988). Core values center on basic human rules of behavior. As Fulghum put it: "Share everything. Play fair. Don't hit people. Put things back where you found them. Clean up your own mess. Don't take things that aren't yours. Say you're sorry when you hurt somebody." These concepts touch on key core values, such as fairness, kindness, responsibility, and respect.
- *Read websites of youth organizations:* These sites may remind you about core values that are important to you, such as thoughtfulness, loyalty, service, health, and community.
- *Read annual reports:* Annual reports and websites of publicly traded companies often provide a business perspective of core values. For example, in an IBM Internet-based "values jam" that asked all employees to candidly express their thoughts and criticisms, values such as dedication to clients, innovation, and trust and responsibility in relationships were highlighted (IBM 2010).

DESCRIBE CORE PURPOSE

As the practice leaders continue to prepare for writing both the vision and mission statements, they will need to take some time to consider the practice's core purpose. As part of this step, they must think about how financial commitments and ethical commitments relate to each other. A description of the practice's core purpose will be the result.

There are many stakeholders in veterinary practice. Members of the profession are responsible to these stakeholders legally, through professional standards, and through personal principles. When ethical dilemmas arise, they usually involve these commitments. With duties to families and employees, to clients and their animals, and to society and public health, is it any wonder that practitioners and other team members struggle with difficult ethical dilemmas on a daily basis? When money is added to the mix, conflicts can arise.

Like it or not, most North American veterinarians practice in "for-profit" companies. The veterinary profession may be driving the highways of duty to animal welfare, society's benefit, and public health, but capitalism fuels the engine. After-tax profit funds the resources required to maintain competent employees, equipment, facilities, pharmacies, and other necessities.

Veterinary practices sustain significant financial burdens. A dual commitment to the advancement of medical knowledge and excellent patient care requires precious investment of time and money. Veterinary professionals must maintain their skill through lifelong learning, high-tech equipment, and specialized facilities. The resulting financial commitments exceed those of many other professions.

The profession will continue to be thirsty for new talent, brilliant young men and women who will succeed those working now as they progress to retirement. They will be necessary if the profession is to meet the demands of a global economy hungry for the wide variety of competencies to which veterinarians lay claim. To attract the best and brightest candidates, the field must offer good compensation and working conditions. Raising practice economic standings in a highly inflationary medical-financial environment requires constant tending of strategies affecting fees, taxes, financial risks, and many other aspects of running a practice.

Think about how you will blend these potentially conflicting objectives. How will you balance the professional and ethical codes with the very real need to generate profit? Write your answers down. For example, you might list specific objectives, such as having a fair fee schedule that supports employee development, investments in leading-edge equipment and education, and a favorable profit return for practice owners (Heinke 2006). These represent the practice's core objectives to attain its primary purpose of providing veterinary care to animals.

If you do not take the financial needs of a thriving practice into consideration during the development of your mission statement, you may end up with a mission statement that is unrealistic financially.

KNOW APPLICABLE LAWS AND CODES OF ETHICS

The practice's nonnegotiable core values must support and blend with the ethical guidelines of the veterinary profession. The American Veterinary Medical Association's Code of Ethics, as well as those of other professional organizations, such as the state veterinary associations, the Veterinary Hospital Managers Association, and American Association of Equine Practitioners, forms part of the practice's governance foundation. Make sure you thoroughly understand the ethical requirements applicable to the profession as a whole and to the practice doctors' specialties or practice areas of special interest.

Every practice owner and manager must also consider the codified veterinary practice acts of the state(s) in which the practice is located and in which its doctors treat patients. A veterinary practice act is the legal statute that guides what each licensed and nonlicensed employee of the practice can and cannot do.

CREATE, AMEND, OR REVISE VISION AND MISSION STATEMENTS

The written practice vision and mission statements collate the four areas you have explored above: (1) the visionary goals of the practice stakeholders, (2) their core values, (3) the core purpose and supporting primary objectives of the practice, and (4) applicable laws and professional ethical codes (see Figure 3.2). The vision and mission statements answer the following questions: "What will the organization stand for?" "What will its reputation be?" "What will its longevity be?"

Ultimately, both the vision statement and mission statement concisely convey the practice's direction with inspirational words. The vision statement defines the practice's purpose through its human values, and its audience is primarily clients and employees The mission statement defines the practice's primary objectives and purpose with an internally facing focus to leaders and owners, including key measures of success.

Unless you are just starting out, the vision and mission statements should express what already exists in the practice, perhaps with a bit of reframing for the audience. Here is a hy-

FIGURE 3.2 CREATING OR REVISING MISSION AND VISION STATEMENTS

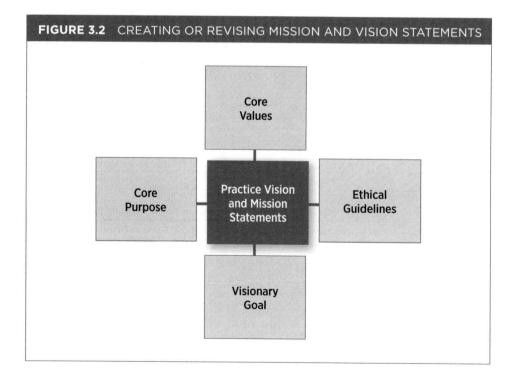

pothetical example of a mission statement. Notice how it focuses on owner and leader goals, including measures of success:

> *To become the trusted community leader in companion animal medical and surgical care, as measured by patient longevity, client retention, and referral numbers, through a fair fee schedule that supports shareholder investment in modern medical technology, compensation supporting employee longevity, and a commitment to lifelong learning.*

Here is a hypothetical example of a vision statement that could be written for this same practice:

> *We help the families of our community live happier and more fulfilling lives by increasing the quality and length of their pets' lives. These goals are accomplished through comprehensive veterinary care encompassing disease prevention, early detection of illness, and advanced treatment capabilities. We dedicate our team to lifelong learning and to exemplary client communication, which supports best care of beloved family members who cannot speak for themselves.*

Practices can be very different from each other, and their vision and mission statements should reflect that. Here is a pair of vision and mission statements that go in a different direction. First, the vision statement:

> *We help families afford pet ownership by providing easy access to vaccination, sterilization, and other basic pet health services.*

The mission statement for this same practice might be:

> *Our mission is to provide highly profitable veterinary services that focus on outpatient disease prevention such as through vaccinations and parasite control. Our community position will be to meet the needs of pet owners interested in minimizing time and money investment through use of short appointments of 10 minutes and by maintaining operational efficiency through referral of patients with apparently challenging medical and surgical problems to other facilities.*

Although these are good examples, no practice manager should simply take a shortcut and adopt these as vision and mission statements. The vision statement for your practice must reflect the true core values and vision of the practice stakeholders. Every team member should know and understand the vision statement as it becomes a guiding principle for day-to-day operations. Similarly, the mission statement should be a clear reflection of owner and leader practice objectives and measurement of progress.

You may wish to take the mission statement one step further by distilling it into a practice motto or marketing slogan. In the first hypothetical practice above, the slogan might be: "The Pet Parent's First Choice for Comprehensive Health Care." In the second practice, it could be "The Pet Parent's First Choice for Affordable Pet Care."

Although the mission statement should be in play every day, a formal reevaluation of the statement should be completed annually. Are owner actions and employee activities congruent with the mission and vision statements and the values they reflect? How do employees and clients perceive the practice? Where is the practice now and where does it appear to be going? A national Gallup Poll survey question might ask, "Do you think the country is headed in the right direction?" The annual process of reevaluating the mission and vision statements is similar, but it asks, "Is the practice headed in the right direction?"

If what actually exists is in conflict with the vision and mission, ask why. Should procedures and policies at the practice be changed to bring them into harmony, or should the statements of guiding principles be revised to reflect the reality of the practice?

Evaluating the Practice's Situation

The next step in strategic planning involves analysis of the practice and its environment. This step is also known as environmental scanning, and it requires evaluation of both external and internal factors as they are perceived to exist and identification of how they might develop and change in the future.

CONDUCT A SWOT ANALYSIS

Here you will complete another helpful exercise. Write down your perceptions of practice strengths, weaknesses, opportunities, and threats. Known by its acronym, SWOT, this strategic planning technique analyzes the practice's internal strengths and weaknesses and identifies external opportunities and threats (see Figure 3.3). An in-depth example of this technique is described in Chapter 13, "Marketing Your Veterinary Practice."

In a strength analysis, describe the attributes of the practice that support your organization's mission, make it unique, and give it a competitive edge. How does the practice create value for clients?

When analyzing weaknesses, describe internal practice issues that detract from the positive attributes. Be specific about the harmful gaps in the practice's capabilities. Only by identifying lackluster performance characteristics can you can develop a plan for change and correction. Some internal factors might be beyond your ability to control, but facing these unpleasant realities is an important part of effective strategic planning.

In opportunity analysis, evaluate the practice's potential by exploring options for perpetuating success. For example, perhaps you could explore service expansion, facility renovation, or the development of better communication techniques between team members or with clients. Encourage SWOT participants to think "out of the box" and dream big, and list all of the ideas mentioned. Even if they are not chosen for immediate action, these valuable ideas may be taken up in the future. They can be measured against the practice mission to determine best fit for objectives to pursue. This part of the exercise is more about brainstorming than about making final decisions.

Use threat analysis to identify external obstacles or challenges. Generally, these "threats" are largely beyond a manager's control. Nevertheless, it is important to recognize them. The strategic plan will have to take them into consideration.

Opinions of practice opportunities and threats may be somewhat subjective. For example, one stakeholder might perceive the practice's lack of overnight hospitalization as an opportunity to provide expanded and needed service, while another perceives the situation as a threat, reasoning that the need cannot be easily met. In these cases, the item can be listed in both areas.

FIGURE 3.3 SWOT ANALYSIS

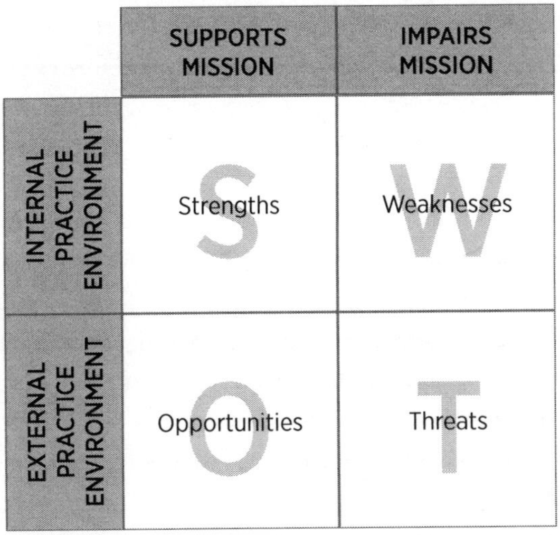

	SUPPORTS MISSION	IMPAIRS MISSION
INTERNAL PRACTICE ENVIRONMENT	Strengths	Weaknesses
EXTERNAL PRACTICE ENVIRONMENT	Opportunities	Threats

ANALYZE EXTERNAL PRACTICE FORCES

A well-designed strategic plan considers a wide variety of external market and competition pressures. These include the following:

- Competitors
- Sales market (clients)
- Supplier market
- Labor market
- Technology
- The economy
- The regulatory environment

Veterinary practice competition (competitive rivalry) may represent an opportunity or a threat. The intensity of competition can be described as high, medium, or low. Your determination of competition intensity can be measured to some extent by how much power you feel you have in pricing services.

Some sources of competitive advantage in the free market include cost, differentiation, and innovation. To see how competitive advantage can be gained through cost control, consider a large company like Wal-Mart: By controlling costs, it drives down prices.

Differentiation has to do with the perceived quality of care, type of service, price levels, and image of your practice. This perception is driven by marketing. Innovation describes the competitive advantage a practice has when others cannot keep up with the new ideas and methodologies it has successfully implemented.

A useful approach to external pressure analysis was developed by Michael Porter (1980). Porter's five-force analysis is more detailed than the SWOT technique. His framework defines different categories of external opportunities and threats within an industry (see Figure 3.4).

Porter's five forces are:

1. Threat of new entrants to the industry
2. Threat of substitutes
3. Buyer (client) power
4. Intensity of rivalry among established practices
5. Supplier power

Evaluate each force in the context of whether it is strong, medium, or weak. Strong forces imply potential threats, whereas weak forces present opportunities to the practice. Consider how situations change over time and use your intuition as to what might realistically happen in the future. Table 3.1 provides a template to use as part of a situational five-force analysis.

Several other tools can help you scan the external macro-environment in which the veterinary practice operates. PEST analysis is a framework using four factors: political, economic, sociocultural, and technological. The political environment includes local, state, and national

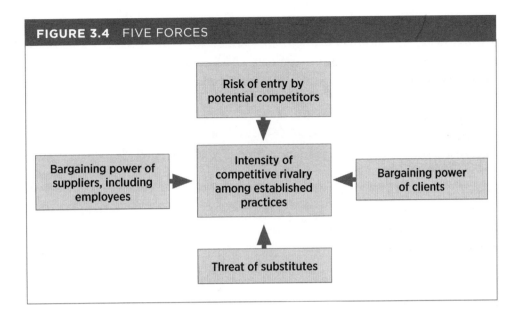

FIGURE 3.4 FIVE FORCES

laws and regulations. Stay aware of regulatory changes, tax law changes, and zoning and environmental law.

The economic environment includes local, regional, and national factors. Economics affect current buying power and future opportunities for investment. For example, a practice owner might choose to close the practice and sell valuable practice real estate for residential real estate development, rather than maintaining it as a veterinary facility. Or, perhaps the practice owner would sell client and patient records to merge operations into another practice, resulting in economies of scale. A third example would be use of fixed, low-interest rate loans to fund an expansion in services or the purchase of equipment that would open up new areas of treatment.

To take the social and demographic environment into consideration, evaluate the type and availability of your employee and client base. Your assessment would include factors such as generational changes and differing attitudes about work, family, play, and companion animal ownership.

The technological environment keeps growing in importance. Be aware of the many influences on the practice stemming from the growth of the Internet. For example, clients have more sources of information about the practice, about your competitors, and about medical diagnosis and treatment. They have more options for purchasing needed items. Communication occurs via venues such as Facebook and Twitter. Veterinary medicine is heavily impacted by other types of technological innovation as well. Advances in patient treatment, new equipment, and specialist availability are examples.

TABLE 3.1 SITUATIONAL FIVE-FORCE ANALYSIS

COMPETITIVE FORCES	FACTORS TO EVALUATE
Potential competitors and barriers to entry	How loyal are your practice's clients?
	How troublesome would it be for clients to switch and use someone else's services and/or products, such as pharmaceuticals?
	Would it require much money (seed capital) to start up a competing practice?
	How hard is it for a new competitor to gain access to distribution channels (supplies, employees, equipment)?
	How long does it take for the employee base to acquire the expertise and skills to provide services in a comparable fashion?
	How difficult would it be for a competitor to gain access to real estate to conduct practice or to provide ambulatory services?
	What possible subset services could a competitor offer (e.g., roving services, specialty services)?
Threat of substitutes	How many of the services offered by your practice have a possible substitute the client could use instead? What are they?
	What is the pricing of comparable substitutes?
	What is the perceived quality of possible substitutes?
	How specialized is your practice, possibly reducing the threat?
	How well has your practice differentiated its services, also possibly reducing the threat?
Intensity of rivalry among established practices	How many close competitors exist?
	What are the sizes of the closest competitors?
	What is the current opportunity for growth in veterinary care in your area?
	How high are the exit barriers? Would high committed fixed costs keep a competitor operating, even at negligible profit or at a loss?
	How diversified are practice competitors?
	How extensively do your direct competitors advertise?
Bargaining power of clients	How many practices are there for clients to choose among?
	Do you depend on only a few or many clients to sustain your sales?
	Are clients using other practices as well as your own?
	How difficult is it for clients to switch to a competitor or purchase products elsewhere?
	Do you have pricing power, or do your clients control what your practice charges?
Bargaining power of suppliers	Are there substitutes for your suppliers' products?
	Do your suppliers serve multiple industries? Does total veterinary-related revenue account for only a small portion of the supplier's total revenue?
	Would it cost the practice much to switch to another supplier?
	Can suppliers compete with what your practice does or sells?
	Can your practice enter or expand into the supplier's business?
	Can your practice negotiate price for supplies and equipment? For software and new technology?
	Current and prospective employees are "suppliers" of labor: How difficult is it to obtain veterinarians, technicians, and others?

FIGURE 3.5 PEST ANALYSIS

POLITICAL	ECONOMIC
Government type Freedom of press Rule of law Bureaucracy/Corruption (De)Regulation trends Professional and ethical rules Social/Employment legislation Likely political change	Business-cycle stage Growth, inflation, interest rates Unemployment, labor supply, labor costs Disposable income and distribution Globalization/Ecology Likely economic change
Population growth/Age profile Health, education, social mobility Employment patterns, attitudes toward work Press, public opinion, attitudes, and taboos Lifestyle choices Likely sociocultural change	Impact of emerging technologies Impact of the Internet Impact of changing communication modalities R&D activity Impact of technology transfer Likely technological change
SOCIOCULTURAL	TECHNOLOGICAL

As you consider political, economic, sociocultural, and technological changes and how they impact the practice, consult Figure 3.5.

ANALYZE INTERNAL PRACTICE ORGANIZATION AND PROCESSES

After evaluating the effects of external forces on your practice and performing a PEST analysis, proceed to an internal analysis of the practice. The next model, the value chain model (Porter 1985), will help you focus on internal strengths and weaknesses of key components of organizational structure and work-process flows.

The overriding emphasis of the value chain model is client satisfaction. By perfecting each step of practice processes, client-perceived value is added to patient care activities. In theory, everything done in the practice must provide client value. When clients value and willingly pay for the services they receive, including good patient-care outcomes, profit results.

In this step, you will therefore evaluate what the practice team does from a value chain–strategy perspective. If employees are doing things that do not add value to the client's experience, they should not be doing them. One management objective is to focus on what your practice does well and keep doing it well. Such effort drives quality and value, thus ensuring client satisfaction and loyalty.

Your primary objective as a manager is to cause the practice to make money. By focusing on excellent service, your team drives client perception of value and willingness to pay for that value (this is called the value proposition). The value chain is illustrated in Figure 3.6.

In the value chain analysis, you will divide the practice into two activity areas:

- The primary operating activities, or those that show the progress of client and patient interaction with the practice
- The support activities, or those governance or managerial activities required to sustain a well-organized and efficiently managed practice

Use the charts supplied in Figure 3.7 to rate your own practice and see where you need improvement.

From your analysis of the practice's value chain, determine which aspects of the organization are the weakest and which are strongest. Each of the weaker links in the chain represents a priority for goal setting. Later you will devise a tactical plan for strengthening each link in the value chain.

DETERMINE CRITICAL SUCCESS FACTORS

In the early 1990s, Dr. Robert Kaplan and Dr. David Norton at Harvard Business School published ideas about an innovative strategic planning and performance management tool. This tool was called the balanced scorecard by process management consultant Art Schneiderman. Kaplan and Norton's first 1992 paper was a popular success and was followed by other *Harvard Business Review* articles and best-selling books by the same authors.

The balanced scorecard theories of process management apply very well to veterinary practice management. The approach enables one to define specific critical success factors and to determine how to track (measure) progress toward them.

When using a scorecard approach, you design a variety of benchmarking criteria that balance the purely financial perspective, which is expounded by much of the practice management literature, by consultants, and by other organizations, with other factors that are nonfinancial. As a management tool, the scorecard helps the practice manager clarify the practice's vision and strategy (which are often rather abstract) and translate them into concrete action. We have modified Kaplan's model for use in veterinary practice, calling it the Veterinary Practice Scorecard (VPS).

The VPS recognizes the financial measures that assure an adequate economic base to drive excellent veterinary care. A balanced scorecard approach guides and measures the practice's progress in providing value through investment in patients, clients, employees, suppliers, processes, and technology.

Knowing the long-term vision and mission of the practice, a manager uses the VPS to plan specific tactics from each of these four perspectives and set goals for them:

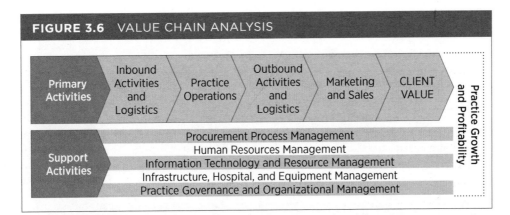

FIGURE 3.6 VALUE CHAIN ANALYSIS

FIGURE 3.7 SUPPORT AND PRIMARY ACTIVITIES: SELF-ANALYSIS WORKSHEET

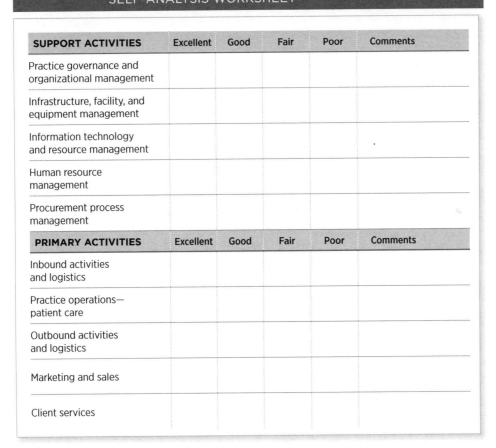

SUPPORT ACTIVITIES	Excellent	Good	Fair	Poor	Comments
Practice governance and organizational management					
Infrastructure, facility, and equipment management					
Information technology and resource management					
Human resource management					
Procurement process management					

PRIMARY ACTIVITIES	Excellent	Good	Fair	Poor	Comments
Inbound activities and logistics					
Practice operations—patient care					
Outbound activities and logistics					
Marketing and sales					
Client services					

- The patient care perspective
- The client perspective
- The learning and growth perspective
- The financial perspective

Each perspective receives equal weight in the analysis. Each has an associated goal and at least one metric that allows for measurement of progress and/or successful accomplishment of the objective. The manager regularly evaluates the practice in this way to ascertain progress as the practice team continues to work toward the VPS-based objectives. The questions to ask when determining the specific VPS objectives you will use appear in Figure 3.8.

The situational analysis process is continual. Practice situations continually evolve and change. A competent manager supports stability by flexing between situational analysis, strategy modification, and change management.

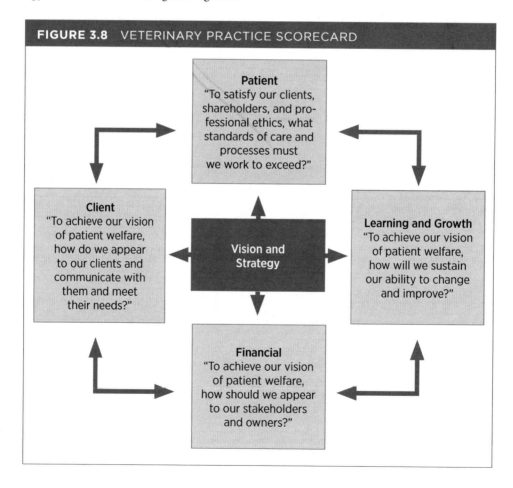

FIGURE 3.8 VETERINARY PRACTICE SCORECARD

Patient
"To satisfy our clients, shareholders, and professional ethics, what standards of care and processes must we work to exceed?"

Client
"To achieve our vision of patient welfare, how do we appear to our clients and communicate with them and meet their needs?"

Vision and Strategy

Learning and Growth
"To achieve our vision of patient welfare, how will we sustain our ability to change and improve?"

Financial
"To achieve our vision of patient welfare, how should we appear to our stakeholders and owners?"

The foregoing tools will help to keep you organized throughout this process, enable you to modify current strategy, and guide you in developing new strategies that prioritize the opportunities that you and other practice stakeholders define. They will also help you optimize practice strengths, identify and rectify or minimize weaknesses, and acknowledge threats and mitigate their risk.

Although external threats tend to fall more outside of your control, it is important to know what they are. However, do not waste energy fearing the threats. Instead, assess how they might impact your practice, and determine the specific actions you can take internally to protect the practice from them.

Excellent capability in strategic thinking is essential when facing large threats, such as an economic downturn or the influence of the Internet on client purchases.

Establishing Goals

There is a purpose to these analysis models: They help you to set goals, formulate strategy, and engage in strategic, tactical, and operational planning. (See Chapter 1 for the difference between the three types of planning.) Here we will see how situational analysis impacts operational, day-to-day planning. It is a formal, stepwise approach that leads seamlessly to strategy formulation.

Say we have evaluated our practice in each area of the value chain and observed that significant weaknesses exist in the primary activity of inbound processes. That is, appointment numbers have fallen, clients often miss appointments or are late, and clients often have to wait to see the doctor after arriving. Although the economy was booming and appointments were plentiful, some of our processes clearly have slipped. We call these lapses policy or protocol drift.

Policy-protocol drift causes a weakening of the value chain. All of the problems appear to be interrelated. (Clients are late because they know they will likely have to wait; when clients are late, the doctor's schedule is further delayed, causing other clients to wait; and some clients even miss their appointments because the appointments take up too much of their time.) We decide to record occurrences of each problem in order to determine a baseline measurement of the current situation. A baseline allows us to gauge process improvement later on.

What we measure for the baseline helps us determine SMART goals in each of the balanced scorecard (VPS) quadrants that will lead to action and incremental improvement. SMART goals are:

- Specific
- Measurable
- Attainable
- Relevant
- Time-bound

As you will see, some of the stated goals may satisfy more than one quadrant. Even though recording them in multiple quadrants may seem somewhat redundant, doing so can show the importance of these goals to ensuring results. The team will be motivated to attain the objectives when they can easily see the reasoning behind the operational changes.

The operational planning objectives in this case might be as follows:

1. *Patient perspective:* If clients miss appointments, the patient is not receiving essential care. The entire team agrees that this is a highly motivating factor to ensure that appointments are kept a high percentage of the time. Also, if a patient has to wait a long time for the appointment, the visit may be more stressful. This also impacts the level of care. (Clients may not pay as much attention to instructions if they feel hurried, for example.)

   » We will measure the number of incoming phone calls from clients or potential clients. We will measure the number of calls that result in a booked appointment. Booked appointments divided by incoming phone calls give a percentage, say 50 percent. Our SMART goal will be to increase the percentage of booked appointments to 70 percent over the next two weeks.

   » We will query the computer database to determine which pets have apparently fallen behind on baseline preventive care, as defined by our medical staff. We will contact all of these clients by snail mail, e-mail, and/or phone calls within the next ninety days. Our goal is to convert 30 percent of these re-contacts to appointments.

   » We will telephone, e-mail, and/or text-message a reminder to all clients twenty-four hours in advance of any appointment.

   » We will measure time of client arrival, time of exam room admit, and time of doctor to patient. Our goal will be to have every client and patient with a technician and/or veterinarian within five minutes of arrival.

2. *Client perspective:* For our practice example, we think clients may be missing appointments because they forget, because they have not been educated to appreciate the importance of keeping appointments, and because, from experience, they have gotten used to the practice not running on schedule.

   » Within the next thirty days, we will develop/modify scripts for employees to briefly and succinctly explain the benefits of preventive care for dogs and cats.

   » We will monitor phone calls to determine if employees need help or retraining to properly inform and assist clients. We will make sure each employee is assessed at least three times in the next week.

   » We will improve our online check-in forms and e-mail communication service so that clients have an alternative and convenient way to make appointments and/or contact our team. Forms will be updated within the next sixty days. E-mail communication will be evaluated within the next ten days, and recommendations for improvement will be made at that time.

» We will telephone, e-mail, and/or text-message a reminder to all clients twenty-four hours in advance of any appointment.

» We will measure time of client arrival, time of exam-room admit, and time of doctor to client interaction. Our goal will be to have every client and patient tended by a technician and/or veterinarian within five minutes of arrival.

» We will employ a three-question exit survey to determine satisfaction with appointment timeliness.

» We will assign two employees to monitor Google Alerts and other Internet communications at least twice per day for any dissatisfied client situations, which will then be promptly handled within twenty-four hours.

3. *Employee perspective:* For our practice example, we believe receptionists may have difficulty handling conversations and knowing how to book appointments for the correct length of time.

» We will interview receptionists this week to ascertain what questions they are having difficulty answering. At the end of each shift, each employee will write down any issues they came across that were challenging to work through. Within the next thirty days, we will develop/modify scripts for employees to briefly and succinctly explain the benefits of preventive care for dogs and cats.

» We will monitor phone calls to determine if employees need help/retraining to properly inform and assist clients. We will make sure that each employee is assessed at least three times in the next week and that follow-up training is completed with coaching.

» We will ask doctors and techs to mark care plans and progress exam requests with the number of five-minute blocks of time that will be needed for the next appointment, so that it is easier for receptionists to book the appropriate amount of time and keep the schedule running on time. Our goal is to have this notation made on 100 percent of care plans and progress exam–appointment requests.

4. *Financial perspective:* We believe that the value chain will be strengthened through the foregoing plan. It is more attentive than our current procedure to client convenience and will help to secure recommended patient care. Employee training and tools to assist in making decisions will improve capabilities and job satisfaction. (These should be measurable through regular communication and feedback from employees, through, for example, regular performance assessments.) These actions should result in increased revenue generated per client and increased average patient visits per year. These are key performance measurements that are regularly assessed. They are impacted by virtually all activities in concert.

» We will employ a three-question exit survey to determine client satisfaction with appointment timeliness.

» We will measure the number of incoming phone calls from clients or potential clients. Our SMART goal is an increase in the percentage of booked appointments to 70 percent over the next two weeks, followed by a reevaluation of the situation and modification of the goal as needed.

» We will query the computer database to determine which pets have apparently fallen behind on baseline preventive care, as defined by our medical staff. We will contact all of these clients by snail mail, e-mail, and/or phone calls within the next ninety days. Our goal is to convert 30 percent of these re-contacts to appointments. We will measure the revenue generated by this conversion.

Operational planning is the short-term, day-to-day type of planning, but these same methods can be used for long-range, strategic planning. Strategic planning looks at the big picture. Table 3.2 provides a template to help you think about how the balanced scorecard will look for your practice when it comes to this type of planning, and it includes suggestions of possible critical success factors. These factors will evolve into specifically stated, measurable goals for each quadrant of the scorecard.

DECIDE ON CRITICAL MEASURES TO EVALUATE PROGRESS OVER TIME

To keep your efforts in evaluating progress balanced and manageable, focus on three key measures for each quadrant of the VPS. These should be top-line measurements that are easy to make and that provide the practice leadership and team with a clear understanding of the progress made.

Have three measures for the long-term strategic plan. These will be "key performance indicators," such as gross revenues, profitability percentage, client numbers, client satisfaction measures, patient numbers, employee longevity, and/or satisfaction measures.

Develop the three measures for each quadrant based on tactical and operational objectives. Measures related to compliance or adherence can help to advance goals established in all four quadrants: client perspective, patient perspective, employee perspective, and financial/owner perspective.

PRIORITIZE GOALS

Once you and the rest of the practice team have developed a strategic-planning and goal-setting mindset, it's easy to use the value chain and balanced VPS framework. In fact, you may think of so many ideas and measurable goals that you cannot pursue all of them. Your objective will then be to prioritize and limit the goals to manageable activities that can be successfully assigned, executed, and accomplished.

TABLE 3.2 CRITICAL SUCCESS FACTORS

Critical Sucess Factors	To My Shareholders (financial perspective)	To My Clients (client perspective)	To My Patients (internal processes or patient perspective)	To My Team (growth, innovation, and learning perspective)
How will our practice differ?				Continual learning
What are critical success factors?	Revenue realization Expanding transactions Improved profitability	Increasing client numbers Client satisfaction Client referrals	Successful care outcomes Patient longevity Patient comfort	Employee knowledge Employee longevity
What are critical measurements of success?	Revenue exceeding inflation by at least 2 percentage points each year Transaction growth of at least 3% each year Profitability improved from current situation by 2 percentage points in next 12 months and by 4 points 24 months from now	Client gains and client attrition (keep accurate count of client numbers) Formal assessments of client satisfaction (at least one per client per year) Client referrals (track referral sources)	Diagnostic codes used 100% of time Track patient demographics/ age for increasing longevity stats Pain assessment and management protocols used in 100% of surgery, dentistry, OA, and cancer cases	Successful completion by employees of at least one learning objective each quarter Decreasing employee turnover rates each year

To narrow down the set of choices, review each proposed goal against the vision or mission statement. Does the idea, plan, or goal fit with the practice's mission statement? If not, should it be thrown out? Or should the mission statement be revised?

Once a goal is deemed to fit with the practice's mission statement, review the goal to see if it is measurable. Restate it in measurable terms, if necessary, and identify which part of the balanced scorecard it pertains to. List it there. If a suggested goal cannot be stated in measurable terms, then it should be omitted.

Use the worksheet in Figure 3.9 to help you rank, design, and assign goals.

FIGURE 3.9 RANKING, DESIGNING, AND ASSIGNING SMART GOALS

RANK/ GOAL	SPECIFY MEASUREMENT	WHO WILL MEASURE?	DUE DATE FOR MEASUREMENT TO BE MADE	DATA SOURCES AND DOCUMENTS FOR MEASURING	DUE DATE FOR REPORTING TO BOARD OF DIRECTORS AND SHAREHOLDERS

Implementing Strategy

Thinking strategically to design tactical and operational plans is one thing. Implementing strategy is quite another. To implement strategy, you will need to communicate with key personnel, and you will need to delegate and establish accountability and reporting requirements. In short, you will need to be a team leader and a communicator rather than a thinker and planner.

You cannot do everything yourself. Thus, having key personnel involved every step of the way may be a good strategy in itself. Many leaders periodically use one- or two-day retreats to focus on communicating goals and ensuring team commitment to them. Sometimes a practice is small enough that the owner can involve the entire team in advancing the operational plan. This is especially true when portions of the plan pertain to client service, expansion of the services offered, or promotion of the practice's service capabilities in the community.

When working with your team, invite members to take on projects. Talk about the practice's core values and the practice vision. Working on the mission statement can bring out the passions of team members for veterinary care, sparking their involvement in goal accomplishment.

Once you have "buy-in," you can then ask team members to stay committed to deadlines and reporting requirements. With accountability comes successful execution.

To implement a strategic plan a practice manager and team must also avoid the pitfalls that can occur. As mentioned earlier, many organizations are not able to successfully implement the strategic plans they establish. Here are some common reasons for failure to achieve a strategic plan, suggested by management consultant Paul Johnson:

- Failure to communicate vision and strategic purpose throughout the organization.
- Leadership failures, both from the top and from the ranks. Everyone must be called upon to step up and lead the effort where they can.
- No plan behind the idea, or inadequate detail about the specific tasks to be done. This mistake is common because, Johnson wrote, "ideas are easier to talk about than to do." Assignments may be unclear or team members may not be sure who is responsible for what.
- Passive management, or the assumption that things will run themselves after being started. Once implementation begins, management must guide the process. While practice leaders must communicate their vision and describe the actions needed to support the plan, management must know how to execute the individual tactics and make team members accountable for following through on assignments.
- Lack of motivation and personal ownership. People want to make a difference. The team must be convinced of the value of the plan and the goals and have a clear vision of the outcome.

By taking concrete steps to avoid these mistakes, you will have a better chance of successfully implementing the strategies you have worked so hard to articulate and plan. Once you have buy-in, team members will be excited to be involved.

ESTABLISH FINANCIAL MODELS TO ALLOCATE RESOURCES

The next strategic step involves financial planning. Financial budgets and plans are important to strategic planning in two main ways: (1) Budgeting can help managers to measure progress toward goals; and (2) good planning and budgeting are needed to fund each part of the strategic plan.

Practice managers generally follow traditional budgeting and accounting practices. They may have little awareness of innovative financial tools. However, some of these financial tools have come to be valuable supplements to or even replacements for the traditional version of a business budget. They can enable practices to become nimble in a changing economy and market. Some examples are rolling budgets, rolling forecasts, flexible budgets, and event-driven budget plans. Be aware of the pros and cons of these financial tools and how they can be used in financial planning.

In addition, some managers break the budgeting process into three sections that correspond to target setting, forecasting, and resource allocation. This type of budgeting can complement a strategic plan. Any practice manager using strategic planning should have a traditional annual budget as well. This budget can help the manager track recent trends in the practice and spot developing trends.

Recent financial history is something of a predictor of expected performance in the next twelve-month cycle, but a strategic plan is a plan to outperform history. So, to measure progress toward the goals of a strategic plan, the manager needs to know where the practice has been financially and understand how different budgetary factors relate to other knowledge, such as the SWOT assessment and the PEST analysis. If you are a practice manager, consider getting input from the practice accountant and perhaps even someone with financial expertise in veterinary practice management. Refer to Chapter 11 for more information on budgeting.

Many practices are moving toward rolling forecasts or budgets that are compared with operating results. The budget of allocated resources plus the SMART measures you developed in the strategic process are your measuring sticks. Powerful and affordable computers, bookkeeping software, and spreadsheet software all assist in real-time development of useful budgets. The more you use spreadsheets and practice data to plan the financial aspects of a plan, the more adept you will become. The process of twenty minutes of brainstorming a project budget of employee hours, the payroll tax effect, and supplies will cause anyone involved to ask questions about fees, volume, marketing, and a whole slew of other considerations that might not have been predicted without such planning detail.

Successful strategy implementation also requires a financial plan, because it often takes money to bring tactical and operational plans to fruition. Managers must be able to predict expenditures with some semblance of reality. Resource allocation to implement a strategic plan may include outlay for equipment, payroll, supplies, and contracted services, for example.

A good example of how strategic planning can drive resource management is in the arena of client communication. Yellow-Page advertising has traditionally been required in veterinary practice. It was a major expenditure, but it was necessary to help prospective new clients find local veterinary practices. The Internet has completely changed strategies for both attracting and retaining clients. Practices must now create flexible communication-promotion budgets that take new forms of communication into account. As a result, marketing budgets have become much more complex.

Capital expenditures now include everything from e-mail reminder systems to consistent branding of websites, e-newsletters, and social-media resources. It is necessary to create a positive Internet presence and to stay up to date with a host of different communication tools.

EDUCATE AND TRAIN TEAM

The process of implementing a strategic plan must include money and time for education and training of all affected team members. This may be little more than including one hour of staff meeting time to explain the vision and goals. On the other hand, it could involve more extensive training time to acquaint every team member with new policies and procedures. Team-member job descriptions may change in ways that require one-on-one or small-group training over several sessions.

Even a short session of training and role-playing can eat up extensive payroll dollars. This is why a culture of "buy-in" to the patient-care-client value proposition is so important. Time is precious, but for the plan to work, sufficient time must be devoted to providing employees with the specific training they need. Role-playing and problem solving are time-consuming activities, and yet they are important factors in this training and can make the difference between failure and success. You will also want to schedule sufficient time for measuring progress and giving feedback.

Communication and follow-up are critical factors to success in tactical plan implementation and operational improvement. The time you spend in these activities may well be critical to ensuring that the team is moving in the right direction. Too much time in training, however, and the employees may become bored or frustrated. As in so many things, finding the right balance for your team is essential: It's a bit like the story of "Goldilocks and the Three Bears." The amount of training must not be too little, or too much, but just right.

You have come a long way already in our journey of practice planning. You will soon discover that there is a cycle in planning: It involves designing, implementing, monitoring, and adapting.

Because you have a plan, you have identified the critical measures of a successful journey. Some of these will change with new information and situations. Others will be very consistent metrics of success at any time.

Regularly measure practice results against your critical measures. Take time to memorialize these results by recording them in meaningful reports. This will give you the opportunity to regularly assess the effectiveness of the activities the practice has embarked upon. What worked, and what did not work? Discuss these issues as a team. Debate your failures and the contributing factors (especially those that can be controlled, or at least partially managed).

While you are measuring and revising your plan, be sure to celebrate successes with your team. Communicating and praising progress builds spirit and optimism. Build from these successes to guide your team as you develop a culture of growth and passion for patient care through client value.

PERSONNEL AND HUMAN RESOURCES

4

Personnel Management

Theories of management have evolved over the past century. In the early 1900s, employers called their theories of management "scientific." Managers felt the best way to improve worker output was to improve the techniques and methods used, such as those embraced by assembly-line production. The manager's function included establishing and enforcing performance criteria based on the needs of the organization and not on the needs of the individual worker. This theory of management is called "the classical school" (Hersey and Blanchard 1982, 84).

Then, in the inaugural issue of the *Harvard Business Review*, published in October 1922, Daniel Starch wrote, "Business and industry consist in the control of human beings who in turn control the physical forces, materials and machines and in that broad sense business is psychological in nature" (Starch 1922). Beginning with this idea, the "human relations movement" entered the management-theory arena. It continued to be popular in the 1930s (Hersey and Blanchard 1982, 85).

According to the "social system school," following the writings of Daniel Katz and Robert Kahn in 1966 and P. Lawrence and J. W. Lorsch in 1967, all parts of the organization are interdependent or interlocking because all are parts within the system. Each part affects and is affected by each other part. A change in any part of the system will result in changes elsewhere.

The "open system school," discussed by B. Aubrey Fisher and Leonard C. Hawes in 1972, recognizes that an organization can be a closed or an open system. The closed system is one with fixed boundaries, whereas an open system has permeable boundaries. Thus, an organization cannot ignore the neighborhood, the economy, and market trends. Like the social system school, the open system school recognizes interdependence and interlocking relationships.

Since then, extensive exploration of how to manage humans in the context of work has occurred. As a result, literature about management theories and their application in the workplace, practical or not, abounds, with related psychological research being conducted. Managing has always been centered on how to get people to get the work done, and managers will continue to need ways to accomplish this primary task as the workplace adapts to a changing world. Thus, research, writing, and testing of management theories will likely continue. New theories will arise, and old ones will be adapted, to explain and influence workplace styles and behavior.

In all of this theorizing, one thing remains clear: Leadership and communication skills are the basis of effective management. Leadership depends on and results from behavior—your behavior as manager and the behavior of the individual or practice team that you are attempting to influence. A manager with solid leadership skills is able to understand what motivates people, to predict how they will respond to leadership, and to direct their behavior to the desired outcome. A manager with good communication skills can motivate and inspire employees, explain tasks clearly and effectively, and foster good communication and interaction in the workplace. Often these two skills are used simultaneously.

Following an introduction to management styles and workplace communication, we will look at two common means of communicating important information in veterinary practice: the team meeting, and personnel and hospital manuals. Other aspects of human resources management, including the employment cycle and employment laws, will be covered in later chapters.

Management Styles

As a manager, you will need to constantly be aware of your managerial and communication style, consciously relying on the methods that will be most effective in directing the team. Managers primarily use four basic leadership styles to varying degrees: directive, supportive, participative, or achievement oriented. The directive style is task oriented. The supportive style is more concerned with people's individual needs than with tasks. The participative style involves consulting with the group in decision making. And achievement-oriented leadership focuses on setting challenging goals. Some managers have an affinity to one style, but generally, leaders utilize a blend of the four styles, emphasizing each at one time or another.

As a manager, you may participate in or have exclusive responsibility for a range of activities:

- Setting the practice goals and objectives
- Determining how to achieve those goals and objectives
- Planning and organizing the work to be done
- Communicating priorities
- Clarifying employee roles and responsibilities
- Directing employees in completing the required tasks at hand
- Reviewing their work
- Making required changes

These steps in the management process can be carried out in any of the four leadership styles. Effective leaders will discern which styles or combination of styles will be more effective for different aspects of management or for their particular workplace situation.

Managers who exhibit a directive style tend to be task oriented. They are more interested in getting results than in discussing how the work is going to be completed. Their communication is direct and practical, without much socializing or chitchat. Effective managers temper directive behavior by implementing people skills or supportive behavior.

Supportive leadership is based on relationships. Supportive managers listen to employees, encouraging them to express their problems, thoughts, feelings, and ideas. A supportive response to this expression includes praise, encouragement, reassurance, recognition, and reward. Managers using a supportive style ask for suggestions, compliment effort, provide feedback, and clearly communicate the hospital's plans and goals to the team.

Participative leadership is based on consulting the employees whom you are leading. This style involves asking for suggestions prior to making any decisions. This is most effective when the employees have a high degree of technical and expert knowledge and add value to the decision-making process. This leadership style is often effective in creating a positive work environment when the employees wish to contribute and appreciate their role in the practice's success.

The achievement-oriented leaders set challenging goals for their employees and then show genuine confidence in their ability to achieve those goals. A key to this leadership style is that the leader must also set challenging goals for himself and lead by example in achieving them. This fosters a practice in which there is an expectation of continuous improvement.

How you implement the leadership styles and how much emphasis you place on each will determine your personal management style. Know your predominant style and then strengthen your effectiveness by flexing into others. For example, a supportive leadership style can often benefit from using a directive style to ensure completion of assignments. Similarly, a directive style will benefit from encouraging employee collaboration and input by adopting attributes of the participative leadership style.

A management style that is primarily directive or achievement-oriented is commonly known as *autocratic* or *authoritarian* leadership. A management style that is primarily supportive or participative is known as *democratic* leadership.

THEORY X AND THEORY Y

How managers adopt one style over another may have as much to do with their ideas about work and motivation as it has to do with their personalities. The ideas behind authoritarian and democratic leadership styles have been explained in *Theory X* and *Theory Y*, respectively. These terms were first popularized by Douglas McGregor in the early 1960s (Hersey and Blanchard 1982, 48). Theory X assumes that people prefer to be directed, are not interested in assuming responsibility, and are motivated primarily by money, fringe benefits, and the threat of punishment.

Theory Y postulates that employees can be self-directed and creative at work if they are properly supported and motivated. Motivation can come from individual desire for recognition, from a sense of self-worth and pride, and from an interest in work well done.

Neither of these theories alone tells the whole story. An effective management style creates a balance between the amount of direction and the amount of support provided. Each employee is different and will require custom modification of your basic management approach, and your ability to adapt to each employee will drive how effective you are at delegating, motivating, and developing others. Some people will respond to the direction and support you provide in a positive way, while others will have an entirely different response.

To select the appropriate style for your practice situation and the practice's culture, think about the needs of your employees and the tasks to be accomplished. How much direction do your employees need to get the job done? How much do you need their input in order to make the practice thrive? Would your employees benefit from more support from you, or do they have plenty of support but lack direction? Choosing an effective leadership style comes down to two basic questions: How motivated are your employees, and how skilled are they?

If your employees seem unwilling or unable to perform their duties, they need more direction. If they are highly motivated and adequately skilled, they do not need much direction but may appreciate a participative leader. Those who are willing but not skilled will need training or mentoring, and those who are skilled but not motivated will need supportive leadership, and perhaps an achievement-oriented leader who will set goals.

MODIFYING YOUR MANAGEMENT STYLE

How people perceive your direction and support ultimately affects their response to you and their behavior at work. You may believe yourself to be a people-oriented, caring person, but your employees might view you as hard-nosed and bossy. Differences between perception and intention are a primary cause of communication breakdown in veterinary hospitals.

Each employee has different perceptions. Communication styles vary. Reaction to workplace stress and job requirements can be markedly different from one person to the next. Employee education, practical experience, age, maturity, and tenure in the practice all have a bearing on individual perception of your management style.

Sometimes an employee will approach you to request a different level of direction and support than you are providing. More often, you will have to discern on your own the needs of employees. To obtain the best work from your team, you must be more adaptable than they are and able to respond effectively to their needs. Knowing your employees and how to effectively motivate them is key.

You should also know yourself. To be an effective manager, you must understand your own natural behavioral tendencies. We are often blind to our own personality traits and management styles, and lacking this self-awareness causes much of the friction that occurs as we try to work effectively with coworkers, employees, employers, partners, and clients. By increasing awareness of your own strengths and weaknesses, it becomes easier to vary your normal behavior style to better meet the communication and interaction needs of the people you are managing.

Improving Team Communication and Interaction

Continual conflict and miscommunication among the team and between employees and management are among the most common complaints made by veterinary practice managers. The entire veterinary hospital team, including its leaders, can benefit tremendously from learning interpersonal skills. The concept of *emotional intelligence*, or EQ, introduced in Chapter 2, is important in learning to manage staff effectively.

A good starting point is to learn as much as possible about human behavior. If you understand why employees say and do what they do in response to workplace stress, clients, and other employees, you can begin to predict behavior, even with a new employee. If you can predict how people will interact, you can communicate in a way that increases the probability of the outcomes you desire. The goal is to create a team that functions smoothly, with people who get their work done by collaborating with others, rather than being divisive.

Think of most human behavior as nothing more than innate and learned reactions to external stimuli. This is true whether the behavior is found in an office manager, a doctor, or a pet owner. In the fast-paced, emotionally charged atmosphere of the veterinary hospital where client demand is high, normal stress-reactive behaviors may not be appropriate. It is up to you to teach your team effective methods for dealing with these behaviors for more productive results. In fact, there are many ideas and tools that can help you in the important responsibility of improving team communications and interactions at your clinic or hospital.

THE IMPORTANCE OF PEOPLE IN THE SERVICE INDUSTRY

Managing an animal hospital is as psychologically and emotionally rewarding as it is demanding, in no small part because it is a people-oriented job. Veterinary medicine is a professional service industry, and so it relies heavily on people, both the people it serves and the people it employs. Positive interaction with veterinary clients is a major part of any successful, reputable, and growing practice.

Trends point toward increasing automation in many businesses, including veterinary hospitals. Computerization, electronic communications, and intense equipment technology development are commonplace. Despite these exciting changes, veterinary hospital employees are still the key to exemplary client service and patient care. Finding and keeping employees with excellent attitudes, enthusiasm for client service, and passion for veterinary medicine will be your biggest challenge as a twenty-first-century practice manager.

Recognizing the importance of managing human resources in a veterinary practice is the first step to improving team communication and interaction with each other and with clients. It begins with the hiring process and continues throughout the management process of planning, organizing, directing, and evaluating.

EMOTIONAL LITERACY

A significant aspect of human resource management resides in people's emotions: how well the manager understands her own emotions and the emotions of others, how constructively she deals with emotions, how well she trains other team members in emotional intelligence skills, and the like. Since instinctive emotional responses can undermine anyone's best intentions when interacting with others, learning and teaching others how to manage emotions is important to employee development. Strong competency in modeling and managing emotions may be considered one aspect of learned "intelligence." These concepts were described in the mid-1990s by Daniel Goleman in his best-selling book *Emotional Intelligence*. This book culminated in popular recognition of researcher ideas about what constitutes intelligence in the context of a person's success.

By suggesting that IQ (intelligence quotient) was not a particularly good predictor of achievement, and that emotional skills were at least equally important determinants of life success, Goleman's postulated emotional intelligence quotient (EQ) became one of several competencies generally recognized as important in managing relationships and leading others.

Emotional intelligence is often described by five levels of competence in which to focus personal improvement:

1. *Self-Awareness:* Recognizing the importance of your emotions and observing them can give you valuable insights into your habituated response to a situation. The more you come to know how your emotions work, the more you can control ingrained emotional responses, keeping them from blinding you and causing you to say or do things that destroy communication, which leads others to erect barriers.

2. *Self-Control:* Reframing stressful situations and managing your emotional triggers enables you to have a greater degree of self-control, improving communication. By regulating your emotions, you can moderate angry responses and maintain perspective and focus.

3. *Self-Motivation:* Using your emotions to motivate yourself increases personal competency in interacting with others in more positive and productive ways. Self-motivation enables you to delay gratification and commit to goals and long-term plans. Practice teams more

enthusiastically follow leaders who demonstrate consistent motivation and commitment to the practice vision.

4. *Empathy:* Recognizing and appropriately responding to the emotions of other people will make those individuals more willing to cooperate and more receptive to direction and change. Empathy includes the ability to discern between another's emotions and your own, not allowing their emotions to replace yours.

5. *Effective management of relationships:* Once the other four emotional competencies are mastered, you can hone your ability to influence, persuade, motivate, and inspire others. By managing the emotions of your team, you will be able to maintain an encouraging and supportive work environment.

Mastering your own emotions and being a student of emotional intelligence will increase your ability to develop an excellent practice team. A testament to your competence as a manager will be found in each employee's ability to develop effective communication skills and to embrace mutual acceptance of various team-member strengths and weaknesses. Understanding emotional intelligence is one tool of many that will serve you well.

In the next section, we explore an offshoot of emotions: behavior. Behavior theory is much like that of emotional intelligence. Behavior and emotions are both learned and habituated responses to external stimuli. Both can be modified through self-awareness and training.

BEHAVIOR STYLES

Our emotions affect our behavior. Both emotion and behavior are typically exhibited in response to the environment and the other people in it. Basic psychology recognizes that all human actions are motivated. People do things (or do not do them) for a reason, and often this reason is based on self-interest. We are genetically programmed to revert to self-interest, particularly when stressed, as a survival mechanism. Often, though, our stress-reactive behavior is instinctual, and in the moment, we are not always aware of our self-preserving motivations.

Although humans all have similar survival mechanisms, each person has a unique personality and life history of experiences, and so interpersonal communications between members of the practice will differ. Scientific attempts to identify and segregate the facets of personality still cause much controversy, even though people have been describing different personality types since ancient times. Hippocrates (c. 460–370 b.c.) first described four types of temperament—choleric, sanguine, phlegmatic, and melancholic—that coincided with the four body "humors"—yellow bile, blood, phlegm, and black bile.

Since Hippocrates' time, many other researchers have described four groupings of personality or behavior. One of the most well-known models was introduced by William Moulton Marston during the 1920s in his book *Emotions of Normal People*. Marston described four basic human behavior styles, which he called dominance, inducement, submission, and compliance.

Marston's model is especially useful because its definition of behavior assumes that an individual's responses are part of the self-preservation instinct. These responses are based on the relationship between two types of perceptions: the individual's perception of his personal power to change the environment, and the individual's perception of the conditions of the environment.

From your perspective as hospital manager, the environment is the veterinary practice. Each veterinary practice's environment will be unique, in part because the people who work within it form a unique combination—the team, those in leadership, and the clients.

Even given the complexities of each person's personality style and the changing impact the environment might have, most people will exhibit the same basic type of behavior they had as children. Over time, the person's responses become fairly predictable as a pattern of behavior unless a significant shift takes place in one or both of the two types of perceptions (Carlson Learning Company 1994, 20). Although maturity and self-knowledge make it possible to change our perception of personal power over the environment, the behavior we most often exhibit is the one most natural and comfortable for us.

Nonetheless, when using behavior style as a tool for working with employees, it is important to understand that no one exhibits purely one behavior style or another. Most people are a complex interaction of each of the four basic behavior styles Marston described—dominance, inducement, submission, and compliance—which are often abbreviated as DISC and are summarized in Table 4.1.

Just as in popular books and articles where people may be referred to as "Type A" (high achieving) or "Type B" (mellow or laid back), discussions based on Marston's work describe people by different personality styles using the letters in "DISC." For example, a person who exhibits a lot of dominance in her behavior style might be referred to as a "D." DISC tools can enable managers to teach team members how to improve interpersonal communications and can help managers understand their own styles of communication.

Dominance (D)

Individuals who exhibit the dominant (D) style perceive themselves as being more powerful than the environment in which they exist, but they also instinctively perceive the environment to be naturally antagonistic or hostile. People who have D tendencies lean toward direct, dictatorial, and domineering communication styles. These individuals tend to have high ego strength and a "can-do" attitude. Individuals with high D characteristics are goal oriented and need results and variety. They are motivated by challenges and enjoy instigating change.

TABLE 4.1 BEHAVIOR STYLE SUMMARY

FACTORS	DOMINANCE Driver, Director	INDUCEMENT Influencer, Expresser	SUBMISSION Steadfast, Relater	COMPLIANCE Conscientious, Analytical
Outward clues	Likes his/her own way, strong viewpoints, quick decisions	Likes being at the center of attention, talkative, passionate	Likes positive attention, helpful, friendly and warm	Likes standard operating procedure, seeks data, asks many questions, methodical and systematic
Communication characteristics	To the point Speaks rapidly Task oriented	Tells stories Expresses opinions Animated	Excellent listener Reluctant to share opinions Speaks slowly, softly	Precise and detail oriented Diplomatic Process oriented
Tends to ask . . .	What? (the results-oriented question)	Who? (the personal influence question)	Why? (the status quo question)	How? (the technical/ analytical question)
What they dislike	Someone wasting their time trying to decide for them	Boring explanations, wasting time with too many facts	Rejection, being treated impersonally, uncaring and unfeeling attitudes	Making an error, being unprepared, spontaneity
Reacts to pressure and tension by . . .	Taking charge, taking more control	"Selling" their ideas or being argumentative	Becoming silent, withdrawing, being introspective	Seeking more data and information
Potential weaknesses	Poor listener May interrupt Lacks patience	Lacks focus Overly collaborative Inefficient	Voice not heard Perceived lack of confidence Overly sensitive	Lacks emotion Overly formal Inflexible, rigid
Best way to deal with them	Let them be in charge	Get excited with them Show emotion	Be supportive Show you care	Provide lots of data and information
Likes to be measured by . . .	Results, goal-oriented	Applause, feedback, recognition	Friends, close relationships	Activity and level of productivity that achieves results
Must be allowed to . . .	Get into a competitive situation Likes to win	Get ahead quickly Likes challenges	Relax, feel, care, and know you care	Make decisions at own pace Not be cornered or pressured
Like to save . . .	Time. They like to be efficient, get things done now.	Effort. They rely heavily on hunches, intuition, and feelings.	Relationships. Friendship means a lot to them.	Face. They hate to make an error, be wrong, or get caught without enough information.

Source: Adapted from Center for Educational Development and Assessment, "Communication Styles," The CEDA Meta-Profession Project, www.cedanet. com/meta/communication_styles.htm, with multiple other resources, including communication styles from Bryan Gillum, CPA, "The Role of a Manager," webinar sponsored by the Ohio Society of CPAs, August 31, 2011, Columbus, Ohio.

Inducement (I)

Individuals who have inducement (I) tendencies are similar to those with dominant traits in that they perceive themselves as having control over the environment. Unlike the D type, inducers instinctively perceive the environment as being friendly and supportive. Rather than dominating a situation, they use persuasive skills and optimism to influence others to act.

Being highly interested in people and influencing others, individuals with I behavior characteristics enjoy meeting and experiencing a wide variety of people. They like expanding their spheres of influence by talking and being with others to work on projects and toward goals. People with this style are most often known as Influencers, and they can be highly inspirational to others through their verbal expressions of optimism and enthusiasm.

Submission (S)

Marston called the third category submission (S). He defined submission as "willingly submitting to the leadership of someone who the person felt was allied for his/her greater good" (Carlson Learning Company 1994, 21). This demeanor of acceptance and acquiescence tends to create an environment of stability. Today, steadfastness is often used as an alternative term for the old behavior category description of submission.

People who have more S personality characteristics tend to be accepting of and loyal to others. They work well with team members because of their cooperative attitudes. Steadfast individuals do not believe they have much control over the environment, but they do look at the environment as being supportive and nonthreatening. While they prefer working with others rather than alone on tasks, they can be rather flexible to meet the needs of the situation, especially when allied with a more direct individual or an influencing type of person. Both D styles and I styles shake things up and cause disruption through change, and with a good foundation of trust and communication, steadfast team members can and will adapt.

Compliance (C)

The fourth broad behavior category is compliance (C). Marston described compliance as a response to a superior force that dominates the situation. Today, the word "conscientiousness" is more commonly used to describe people who have a C behavior style. Cautiousness is also used to describe this personality type, which is careful to check out the rules and to control compliance with them.

Team members with a predominance of conscientious behavior attributes emphasize quality control and attention to facts and details. They are motivated by their concern for correctness and quality of work. Because C individuals tend to view their control of the work environment as being negligible, they may also naturally view any particular situation as being potentially antagonistic or hostile, especially if a proposed change appears to threaten standards of quality.

READING BEHAVIOR

Notice a few patterns that provide insight into Marston's four basic behavior styles. People who have styles leaning toward D or C characteristics may perceive their situations as potentially antagonistic environments that require either self-protective aggressive or defensive responses. Team members who have more I or S characteristics, however, tend to act in a more open and accepting manner. They normally perceive the work environment to be supportive, assuming the other people in it have not become too domineering or critical.

Many times, you can guess a person's primary style simply by observing facial expression and body language. For example, arms folded over the chest and a rather closed expression on the face could indicate that you are dealing with either a D or C type. Someone who has a warm, expressive countenance and open, unguarded body language may have a predominantly I or S type behavior style.

Individuals who show D or C behavior characteristics tend to be more task oriented than relationship oriented. Their primary goals are to obtain objectives and get the job done. Individuals who have more I or S behavior characteristics, in contrast, tend to be more interested in people and in sharing experiences with others. They preferentially emphasize relationships over tasks.

You can now start to recognize the value in understanding your employees (and yourself) in terms of these characteristics and tendencies could be helpful in avoiding common misunderstandings. For example, it is not unusual for someone with a preponderance of dominance characteristics to clash with an individual whose natural behavior emphasizes conscientiousness.

The D may be very direct, blunt, and to-the-point without giving much detailed information. The D wants to accomplish a task by the shortest line of action possible. But the C individual tends to be defensive in the face of blunt and direct communication, which can easily be perceived as criticism. An employee with a conscientious style is motivated to do things right the first time, which means collecting additional details and clarifying understanding by asking questions. The domineering employee may be frustrated by lots of questions, which can be misperceived as questioning authority and even as combative.

When the C-style employee perceives the D employee's direct communication style as hypercritical, expect the conscientious employee to adopt a defensive attitude. After all, highly driven by conscientiousness and quality of task completion, the C-style employee has worked hard to make sure everything is done correctly. Wouldn't you be greatly offended by the perceived criticism? Yet the D-style employee may be clueless, unaware that the communication seemed offensive, because for a D, directness is natural.

If only both C and D had understood their own and the other person's tendencies! This conflict might have been averted before feelings were hurt.

USING BEHAVIOR TYPING

As a practice manager, you should understand the fundamentals of using behavior typing as a management tool in your practice. The DISC system described above is one method. You can also use the Myers Briggs Personality Inventory or its simpler cousin, Kersey Bates. Other methods are described in books on psychology and management, on Internet management training websites, and the like. You can draw from psychology classes or workshops you have attended as well.

Many questionnaires and other methods of determining a person's behavioral tendencies, called *behavior typing instruments* or *instrumented behavior assessment tools*, have been developed in conjunction with these systems, and learning about communication and management by using these systems is called *instrumented learning*. (Additional skills related to DISC and behavior typing are discussed further in the next section of this chapter, "Behavior Recognition Skills." See also the section entitled "Additional Resources" at the end of this book.)

Instrumented learning is a powerful tool. Because you cannot change how people react to situations any more than you can change their core traits, you must learn how to deal with the behavior exhibited. Any person at any stage of life can always learn more about how his actions affect others and how to develop self-awareness aptitude and self-control competencies. Each of us has the power to modify our behavior to best fulfill cohesive teamwork objectives. Your job as a human resource manager is to provide training and education that will help each member of the team learn the same skills. You can adapt your approach to fit each person's need as closely as possible.

Instrumented learning can help employees see a situation through their coworkers' eyes. Two people often perceive the same situation in totally different ways, and this can very easily become a barrier to cooperation. Called *situational perception*, this phenomenon influences how people interpret social interactions. If you teach your employees to understand the differences in individual perception, barriers break down. Improved communication and acceptance result, as each understands what the other person is trying to accomplish in the situation.

Additionally, we tend to be more aware of our individual strengths than we are of our limitations. Some people are fairly blind to their own limitations, but may still be open to developing increased self-awareness of habituated behavior and instinctive responses that may not be effective in working with others. Sometimes employees overplay their strengths, which can result in less effective outcomes, in conflict with coworkers, and in communication troubles with clients. Using instrumented behavior assessment tools with each employee helps individual employees to understand their weak areas and to learn how to change long-ingrained habits of behavior and overcome them through conscious effort.

It's important to remember that each behavior style adds value to the practice team. There is no such thing as a "good" or "bad" behavior style in the DISC model. Of course, there can be totally inappropriate behavior, such as excessive displays of anger, or overuse of sarcasm or foul language, that clearly should not be condoned in a healthy workplace. Emotional intelligence training is a useful tool in these situations.

Each person brings special behavior attributes and strengths to the workplace that others may not have. For example, one doctor with an inducement style may be a great rainmaker because of his extensive relationship building in the community. He may be genuinely interested in getting to know many people from all walks of life, and this brings in clients. A technician with high dominance and conscientious characteristics may be great at heading up emergency surgical case management because she can make quick decisions, direct others, and coordinate a large number of activities that must happen rapidly. A receptionist with high steadfastness characteristics may be able to work in a friendly, calm, and consistent manner with clients of all kinds while managing cordial relations with demanding doctors and technicians.

Veterinary practices tend to become more efficient and, as a result, more profitable when the individuals within the organization, especially the managers, become highly effective through learned appreciation of the differences in each other's behavioral styles. Diversity brings strength; differences in behavior styles are healthy and help to meet the needs of the practice as well as the clients and patients. Appreciation of differences instead of criticism becomes an important step in improving your ability to interact and lead the people around you.

BEHAVIOR RECOGNITION SKILLS

A variety of tools are available to help you learn about behavior styles in the workplace. Commercially available systems identify behavior styles and teach employees why they act and speak the way they do. Most of these systems use self-administered online platforms. Some can provide feedback about a person's preferred or natural behavior style following a questionnaire that takes about twenty minutes. Ultimately, the knowledge gained from consistently using behavior typing instruments helps facilitate employee training, workplace interaction, and client service. In turn, a more enjoyable and profitable practice environment results.

These instruments provide insight into how people uniquely think and react in given situations. When team members understand themselves better, they begin to recognize behavioral styles in other people, which helps them to communicate more effectively. For example, a receptionist who has learned about behavior styles becomes more aware and accepting of the varying personality types and discovers that she is better equipped to deal with clients on an individual basis.

Another benefit of these instruments is highlighting attributes that allow you to place people in positions that emphasize their best abilities. As a part of personnel management protocol, consider evaluating individuals who will be working together. Use the results of the evaluations to develop strategies for team building and to reduce communication conflicts. This can increase overall work effectiveness because relationships are improved among individuals within the practice unit.

Behavior typing instruments are designed not to provide a way for you to manipulate employees, but to help you understand how to create the greatest harmony. Your objective is to help individuals understand their work tendencies and recognize how their individual styles can affect others. The wide variety of available employee learning tools can help you as a manager to leverage the diverse wealth of people skills and styles in the practice in order to accomplish envisioned practice goals.

Whichever behavior-typing tools you use, plan to follow up administration of the typing instruments with exercises that highlight the various types. Such exercises can be fun and informative. For example, you might group team members together who share the same style and give all of the groups the same assignment. You could describe a hypothetical situation that involves some sort of problem and have each group discuss the scenario and report back to the larger group about how they would solve it. You might say, for instance, "You are planning a special event but can only accommodate twenty people. How will you decide who to invite?" Or, you might simply pose a question that involves brainstorming. For instance, "List all the things you can do with an orange."

During the follow-up discussion, note the different outcomes. You will find that people with different personality types think differently. These exercises underscore the value of knowing the people with whom you work and appreciating different ways of thinking. Having different perspectives and a variety of proposed answers in a real-life situation can often be helpful.

You will also want to apply the information obtained from these instruments to the everyday veterinary hospital setting. Potential application areas are:

- Teaching self-awareness and self-management.
- Improving peer relationships and team building.
- Implementing performance coaching.
- Matching individuals with positions based on behavioral strengths
- Easing frustration and conflict between team members.
- Improving client service and pet care through effective communications.
- Teaching and coaching listening skills.
- Developing management strategies for communicating, delegating, and motivating based on the personal preferences of the person you are managing.
- Coaching associate veterinarians, receptionists, and technicians in a client service environment.
- Identifying how a potential partner tends to manage, including communicating, delegating, directing people, developing people, decision making, managing time, problem solving, and motivating others.

When you begin to implement behavior training in your practice, you will find that its application extends far beyond employee interaction and team building. It applies, for example, to the reception area and examination room, since clients as well as employees have their own behavior styles. When doctors and other team members understand behavior styles, it is much easier for them to communicate more effectively with clients, responding to each client's communication needs.

Ultimately, your goal is to develop your veterinary practice into a healthy, productive, positive-thinking culture. This means recognizing that what is helpful for one person may be difficult for another. As one doctor has put it, in managing a veterinary practice, we do not necessarily want to follow the Golden Rule: "Do unto others as you would have them do unto you." Once you understand natural behavior preferences, you can begin to appreciate that the best way to build relationships is to treat others as they would like to be treated, based on their perception of the environment and of themselves. When communicating with others as they would prefer rather than as you would prefer, you are practicing the "Platinum Rule" of human relations (Russell 1996).

You will be responsible for many important tasks as an animal hospital manager. None will have greater impact on your overall success and effectiveness than the task of managing personnel. How you control and adapt your behavior to develop a management style, and how successfully you delegate responsibility but retain oversight and accountability, will be major factors in this task. Ultimately, your leadership and management skills will support the growth, profitability, and success of your veterinary practice.

For a more complete study of management styles and theories, consult the following resources, which are referenced in full in the "Additional Resources" section at the end of the book:

- Chapter 1, "Leadership Makes a Difference," of Dennis McCurnin's *Veterinary Practice Management*
- *The Miracle of Personal Leadership*, by Ray Russell
- *Management of Organizational Behavior*, by Paul Hersey and Kenneth Blanchard
- *Leadership and the One Minute Manager*, by Kenneth Blanchard, Patricia Zigarmi, and Drea Zigarmi
- *Ethics 101: What Every Leader Needs to Know*, by John C. Maxwell

COMMUNICATION STYLES

Let's apply what you have just learned about behavior to some communication basics (see Figure 4.1). The communication styles that correlate with the behavior preferences we just discussed are these:

- Dominant—Direct communication style
- Influencing—Spirited communication style

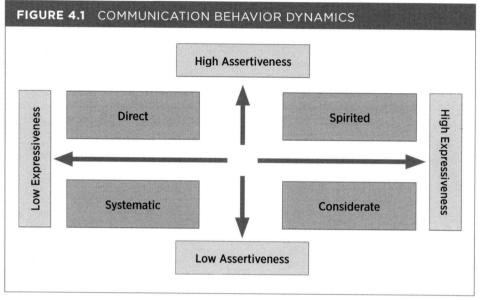

FIGURE 4.1 COMMUNICATION BEHAVIOR DYNAMICS

Adapted from materials by HRDQ, HRDQstore.com

- Steadfast—Considerate communication style
- Conscientious—Systematic communication style (Gillum 2011)

Communication breakdowns are common among human beings. Here are some apt aphorisms to remember when it happens in your practice, quoted from the Finnish communications researcher Osmo Wiio (1978), who adapted "Murphy's Law" for this purpose:

- If communication can fail, it will.
- If a message can be understood in different ways, it will be understood in just that way which does the most harm.
- There is always somebody who knows better than you what you meant by your message.
- The more communication there is, the more difficult it is for communication to succeed.

The point is to keep honing your communication skills while maintaining awareness that interpersonal communication is complicated by many variables outside of your control. Remain calm when failures occur. Try not to take it personally. American philosopher and psychologist William James noted that "whenever two people meet there are really six people present. There is each man as he sees himself, each man as the other person sees him, and each man as he really is."

Granted, communication is complicated. Table 4.2 summarizes a simplified perspective, using the four behavior styles. At the end of this chapter, we've included a handy reference to help you identify behavior and communication characteristics based on the four DISC styles.

TABLE 4.2 FOUR BEHAVIORAL STYLES

STYLE	CHARACTERISTICS	POTENTIAL WEAKNESSES
Direct (Dominant)	To the point Speaks rapidly Task oriented	Poor listener May interrupt Lacks patience
Spirited (Influencing)	Tells stories Expresses opinions Animated	Lacks focus Overly collaborative May be inefficient
Considerate (Steadfast)	Excellent listener Reluctant to share opinions Speaks slowly using soft tones	Voice not heard Lacks confidence Overly sensitive
Systematic (Conscientious)	Precise and detailed oriented Concise Process oriented	Lacks emotion Overly formal Inflexible/rigid

Source: Adapted from Bryan Gillum, "The Role of a Manager," webinar sponsored by the Ohio Society of CPAs, August 31, 2011, Columbus Ohio.

Before we leave the subject of communication styles, it's useful to reflect on the spectrum of assertiveness suggested by Figure 4.1, "Communication Behavior Dynamics." Communicators can be classed in a similar way, but with characteristics suggesting passive, assertive, or aggressive styles. The grid shown in Table 4.3 is referenced by many management training resources and attributed to Christopher L. Heffner, MS.

Finally, it is worth highlighting two communication skills important to the workplace that can be learned by anyone, regardless of communication style. One is simply being considerate and listening to others. Although it may be true that someone with a steadfast S style of communication tends to be more naturally considerate than others, and that both S and C types are naturally better listeners, that does not mean that other types of managers and employees cannot learn to be considerate, or good listeners.

Listening is perhaps the most important communication skill of all, and it is essential for managers and employees of all types to consciously develop it. It may not always be easy to learn to listen. Listening is about more than hearing words; it involves sensing the feelings that accompany the words, being aware of nonverbal messages, and considering the experience of the speaker, for example.

A second skill worth highlighting is the "I"-statement used by the assertive communicator. What is an "I"-statement? It is a statement by which the speaker shares his feelings or needs. When you use an "I"-statement, you disclose how you feel and how the situation is affecting you. By starting your disclosure with "I," you will be talking about yourself. This stands in sharp contrast with a "you"-statement, which tends to deliver blame or accusation. An "I"-statement, for example, would be, "I am really worried that our report won't be finished on

TABLE 4.3 PASSIVE, ASSERTIVE, OR AGGRESSIVE COMMUNICATION STYLE

	PASSIVE	ASSERTIVE	AGGRESSIVE
Definition	Communication style in which you put the rights of others before your own, minimizing your own self-worth.	Communication style in which you stand up for your rights while maintaining respect for the rights of others.	Communication style in which you stand up for your rights but violate the rights of others.
How this style makes others feel	My feelings are not important. I don't matter. I think I'm inferior.	We are both important. We both matter. I think we are equal.	Your feelings are not important. You don't matter. I think I'm superior.
How others "hear" the communication style	Apologetic. Overly soft or tentative voice.	"I"-statements. Firm voice.	"You"-statements. Loud voice with aggressive tone.
Nonverbal characteristics of the communication style	Looking down or away. Stooped posture, excessive head nodding. Accepting of the outcome despite it not meeting one's own needs.	Direct gaze. Relaxed posture, smooth and relaxed movements.	Staring, narrow eyes. Tense, clenched fists, rigid posture, pointing fingers.
Potential consequences	Lowered self-esteem. Anger at self. False feelings of inferiority. Disrespect from others. Pitied by others.	Higher self-esteem. Self-respect. Respect from others. Respectful of others.	Feeling guilty. Anger from others. Lowered self-esteem. Disrespect from others. Feared by others.

Source: Adapted from Christopher L Heffner, MS, "Communication Styles," Center for Educational Development and Assessment, "The CEDA Meta-Profession Project," www.cedanet.com/meta/communication_styles.htm.

time without your part completed." A "you"-statement in the same situation would be, "You are late with your contribution to the report. You will make us all late."

Communicating Through Team Meetings

To efficiently communicate with your team, you will need to rely on oral and written communications. This section discusses team meetings, an indispensible part of personnel management. Most animal hospitals have a number of employees and fairly complicated employee scheduling needs, so it is rare for all employees to be on the premises at the same time. How will you, the manager, communicate to employees new information about hospital policy and operations, pricing, techniques, wellness care recommended by the doctors, compliance initiatives, or seasonal marketing programs to increase the hospital's business? One way is through well-organized team meetings. The team meeting is an important forum in which to apply the concepts you have learned relating to management styles and communication.

Your primary goal in structuring team meetings is to make them as beneficial as possible for both your team and the hospital. Don't limit yourself to one type of meeting. The structure of the meeting should depend on the people involved and the purpose of the meeting. Meetings can be a formal time for all employees to convene at once, or they may be structured for a departmental or specific group effort, with as few as two people involved. Meetings can serve a variety of purposes:

- Team building
- Maintaining routine communications
- Enhancing accurate dissemination of information
- Informing employees about changes in hospital policies and procedures
- Ensuring quality, as in peer review sessions
- Learning techniques for improving and maintaining a constant level of client service
- Group brainstorming for practice improvement or troubleshooting
- Acquiring information that enhances patient care
- Maintaining compliance with regulatory requirements, such as workplace safety

As practice manager, you are charged with the heavy responsibility of assuring that team meetings achieve their goals. A lack of planning can result in too many meetings without clear agendas, so that people become fidgety and decisions are hurried. When too many employee hours are consumed in meetings, payroll budget overruns will result in financial detriment rather than profit enhancement. Often, when time is set aside for team meetings, it means time taken away from client appointments. But when hospital doors are locked and phones are unanswered too often, client needs are deferred. Too much breach of client convenience causes irritation and potential client loss.

Considering the amount of information dissemination and training that must occur in a rapidly changing practice environment, deciding how much time to allocate to meetings and to the necessary work of the day can be a big challenge. (See textbox on "Planning an Effective Meeting.")

There are times when you need to gather as many employees as possible to exchange general information and conduct hospital-wide training. Coordinating these general-interest team meetings can be challenging, especially if you have a large practice team. Here are some ideas to help you hold general team meetings that will accomplish these purposes:

Hold Meetings Regularly. Hold meetings approximately once a month or once a quarter, depending on veterinary practice size. Larger hospitals tend to have more departmental meetings than general-interest meetings. The lunch hour seems to be a good time for many

Planning an Effective Meeting

When planning meetings for your team, consider these criteria:

- **What is the purpose of the meeting?**
  - » Identify your goals. Consider whether a meeting is the best way to obtain these goals. Decide whether the meeting will be informational or for decision-making purposes. Here is a selective list of specific meeting purposes:
  - » Training in medical or surgical technique
  - » Training in product use
  - » Discussion of customer service issues
  - » Review of hospital procedures
  - » Update of workplace safety issues and OSHA compliance training requirements
  - » Introduction of new marketing information
  - » Review of important information for general dissemination, such as fee increases, schedules, case reviews, etc.
- **Who should attend the meeting?**
  - » Although the tendency is to invite every employee, try to invite people on a "need-to-know" basis. Does it make sense for a bookkeeper or maintenance person to attend an extensive discussion of a new anesthetic monitoring procedure? Try to include only those people whose presence is essential.
- **How long should the meeting last?**
  - » Multiply the number of people in the meeting by hourly wage rates and by the time expended. Then, multiply this figure by 1.3 to come up with a realistic payroll cost assessment for running the meeting. When you start computing the payroll dollar expenditure, you will be much more selective about who attends and how long the meeting lasts.
- **When should the meeting be held?**
  - » Determine the most convenient times for the greatest number of people. Also consider client convenience and patient care. Meetings are generally more productive in the morning than in the afternoon.
- **What will be accomplished?**
  - » Have an agenda. The agenda should include the names of participants and the time, place, and order of business (Thill and Bovee 1996, 422). If several topics or a complicated issue will be covered, allocate to each person a limited amount of time to

CONTINUES >

> PLANNING AN EFFECTIVE MEETING, CONT.

speak, say five minutes. Keep on schedule. You might even use a stopwatch to time segments of the meeting or speakers. This allows participants to pay attention to what others are saying, since they know they will each have their own chance to speak.

- **Will people be listening?**
    - » Short meeting agendas keep team meetings from getting too boring. If one person controls all the talking, people tune out quickly and everyone's time is wasted. Keep the meeting entertaining. Try using humor or anecdotes to get a point across (Crossen 1997).
- **Who will make sure that decisions are implemented?**
    - » Assign a meeting secretary to take minutes. A summary of these notes should be distributed to team members within a few days of the meeting. File your copy in a meeting notebook that you can reference later to ensure follow-through. (You can also harvest old ideas from this notebook later on, when they may seem like new ideas.)
    - » Establish a schedule for any agreed-upon tasks formulated at the meeting. Assign one person to accomplish each task and give each person a deadline for reporting results.

practices (employee time paid, with lunch hosted by the employer, and, if required by state law, other break time allowed), but some use the early-morning hours. If possible, hold the meeting away from the practice to minimize interruptions. Wherever the meeting is held, either close the hospital for the duration of the meeting, leave one employee to cover (this role should be rotated among employees), or have an answering service take calls.

Consider Supplying Food. If food and drink are provided, the hospital should pay for them. Keep in mind, however, that although having food may produce better attendance, it will also prolong the meeting and make it less efficient. People will not be paying as much attention as they would otherwise.

Pay for Attendance. Pay employees at their usual rates for the time spent at the meeting. This includes employees who are not scheduled to work at that time; they should be reminded of the meeting and encouraged to attend.

Hold Mandatory Meetings. Some meetings, such as those for workplace safety training, may be mandatory. Make sure that employees know they must attend and be on time. Warn employees they will suffer a penalty if they are late or absent. A written warning or reprimand may be used. Some practices dock or fine employees who don't attend or whose tardiness delays a mandatory meeting.

Be Punctual. Always start meetings on time and end on time, and do not delay meetings for those who are tardy, except in emergencies. This practice encourages employees to be prompt.

Follow an Agenda. Each meeting must have an agenda. Before the meeting, distribute the agenda or post it in a central place. If your employees are well-wired through the hospital Internet service, you can post a link to the agenda in a text message or e-mail. You might consider delegating the job of setting the agenda, organizing the meeting, and chairing the meeting, rotating this responsibility among team members. The meeting agenda can include introduction of new team members or new office procedures and an opportunity for each team member to voice any concerns. However, don't let meetings turn into complaint sessions. The meeting should be a forum for ideas rather than for complaints. When team members have concerns, they should also suggest ideas for correcting the perceived problems.

Get Others Involved. Seasonal topics (e.g., a meeting on educating clients about heartworm, fleas, and ticks), should be presented by knowledgeable team members. Periodically, invite guests, such as representatives of pharmaceutical companies or other suppliers, to give informative presentations. A bulletin board, suggestion box, or e-mail system can allow employees to suggest items for the agenda or speakers for the next meeting.

Also, make sure to keep meeting minutes and distribute them to those in attendance as well as to those unable to attend. The success of a meeting will depend on the leader's communication effectiveness and preparation. The meeting will also generally be productive if the appropriate participants have been selected. The meeting leader may be responsible for any or all of the following:

- Pacing the meeting
- Appointing a note taker
- Following the agenda
- Starting and ending on time
- Stimulating participation and discussion
- Summarizing decisions, actions, and recommendations the group makes
- Reviewing main points at the end of the meeting
- Setting the time and date of the next meeting
- Circulating the minutes (Thill and Bovee 1996, 423)

Well-planned meetings are an excellent way to maintain solid communication with employees. If meetings are productive, your team will be better informed and more effective with clients.

HONORING SCHEDULED MEETINGS AND OTHER APPOINTMENTS

Success in any business relationship can be ensured by respecting coworkers and clients. Respect can be given and measured in many different ways. One of the most important of these in a veterinary practice is punctuality. In today's competitive environment, the practice manager who remembers and keeps appointments will be considered a much better employer than one who is habitually late. The veterinarian and other team members who keep schedules on time will be judged a much better value by discriminating clients.

We all know that it is impossible for veterinary clinics to always run according to schedule. Hospitals in which team members promptly and courteously inform clients of scheduled delays will be more highly appreciated than those adopting a more nonchalant attitude.

Punctuality in appointments shows respect, not only when dealing with clients, but also in employee relations. If you arrange a specific time to meet with employees in regard to work matters, it behooves you to keep the appointment. Not keeping an appointment may be interpreted as nonverbal communication. For example, if you delay a meeting with an employee because you want to finish some routine duty, you give the nonverbal message that the employee is less important to you. Although the message may be unintended and even untrue, the employee will feel that the duties that kept her waiting were more important to you than the meeting you had previously scheduled. If this unintended slight is just one of many small incidents, you might have a problem in the making. Taken as a whole, these "small incidents" can be devastating to team morale.

As a corollary, coworkers who schedule appointments with or for their employers and fellow employees must make sure that all parties have the pertinent information. When team members miss meetings or appointments or are late because of miscommunications, it may be a sign of management problems. The astute practice manager heeds such failures and makes immediate changes to protocol that assure accurate scheduling communication.

In today's rushed society, where time is money, punctuality may be one of your most important tools for crafting success in veterinary practice. It shows respect for both clients and employees.

Policies, Procedures, and Operations Manuals

Personnel and operations guides are important sources of information that can effectively and consistently communicate the hospital's policies, procedures, and systems to employees. These guides give employees the answers to questions they didn't necessarily ask when they were hired. They serve as references to specific questions that arise as their duties become more clear. As important components of a hospital's communication methods, they must be professional in appearance and carefully prepared.

In veterinary hospitals, at least two major areas require documentation:

1. Hospital operations and procedures (see textbox on "Suggestions for Hospital Procedures Manual")

Suggestions for Hospital Procedures Manual

Job Descriptions for All Positions
- Reception Procedures
  - » Welcoming Clients and Hospital Visitors
  - » Answering and Managing Incoming Telephone Calls
  - » Scheduling Appointments
  - » Turning Phone Shoppers into Clients
  - » Handling Emergencies in Reception
  - » Communicating Vaccination and Preventative Care Protocols
  - » Managing Requests for Prescriptions and Refills
  - » Communicating Hospital Credit Policies
  - » Dealing with Challenging Situations
  - » Handling Abusive or Criminal Activity
  - » Handling Confidentiality of Client and Patient Information of All Types (Personal, Financial, Medical, and otherwise)
- Accounting Procedures
  - » Managing Hospital Credit Policies and Collection Procedures
  - » Handling Money
  - » Client Invoicing Procedures
  - » Employee Invoicing Procedures
  - » Vendor Contract Procedures
  - » Vendor Payment Procedures
  - » Inventory Management Procedures (Ordering, Receiving, Stocking, Auditing)
  - » Financial Reporting Procedures
  - » Budgeting and Other Financial Planning Procedures
- Hospital Procedures
  - » Handling Client and Patient Flow
  - » Effectively Managing Exam-Room Communications
  - » Using Care Plans, Estimates and Release Forms
  - » Outpatient Appointment Procedures
    - ∘ Preventive Care Appointments
    - ∘ Interventive Care Appointments
  - » Hospitalization Procedures
    - ∘ Admittance Procedures
    - ∘ Visitation Procedures
    - ∘ Discharge Procedures

CONTINUES >

> SUGGESTIONS FOR HOSPITAL PROCEDURES MANUAL, CONT.

- » Surgical Suite Scheduling, Procedures, and Protocols
- » Radiology and Imaging Procedures and Protocols (Safety Policy Reference)
- » Laboratory Procedures
  - ◦ Reference Laboratory Procedures
  - ◦ Internal Laboratory Procedures
- » Patient-Care Procedures
  - ◦ Nursing Protocols and Procedures
  - ◦ Biosecurity Protocols and Procedures
  - ◦ Husbandry Procedures
  - ◦ Feeding Procedures
- • Kennel and Grooming Protocols and Procedures
- • Janitorial, Cleaning, and Sanitation Procedures
- • Equipment and Facility Maintenance Procedures
- • IT Procedures
  - » Social Media, Texting, E-mailing Procedures (Referencing Employee Use of Internet and Equipment Policy)
  - » Password Procedures (Referencing Policy for Password Security)
  - » Data Backup Policy and Procedures
  - » VPIMS Use Procedures
  - » Other Software Use Procedures
  - » Time Clock Use Procedures
  - » Hardware and Software Maintenance Procedures
- • Sample Hospital Forms

2. Employee policies, procedures, and guidelines (see textbox on "Suggestions for Employee Guidelines and Policy Manual")

Every veterinary practice should consider establishing and maintaining documents that outline the policies and procedures under which the business operates. The employee policies and guidelines manual gives employees information pertinent to their employment with the practice. The hospital operations manual presents information about how to perform duties associated with client service, animal care, facility maintenance, and other business protocols. These manuals can be a useful tool for training and communicating with your team, promoting greater understanding among your team, and fostering teamwork.

Suggestions for Employee Guidelines and Policy Manual

- Veterinary Practice General Overview
  - » Welcome to Our Veterinary Practice Team
  - » Management Philosophy
    - ◦ Mission Statement, Vision Statement, and Core Values
  - » A History of the Veterinary Practice
  - » The Practice's Purposes and Goals
  - » Description of Expected Employee Attitude and Cooperative Effort Through Teamwork
  - » Organizational Chart
- Employment Policies
  - » Immigration-Law Compliance
  - » Equal Opportunity
  - » Anti-Harassment
  - » Employee Pregnancy
  - » Employee Illness
  - » Family and Medical Leave
- Personnel Guidelines
  - » Personnel Records
  - » Salary and Wages
    - ◦ Payday, Paychecks, Advances
    - ◦ Tax Withholding, Garnishments, Levies, Attachments
  - » Employee Benefits
    - ◦ Paid Time Off: Vacations, Sick or Personal Leave, Holidays
    - ◦ Uniforms
    - ◦ Health and Other Insurance
    - ◦ Pensions, Profit Sharing, and Retirement Savings Programs
    - ◦ Continuing Education
    - ◦ Licenses, Dues and Subscriptions
    - ◦ Other Qualified Business Expense Reimbursements
  - » Trial Period, Training, Evaluation, and Promotion
  - » Work-Scheduling Policy, Work Breaks, Absences, and Tardiness
  - » Leaves of Absence, Jury Duty, Maternity Leave, Military Leave, Voting Time
  - » Hospital Communications and Staff Meetings
  - » Hours of Business
  - » Grievance Procedures

CONTINUES >

> SUGGESTIONS FOR EMPLOYEE GUIDELINES AND POLICY MANUAL, CONT.

- » Disciplinary Procedures
- » Termination Procedures
- Code of Conduct
  - » Courtesy
  - » Confidentiality
  - » Integrity and Honesty
  - » Personal Appearance, Dress Code, and Name Tags
  - » Hospital Appearance
  - » Professional Relationships
  - » Mistakes
  - » Quality of Client and Patient Care
  - » Supplies and Equipment
  - » Keeping Informed
  - » Telephone and Internet Usage
  - » Employee Pets at Work
  - » Authorized Use of Facilities
  - » Smoking
  - » Substance Abuse
  - » No Solicitation Policy
- Safety Procedures
  - » OSHA Right to Know
  - » Ergonomics Standards, Policies, and Procedures
  - » Building Security
  - » Computer Security
  - » Emergency Evacuation
  - » Reporting Accidents and Personal Injury

EMPLOYEE POLICIES, PROCEDURES, AND GUIDELINES MANUALS

Employee manuals can help solve workplace problems fairly because they clarify policies. Hospital protocol clearly communicated in a written format allows you to give a consistent management response to employee questions. This reduces misunderstanding and increases employee compliance with rules. Employee complaints may be mitigated before they become serious, reducing the risk of lawsuits.

Care must be taken in writing and using these manuals. Before a manual is written, your hospital must be prepared to be bound by its own published procedures and standards. A court may consider a manual to constitute a contractual agreement, even when a signed contract does not exist. Violation of the terms of the manual could be considered breach of contract (Tannenbaum 1989, 304). Ask the practice's attorney to review the manual before you print, distribute, or use it. The attorney will check that all statements and information are in current compliance and agreement with laws and regulations.

You can secure additional legal protection if you clearly state in large print at the front of the manual that it is not a contract. After new employees read the manual, they should be asked to sign a statement, prepared and reviewed by the practice's attorney, stating that they have read the manual and understand that it does not constitute a contractual agreement.

One advantage of a written manual is that it enables management to periodically and formally evaluate policies and procedures for effectiveness and legal compliance (Osborne 1995, 4.03). Update the manual as needed, and have the lawyer review the modifications. After many changes and updates are made to the manual, all employees should read the changes and sign the statement again.

When compiling a policies and procedures manual, you will first need to decide what subjects must be included and what subjects should be left out. Any topic that concerns

Intranet File Management

Virtualization of documents by maintaining well-organized server directories will help support your efforts to keep manuals up to date. A hospital intranet uses network technologies to facilitate information sharing among employees. Typically the intranet is firewall protected but does allow employee access via the Internet. The simplest type of intranet uses an internal e-mail system. A sophisticated intranet that supports dissemination of hospital policy and procedure could include a message-board service, a private website, links to payroll information, databases, client and employee forms, and practice news. It is even possible to have a practice social network for employees and/or clients.

There is little that is more aggravating than not being able to locate an electronic policy or procedure document that you know you created and need to update. When updating any form, it is important to adopt standard operating procedures about:

- Directory and file-naming conventions
- Network location via directory and file organization
- Revision date of the document (usually at the bottom)
- Initials of the person(s) who created and/or revised the document or form

employee-employer relationships is suitable for discussion. The following questions will guide you in deciding what to include in an employee policy and procedure manual:

- What do you want your employees to know about your hospital?
- What accomplishments bring the most pride to your veterinary practice?
- What conduct do you expect of your employees?
- What rules must be followed?
- What problems have occurred in the past that you would like to avoid? (Osborne 1995, 4.05)

AAHA Press publishes a useful reference entitled *AAHA Guide to Creating an Employee Handbook*. Available in book or computer disk form, this guide covers many subjects that you might include in an employee policies and procedures manual and suggests appropriate format and wording.

HOSPITAL OPERATIONS AND PROCEDURES MANUAL

This valuable reference source explains various aspects of hospital activities, ranging from client service to proper sanitation procedure. The detail of explanation in the manual depends on a number of factors, including the age of the practice, the operation size, and the dedication of management to organization and employee training and direction. Generally, the bigger and more complex a practice, the greater the need for detailed information about where to find things, how and when to perform certain work tasks and duties, and what to do in the event of emergencies or other more mundane occurrences.

Often the need for a hospital operations and procedures manual comes to the attention of administrators when avoidable mistakes are made repeatedly and management becomes increasingly concerned about workplace and employee safety. It can be frustrating, for instance, when employees forget to complete chores or when important maintenance tasks are delayed. When needed pieces of equipment are not working properly, delays occur and patient care can be impaired. People may not be able to locate supplies, forms, equipment, or records from shift to shift because things have not been put back where they belong, orders have not been placed, or supply areas not restocked. Patient reminders might not be mailed on time because a documented system is not in place. Computer back-ups might be made incorrectly or not at all—a potential crisis situation if the computer system crashes.

Another reason to create a hospital operations manual is to ensure quality control and provide a means for quality assessment. The hospital manual not only gives instructions on the correct way to complete a task or procedure, it also provides a benchmark to measure how employees are living up to established standards. A good example is reception area appearance, which is an important part of presenting the quality of overall veterinary care to clients. The manual would give instructions on how and when to check floors for urine and trash, straighten up magazines, water plants, reorganize the bulletin board, dust product displays, and assess the area for damage to walls and furniture. Often a series of checklists evolve as part of the manual, and these can serve as guidelines for use on a daily, weekly, or monthly basis.

Creating checklists is an art unto itself. Well-designed checklists can greatly improve patient care outcomes, workplace safety, client service, and more. A wonderful reference and compelling read for any practice manager and any veterinarian is *The Checklist Manifesto: How to Get Things Right* by Atul Gawande. The author of this book also has a website that provides useful information on creating checklists (see gwande.com/the-checklist-manifesto).

In larger practices, the hospital operations manual often becomes segmented into multiple volumes as the level of detailed instruction increases as a result of employee training and documentation requirements. One manual might be geared to reception and front-desk operations. Another might be for facility and equipment maintenance. A third manual could be developed for kennel oversight, sanitation procedures, animal handling and safety issues, feeding instructions, and pet-monitoring requirements. A manual geared to exam-room protocol would explain how exam rooms must be cleaned, detail what supplies to stock and when to check for reordering, describe animal-handling and client-safety issues, and outline patient examination guidelines.

One good starting point for a hospital operations manual is to compile all existing job descriptions. If a job description does not exist for a particular position, create one (see Chapter 5). Job descriptions should clearly outline specific task responsibilities, perhaps in a bulleted list. Each bullet then serves as the starting point for more detailed information about the correct way to compete the task in accord with management requirements. Once written, these instructions become concrete and uniformly communicated rather than vaguely understood through word of mouth or trial and error.

At the beginning of this book, we explored the definition of management as, in part, "working with and through individuals and groups to accomplish organizational goals" (Hersey and Blanchard 1982, 3). This rather clinical statement doesn't really get at the emotional aspects of management that are involved when you are working with people and animals. It should be obvious that fulfilling this definition of management is no small or simple task. Instead, it becomes a wonderful career-long endeavor to structure the perfect team of congenial, productive, and satisfied veterinary-care providers.

In your efforts to reach this dream, be a diligent student of human nature. Constantly search for new, creative ways to communicate and teach. Seek out the information you need. Know your limitations, but challenge yourself.

Never hesitate to seek professional assistance in dealing with the intricacies of law, compensation, and employee management issues. The practice's attorney and certified public accountant are good resources. Don't get discouraged when you think you have finally resolved a problem, only to have it pop up again. This is a normal course of events when working with people in business.

Working successfully with your team and with clients will be both one of the most enjoyable and one of the most challenging aspects of veterinary practice. You will celebrate the lifelong relations and friendships you discover in your work. The more you learn about human behavior and understand the people with whom you share a large part of your time, the more at ease you will be in leading and coaching them.

Yet you will temper your support with direction. As you listen to coworkers, you will avoid the temptation to act as a crutch for them. You will strive to be fair, remembering that your first loyalty and obligation is to the practice. To be effective at management, you may have to keep yourself somewhat distanced from employees so you can make rational and prudent decisions. There is a fine line between maintaining your authority and losing it in personal involvement. Practice management is an art that requires a delicate balance between the interests of owners, employees, clients, and animals.

5

The Employment Cycle

A big part of human resource management is orchestrating the required employees to meet client demand for veterinary services. These extensive responsibilities encompass all four steps in the management process: planning, organizing, directing, and evaluating. In the employment cycle, these stages translate roughly into planning employee acquisition, hiring, conducting orientation and training, and engaging in performance evaluation.

But there is no line of demarcation separating the four steps of the management process into these four stages of the employment cycle. Your organizational skills will be required in planning employee acquisition, training, and evaluating employees. You will also direct at every stage of the cycle, and you will evaluate at every stage. For example, you must be able to judge who is a good candidate for a position, based on the criteria you have set and the information you have collected.

This chapter explores the employment cycle in a veterinary hospital, from hiring and training through conducting employee performance reviews.

Planning Employee Acquisition

Hiring people for veterinary hospital employment is often a hit-or-miss proposition. Often a practice manager isn't even sure an additional person is needed; the need has been determined by the hue and cry of other employees: "We can't do any more! You need to hire someone to help us!" What that new person will accomplish and how existing staff will continue to be effective and efficient in their own work should be defined before placing the employment ad.

Hiring new staff involves recruitment, screening, and selection. Before you hire anyone, however, it is important that you plan carefully for the expansion. Two key ingredients in a complete plan for staff acquisition are the budget and the job description.

BUDGETING FOR STAFF ACQUISITION

The first step in the planning process is to develop or review a formal practice budget. Although often ignored, this step is a crucial part of ensuring adequate and cost-effective staffing. The budget—based on historical financial data, including detailed payroll analyses—should forecast client activity and demand, patient load, veterinary services, and product types. Staff hours worked, distribution of duties, and hourly pay rates are considered, and total staff costs are determined. Often, the practice's accountant or consultant works with management in deciding how the practice unit should be budgeted for the coming year.

During this planning phase, you should have quite a bit of discussion about the capabilities of the current staff, as well as capacity. The people you have may have drifted into occupying their time with duties that are redundant or not important. By realigning employee skills with prioritized work, you may find more capacity than previously known, alleviating the false urgency to hire another warm body.

Compute the number of hours of work anticipated from each employee and the expected hourly rates of pay, and compare these figures with the budget figures. Here is where a manager's competent use of computer spreadsheet programs shines. Once you have established a detailed model, it is a relatively straightforward process to update it at the next planning or monitoring date. If your practice has extended hours that lead to expected overtime situations, then you should carefully track and plan for this cost, too, as these costs added to the existing employee base salaries and wages can greatly inflate overall employment costs beyond what you might have mentally calculated.

Practice benefit programs should also be computed and projected as best you can. For example, group health insurance premiums have ratcheted up at double-digit annual increases. Besides the premium variable, your payroll plan should include determining who qualifies for participation, the amount the practice will subsidize, and the effect of any new hires. Also consider the effect of any qualified retirement plans and the practice's estimated funding liability, as well as the estimated number of participants. Finally, see the section entitled "Compensation Issues" later in this chapter, as the questions raised there will also impact employment-cycle planning.

With all this information, you now have a detailed analysis by employee and payroll dollar commitment for each type of worker payment and benefit. Considering that the total costs of a veterinary practice's labor force (veterinarian and support staff compensation) will be 38 to 45 percent, and up to 45 to 55 percent of gross income including benefits and taxes, in the author's experience it is important to have this level of detail to supplement the overarching practice operating budget. Once the pieces are organized and compared, you can determine the excess projected capital resources available for additional staff hires, increased wage incentives for existing staff, or both.

In other words, through the budgeting process you can establish how many additional employee work hours the practice should be able to pay for, if any. These additional hours can be gained by expanding the hours of existing part-time staff, by hiring new employees, or even by hiring temp employees as needed for seasonal fluctuations.

When considering employee acquisition, consider necessary experience level, the marketplace, and unemployment levels. When unemployment is high, you generally have a lot more flexibility when it comes to starting wages. This must be balanced against too weak of a compensation package, which can leave employees dissatisfied and simply waiting around for another job opening somewhere else. An economy with low unemployment generally requires higher starting wages to attract talent. Estimate an hourly rate of pay and the number of hours required. All of these factors help in finding the right person for the position.

DEFINING THE JOB AND ITS REQUIREMENTS

The second step in planning staff acquisition, a step that is as frequently bypassed as formal budgeting, is to create complete, accurate job descriptions. Job descriptions are outlines of the duties and responsibilities of each position in the hospital (Eppinger 1997, 6), and they are useful tools in recruiting and selecting new employees, training new employees, streamlining work, reviewing performance, and determining salary. The description serves as an initial screening device that quickly defines the job, tells the prospective employee what will be expected, and stimulates questions that can be addressed during the interview process.

If job descriptions already exist, they should be reviewed and updated as necessary to reflect actual job requirements. When you have identified a specific hiring need, create or review and update a job description before placing an advertisement.

Usually, job descriptions exist for each major job function within the hospital, including veterinarian, office manager, veterinary technician, veterinary assistant, kennel or barn attendant, receptionist, maintenance personnel, and bookkeeper. Job titles and functions vary from hospital to hospital. Sometimes employees share duties that span several different job descriptions, like a technician who also manages inventory purchasing. So remember that titles and functions discussed here might require adaptation or modification for your practice.

Begin the job description with a big-picture view of responsibilities. What are the expectations for this person? What types of change should the employee be effecting within the organization, if any? Include information regarding the authority that the team member will have. To whom does the employee report? Who reports to the employee?

A good job description provides a fairly detailed list of specific responsibilities, segregated categorically (administrative, patient care, etc.). Compose a complete wish list. Do not limit the job description to what previous employees in that position may have accomplished.

Often you may ask an employee to perform a task that is not included in that person's job description. It is discouraging to hear the comment, "That's not in my job description." For this reason, you will want to incorporate into each job description some flexibility to allow for changes in duties. Many job descriptions include a general description, such as "Any other task that is assigned or required by your supervisor. Any employee is expected to willingly assist a coworker when requested."

Another disclaimer suitable for inclusion in a veterinary hospital job description reads as follows: "Every employee works for Animal Hospital X as a whole, not only for a particular supervisor or department. Accordingly, employees are expected to act in the best interest of the hospital, even if doing so requires actions or responsibilities not listed in the above job description. This job description is provided for informational purposes only and is subject to revision by management when client need and patient-services requirements change" (Osborne 1995, 9.52).

If your practice does not have job descriptions, there are several good ways to get started in creating them. When establishing any hospital system, remember that many other hospital managers have already grappled with the same issue; there is no need to reinvent the wheel. Look for resources that give you general examples that can then be customized:

- A "Forms Bank" that includes sample job descriptions, in addition to many other management forms and practice marketing ideas, is available from the VHMA (see "Additional Resources").
- A helpful guide to veterinary practice job descriptions is *Job Descriptions and Training Schedules for the Veterinary Team* by James F. Wilson and Karen Gendron (2005).
- Figure 5.1 includes a sample job description.

Your staff can help you integrate sample job descriptions into your practice. Ask employees to write their own job descriptions, listing the duties they currently perform daily, weekly, or at other intervals, as well as any special assignments or responsibilities. Give them a limited time, perhaps one week, in which to complete the list. Compare each list with sample job descriptions from other sources and with your own knowledge of the job. Watch for duty descriptions that seem unnecessary or that could be streamlined, for instance, by reassigning it to another employee or combining it with another duty. Keep in mind that employees may omit tasks that they do not like to do.

As you customize job descriptions for your practice, make sure they have the following elements:

Position Title. Even if the practice has only a few employees, assign a title to every position. A formal job title establishes job identity. In a larger hospital, titles help define the hierarchy.

Summary. Provide a brief overview of the position, including major goals and objectives.

List of Duties and Responsibilities. List job duties in order of descending priority. Break higher-level positions into functional areas and categorize specific duties in each area.

FIGURE 5.1 JOB DESCRIPTION TEMPLATE FOR VETERINARY RECEPTIONIST

PAGE 1 SHOWN

˅

FULL FORM INCLUDED ON COMPANION WEBSITE

JOB TITLE: VETERINARY RECEPTIONIST

Exempt or Nonexempt Status: Nonexempt

General Description of Position: Duties include, but are not limited to, representing the practice with professionalism, courtesy, and a positive attitude; greeting clients, patients, and visitors; answering telephone, answering questions, promoting practice services and products, making appointments, transferring calls, and taking messages; proficiently using computers, invoicing, and record-keeping software, word-processing software, e-mail, and more; preparing patient records; preparing invoices; maintaining an organized and clean reception area; assisting clients with animals, children, and packages.

Key Competencies:

- Verbal and written communication skills (English/Spanish)
- Professional personal presentation
- Client service orientation
- Information management
- Organizing and planning
- Attention to detail
- Initiative
- Reliability
- Stress tolerance

Job Requirements/Skills: Able to perform several tasks concurrently with ease and professionalism. Able to read, write, speak, and understand English well. Speaks in an articulate manner and with a pleasant telephone voice. Able to operate a multiline telephone. Able to operate computer system and software in Microsoft Windows environment. Type 45 words per minute. Able to apply basic math skills to count money, make change, record patient weights, prepare prescriptions, and more. Able to use 10-key adding machine, fax machine, copier, credit-card processor, cash register, printers, and other office equipment. Familiar with veterinary medical terminology and knowledgeable about hospital procedures, policies, and services.

Reports to: Head Receptionist (or Practice Manager).

Supervises: No one.

Essential Functions:
- General Duties:
  » Performs opening and closing procedures pursuant to checklists.
  » Keeps reception area (all client and employee areas, public restroom, foyer) and outside client walkways clean, organized, and litter-free.
  » Immediately cleans up urine, feces, vomit, hair, and other patient debris.
  » Keeps trash receptacles and cigarette ash and litter bins empty and clean.
  » Keeps glass clean.
  » Restocks office, printing, client education, and janitorial supplies.
  » Restocks and organizes retail products.
  » Notifies maintenance of problems such as light replacement, repairs, painting, heating/AC, telephone, Internet or other IT, plumbing, etc.
  » Checks and maintains Facebook page.
  » Deals with queries from general public.
  » Receives mail and deliveries. Sorts mail and delivers to employee mail boxes.
  » Performs light clerical duties such as envelope stuffing, typing, preparing marketing materials, sending thank you and sympathy cards.
  » Rearranges and coordinates reception area for special promotional events such as for dental health, senior care, flea and tick season, etc.

Adapted from James Wilson, DVM, JD, and Karen Gendron, DVM, Job Descriptions and Training Schedules *(Priority Press, 2005)*; Catharine T. Eppinger, Creating Job Descriptions for Your Veterinary Support Staff *(AAHA Press, 1997)*

Describe what has to be done to fulfill each duty. Establish parameters or monitoring criteria so the employer and employee know when the job is done. Among the list of essential duties, provide descriptions not only of skilled or specialized duties, but of physical duties, including the amount of time and stress involved. Secondary duties that may be required under certain circumstances should be listed as well. For example, if the employee is expected to be able to lift a 50-pound dog, say so in the job description.

Description of Necessary Skills and Qualifications. Describe any special skills the job requires, including requirements for experience, special knowledge, or education. List personal qualities that are a help or a hindrance in the job if the presence or absence of such characteristics is necessary for adequate job performance. For example, a job description for kennel assistant might include the following: "This job requires handling a wide variety of breeds and types of dogs and cats. A person who is afraid of or tentative around unfamiliar animals should not work in this position." Although this may sound obvious, many managers can attest to the wasted time they have spent in hiring and training people who are afraid of some animals!

Description of Accountability. Establish the boundaries of authority for the position. To whom does this employee report? Who will determine how well the employee is functioning? How much authority is assigned to the position? (Stockner 1983; Osborne 1995, 9.03–9.04)

The resulting job description will represent your dream employee. Eventually, you will use it when conducting performance reviews. The employee can be continuously measured against the job description to identify gaps in performance.

Job descriptions are an important tool in the hiring process. Give a copy of the appropriate job description to every qualified applicant. The job description will provide a point of departure in interviews as you and the applicants compare the position requirements with their skills and abilities to see if they are a good match.

The inability to perform the essential duties could cause a prospective employee to be deemed unqualified for the position. It is important to keep in mind that in the case of an otherwise qualified person who has a disability, the employer may be required to make a reasonable accommodation that removes the disqualification. This subject is covered in more detail in Chapter 6 under the heading "The Americans with Disabilities Act." Although the Americans with Disabilities Act (ADA) does not require written job descriptions, a hospital using them should assure that each description represents a current and accurate profile of the job functions you expect employees to perform.

A job description is also helpful for training because it serves as a roadmap of topics that should be covered during orientation. More detailed descriptions can also help. Ask experienced employees to write down detailed explanations of each duty listed in their job descriptions. The resulting reports can become a part of the hospital's operations and training manuals.

Job descriptions should be reviewed at least once annually—more often in the event of staff reduction or staff growth. The budgeting meeting or a management retreat is a good time to schedule this task.

Hiring

Now that you've planned for staff acquisition, you are ready to organize and direct the hiring process. The process of hiring a new employee involves three basic steps: recruitment, screening, and selection.

RECRUITMENT

Good times for the economy can mean difficult times for job recruiters. Low unemployment makes it challenging to attract applicants to entry-level jobs. Down economic times provide employers with opportunities when it comes to recruitment. When unemployment is high, advertising a job opening typically produces a large number of qualified applicants. It will likely also yield a large number of unqualified applicants, which will require your skill in excluding them from the potential interview pool.

Establish protocols to explore all potential recruiting options to keep up with hospital needs. If you have planned adequately, you will know when additional employees will be needed. Start the recruitment process early if it seems that finding a good match for the position might be difficult. A practice's protocols when it comes to hiring can make the difference between finding the best candidate for the job and ending up with a candidate who is not ideal. With job postings bound to attract a large number of applicants, it is important to execute the employee recruitment and hiring process flawlessly from start to finish to ensure the hiring of an applicant who is a great fit to the team.

If the applicant pool seems small, be open to candidates with a variety of life experiences. Sometimes having to train a personable, willing employee on the job is acceptable, given the difficulty of finding someone who already fits the needs of the practice exactly.

Don't overlook resources you already have close at hand, such as team members with hidden and not-so-hidden talents and experiences. Over time, it can be easy to lose track of past-hire competencies and capabilities, since people often apply for veterinary practice positions that do not necessarily match all of the education they have. You might have advertised for a receptionist and hired an animal lover with strong marketing or organizational skills two years ago.

A valuable exercise is to read through the résumés already in your practice's employee files. You might also ask your team members to brush up their résumés and give you copies to reread with a fresh eye. Advertise the job internally before paying for outside ads. Perhaps promotion from within will save you time and provide a good match to the job you thought to fill.

Even if you choose to evaluate your existing employees for a possible new assignment, you might want to take the next logical step in recruitment, writing an advertisement for the available position. This helps you distill your vision and expectations of the position duties and worker attributes.

How the job position is announced depends to a great extent on the job title and position requirements. Base your advertisement on the criteria established by the job description; look at the major responsibilities and highlight them in the ad.

The advertisement can narrow the field by stating the probable range of compensation. Or, if you don't want to limit the number of applications, consider asking the applicants to define the compensation they expect, perhaps with a statement such as, "Please state your salary or wage requirement when applying for this position." This will also identify candidates who can take directions, since many will not give you this information even though it was requested. The figures provided by those who do comply will indicate what the market seems to be for people responding to the ad. If stated wage ranges are significantly higher than expected, reevaluate the ad. Possibly the ad has not been worded to attract the right pool of applicants or has been placed under the wrong help-wanted job heading.

As you are writing the advertisement, consider where you will place it. The title and requirements of the position will determine where you place the ad. For example, you would typically not advertise for a veterinarian or a veterinary technician in a small local newspaper. You would probably not advertise for a receptionist in the classified section of a professional journal.

Consider also that each medium will have its own requirements. A newspaper ad might be much shorter than a job announcement in a professional journal. Keep in mind that Internet options for ad placement are evolving and changing every day. Virtually all of the traditional print venues, such as professional journals and local newspapers, also have online placement, giving more bang for the advertising buck. You may be allowed higher word counts online than in print, which means you can fit in more of the job description. You may need to compose two versions of the ad, one for the online version and one for the print version of the same publication, because of the different word-count requirements.

In deciding where to place the ad, identify the venues that your potential recruits will be most likely to look at. Although you will probably consider common recruitment-ad placements such as newspapers and journals, try to come up with creative alternatives for reaching the perfect employee. People who are well suited to and qualified for your hospital's positions might not even be looking for a job and so wouldn't be reading the classified ads, either in print or on line. Somehow you have to catch their attention through other venues. Think about getting the word out in places where these prospective employees might be more apt to hear about the job.

State and local veterinary association newsletters (print and web-based) are logical places for veterinarians and veterinary assistants and technicians to look. The Veterinary Information Network (VIN) is good place to recruit doctors of veterinary medicine. Craigslist seems to work well for local market advertising. Keep in mind, too, that anyone who sees an interesting electronic ad can tweet or e-mail a link to it to a friend, so quick dissemination through virtual social networks is potentially the new norm.

There are many resources, formal and informal, that may be of help in your recruitment process. These range from personal recommendations to full-service agencies that help with the entire hiring process. Consider the following as you plan any staff expansion:

Placement Services. The American Veterinary Medical Association (AVMA) maintains a large database in its online Veterinary Career Center. The site includes job-seeker resources and employer resources, including listing notifications through Twitter and Facebook. Any job related to veterinary medicine can be posted.

Employment Agencies. Whether run by the government or private concerns, these agencies are primarily used to obtain secretarial help or unskilled labor.

Professional Recruiting Agencies. The services of these agencies include placing ads, evaluating résumés, and handling preliminary interviews. The placement fee is typically a percentage of the employee's first year salary, ranging from 25 to 40 percent. This is a sizable fee, so many employers hesitate to engage a professional agency except for very high-end, specialized positions. Placement services specializing in the veterinary industry are becoming more common, especially with the increasing popularity of the Internet. (For example, see My Veterinary Career at www.myveterinarycareer.com.)

Temporary Services. You can hire temporary personnel for hours or days on an as-needed basis. You might consider a temp service for basic bookkeeping, filing, transcription, preparation of bulk mailings, or other secretarial services. Occasionally, you might be so impressed by temporary workers that you hire them as permanent employees.

High Schools and Trade Schools. Stay well-acquainted with placement offices, guidance counselors, and faculty. If they know who you are, they may steer appropriate applicants your way. Put key contacts on the practice's mailing list and keep them updated with practice newsletters and brochures so they can be shared with students. Local trade schools and community colleges increasingly provide valuable exposure and inexpensive posting options through online job boards.

Professional Schools. Veterinary colleges and technician programs commonly provide a variety of options for recruiting graduates, including job listings, job boards, and onsite interviews. As with trade schools, your relationships with faculty can help cue you to an excellent prospect months or even years before graduation. Faculty can also invite practice veterinarians and technicians to give presentations to students about practical aspects of private practice. Find out about career-day events, and be there with information that sets your hospital apart.

Current Employees. A member of your own team may know someone who would be a worthy candidate. If you have employees going to school as well as working, keep them primed to look for classmates with desirable attributes, such as punctuality, personality, and intellectual competency. Train your team's working students how to use practice business cards to steer good candidates to the practice website and you. One word of warning here: Be wary of hiring family members or close friends of employees.

Personal Contacts. Keep your eyes open. Wherever you are—dealing with local merchants, eating in restaurants, or visiting the podiatrist or dentist—be alert to exceptional customer service. Always have your business card ready to hand out, accompanied with a friendly, "If you are ever thinking about a change of scenery, please consider giving me a call."

Other Practices. A neighboring hospital may have surplus help. Call the practice manager or owner to find out if they have personnel they would like to send your way. Another word of warning, however: You may be hiring someone else's problem. However, you may find someone who didn't work well in the other hospital but fits very well into your practice.

Vendor Representatives and Salespeople. Pharmaceutical-supply company representatives are well connected with many practices. Representatives have large territories and work for national or regional companies. They might know when a well-qualified individual is relocating to your practice's catchment area. Your representative may be able to give you a confidential lead about an employee in another practice who is interested in finding a different job.

Professional Networking. Stay well-connected with practice managers and veterinary practice owners in other regions or communities. They may have employees who will be relocating to your area. You can also network locally by attending local veterinary association meetings and chamber of commerce events. Networking happens everywhere: at the grocery store, barber shop and hair salon, and gas station. You have many options to talk up your practice and find out about what other people are doing in your community that will lead to a potential good employee, and perhaps several good new clients, too!

Clients. A client or a client's teenaged child may be well qualified for a job, so be sure to include appropriate job announcements in the hospital newsletter. A third word of warning: If the employment doesn't work out well, it may be difficult to fire that person. The practice could lose both an employee and a good client. Be careful to communicate expectations through a candid conversation before extending a job offer.

Newspaper Advertising. Newspapers used to be the most common source of advertising for nonprofessional employees, and online versions continue to be quite useful, as do print ads in small local papers. Use the job description as the basis for the ad. Keeping the advertisement specific will help you to eliminate unqualified applicants. Newspaper job advertisements may carry the name and address of the prospective employer or may be blind, giving only a box number, telephone number to call, or e-mail address. Some sources suggest that response rates decline by as much as 50 percent when advertisers use box numbers rather than telephone numbers or addresses (Isadore 2011).

Professional Journal and Publication Ads. If the advertised job is a professional or management position, place the advertisement in the appropriate professional journal. Reading a journal regularly will help you determine whether the audience includes the kinds of individuals you are targeting.

Association Newsletters. Local, state or provincial, and regional veterinary and technician association newsletters often provide space for employment ads. Since these target a group in closer proximity to your practice, they may be more likely than national publications to attract the applicants you seek, and the cost of advertising is likely to be lower. If your practice is seeking a manager or hospital administrator, consider the VHMA newsletter and the AAHA Managers Job Bank.

Other Newsletters. Newsletters for local dog and cat clubs and breed associations might allow space for ad placement. Other local animal organizations, including humane societies, could also be a way to reach good employee prospects.

Marquis Advertising. If your practice has an outside advertising marquis sign, consider placing a notice there, even something as simple as "Now hiring." If you don't have a marquis, engage the local sign shop to make a small sign, like those that real-estate agents place on the lawns of properties for sale. If the message is general, this sign can be put out whenever it is needed.

Website/Internet Advertising. Consider placing employment positions on your website. A "now hiring" link on the homepage can take interested parties directly to the pertinent virtual page. Facebook and Twitter are options, too. See the marketing chapter for more on social-media venues for marketing the practice. Link your homepage to the website of your community to provide a broader audience.

SCREENING

Now that your recruitment efforts have resulted in a long list of applicants from which to choose, the next step is to screen the candidates who have applied for the job. First, you will eliminate any candidates who do not meet the requirements stated in the job description. Then, by analyzing the information at hand, determine which of the remaining candidates seem the best qualified. To judge accurately among many candidates, try to get the same type of information from each applicant and follow the same steps in each case. Your goal at this point is not to settle on one candidate, but to determine which ones you would like to consider and interview.

Several sources of information about candidates can help you narrow the field before the interviews begin. These include letters of qualification, résumés, letters of reference, Internet searches, and telephone conversations with candidates.

Letter of Qualification. Ask all candidates to provide letters stating their qualifications for the position and reasons for wanting the job. This request could be made at the outset, through the ad copy, or after the prospective employee has applied for the job. If writing is an important duty in the position, a letter of qualification is particularly valuable as an example of the candidate's writing, grammar, and spelling skills. Given that many letters are now submitted electronically by e-mail attachment, you should also have some evidence of computer competency and etiquette.

Résumé. Depending on the position, you may ask for a résumé. Résumés are most valuable for professional or technical positions where prior education or experience is required or desired. In examining both the letters of qualification and the résumés, look for applicants who know what they are looking for and aren't afraid to say it. Vague statements about goals and objectives may indicate a lack of commitment. Of course, you must also understand the position. Someone responding to a kennel attendant position is not likely to consider it a lifelong career opportunity. Don't make notes on the résumé or other documents received from the applicant. Keep any notes on a separate piece of paper. Also, presume that anything you write could eventually be held against you as evidence in a court of law. Understand that the threat of claims of discrimination in hiring requires good defensive tactics in all phases of the hiring process.

Letters of Reference. Letters of reference may be voluntarily provided by the applicant as part of the résumé package or requested before the interview. If the prospective employee will be responsible for handling finances (for example, as a bookkeeper), ask for a financial reference as well. An example of a potentially good financial reference would be a certified public accountant or banker who is familiar with the applicant's work and character.

Telephone Calls. Usually, letters of reference are written by past employers. You may want to follow up with a phone call to the author of each letter; this will allow you to ask any questions and will give the authors the opportunity to express any reservations they might have been unwilling to put into writing. A reference may have asked the candidate to write her own letter, simply glancing at it before signing. Other letters are written to smooth a difficult termination. Be aware that even with phone calls to those who supplied the references, you may not get all the information you would like. Fearing litigation, past employers may be reluctant to tell you much of anything. Nevertheless, it makes sense to call references in case a glowing report comes through. If you call a reference for one candidate, you should do the same for all.

Internet Searches. While using the Internet to search information about prospective employees may be the norm nowadays, you should be aware of the possible pitfalls of researching candidates in this way. A manager might view Internet searches as a straightforward solution to finding out about candidate backgrounds, because the Internet is a public arena and much of the information is voluntarily posted by the people for which managers seek information. However, some attorneys suggest that Googling prospective employees is a risky move.

Discrimination in hiring practices is illegal. In theory, a plaintiff's attorney could cross-examine a veterinary manager to show that some of the information found during Internet searches, such as a disability or the existence of multiple young children and other apparent family obligations, was used to make a decision against offering the individual a job. Such allegations would be particularly difficult to contradict if the candidate could show he was as qualified as the person ultimately hired for the advertised position.

Some specific websites appear to be rational sources for investigation and exploration of a candidate's pedigree. LinkedIn, for example, is explicitly designed to feature the work history and qualifications of people in the workforce. It seems reasonable to assume that using such a recognized work-related social-media site would not lead an employer afoul of the law. If a candidate added personal information such as family members or other data unrelated to her qualifications as a worker, the disclosure appears to be parallel to the person verbally volunteering the information during an interview.

The Internet creates a shifting landscape of risks and opportunities in job hiring, and understandings of how existing employment laws might apply to this source of information is evolving. Before embarking on Internet searches about candidates who have applied for a new job opening, a manager should query the practice's attorney for a current opinion about any limits that should be set. You might ask the attorney to provide this opinion in writing, as this document may become evidence of practice effort to take the high road, should questions later arise.

Reviewing Résumés

Review all résumés with an open mind. Your ideal employee could be hiding behind job experience that appears irrelevant, or you may find precisely what your practice needs in other transferable skills that an applicant has obtained.

Divide the submitted documents into three categories: definitely interview; definitely reject; potential interview. Once you cycle through all of the candidate résumés, revisit the "definitely interview" category and make sure that only the best of the best are being considered. Respond immediately to the "definitely rejected" résumés, in a polite and considerate way. Be cognizant that your communication will reflect on the practice's image.

Hold potential interviewees' documents until after the first round of interviews is completed; you may have to consider some of these candidates if you do not find the right candidate in the top tier.

Then, respond to the "definitely interview" candidates (see next section). Schedule the first interviews as soon as possible to ensure you retain their interest. If you wait, these quality job-seekers may find employment elsewhere.

Calling Candidates

A telephone conversation can inform you about a candidate's telephone style, which is especially important when the position entails talking with clients or others on the telephone (e.g., reception). This conversation does not have to be a formal interview. For example, you can call the candidates or ask them to call you to confirm information on their application form, or even call to schedule the interview. It is best if you call the candidates, rather than having them call you, so that you can catch them unaware and get a true example of their telephone presence. Even answering-machine recordings can give you some hints about personality, professionalism, and other traits. Listen carefully to determine the candidate's level of poise and voice projection.

You can also use the telephone call as an initial, informal interview. Face-to-face interviews can be time consuming, and you may spend a lot of time talking with people who will not be good candidates. Telephone interviews are a great way to help you narrow the field of applicants so that you can concentrate on only the best candidates in the face-to-face interviews.

Here are some questions to pose in a telephone interview:

- Are you currently employed? If not, why not?
- What position are you expecting to fill?
- Do you have any experience working for veterinarians? If so, please describe it.
- What size and type of veterinary hospital are you interested in working for?
- How long have you been working at your present job? Why do you want to leave it?
- Where did you receive your training?
- Are you licensed? (where applicable)
- When would you be available to begin work?
- What is your salary requirement? (Osborne 1995, 2.08)

In a telephone interview, listen for the applicant's level of energy, enthusiasm, and overall interest. Since he took the time to apply, the candidate should be able to articulate basic knowledge of the job and the practice. A truly interested candidate will have thoroughly investigated the practice's online presence and information about it (unless your ad did not identify the practice name).

The Interview

After reviewing all of the other evidence, you will interview the candidates that you have chosen as the best prospects. The interview process can include scheduling interviews and tours, designing an interview checklist, choosing interview questions, administering tests, calling references and reviewing credit checks, and perhaps conducting second interviews. Your interview process should be consistent across the candidates. Be methodical with interview questions, administered tests of skills and aptitude, and how you summarize your assessment of each person (see Figure 5.2).

Make sure to spend adequate time preparing questions for your candidates. Questions more specific to the candidate can evolve from your review each of the candidates' résumés and corresponding documentation. What stands out? What does not make sense? Your questions can probe for specifics: metrics, accomplishments, and examples.

Prepare several behavioral questions relating to problem solving and analytical ability, anticipatory thinking, motivation, interpersonal skills, attitude, flexibility, and leadership. Ask questions regarding the candidates' expectations in order to gain insight into their work ethic and level of integrity as well as to determine if they would be a good fit with the practice. Ask candidates to label five of each of the following: their strengths, weaknesses, likes, and dislikes. When you review their responses, you will consider whether you have the means to mentor and develop their weaknesses, and you will identify how their strengths will benefit the practice. (Sample questions appear later in this chapter.)

After you have completed the first round of interviews, you will also compare responses across candidates to determine which candidates would best meld with the operating philosophy of the practice.

Decide what skills will be tested, such as computer usage, technical skills for animal handling and treatment, math skills (dosage calculations, for example), and typing and writing (patient record preparation). If permitted in your state, plan on whether you will use behavior typing assessments such as DISC at the first or second interview. (See Chapter 4 for more information.) If these are not legal in your state as an interview tool, see if a behavior instrument can be used after tendering an employment offer. The least risky option is to use this type of analysis after employment is offered and accepted.

Below are some additional factors to organize when interviewing job candidates.

Scheduling and Preinterview Testing. Schedule the initial interviews to last about thirty minutes. Once you have scheduled the interviews, confirming that these candidates are still interested, write a short note to those applicants who will not be invited to interview. Keep the note neutral, brief, and to the point. There is no need to explain your decision, simply state the facts. For example, "We appreciate your recent application with our hospital. We regret that we cannot offer you an interview at this time."

FIGURE 5.2 INTERVIEW CHECKLIST

INTERVIEW CHECKLIST

Applicant Name _____ Date _____

Position Desired _____ Interviewer _____

Overall Impression ❑ Poor ❑ Below Averge ❑ Average ❑ Very Good ❑ Excellent

Based on the requirements of the current position opening, check the appropriate box in each category, then make additional comments and recommendations below.

EXPERIENCE	JOB KNOWLEDGE	EDUCATION	MOTIVATION	EXPRESSION	APPEARANCE
Background experience does not relate to current position opening. ☐	Has little to none as pertains to this position. ☐	Has no relevant education background. ☐	Appears apathetic, indifference, disinterested. ☐	Demonstrates uncommunicative, confused thoughts, poor vocabulary. ☐	Indifferent to attire and grooming, sloppy, unkempt. ☐
Has little relative background experience. Needs much training. ☐	Will need considerable training. ☐	Has weak educational background. ☐	Has little interest in position. ☐	Is poor speaker; hazy thoughts, ideas. ☐	Careless in attire, poor grooming. ☐
Has some relative background experience, needs some training. ☐	Has basic, but will learn on the job. ☐	Has some relative educational background. ☐	Has sincere desire to work. ☐	Speaks well, expresses ideas adequately. ☐	Is functionally dressed, neatly groomed. ☐
Possesses adequate background experience, needs little training. ☐	Is well versed in position, little training needed. ☐	Has strong educational background. ☐	Has strong interest in position, asks questions. ☐	Speaks, thinks clearly, with confidence. ☐	Is well groomed. ☐
Background experience is perfect match to job requirements. ☐	Is extremely well versed, able to work without further training. ☐	Has excellent educational background. ☐	Is highly motivated, eager to work, asks many questions. ☐	Speaks clearly, concisely with confidence, ideas well thought out. ☐	Is immaculately attired and groomed. ☐

Additional Comments and Recommendations
_____
_____
_____
_____
_____
_____
_____

Should we interview further?   For what position?   Refer to: (Manager of position)   Department?
_____   _____   _____   _____

Adapted from materials by Amsterdam Printing and Litho Co.

The interviews should be conducted in quiet surroundings so that you can give full attention to each person. Request that other staff not interrupt your meeting and that no calls be put through.

Each candidate should have already completed an approved, legal application for employment (see Figure 5.3). If the position requires writing or filing, administer a spelling and grammar test, perhaps including some veterinary medical terminology. Computer use skill tests are also appropriate, including the ability to type and use word-processing programs, use e-mail, and navigate common operating systems.

Interview Style and Questions. The interview should be a relaxed dialogue, with the candidate doing most of the talking. Don't try to fill in gaps in the conversation. A lengthy pause may inspire the candidate to jump in and reveal information you might not have learned otherwise.

Do give each candidate a brief summary of the position. Read the job description together or allow the applicant five minutes alone to review it. Then you can address questions about the position and the hospital.

During the interview, ask open-ended questions instead of questions that require a yes or no answer. Also avoid asking leading questions, such as, "Are you willing to work overtime?" These lead the candidate to the answer you are seeking. It is much more valuable to ask questions such as, "Why do you want to work here?" or "What hours are you available to work?" As you listen, pay close attention to the candidate's appearance, diction, use of grammar, and personality.

Here are some other possible interview questions:

- "Tell me about yourself." The answer may identify likes, dislikes, and prejudices.
- "What jobs have you held and what were your duties?" The answer will help to identify skills.
- "What attracted you to this position?" The answer will help to determine interest in the position.
- "Have you ever been discharged from a position?" The answer will help to determine the reliability of the candidate.
- "How does this position fit into your long-range goals?" The answer should tell you about motivation and dedication.
- "Why are you leaving your present position?" This answer may reflect the suitability, loyalty, and commitment of the candidate.
- "What did you do when things were slow at your prior job?" The answer shows the candidate's self-motivation for being helpful and valuable to the company.
- "What did you do when you were uncertain of supervisor communications or expectations?"

PAGE 1 SHOWN
⌄
FULL FORM
INCLUDED ON
COMPANION
WEBSITE

FIGURE 5.3 APPLICATION FOR EMPLOYMENT

APPLICATION FOR EMPLOYMENT

(Please print clearly)
An Equal Opportunity Employer

Our practice does not discriminate on the basis of race, religion, national origin, color, sex, age, veteran status, disability, or any other status protected by applicable law or regulation. It is our intent that all qualified applicants be given equal opportunity and that selection decisions be based on job-related factors.

Date _____

Name _____
Last   First   Middle

Present address _____ Phone _____
No.   Street   City   State   Zip

Position applied for _____ Email address _____

Employment you are seeking ☐ Full-time ☐ Part-time Specify days and hours if part-time _____

Were you previously employed by this organization? _____ If yes, when? _____

List any friends or relatives working here, other than spouse _____
Name(s)

If your application is considered favorably, on what date will you be available for work? _____ 20 _____

Are there any other work experiences, skills, or qualifications that you feel would especially qualify you for employent here? Please add any additional comments you think are important for us to consider. Use an additional sheet of paper if necesary
_____
_____

If hired, can you furnish proof you are eligible to work in the United States? ☐ Yes ☐ No

Have you ever been convicted of a felony? ☐ Yes ☐ No
A yes answer does not automatically disqualify you from employment since the nature of the offense, date, and the job for which you are applying will be considered.

If yes, please explain _____

Have you previously applied here? ☐ Yes ☐ No

If yes, when? _____

Have you worked for any entity under a different name? ☐ Yes ☐ No

If yes, give name _____

If you are applying for a position with minimum age requirements, you may be required to submit proof of age.

For jobs with minimum age requirements: Are you 18 years of age or older? ☐ Yes ☐ No

For driving positions only: Do you have a valid driver's license? ☐ Yes ☐ No

Driver's license number _____ Type/Class of license _____ State _____

Has your driver's license been revoked or suspended in the last 3 years? ☐ Yes ☐ No

AAHA
© 2010 AAHA

The answer helps ascertain the candidate's maturity level in initiating productive collaborative conversations.

- "Thinking of a time when you had a conflict with a coworker, what did you do?" The answer may provide indications of the candidate's ability to work through conflict in an effective and professional way, and whether less desirable behavior like triangulation or pot-stirring might be evident.
- "Talk to me about what your process was for _____". This answer gives information about the candidate's ability to articulate processes and communicate effectively, and also checks the accuracy of her résumé-claimed knowledge and skills. In other words, does the candidate really have the knowledge she claims to have?
- "Tell me about your personal core values," or, "What are your three essential personal values that are unbreakable?" This answer speaks to the values that form the core of what the applicant believes and what actions will follow, especially in difficult situations and when ethical dilemmas arise. Listen for descriptive words like compassion, honesty, truthfulness, respect, friendship, work ethic, and so on. Ideally, these values will match up with the practice's core values.

Also ask some problem-solving questions to determine how the candidates think on their feet. For example:

- "If a doctor had left for the day and had not spoken to you about specific instructions on how to care for a particular patient, what would you do?"
- "If a client asked how to give a medication, what would you do?"
- "If a person called with a pet who had vomited a little bit during the night, what would you do?"

Some of your questions should help you to determine whether the candidate will have any trouble with some physical or emotional aspect of the job. For example, if the position involves handling animals, discuss various aspects of animal care, such as the candidate's fitness, both physically and emotionally, to carry out job responsibilities, particularly with reference to euthanasia and patient pain. One way to lead into such a discussion is to address each of the essential functions listed on the job description and ask the prospective employee about performing them. If the candidate mentions a disability that could prevent him from fulfilling the essential duties, it will be your responsibility, together with the candidate, to determine whether he could perform the duties if you provided a reasonable accommodation (see discussion of the ADA in Chapter 6).

Application and Interview Checklist. As previously stated, there are many laws and regulations designed to reduce or eliminate employment discrimination. Ensure the questions that you ask relate only to the job you are trying to fill and whether the candidate can perform the job functions necessary. Educate all team members who will be a part of the interview process about questions that can and cannot be asked. For example, interviewers are not permitted to ask certain questions relating to nationality, religion, age, marital and family status, gender, sexual orientation, or health and physical abilities. (See Table 5.1 for more information.)

These laws also apply to questions that can and cannot be asked on application forms. Make sure you are familiar with current federal and state law, and keep abreast of changes as additional laws are passed. Legal interpretations of the law may also change. When in doubt, call the practice's retained employment attorney.

The interviewer should use a form to guide the interview and to provide a space for notes on selected issues. If several candidates are to be interviewed, use the same form with each so that you can compare the candidates. Complete the form immediately after the conclusion of each interview. That way, you will be less likely to forget your impressions or confuse the candidates.

Tour of the Facility. After each interview is completed, give the candidate a tour of the hospital, introducing present employees and pointing out aspects of hospital operations relative to the job position. For example, a prospective surgical technician would be most interested in the surgery suite and patient prep and recovery areas. Remember that your best candidates will be able to find any number of jobs. If they couldn't, they wouldn't be your best candidates. You may have to convince them that they should be working for you. The best way to do this is with a pleasant interview experience and a tour that shows a nice, well-equipped place to work and happy, congenial coworkers.

During the tour, you can continue to pick up cues about the candidate. Watch body language and observe how the person responds to others. Look at facial expression, body carriage, and eye contact. Does the applicant smile readily and extend a hand in greeting? Try to gauge energy and attention levels and notice how the person comports herself.

A quick test is to observe what the person does when something is out of place, like a patient history card that has fallen to the floor. If the candidate picks it up without a second thought, he is a self-thinker, helpful, and neat. The candidate who voluntarily wipes up animal urine or feces in the treatment area while you stop to talk with a staff member is exceptionally observant and helpful.

Concluding the Interview. At the conclusion of the interview and/or tour, give the candidate a specific date when you will have made your hiring decision. If it is obvious that the candidate does not have the necessary skills to meet the job requirements, you may want to say so at this time, rather than call later. If you have several good candidates to interview, resist the temptation to hire until you have completed all of the interviews. In a tight labor market, however, you may have to move fast in order to hire a good employee. If you know you have found the right person, don't dally! Tomorrow your best candidate may accept another job offer.

TABLE 5.1 LAWFUL AND UNLAWFUL INTERVIEW QUESTIONS

SUBJECT	LAWFUL QUESTIONS	UNLAWFUL QUESTIONS
Age	*Are you 18 years of age or older? If not, state your age. Do you have a work permit? If hired, can you provide proof you are of legal age to work?*	How old are you? What is your date of birth? What are the ages of your children? When did you graduate from high school?
Arrests and convictions	Application can ask if a person has been convicted of a crime if (1) the form indicates that a conviction is not an automatic bar, and the seriousness of crime and date of conviction will be considered, and (2) the question reasonably relates to performance of the position.	*Have you ever been arrested?* Questions regarding a person's police records are illegal.
Marital or family status	There are no legal questions regarding marital or family status. If you need to know if a person can work overtime or weekend or late shifts, ask: *Is there any reason why you will not be available for overtime or weekend work?*	*Do you wish to be addressed as Miss? Mrs.? Ms.? Are you married? Single? Divorced? Separated?* Questions about applicant's spouse or children.
Disability/medical conditions/illness	*Are you capable of performing the essential functions of the position with or without reasonable accommodation?*	*Do you have a disability? Have you ever been treated for any of the following diseases . . . ? Do you now or have you ever had a problem with alcohol or drugs?*
National origin	None	Inquiry into the lineage, ancestry, national origin, descent, parentage, or nationality of applicant or applicant's parents.
Race or color	None	Questions about complexion or eye, hair, or skin coloring.
Religion	There are no legal questions regarding religion. If you need to know if a person can work weekends, ask: *If hired, are you available to work Saturdays or Sundays on an as-needed basis?*	Questions about observance of religious holidays or religious affiliation.
Sex	None	
Address or duration of residence	*How long have you been a resident of this state or city?*	
Birthplace	None	Requirement that applicant submit birth certificate or naturalization or baptismal record.
Citizenship	*Are you a citizen of the United States? If not a citizen, do you intend to become a citizen of the United States? If you are not a citizen, have you the legal right to remain permanently in the United States? Do you intend to remain in the United States?*	*Of what country are you a citizen?* If the applicant is a naturalized or non-native-born citizen: *When did you acquire citizenship?* If applicant's parents are naturalized or non-native-born citizens: *When did your parents acquire citizenship?* Requirement that the applicant produce naturalization papers or first papers.

CONTINUES >

> TABLE 5.1

LAWFUL AND UNLAWFUL INTERVIEW QUESTIONS, CONT.

SUBJECT	LAWFUL QUESTIONS	UNLAWFUL QUESTIONS
Driver's license	*Do you possess a valid driver's license?*	Requirement that the applicant produce a driver's license.
Education	Inquiry into the applicant's academic, vocational, or professional education and the public or private schools attended.	*Are you a high school graduate?*
Experience	Inquiry into work experience.	
Military experience	Inquiry into the applicant's experience in the U.S. armed forces or state militia.	*Did you receive a discharge from the military other than honorable discharge?* Inquiry into the applicant's military experiences beyond that in the U.S. armed forces or state militia.
Organizations	Inquiry into applicant's membership in organizations that the applicant considers relevant to the job performance.	*List all clubs, societies, and lodges to which you belong.*
Photograph	None	Requirement or suggestion that applicant attach a photograph to employment form at any time before hiring.

Sources: Adapted from Sheldon London, How to Comply with Federal Laws: A Complete Guide for Employers Written in Plain English, *rev. ed. (Rochester, NY: Vizia, 1998), 207; American Institute of Certified Public Accountants (AICPA),* Management of an Accounting Practice Handbook *(New York: AICPA, 2005 revision), Exhibit 214-3, Chapter 214, 61-62.*

References

After you have chosen one or two top candidates, it is a good idea to call their references. If you haven't already done so, ask the candidate for contact information at the interview (if they have it handy, this may be another indication that they know how to think ahead). In particular, ask for the names of employers, especially the current or most recent one. Tell applicants you plan to telephone the listed references, and obtain their written permission to do so.

Even with written consent, it may be difficult to obtain useful information from a reference. Traditionally, the law protected employers who gave employment references to subsequent employers. Such references, if made in good faith, were subject to immunity from defamation liability. Now, because more defamation lawsuits have been filed against former employers who have provided information to potential employers, many people are reluctant to say anything at all about candidates, either positive or negative.

To make things more complicated, even refusal to give a reference can get an employer into trouble. Some courts have opined that occasions do arise when an employer has a duty to do more than just give a "no comment" reference. If a past employer refuses to give negative information about a former employee, that employer may be held responsible for violent or illegal acts committed by the person in the employ of the new employer. This is called a "negligent referral." Employers are in the uncomfortable position of trying to avoid defamation claims from former employees while also avoiding claims of negligent referral from subsequent employers. Be aware of these risks, since you may also be called as a reference for a former employee. (For more information, see the textbox entitled "After the Termination: How to Handle Referral Calls," which appears later in this chapter.)

Calling former employers does at least allow you to verify that applicants worked where and when they claim to have worked. If the reference is a former employer, ask about the circumstances of the candidate's departure from that position. Also ask, "Would you willingly rehire this person?"

The person who conducts the interview should be the person who calls the candidate's references. This allows for any inconsistencies between what the reference says and what the candidate said to be revealed. When calling references, use a form to guide you in your questions (see example in Figure 5.4). A standard form helps you to keep your questions consistent for each reference called.

Here are some more guidelines for checking references:

- All references should be checked before (not after) extending an offer of employment.
- Reference-checking procedures should be uniformly applied to all candidates. If references are checked on one candidate, they must be checked on all.
- All questions should be job related.
- All opinions expressed by the person supplying the reference should be substantiated by facts. Seek confirmation from her when you hear a negative opinion.
- Don't take a bad reference at face value. Ask to speak to another person in the organization to verify the information. Personality conflicts, among other factors, can give rise to negative references.
- Don't express an opinion when responding to a negative comment from the person supplying the reference. Your job is only to collect facts.
- The best source of information is the applicant's most recent employer or supervisor (Osborne 1995, 2.19).

Credit Checks

Credit checks can be used to confirm employment with prior employers whom you are unable to contact. Because credit checks identify current and past credit information and list late payments, some employers believe that credit scores can also indicate how the potential employee handles obligations. Remember that credit reports may be inaccurate, however, and that credit checks require the written consent of the person being checked. Also keep in mind

FIGURE 5.4 QUESTIONS TO ASK A REFERENCE

PRE-EMPLOYMENT REFERENCE CHECK

Date _____

Company Name
1234 Street
City, State, Zip Code
Attention:

The applicant named below has told us that he/she previously worked for your company. We would appreciate your supplying us with as much of the information requested below as possible. Any information you may give will be treated confidentially. A quick reply will be greatly appreciated.

Sincerely yours,

_____ Title _____

Company Name
1234 Street
City, State, Zip Code

Applicant's Name: _____

Dates in Your Employ: From _____ To _____ Salary: $ _____ Per _____

Position Held: _____

Is the information listed above correct? Yes _____ No _____ If no, please supply the correct information below.

_____

_____

Why did applicant leave your company? _____

Would you re-employ? Yes _____ No _____ If no, why not? _____

_____

Please circle the word that best describes the applicant on the following characteristics:

Quality of Work	Poor	Fair	Average	Very Good	Excellent
Quantity of Work	Poor	Fair	Average	Very Good	Excellent
Job Knowledge	Poor	Fair	Average	Very Good	Excellent
Attendance*	Poor	Fair	Average	Very Good	Excellent
Dependability	Poor	Fair	Average	Very Good	Excellent
Cooperativeness	Poor	Fair	Average	Very Good	Excellent
Ingenuity	Poor	Fair	Average	Very Good	Excellent

*If attendance was "poor," is there a question of need for reasonable accommodation?

Date _____ Signed _____

Title _____

that many otherwise hardworking and responsible people have had financial difficulties. Their credit scores may reflect problems outside of their control, such as a spouse losing a job from company downsizing.

Second Interviews

After the first interview is completed, your top candidate may be obvious and you may be ready to offer this individual the position. If the choice is not yet clear, you may have to decide who to invite for a second interview. As with first interviews, it is considered professionally courteous to promptly notify any applicants who will not be invited for second interviews. Again, do not elaborate on your decision. Keep it simple. For example, you can say, "We appreciate your recent visit to our hospital to interview for the position of kennel supervisor. We regret we cannot offer you a position at this time."

The second interview may include additional testing. If you did not do so in the original interview, you may want to consider a personality-style or behavior-typing instrument (discussed in Chapter 4) to gain a deeper understanding of probable behavior based on how candidates would view themselves in their work environments. The results may help you to determine which styles might be compatible with existing team members and which behavior traits are best suited to the position.

If this type of assessment is used prior to an offer of employment, it must be given to all candidates and should be used in conjunction with other tests (typing, spelling, animal-care knowledge, etc.). You should be able to show that the assessment was only one of many criteria used to select a candidate for the position. If the personality instrument identifies any trait or condition that could be considered a disability or caused by a disability, this result should not be used as a reason for not employing the individual. In any case, because law and precedent vary from state to state, do ask the practice's employment attorney whether such assessments should be avoided as a prehiring technique in your area.

Behavior preference profiles may be more valuable after employment. As we saw in Chapter 4, an individual's perceived control of and relation to the hospital environment can affect the profile outcome. The most valid and helpful results may be those obtained after a new employee has worked in your hospital for a while.

Our experiences have shown that prospective employees tend to be impressed that an employer is sincerely interested in their personal styles and how they would work most successfully with others. Some managers obtain personality-style profiles for candidates who have been offered positions but have not yet accepted them. Explain that the practice culture embraces and supports employee growth and development, including training in healthy interpersonal relationships and leadership. To accomplish this, the practice regularly uses personality and behavior typing with all employees.

After sharing the results with the potential employee, you can sit down together and review how he would work with others in the job position. You can review the person's strengths and weaknesses relative to the job requirements and identify potential behaviors that might produce some stress as the new employee adapts. As before, discuss with the attorney how you plan to use a behavior-assessment tool before beginning the hiring process so that you can plan for any foreseeable problem that might arise.

For example, say you have offered a technician position to a candidate and she has not yet decided whether to accept it. Personality testing reveals that this candidate has very pronounced dominance characteristics. She would be required to work directly with and under the supervision of a technician who also has very high D-type behavior. You could warn the candidate that she would have to be willing to take directions and follow through with tasks, even though that might not be her natural tendency. With this information, the candidate can make a more considered decision. If she accepts the job, her employment will have a greater chance of success because she has the information she needs to modify her behavior and establish a good relationship with her supervisor from the start.

The second interview should also include frank discussions about salary, including opportunities for raises and other advancement. Eligibility for overtime pay and available pretax benefits should be specified. Make sure you discuss hours of required work, including weekend and holiday duty. Be forthright and consider formally documenting expectations, so that there is no confusion later on either side.

SELECTION

The last step in the hiring process is the selection of the best candidate for the position. You should have the following information on each remaining candidate: a completed application form, names of references, a completed interview form, and other materials, such as a behavior profile and other tests.

If you are filling a position that requires professional credentials and licensing, such as veterinarian or technician, you should also make sure that all licenses, registrations, and accreditations are valid and current. Don't make the mistake of offering a job to someone who is not licensed to do it. A degree doesn't guarantee that someone is licensed or registered to practice in your state.

After you have completed the entire process and have made your decision, rank the candidates from your first choice on down. Consider each of the following characteristics:

- Prior training and education
- Apparent technical skills and aptitude
- Overall attitude, degree of enthusiasm, and energy level
- Demeanor and physical presentation

- Verbal and communication skills

You may think of other observations that you will include when making your ranking.

Call your top candidate and offer the position before you make any other calls. Never call other candidates to inform them that the position has been filled until you have completed the hiring process. Your top candidate may not want the position or may have accepted another.

You may also find that the person you have selected wants to negotiate the salary you have offered or some other part of the employment package. Be prepared for this; either make a counteroffer or arrange to continue the discussion after you consult with others in the practice.

After your job offer has been accepted, call the remaining candidates and inform them that the position has been filled. It may be a good idea to ask the best among these candidates, "If another position becomes available, would you be interested?" By keeping the files of interested candidates, you could very well eliminate having to go through the entire process the next time you need a new employee. Before making such an offer, however, be sure to ask your legal counsel if this type of question could have any legal consequences.

You may choose to extend or confirm an offer of employment in writing by using the practice's attorney to create an offer letter that lists many of the terms of employment. An offer letter would be more common to hiring for employees at the higher levels, such as for associate veterinarian. Offer letters are often used when a written *employment agreement* will result. This agreement lists terms of employment, duties, and compensation. (See textbox, "Employment Agreements.")

Employment Agreements

For most practices, hiring for professional and managerial positions, such as doctor of veterinary medicine or practice manager, involves an employment agreement. Employment agreements are beyond the scope of this book, but you should be aware of them. Employment agreements can be written or oral. Written agreements formalize the terms of employment, the compensation elements, and the duties and responsibilities of the new employee. They often include restrictive covenants prohibiting the employee from competing with the practice, divulging confidential information about the practice, or soliciting clients or other employees after termination of employment (Salzieder 2007, 450).

Use the practice's attorney to write any legal documents such as a written employment agreement. The attorney's expertise ensures that all provisions of the contract comply with the laws of the practice's jurisdiction and accurately describe the intended agreed-upon terms between employee and employer. As a general rule, written employment agreements should be provided to the prospective employee to read and sign before the employee begins any work for the practice.

Conducting Orientation and Training

Your hospital now has a new employee. What happens next? Too many times, the answer to that question is "nothing." Providing new employees with adequate training is essential in the development of a good working relationship. A standard orientation procedure not only helps new employees get acclimated but also shows them that your hospital is well organized. It sets a tone of professionalism that they are likely to follow.

Welcoming a new employee is like having a guest into your home. You are the lead hostess helping the new employee feel like part of the practice family.

ON-BOARDING

Implementing and using a plan to start a new employee out effectively with a prepared welcome, orientation, and training schedule is called *on-boarding*. A good on-boarding plan will help the employee feel welcome and enable him to be productive immediately. An on-boarding plan starts with the practice welcome letter, outlines the first day on the job, and establishes a schedule that helps the employee succeed in the job and in working with others as quickly as possible. In one on-boarding plan covering the first 120 days of employment, the manager was required to include one new learning objective for each day (Heathfield n.d.).

Shortly after the employee has accepted the job, follow up with a brief e-mail or note to confirm the conversation and express the practice teams' excitement about the candidate's hire. In the welcome letter, also provide a line of communication for the new hire to use for questions or additional information.

A welcome letter can include other types of information that will be helpful for the employee to know in advance of the first day on the job. Think back to your first day of a new job and all the questions you might have had, ranging from what to wear to where to park. You can provide some basic information to the employee ahead of time that will greatly ease such worries.

The welcome letter typically includes confirmation of the first day of work, time to report, and dress code. You may wish to send the employee policy manual with this letter. The employee may appreciate being able to read the information in advance and can then come prepared with any questions she has.

Encourage the employee to check out the practice website to become familiar with the faces and names of the other employees. Or, provide a list of employee names and job titles with a picture of each team member. Some practices maintain a bulletin board that has pictures and names of all employees for easy reference as well, which can be helpful especially to new employees. If your practice has an intranet, give the employee early access to it so he can browse internal information and gain familiarity with training materials, other employees, and events.

Some practices set up an orientation in advance of the first formal work-day. In a one-hour orientation, you can:

- Review a summary sheet of employee handbook highlights and send the complete manual home with the employee
- Provide a written work schedule for the first two weeks of employment
- Provide a uniform so that on the first day the employee already looks like part of the team
- Inform the employee that the practice will plan lunch for the first employment day
- Introduce the employee to her assigned trainer
- Show the employee where to park
- Have the employee complete required employment paperwork.

ASSIGNING ORIENTATION TASKS

Your next step is to assign different aspects of orientation and training to the people responsible for them. This step should be taken well before the new employee arrives at work so that orientation and training can be handled efficiently and effectively. If this is a new position, you as the manager may provide training. Otherwise, coworkers who hold similar positions or the person who is leaving this position might be the best trainers, as long as they are not disgruntled employees.

Remember, this is your opportunity to mold a new employee from the very beginning. From day one, it is critical that you teach the employee the correct way to fulfill his duties, the expected attitude, and the overall culture of the practice. Your communication of the practice's expectations of an employee's level of patient care and efficiency starts with the first day of training; it is much easier to develop your employees properly from the start than to try to correct and change them later on.

Famed quality pioneer W. Edwards Deming believed that a company could not generally attribute poor quality and a lack of efficiency to employees individually. Instead, failures are caused by the system as a whole. Management bears responsibility for correcting and maintaining the system (Stevenson 2009, 409). A poorly or improperly trained employee is the fault of management.

Too often, employees are poorly or inadequately trained, resulting in a frustrating situation for everyone involved. A properly planned and executed training system will result in competent employees that fit the practice's ideal culture and pursue quality and efficiency in their work.

Never allow new-employee training to be done by employees who are disgruntled, employees you plan to fire, or employees who have done an unsatisfactory job. This would only ensure another unsatisfactory performance.

As you decide who will train the new employee, remember that experience is critical. Whoever conducts the orientation must know the job thoroughly.

Before the new employee's first day, inform the rest of the staff about the hiring decision and give them pertinent information about their new colleague—name, start date, and job title. Ask an employee, preferably someone with whom the new person will be working closely or someone with a similar position, to be a companion for the newcomer at lunchtime, at least on the first day. This will prevent the employee from feeling isolated and will provide another set of "ears" during the important period of training and team integration.

Consider whether or not a formal mentoring process is right for your practice's culture and environment. Mentor programs are designed to help new employees adapt to the practice's cultural and social norms.

For an orientation checklist, see Figure 5.5. For more ideas about setting up mentorships, see textbox, "Mentor Programs."

THE FIRST DAY

Even if you will not be directly responsible for the new employee's training, as manager you will have responsibility for creating, sharing, and monitoring the on-boarding schedule. As the ideal host, be prepared to personally conduct some important introductory tasks.

Mentor Programs

Here are some guidelines for a mentoring program (Tapper n.d.):

- The mentor is not the trainer, but an experienced, knowledgeable employee who helps cement the employee to the practice by quickly forming a trusted relationship with the newbie and maintaining a caring, listening ear. The mentor helps to ensure that the new employee is comfortably fitting in. The ultimate mentor is one with whom the employee feels comfortable discussing any work issues that arise.
- The mentor privately meets with the employee at least once a day during the first two weeks of employment to find out how work is going. Questions to ask include: Is training adequate, too much, not enough? Are you overwhelmed? Are you being accepted into the team? Do you like your position?
- The mentor continues initiating regular interactions over the next three to six months of employment and may periodically take the employee out to lunch.
- With good lines of communications, the mentor may discover work issues that can and should be adjusted, which might otherwise lead to the loss of a new, yet valuable employee.

FIGURE 5.5 ORIENTATION CHECKLIST

PAGE 1 SHOWN
⌄
FULL FORM
INCLUDED ON
COMPANION
WEBSITE

NEW EMPLOYEE ORIENTATION CHECKLIST

Name of New Employee: _____

Position: _____

Start Date: _____ ❑ Full-time ❑ Part-time ❑ Temporary

Name of "Buddy": _____

Initial and date each blank when task is completed.

1. Pre-arrival Preparation:
   - ❑ Send a letter confirming employment and indicating start date, position, time and place to report, salary, and overtime compensation, if applicable. See sample letters in c:\ _____ .
     Include:
     - ❑ Hospital brochures
     - ❑ Hospital magazine/internal newsletter/client newsletter
     - ❑ Administration memoranda
     - ❑ Other non-confidential information to acquaint new employee with the hospital
     - ❑ Sample confidentiality agreement (c:\ _____)
     - ❑ Non-compete agreement, if veterinarian or management position
     - ❑ Licensing compliance affirmation (c:\ _____)
     - ❑ Copy of employee manual
     - ❑ Job description
   - ❑ Prepare memo advising staff and clients of new employee's arrival. Copy to new employee.
   - ❑ Determine any other announcements to be made.
     - ❑ News releases
     - ❑ Home page
     - ❑ Newsletter
   - ❑ Set up personnel file. Employee will fill in general information on first day.
     Add to file:
     - ❑ Résumé
     - ❑ Application
     - ❑ References
     - ❑ Any notes or other information related to interview
     - ❑ Copy of employment offer letter, if one was sent
     - ❑ Copy of acceptance letter
     - ❑ Copies of any documents sent with acceptance letter
   - ❑ Coordinate with various internal departments to prepare for new employee's arrival.
     - ❑ Telephone—update all phones for intercom address
     - ❑ Publications—add to circulation stamp for brochures, newsletters, and magazines
     - ❑ Purchasing—business cards
     - ❑ Payroll
     - ❑ Network administrator—passwords, E-mail, provider listing, etc.
     - ❑ Personnel roster, organizational chart
     - ❑ Staff scheduling
     - ❑ Facility security—key and password assignment

2. First-Day Welcome and Introduction to Hospital:
   - ❑ Greet new employee in reception area
   - ❑ Introduce to receptionists
   - ❑ Introduce employee to hospital administrator and owners, and other employees.

3. Orientation Meeting:
   - ❑ Overview of Hospital
     - ❑ Philosophy
     - ❑ Services

Be at the hospital early to greet the new employee when she arrives on the first day. Show the new employee where to store personal items such as a coat, lunch, or purse. Show her where to punch in. If a locker or personal space is available, assign one. If uniforms are to be provided, distribute them now, or, if this has not been done previously, obtain the new employee's size and order them.

One of the first tasks to complete soon after arrival is paperwork. The new employee must complete the necessary personnel forms that regulations require the hospital to have on file. To be efficient, and because documentation and supporting information is extensive, inform the employee in advance what she must bring the first day of work. (See textbox, "Regulatory Employment Documentation.")

Additional information about personnel files appears later in this chapter. See also Chapter 6 for information about employment laws.

Introduce the new employee to the rest of the hospital staff. If any team members are absent, arrange an introduction as soon as possible. The practice team should know about the

---

Regulatory Employment Documentation

In the United States, the forms to complete and documentation to collect include:

- **Form W-4—Employee's Withholding Allowance Certificate:** This reports federal income tax withholding information (see Figure 5.6).
- **State income tax withholding forms:** States with income tax withholding requirements require this form; use the department of revenue website for your state to check for new requirements and obtain forms.
- **Form I-9—Employment Eligibility Verification form:** The I-9 must include copies of documents required for identity confirmation (see Figure 5.7). It establishes the employee's eligibility to legally work in the United States. This document needs to be stored separately from the rest of the employee's personnel file.
- **Medical and retirement forms:** These include signed application forms for employee benefit programs, including group health and life insurance, and any forms needed for the practice-sponsored retirement plan, if any.
- **Copies of professional credentials and licenses, where applicable:** This would Include state-required evidence of current license renewal.
- **Personal information:** Full name; permanent address; telephone number; name, address, and phone number of person to contact in an emergency

FIGURE 5.6 FORM W-4

PAGE 1 SHOWN

⌄

FULL FORM
INCLUDED ON
COMPANION
WEBSITE

Form W-4 (2011)

Purpose. Complete Form W-4 so that your employer can withhold the correct federal income tax from your pay. Consider completing a new Form W-4 each year and when your personal or financial situation changes.

Exemption from withholding. If you are exempt, complete **only** lines 1, 2, 3, 4, and 7 and sign the form to validate it. Your exemption for 2011 expires February 16, 2012. See Pub. 505, Tax Withholding and Estimated Tax.

Note. If another person can claim you as a dependent on his or her tax return, you cannot claim exemption from withholding if your income exceeds $950 and includes more than $300 of unearned income (for example, interest and dividends).

Basic instructions. If you are not exempt, complete the **Personal Allowances Worksheet** below. The worksheets on page 2 further adjust your withholding allowances based on itemized deductions, certain credits, adjustments to income, or two-earners/multiple jobs situations.

Complete all worksheets that apply. However, you may claim fewer (or zero) allowances. For regular wages, withholding must be based on allowances you claimed and may not be a flat amount or percentage of wages.

Head of household. Generally, you may claim head of household filing status on your tax return only if you are unmarried and pay more than 50% of the costs of keeping up a home for yourself and your dependent(s) or other qualifying individuals. See Pub. 501, Exemptions, Standard Deduction, and Filing Information, for information.

Tax credits. You can take projected tax credits into account in figuring your allowable number of withholding allowances. Credits for child or dependent care expenses and the child tax credit may be claimed using the **Personal Allowances Worksheet** below. See Pub. 919, How Do I Adjust My Tax Withholding, for information on converting your other credits into withholding allowances.

Nonwage income. If you have a large amount of nonwage income, such as interest or dividends, consider making estimated tax payments using

Form 1040-ES, Estimated Tax for Individuals. Otherwise, you may owe additional tax. If you have pension or annuity income, see Pub. 919 to find out if you should adjust your withholding on Form W-4 or W-4P.

Two earners or multiple jobs. If you have a working spouse or more than one job, figure the total number of allowances you are entitled to claim on all jobs using worksheets from only one Form W-4. Your withholding usually will be most accurate when all allowances are claimed on the Form W-4 for the highest paying job and zero allowances are claimed on the others. See Pub. 919 for details.

Nonresident alien. If you are a nonresident alien, see Notice 1392, Supplemental Form W-4 Instructions for Nonresident Aliens, before completing this form.

Check your withholding. After your Form W-4 takes effect, use Pub. 919 to see how the amount you are having withheld compares to your projected total tax for 2011. See Pub. 919, especially if your earnings exceed $130,000 (Single) or $180,000 (Married).

	Personal Allowances Worksheet (Keep for your records.)	
A	Enter "1" for **yourself** if no one else can claim you as a dependent	A _____
B	Enter "1" if: { • You are single and have only one job; or • You are married, have only one job, and your spouse does not work; or • Your wages from a second job or your spouse's wages (or the total of both) are $1,500 or less. } . . .	B _____
C	Enter "1" for your **spouse.** But, you may choose to enter "-0-" if you are married and have either a working spouse or more than one job. (Entering "-0-" may help you avoid having too little tax withheld.)	C _____
D	Enter number of **dependents** (other than your spouse or yourself) you will claim on your tax return	D _____
E	Enter "1" if you will file as **head of household** on your tax return (see conditions under **Head of household** above) . .	E _____
F	Enter "1" if you have at least $1,900 of **child or dependent care expenses** for which you plan to claim a credit . . .	F _____
	(**Note.** Do **not** include child support payments. See Pub. 503, Child and Dependent Care Expenses, for details.)	
G	**Child Tax Credit** (including additional child tax credit). See Pub. 972, Child Tax Credit, for more information.	
	• If your total income will be less than $61,000 ($90,000 if married), enter "2" for each eligible child; then **less** "1" if you have three or more eligible children.	
	• If your total income will be between $61,000 and $84,000 ($90,000 and $119,000 if married), enter "1" for each eligible child plus "1" **additional** if you have six or more eligible children	G _____
H	Add lines A through G and enter total here. (**Note.** This may be different from the number of exemptions you claim on your tax return.) ▶ H _____	
	For accuracy, complete all worksheets that apply.	• If you plan to **itemize** or **claim adjustments to income** and want to reduce your withholding, see the **Deductions and Adjustments Worksheet** on page 2. • If you have **more than one job** or are **married and you and your spouse both work** and the combined earnings from all jobs exceed $40,000 ($10,000 if married), see the **Two-Earners/Multiple Jobs Worksheet** on page 2 to avoid having too little tax withheld. • If **neither** of the above situations applies, **stop here** and enter the number from line H on line 5 of Form W-4 below.

------------------------------- Cut here and give Form W-4 to your employer. Keep the top part for your records. -------------------------------

Form **W-4** Department of the Treasury Internal Revenue Service	**Employee's Withholding Allowance Certificate** ▶ Whether you are entitled to claim a certain number of allowances or exemption from withholding is subject to review by the IRS. Your employer may be required to send a copy of this form to the IRS.	OMB No. 1545-0074 20**11**

1 Type or print your first name and middle initial.	Last name	2 Your social security number

Home address (number and street or rural route)	3 ☐ Single ☐ Married ☐ Married, but withhold at higher Single rate.
City or town, state, and ZIP code	**Note.** If married, but legally separated, or spouse is a nonresident alien, check the "Single" box. 4 **If your last name differs from that shown on your social security card, check here. You must call 1-800-772-1213 for a replacement card.** ▶ ☐

5	Total number of allowances you are claiming (from line **H** above **or** from the applicable worksheet on page 2) . . .	5
6	Additional amount, if any, you want withheld from each paycheck	6 $
7	I claim exemption from withholding for 2011, and I certify that I meet **both** of the following conditions for exemption.	
	• Last year I had a right to a refund of **all** federal income tax withheld because I had **no** tax liability **and**	
	• This year I expect a refund of **all** federal income tax withheld because I expect to have **no** tax liability.	
	If you meet both conditions, write "Exempt" here . . . . ▶	7

Under penalties of perjury, I declare that I have examined this certificate and to the best of my knowledge and belief, it is true, correct, and complete.

Employee's signature
(This form is not valid unless you sign it.) ▶   Date ▶

8 Employer's name and address (Employer: Complete lines 8 and 10 only if sending to the IRS.)	9 Office code (optional)	10 Employer identification number (EIN)

For Privacy Act and Paperwork Reduction Act Notice, see page 2.   Cat. No. 10220Q   Form **W-4** (2011)

Department of the Treasury, Internal Revenue Service

PAGE 1 SHOWN

˅

FULL FORM
INCLUDED ON
COMPANION
WEBSITE

FIGURE 5.7 FORM I-9

OMB No. 1615-0047; Expires 08/31/12

Department of Homeland Security
U.S. Citizenship and Immigration Services

**Form I-9, Employment
Eligibility Verification**

Read instructions carefully before completing this form. The instructions must be available during completion of this form.

ANTI-DISCRIMINATION NOTICE: It is illegal to discriminate against work-authorized individuals. Employers CANNOT specify which document(s) they will accept from an employee. The refusal to hire an individual because the documents have a future expiration date may also constitute illegal discrimination.

Section 1. Employee Information and Verification *(To be completed and signed by employee at the time employment begins.)*

Print Name: Last	First	Middle Initial	Maiden Name

Address *(Street Name and Number)*	Apt. #	Date of Birth *(month/day/year)*

City	State	Zip Code	Social Security #

I am aware that federal law provides for imprisonment and/or fines for false statements or use of false documents in connection with the completion of this form.

I attest, under penalty of perjury, that I am (check one of the following):

☐ A citizen of the United States
☐ A noncitizen national of the United States (see instructions)
☐ A lawful permanent resident (Alien #) _____
☐ An alien authorized to work (Alien # or Admission #) _____
  until (expiration date, if applicable - *month/day/year*) _____

Employee's Signature	Date *(month/day/year)*

Preparer and/or Translator Certification *(To be completed and signed if Section 1 is prepared by a person other than the employee.) I attest, under penalty of perjury, that I have assisted in the completion of this form and that to the best of my knowledge the information is true and correct.*

Preparer's/Translator's Signature	Print Name

Address *(Street Name and Number, City, State, Zip Code)*	Date *(month/day/year)*

Section 2. Employer Review and Verification *(To be completed and signed by employer. Examine one document from List A OR examine one document from List B and one from List C, as listed on the reverse of this form, and record the title, number, and expiration date, if any, of the document(s).)*

List A	OR	List B	AND	List C
Document title:				
Issuing authority:				
Document #:				
Expiration Date *(if any)*:				
Document #:				
Expiration Date *(if any)*:				

CERTIFICATION: I attest, under penalty of perjury, that I have examined the document(s) presented by the above-named employee, that the above-listed document(s) appear to be genuine and to relate to the employee named, that the employee began employment on *(month/day/year)* _____ and that to the best of my knowledge the employee is authorized to work in the United States. (State employment agencies may omit the date the employee began employment.)

Signature of Employer or Authorized Representative	Print Name	Title

Business or Organization Name and Address *(Street Name and Number, City, State, Zip Code)*	Date *(month/day/year)*

Section 3. Updating and Reverification *(To be completed and signed by employer.)*

A. New Name *(if applicable)*	B. Date of Rehire *(month/day/year) (if applicable)*

C. If employee's previous grant of work authorization has expired, provide the information below for the document that establishes current employment authorization.

Document Title:	Document #:	Expiration Date *(if any)*:

I attest, under penalty of perjury, that to the best of my knowledge, this employee is authorized to work in the United States, and if the employee presented document(s), the document(s) I have examined appear to be genuine and to relate to the individual.

Signature of Employer or Authorized Representative	Date *(month/day/year)*

Form I-9 (Rev. 08/07/09) Y Page 4

Department of Homeland Security, US Citizenship and Immigration Services new employee and should be prepared to give her a friendly welcome. The employee who has agreed to be a lunch companion and/or mentor should make a special effort, inviting her to lunch and setting a time and place to meet.

Next, retire with the new employee to a quiet area of the hospital. Together, review the job description. Ask questions to find out where additional clarification of duties might be necessary. If any terms, such as medical terminology, seem confusing to the newcomer, encourage her to keep an ongoing list of unfamiliar words and phrases. Use this list as part of your training meetings over the next several weeks. Give the new employee a copy of any reference materials you have developed for hospital staff, such as a glossary of terminology and commonly used abbreviations.

Review policies and procedures in a logical sequence. Provide written instructions or a copy of the hospital policy and procedure manual for later reference. If the employee has been hired for a trial period, make sure she understands the terms of the trial. Explain how you will determine whether employment will be continued when the trial period is over.

Discuss the newcomer's expectations. Find out what she expects within the first thirty days of employment and what type of feedback she is seeking. Talk about performance standards and reviews. Describe your management style and ask how it compares to her prior work experiences. Now is a good time to compare your behavior profile with the employee's, so that the two of you can anticipate any communication problems and begin to work out solutions.

Provide information on wages or salary, benefits, personal conduct, general organization of the practice, management goals and philosophy, and other pertinent issues in writing. Discuss each point and address questions.

Provide information about hazardous materials and ergonomic risks in the workplace, as required by the Occupational Safety and Health Administration (OSHA). Important personal-safety training in the veterinary practice setting relates to the employee's abilities in handling and being around animals. Maintain good training resources about normal animal postures and body language. You may assume that someone who has sought a position in a veterinary practice naturally knows about how animals behave. But many do not, especially in reading an animal's level of anxiety in unfamiliar surroundings where it may instinctively feel threatened and react accordingly. Video clips and training can be used to educate new employees and refresh the knowledge of old ones. This kind of training can save people and animals from avoidable injuries, including potentially devastating bite wounds.

Before proceeding to on-the-job training, you should be satisfied that all hospital policies and procedures are understood by the new employee.

ON-THE-JOB TRAINING

The person assigned to train a new employee should be the individual with the highest level of knowledge of the position. How long training for any particular job function lasts will depend on how complicated the task is and how much time the individual needs to gain knowledge and skill. The key is to encourage hands-on learning, in addition to explanatory and illustrative methods.

The trainer should first find out what the new employee already knows about the position and what skills he already has that can immediately be used. The trainer should stress and repeat key points, provide clear and complete instructions, allow for questions and hands-on practice, and teach only what can be mastered in the time allowed.

You can easily overload a new employee with too much information. Some trainers make the mistake of over-explaining a procedure without allowing the new employee to observe or try the procedure. If you merely lecture a person on how to complete a procedure, he will promptly forget how to do it. Allow the employee to try doing it and ask questions. One doctor quotes an ancient proverb to make this point: To hear is to forget, to see is to remember, to do is to learn.

Another key attribute of a successful training program is variety. Most training information can be presented in several different formats—textual material, videos, lectures, interactive computer programs, and so on. (See the "Additional Resources" section at the end of this book for selected resources.) Journals or magazines that feature articles pertinent to the new employee's position can be useful adjunct training tools. Also consider using training videos. Videos that provide training for a variety of skills can be purchased from organizations such as the American Animal Hospital Association or private companies (for example, Animal Care Technologies [ACT] and Lifelearn). Much of the current quality content can be accessed on line, making it convenient to train from a variety of physical locations, including at home.

On-the-job training can also be aided and assisted by digital image presentations (such as PowerPoint) assembled by your hospital staff for the purpose of training new team members. Short video clips made using a smartphone or flip video recorder are easy to produce and upload for Internet access and training. They can be integrated with a practice intranet or through a private website portal. Use visual presentations to show a new employee how to complete specified tasks, such as phone answering, surgery pack preparation, and kennel cleaning.

Prepared presentations of videos or digital images can be particularly helpful in illustrating situations that do not occur frequently but may still be important to understand. Presentations made for this purpose are available from veterinary organizations and others in the business of employee training. For example, understanding how to correctly restrain animals for examination and treatment can be gained through live demonstrations on available patients. But a video would be very useful to teach interpretation of various animal body postures and how to correctly approach, capture, and restrain a very nervous or aggressive animal.

One drawback with videos is that they do not provide much opportunity for interaction. In small doses, such as one-minute YouTube clips, they can be entertaining and will help any employee refine skills and build knowledge. Longer training sessions by video may be somewhat less effective. Attention spans appear to be dwindling across all generations. Do not expect a new employee to know how to do his job effectively after merely watching hours of video demonstrations. No matter how interesting the format, people will get bored with training that is based exclusively on videos, and more importantly, they will miss the powerful learning gained from hands-on experience.

Interactive computer programs available on DVD or through the Internet are also training methods you can explore. These programs require users to think about and respond to the program's queries, and so knowledge retention rates may be higher. Nonetheless, human interaction and direct hands-on experience are the most effective ways of teaching.

Continuing education for new and existing staff should be a well-defined part of your personnel program. In-house presentations, classes at local community colleges, veterinary association meetings, and specialized conferences are all useful.

The amount of training necessary for new employees to become effective on the job varies tremendously from person to person and from position to position. Do not ask a new employee to take primary responsibility for assigned duties until he has demonstrated a full understanding of the position and the responsibility.

To make sure that a new staff member becomes capable and comfortable with a task, check the employee's progress as he completes each step of the activity. As the employee becomes more comfortable, you can gradually relax supervision, checking on him less frequently. Tests can also indicate what the employee knows. When the employee does "go it alone," be sure to check in daily to see how things are going from his perspective.

Encourage the new employee to ask questions throughout the training. Make sure he knows who to go to for help. The employee should consistently be using the same person as a resource. If the trainee is asking a lot of different people the same questions, problems may be brewing that could be hard to catch. Repeatedly asking the same question indicates that the trainee needs further hands-on, one-on-one training in that area.

Most new employees prefer having one person in charge of their training who has a thorough understanding of the job, rather than multiple people telling them what to do. In addition, they feel more comfortable directing their questions to someone they can view as a peer, rather than to those with more authority.

Of course, reporting to only one person can be a problem if the trainer does not have the best answer. If you have not chosen the trainer carefully, you may end up with a trainer who has little knowledge of the job or even less knowledge than the new person. Make sure the trainer reports to you regularly and directs any unanswered questions to you. Don't end up with the blind leading the blind.

When the new team member appears to be comfortable with the position, start expanding his knowledge of other staff positions. Employee cross-training is valuable. Cross-training

The Benefits of Cross-Training

In its simplest form, cross-training consists of identifying essential operational tasks and training them across enough employees to cover the practice. These tasks must be handled, even if a key responsible employee is absent from work. In a cross-training program, alternate employees are chosen and trained to take on critical tasks when the need arises. The benefits of cross-training are many. For example:

- Employee knowledge of the practice as a whole and the roles of others within the practice grows.
- When staff members are ill or absent for other reasons, such as vacation time, client service and wait times do not have to decline.
- Cross-training places another level of employee accountability into the system, helping to reduce the occurrence of fraud and theft.

To ensure the program's success, clearly communicate to employees that cross-training is intended to help them improve their job satisfaction. It is not a threat to job security. (For more information on establishing and monitoring a cross-training program, see Gill 1997; Love 1998; Reference for Business n.d.; Reh n.d.; Rogerson 1993).

teaches more than one team member how to do a particular job, which is helpful in case of sickness, vacation, or emergency. Cross-training also allows employees to better appreciate the value of their coworkers, because they each understand the stresses and responsibilities of other jobs within the practice. (See textbox, "The Benefits of Cross-Training.")

CONCLUDING THE TRAINING

Establish a date by which the formal training period will be concluded. The length of the formal training period will typically be between sixty and ninety days after the hire date. During this period, the employee should be receiving feedback about her performance. For example, you might meet with the trainee daily throughout the transition period to review her work for the day and to respond to questions and concerns. This makes it easier to provide additional training or support if the work suffers for any reason.

At the end of formal training, review the new employee's performance. If the review is not satisfactory, employment should not be continued. Again, if you have been meeting regularly with the new employee and/or the trainer, the employee should have had sufficient constructive warning about any deficiencies, and employment termination should not come as a surprise to anyone. If your team and you have devoted enough time and provided proper training to the employee and have enough information on her performance to sufficiently evaluate it, do not hesitate to end a dissatisfactory relationship.

If the performance review is satisfactory, then use the review meeting to discuss expectations for the next six to twelve months. Ascertain if there are any tasks about which the employee still feels unsure. Plan with the employee how she can become more proficient in weaker areas of job responsibility. Establish follow-up dates to further evaluate the progress being made.

Document all points discussed in this review meeting for inclusion in the employee's file. Both you and the employee should sign off on the review notes. Check prior notes to determine if any other administrative tasks need to be taken care of at this time, such as adjusting the pay from the training to the regular rate, ordering employee business cards, or changing the employee's title and name badge.

Engaging In Performance Evaluation

In the employee evaluation process, the hospital manager measures and shapes employee performance (McCurnin 1988, 57). There are many acceptable ways of performing evaluations, but all involve utilizing good communication skills and knowing your goals and objectives for shaping employee performance. For the purposes of this book, employee performance evaluation consists of three basic approaches: formal performance reviews, coaching conversations, and corrective-action discussions.

Formal performance reviews and coaching conversations give employees an opportunity to find out how satisfied their employers are with their job performances. They also provide employees with a forum in which to talk about their job satisfaction and goals. Corrective-action discussions address unacceptable behavior and work-performance issues that have not improved through coaching and/or formal evaluations.

Managers and employees alike often dread performance evaluations. Some believe the reviews are irrelevant and a waste of time. Others are uncomfortable with the process of a face-to-face discussion of individual performance. Part of this discomfort may be related to the reviewer's own fear of criticism and desire to be liked. Corrective-action discussions or negative reviews can stem from problems that should have been addressed earlier and were not, which in turn are indicative of prior communication breakdowns. Few people enjoy having difficult conversations, so it is not surprising that communication is often procrastinated.

Often, both the manager and the employee feel that the evaluation places them in an adversarial situation. In a properly executed performance evaluation, however, nothing could be further from the truth. A performance evaluation can have a positive effect, both on the practice and on the human relations within that practice. The key here is that the manager must demonstrate that most important skill of management: the ability to communicate.

Your challenge as the practice manager is to make coaching conversations and formal performance reviews relevant and useful to the hospital and its employees. No human being and no employee is perfect. It is a manager's responsibility to increase the practice team's strengths and minimize its weaknesses by helping each member improve and mature over the term of employment.

If employees are to grow professionally, they need to know what they are doing well and what can be improved. If a practice is to prosper, it needs to understand the strengths and weaknesses of its employees. This means that the performance evaluation process is important to both the employer and the employee.

Complete a formal performance evaluation at the end of the trial employment period or no more than ninety days after hiring a new staff member (see previous section, "Concluding the Training"). Be sure to base evaluations on the detailed job descriptions described earlier in this chapter. Aim to have follow-up evaluations at least once a year thereafter.

More frequent evaluations (coaching conversations) encourage open communication. It is better to address poor performance soon after it occurs than to wait until months later to bring it to the employee's attention. And it is equally if not more important to praise superb performance and work effort when it happens. Neither negative nor positive feedback should wait until formal performance review dates.

As a general rule, your management goal is for all employees to experience formal performance reviews that are helpful, positive, and motivating. There should be little, if any, surprise feedback in them. If you have been a good coach of expected behavior, correcting mistakes in performance as they occur in order to keep the employee on track, you'll have little anxiety about giving formal performance reviews.

Performance reviews should not coincide with wage and salary reviews, however. Associating formal performance reviews with wage and salary reviews can diminish the value of the performance review. The one exception is the case of the new employee who is scheduled to receive a wage or salary increase at the satisfactory conclusion of a trial period (Stockner 1983).

BEFORE THE EVALUATION

Prior to doing a formal performance review, the manager should recall what it is like to go through such an evaluation. This exercise gives the manager perspective on how to effectively handle the task of evaluating other staff members.

The manager should thoroughly prepare for the review in advance by reading the employee's file and any other documents that gauge performance. For example, if you are meeting with a veterinary technician or veterinary nurse, you might want to read recent patient charting notes completed by that individual. Complete an evaluation form for each employee before the performance review meeting. See Figure 5.8 for a sample evaluation form. The

FIGURE 5.8 EMPLOYEE EVALUATION FORM

PAGE 1 SHOWN

˅

FULL FORM
INCLUDED ON
COMPANION
WEBSITE

EMPLOYEE EVALUATION FORM

Name:_____ Date:_____

Department:_____ Job Title:_____

Purposes of this Employee Evaluation: To take a job-related personal inventory, to pin-point weaknesses and strengths, and to outline and agree upon a practical improvement program. Periodically conducted, these evaluations will provide a history of development and progress.

Instructions: Listed below are a number of traits, abilities, and characteristics that are important for success in practice. Place a checkmark on each rating scale over the descriptive phrase which most nearly describes the person being rated. (If this form is being used for self-evaluation, you will be describing yourself.)

Carefully evaluate each of the qualities separately.

JOB KNOWLEDGE
The information concerning work duties which an individual should know for a satisfactory job performance
❏ Is poorly informed about work duties.
❏ Lacks knowledge of some phases of work.
❏ Is moderately informed; can answer most common questions.
❏ Understands all phases of work.
❏ Has complete mastery of all phases of job.

QUANTITY OF WORK
The amount of work an individual does in a work day
❏ Does not meet minimum requirements.
❏ Does just enough to get by.
❏ Performs volume of work satisfactorily.
❏ Is very industrious, does more than is required.
❏ Has superior work production record.

QUALITY OF WORK
The correctness of work duties performed
❏ Makes frequent errors.
❏ Is careless; makes recurrent errors.
❏ Is usually accurate; makes only average number of mistakes.
❏ Requires little supervision; is exact and precise most of the time.
❏ Requires absolute minimum of supervision; is almost always accurate.

INITIATIVE
The desire to attain goals, to achieve
❏ Has poorly defined goals and acts without purpose; puts forth practically no effort.
❏ Sets goals too low; puts forth little effort to achieve.
❏ Has average goals and usually puts forth effort to reach these.
❏ Strives hard; has high desire to achieve.
❏ Sets high goals and strives incessantly to reach these.

PERFORMANCE UNDER PRESSURE
The ability to withstand pressure and to remain calm in crisis situations
❏ Cannot handle pressure; utterly incapable of performing job during crises.
❏ Occasionally "blows up" under pressure; low tolerance for crises.
❏ Has average tolerance for crises; is usually calm.
❏ Tolerates most pressure; has very good tolerance for crises.
❏ Thrives under pressure; really enjoys solving crises.

VHMA Career Center is also a good resource. In its member sample document library, there are sample job descriptions as well as sample evaluation forms. Customize each evaluation form to meet the requirements of the position. Refer to the position's job description to see if any additional criteria should be evaluated.

Consider letting the employee review his evaluation results before the actual meeting. This gives him time to address perceived problems and suggest ideas for improvement. It may also help to alleviate some of the employee anxiety that is inherent in the performance review process. Another way to encourage employee self-evaluation is to ask the employee to complete the same evaluation form that you use for reviews. The form should be completed about a week before the scheduled meeting and before you share the evaluation you have made. Using the same form allows both of you to think about the same aspects of performance. Read the employee's self-evaluation before the meeting so that you can identify any differences between your observations and respond to them at the meeting. (See Figure 5.9.)

Just before the meeting, read the employee's behavior-style profile. Think about how you can best communicate with the employee, keeping his behavior style in mind, and adapt your style accordingly. This technique will make it easier for the employee to understand the performance you are trying to help him achieve.

THE EVALUATION MEETING

Conduct performance reviews in a private setting and ensure that you will not be interrupted. First, discuss the evaluation forms with the employee, comparing your evaluation with the employee's self-evaluation. Read your evaluation to the employee, pointing out areas of agreement.

In cases of ongoing major concern about the employee's performance, provide specific examples and documentation. Keep in mind that you should be addressing problem issues as they arise, not letting them compound and stockpile for a massively negative review. Contemporaneous feedback enables an employee to take corrective action and meet expectations on an ongoing basis. Examples of issues that should be proactively addressed before the formal review ever occurs are patterns of persistent tardiness, protracted personal phone calls, and incomplete or illegible patient nursing notes. If the employee hasn't resolved deficiencies adequately, then they can be redocumented and presented to the employee again during the formal performance review.

Compare the employee's performance to the job description. Don't fault the employee for not performing tasks that are not in the job description, but do bring to the employee's attention instances in which she did not complete duties that were assigned outside the scope of the job description. Ask the employee to comment on your assessment: Does the employee agree with the assessment? Does she disagree with it? If the latter, why?

FIGURE 5.9 EMPLOYEE SELF-EVALUATION FORM

INCLUDED ON
COMPANION
WEBSITE

EMPLOYEE SELF-EVALUATION

Employee Information   *Please Print*
                        Name:_____
                        Date:_____
                        Job Title:_____
                        Department:_____Length of Time in Job:_____

Instructions: For each of the twelve work factors rate yourself excellent, very good, average, fair, or poor, using these rating definitions, and check the appropriate box.

Excellent means I am unquestionably above acceptable employee standards and that my performance consistently exceeds job requirements.

Very Good means I am above acceptable employee standards and that my performance usually exceeds job requirements.

Average means I meet acceptable employee standards and that my performance of job requirements is consistent.

Fair means I must improve to meet acceptable employee standards and that my performance of job requirements is inconsistent.

Poor means I am definitely below acceptable employee standards and that my performance of job requirements is consistently deficient.

WORK FACTORS	Poor	Fair	Average	Very Good	Excellent

_____   **Job Knowledge** means how well I understand the fundamentals, skills, methods, and procedures required in my present job.

_____   **Quantity** means the amount of work I produce in my work day.

_____   **Quality** means the accuracy and completeness of my work.

_____   **Initiative** means my desire to seek new assignments and additional duties.

_____   **Performance under Pressure** means my ability to withstand pressure and to remain calm in crisis situations.

_____   **Dependability** means my ability to do required jobs well with a minimum of supervision.

_____   **Attendance** means my punctuality, conforming to work hours, and maintaining an acceptable attendance record.

_____   **Ingenuity** means my ability to find new and better ways of doing things and to be imaginative.

_____   **Interpersonal Relationships** means my willingness and ability to cooperate and communicate with my co-workers, subordinates, supervisors/managers, customers, and other outside contacts.

_____   **Courtesy** means my polite attention given to other people.

_____   **Policy Adherence** means how well I follow company rules and regulations.

_____   **Overall Evaluation** means comparing myself with other employees with the same length of service in my present job.

I scored highest on:_____ I scored lowest on: _____

This is what I can do to improve my job performance:
_____
_____

This is how the company can help me improve my job performance:
_____
_____

_____   _____
Employee's Signature   Date

Next, suggest how the employee can improve her performance and correct problem areas. Praise performance that exceeds expectations. Be specific and provide detail when commending performance. Allow the employee to ask questions and give comments on working conditions, chances for advancement, and overall job satisfaction.

Strive for a candid conversation during the review session. Both of you should be actively engaged and participating. Think of this time as focused collaboration and problem solving with the employee about her job performance. Share ideas and perspectives. Having the following guidelines will help you, and so will frequent practice in conducting evaluations.

- Define what you hope to accomplish with the employee by preparing in advance. This will prevent you from becoming distracted during the review or forgetting to address the important issues.
- Keep your comments constructive. Use neutral, factual observations and describe patterns of behavior, especially when it is recurring behavior that impairs the employee's performance.
- Focus on performance rather than personality. Discuss behaviors or results. Your goal is to help the employee learn and agree to change behavior, not to alter who the employee is as a person.
- Give examples of superior performance. Express appreciation and recognition of employee strengths.
- Assure employees that effort is important. Mistakes can happen as they try to learn new things and to excel, and they are forgivable as long as the employee is trying to improve.
- Suggest how employees can overcome obstacles to success. Engage the employee on her own ideas for possible solutions.
- Suggest alternatives to current detrimental behaviors. Explain the importance and effect of behavior on team members.
- Give specific examples of how assignments or circumstances could have been handled in areas where the employee demonstrated weakness.
- Define required performance changes and set deadlines for those changes. Don't fail to follow up at the agreed time.
- Obtain the employee's commitment to the required performance changes.
- If termination is being considered, provide adequate time for the employee to correct the situation (usually thirty days).
- End on a positive note by thanking the employee for working with you to resolve any problem. Express your willingness to help her succeed, as well as confidence in the employee's ability to make changes. Congratulate the employee on desirable behavior and encourage continued effort in all areas of task and job-performance success.
- Protect the hospital against claims of discriminatory performance reviews by conducting them similarly across all employees.

- Create and maintain contemporaneous documentation for defense against possible claims of wrongful discharge (Osborne 1995, 9.03, 9.07–9.08).

Retain written documentation and evaluation forms in the employee's personnel file. Complete records protect the practice in the event of any employee complaint. Make sure evaluations are dated and signed by both employee and employer when they are prepared and when they are completed.

CORRECTIVE-ACTION DISCUSSIONS

As previously discussed, you do not want to procrastinate having candid employee conversations when there are clear problems in work performance or behavior. Waiting until the time of the usual formal performance review will allow behavior incongruent with management expectations to habituate. It then becomes much more difficult for you to bring up the topic of the behavior with the employee, and more difficult for the employee to change the behavior.

Sometimes managers don't address behavior in a timely fashion because bothersome issues appear to be only small breeches of behavior expectations. They do not seem to rise to the level of a time-out. Most managers also do not like to single out small transgressions. After all, who wants to be known as a nitpicker, a micromanager, or something worse? And yet, repetitive occurrences make for a pattern, and a manager must address it before the behavior gets out of hand.

Try the "rule of three," described by Peter Bregman (2009). If a situation is enough to catch your attention and annoy you, take notice. The second time it occurs, mentally bookmark the occurrence as a repeat offense and perhaps the start of a pattern. Plan your words in the event of a third occurrence. The third time, speak with the employee: "I've noticed something three times and I would like to discuss it with you."

As Bregman explains, by the third occurrence both manager and employee know the behavior is a trend. Using the rule of three, you will be able to speak up with confidence and authority, knowing it is reasonable to have a corrective-action discussion with the employee. Do not procrastinate. The conversation will not get any easier if you delay.

There is a difference between corrective-action discussions and positive collaborative communications that happen during coaching conversations. Serious performance issues call for corrective-action discussions, which address behavior that cannot be tolerated. Corrective action is also needed if the employee has not lived up to agreements made in prior performance discussions.

Keep these discussions firm and direct. The tone should be adult to adult, not parent to child. Be clear that the employee bears total responsibility for the correction. Succinctly explain the consequences of not correcting the problem.

Dr. Marie McIntyre, a management and career consultant who has a website called "Your Office Coach," describes a useful A-B-C-D-E-F formula for structuring a corrective action meeting with an employee:

A = Awareness. Describe the problem in terms that leave the employee with a clear understanding of what the problem behavior is, how it affects team members, and that it must stop immediately. Some folks are plainly oblivious to the disruption or difficulties they cause. Do not assume the employee knows of the problem before you describe it.

B = Behavioral Expectations. Explain the specific improvement the employee must make and describe acceptable behavior. Do not be vague. For example, instead of saying, "be more cooperative," tell the employee how, when, and with whom he is to be cooperative.

C = Consequences. Before beginning the conversation, know what consequences you will describe to the employee if he does not make immediate changes. Consequences can range from work reassignment, to a demotion, to termination. Tell the employee exactly what will happen next if the behavior is repeated.

D = Decision Confirmed. Ask the employee if he is able and willing to change his behavior. You can ask for an immediate decision or you can allow the employee to think about his answer overnight. Your goal is to have the employee commit to changing either right away or the following day.

E = Employee Involvement. When the employee makes a commitment to change, he must write an action plan specifying the steps he will take in order to make the change successful.

F = Follow Up. Set a definite time when you will meet with the employee again to assess progress. Assuming the employee has been successful at that time, praise the improvement and express appreciation for the effort. If no significant progress has been made, then you must follow through and enforce the consequences you previously defined.

Remember, poor performers will drain your energy. They also hurt the morale of good employees. As Dr. McIntyre wrote, "It's been said that 'A paycheck doesn't buy someone's soul, but it does rent their behavior.' When faced with serious performance issues, you need to change the terms of your 'rental agreement' as soon as possible!"

RECOGNIZING AND DEALING WITH "BURNOUT"

Over time, circumstances change, at home or at work, and any staff member can suffer from burnout. Burnout is characterized by prolonged feelings of unhappiness, frustration, depression, or anger, usually caused by chronic stress, especially in the workplace. When burnout occurs in a veterinary hospital, the bonds between team members, or between team members and clients, can easily deteriorate.

Burnout can result from long hours, unrealistic job expectations, compassion fatigue, conflict with other team members, boredom, lack of challenge, financial pressures, personal troubles outside of work, and other reasons. Burnout can cause a veterinarian, nurse, or any other staff member to lose the ability to relate well, either to animals or to people. People who are burned out may still be technically proficient and able to complete surgeries and treatment, but they just aren't able to effectively empathize with others. Symptoms of burnout can result in unacceptable behavior and bad attitudes that may be contagious to other people on the team.

As a hospital manager, you should be aware of the signs of stress and burnout. A key hospital employee exhibiting these signs can have a profoundly negative effect on the attitude and enthusiasm of every other employee. Clients ultimately pick up on the discord. You can reduce the magnitude of such problems before they occur if you learn to recognize the early signs of burnout and act quickly.

Signs that may indicate a problem with burnout include:

- Arriving late at work
- Missing days, calling in sick more often than usual
- Paying less attention to appearance—neatness, hygiene, and hair care may suffer
- Lacking a sense of humor
- Complaining of overwork, exhaustion, boredom, or depression
- Signs of apathy or aloofness
- Inappropriate anger—may include yelling, arguing with clients or other employees, throwing things, slamming doors, or engaging in abusive behavior toward animals
- Lower productivity and diminished quality of work
- Inattentiveness to details, lack of follow-up on assignments or necessary work requirements, failure to return calls
- Preoccupation with nonproductive busywork, such as "researching" cases on the Internet
- Making mistakes more frequently than usual

Make sure that your team understands these signs and can identify feelings in themselves that might indicate a problem. Employees who recognize the signs of burnout in themselves can take the earliest action. Here are some suggestions for relieving one's own burnout suggested by the National Association of Veterinary Technicians in America (1998):

- *Set realistic goals:* Don't try to do too much in too little time. Prioritize work to get the most important and challenging assignments done first. Having the tough work done first allows you to better enjoy your favorite parts of the job, rather than having what you dread hanging over your head.
- *Set limits:* It's okay to say no occasionally. Learn to delegate portions of your work, if possible; to ask coworkers for help; and to be thoughtful in making such requests.
- *Exercise:* Working out is a proven stress reducer.
- *Relax:* Practice relaxation techniques. Take a few minutes to close your eyes, relax the muscles in your neck and shoulders, and breathe deeply.

- *Meditate or pray:* Reconnecting with your spiritual self can make a big difference in how you feel about life and work.
- *Listen to your body:* If you always feel tired and run down, you may need a break. Take a vacation. Vacations and personal time are important for mental and physical health.
- *Treat yourself:* Schedule time to do something you enjoy: going to the movies, eating at a nice restaurant, hiking, getting your hair done. Whatever you do, try to let go of your worries for a while.

Unfortunately, in many cases relaxation exercises, entertainment, and excursions only go so far, since the causes of burnout may be complex. Individuals may have to identify and address the underlying reasons to effect a long-term solution. The employee may need to obtain outside counseling, particularly since signs of burnout may be superimposed over depression or other medical issues for which the employee should seek help.

It is important to identify whether practice dynamics are leading to distress. Burnout can occur when an employee's personal values, morals, or ethical standards are in conflict with those exhibited at the practice. For example, if the business or personnel practices are in conflict with an individual's moral sensibilities, this can cause an employee to feel that she is making too many compromises. This can include perceived unfairness in how a coworker is treated or paid. In addition, expectations of economic advancement far higher than actual compensation can cause burnout. It is also important to understand the difference between burnout and compassion fatigue, which is discussed at the end of Chapter 12.

Burnout in veterinary practice can be prevented by going into the work with realistic expectations, gathering enough information about a practice before accepting a position there, and realigning one's personal views to the realities of the veterinary profession. If, after having done all this, an employee still feels that her philosophy of veterinary care does not align well that of the practice, it may be time to move to another practice. This may be a difficult decision, and as manager you may have to suggest it yourself, both for the good of the employee and for the good of the practice. Finding a practice that fits the philosophy and expectations of the employee will be a far better solution to burnout than "sticking it out" until ethical compromise or financial burden forces her to completely abandon the profession (McCafferty 1999).

If a person is exhibiting advanced signs of burnout, you may need to intervene promptly. For example, abusive behavior toward coworkers could have a devastating effect and should not be tolerated for any length of time. Abuse of an animal is clearly cause for immediate discharge.

If the situation is gradually escalating, use the corrective-action steps described in the previous section. Don't delay. Document all warnings in the individual's personnel file. Employees with burnout may need a paid day off to reconsider their position with the hospital. Any individual working in any capacity in an animal hospital must have an appreciation for the human–companion animal bond. Those who are insensitive to or skeptical of this bond should not be employed in any capacity.

If you become aware that the practice owner is having a problem with burnout, anger, or abusive behavior, and if talking directly with this person is not possible, you will have to tell someone else about the problem and enlist their help. Are you aware of any confidants or business counselors, such as the practice's attorney or accountant, who could be approached confidentially? The practice's co-owner might be an appropriate source of help. In all cases, no matter who is showing signs of a problem, be judicious and discreet in choosing someone with whom to discuss the matter.

COMPENSATION ISSUES

The evaluation and review process is often closely linked to compensation issues. Even if you do not tie the annual performance review directly to the salary review, the two do go hand in hand. The best determination of increases is through an integrated approach of individual assessment and overall practice financial health. Here we will look at both of these elements and how they are related.

Employee management difficulties arising from compensation issues can be challenging for managers and employees alike. Finding and keeping an effective balance between fair compensation and a good profit takes knowledge of the market, an understanding of finance, and awareness about how management is perceived within the practice. You want to be perceived as fair in making decisions about how team members are paid. Skillful communication is required to both reward and inform employees. When economic pressures and market volatility hinder practice revenues, negotiating compensation can be particularly difficult.

When labor markets are tight, it can be difficult to attract top-notch staff members, and wage inflation can result. Conversely, quick reversals in the economy lead to a relatively large number of capable people seeking employment, but it may be difficult for them to see that their value on an hourly basis may be diminished because of a variety of negative economic pressures.

To successfully balance these pulls on the labor market and compensation, managers will need to consider several factors: the practice compensation budget, ancillary payroll costs, benefit program costs, and salary reviews and increases.

The Practice Compensation Budget

In our discussion of planning for staff acquisition earlier in this chapter, we reviewed the ultimate starting point for hospital staffing: the practice budget. Your practice must have some sort of budget for salaries, wages, and benefits. The cost of all expenses related to maintaining competent employees delivering veterinary care is significant. Poor management of these costs and the activities leading to accumulated payroll hours can easily sink a practice financially.

There are several possible scenarios for the level of authority granted the veterinary practice manager on salary and wage decisions. The budget may provide salary and wage ranges or other guidelines for hiring employees for specific positions. Alternatively, the budget may simply indicate a single salary and wage pool for all salaries and wages, and you, as the manager, allocate salaries at your own discretion within this limit.

Or, you may have no authority to decide on a wage level for any particular employee. In this case, you may still be relied upon to give a recommendation, subject to approval. In the worst-case scenario, you may have no guidance at all. This last circumstance is most difficult, particularly if you have no clear measure of the capital resources available to the practice. If this is the case, start planning how you can work with the practice owners and financial advisers to establish the parameters of the practice's payroll budget. Payroll summated with ancillary employment costs, such as employer payroll taxes, qualified benefit programs, and workers' compensation coverage, can easily consume 50 percent of every revenue dollar earned.

Whatever the state of the practice budget, your job is to explain salaries, hourly wages, and other forms of compensation to employees. This can be done with verbal or written contracts. Some practices supply written contracts for all employees, but most practices establish contracts only for certain employees. Written contracts should be established with any individual who has significant responsibilities to clients and the practice. The individuals with professional and fiduciary responsibility include veterinarians and practice administrators or managers.

Ancillary Payroll Costs

The ancillary elements of employee compensation other than salary may add as much as 25 to 30 percent to the total cost of hiring an employee. Employees are often unaware of these factors and frequently consider only their wage or salary as their compensation.

Factors in employee costs vary, depending on the practice and the position. Payments made by the practice on behalf of veterinary hospital employees can include the following:

- Hourly wages or weekly, monthly, or annual salary
- Bonuses or incentive pay
- Employer's portion of Social Security and Medicare payments
- Employer's unemployment, disability, and workers' compensation taxes
- Applicable local, state, or provincial taxes
- Sick pay and pay for personal days off
- Vacation and holiday pay
- Health insurance and major medical plan costs
- Employer contributions to health savings accounts and qualified medical reimbursements
- Employer contributions to pension, profit-sharing, and retirement plans

- Professional, legal, and accounting fees related to the maintenance of various employer-sponsored employee benefit plans
- Life insurance premiums
- Uniform allowances
- Professional dues and subscription costs
- Continuing education tuition or assistance
- Cost of veterinary care for employee-owned animals
- Bonding and malpractice insurance premiums, where applicable

Owners generally want this information to be clearly communicated to employees, and you might provide it during annual wage and salary reviews. However, be careful how you categorize these costs. Listing some personnel costs as compensation may cause tax problems. Check with the practice's attorney and accountant before including extensive descriptions of "additional compensation" in contracts or employee manuals. Better yet, ask the practice attorney to assist in writing and reviewing contracts and employee manuals.

Wage/Salary Reviews and Increases

Employees generally expect an annual wage and salary review. This review establishes what raises will be given, if any, when they will become effective, and to whom they will be awarded. As mentioned above, salary increases are best determined through an integrated approach that takes individual assessment and overall practice financial health into consideration.

To conduct a salary and wage review, you first need to familiarize yourself with the practice's budget for the prior year and determine how the practice fared in comparison with the projections. If your practice's budget is organized by department (reception, kennel, technicians and assistants, etc.), then so much the better. You should also determine any hiring and wage trends that became apparent during the past twelve months. If unemployment is low, entry-level wages may have escalated rapidly in order to remain competitive. Higher entry wages for new employees may affect your decisions about increases for individuals who have been with you longer. Meanwhile, higher unemployment increases the flexibility of starting wages and reduces the pressure for large wage increases.

Other compensation review factors include merit, effort, attitude, and any new credentials obtained by employees during the year. Quantify any new, existing, or modified benefit plan expenses, because these affect the overall value of the compensatory package for any employee. In most cases, final decisions about wage and salary adjustments will be made through consensus between key management personnel and other decision makers, such as owners, who ultimately bear the financial risk of compensation adjustments.

After final decisions about raises are made, schedule time to meet with each employee. Briefly discuss the employee's wage, bonus, and benefit history and propose the suggested new salary or wage. It may be advisable to present the overall rate of increase. Review the entire compensatory package with the employee to make sure the individual understands that its value does not reside exclusively in the hourly wage. Benefits such as health insurance and retirement plans add important additional value to the compensation arrangement for the coming year.

Health insurance premiums are rising at a rapid rate, a trend expected to continue for at least the near future and greatly impacting small businesses (Pear 2011). It is not unreasonable to explain health insurance cost increases to employees. If your practice provides health insurance, any increase in premiums paid by the practice should be considered part of a raise.

Just because a wage and salary review occurs does not mean that salary or wage increases must be given. Employees should understand that they are paid fairly for the work they do. A long tenure, in and of itself, is not enough to merit a raise. Employees must continue to provide value to the practice to earn their current salary, and they must excel in their work to be eligible for any increases that might be given.

The practice has several options when it comes to granting wage or salary increases, including no compensation increases for anyone, selective increases to employees of merit, or a percentage or set amount of increase to everyone. The decision is usually based on fiscal constraints identified either by the hospital budget or by perceived or actual cash flows. Practice philosophy is also a factor in the decision.

The decision to grant no increase to any employees will probably be based on hard, cold financial facts. While your staff may be supportive of such a decision during hard times, a long-term policy of not offering raises can certainly make employees feel they have actually lost buying power because of general inflationary effects in the economy.

Granting increases to some employees but not to others can produce some obvious morale problems. Some employees may suspect favoritism. If the practice manager has not been very good about completing performance evaluations, some employees may not understand why they were left out of an increase. However, selective raises can be an effective motivational device when performance reviews have been given and the reasons are clearly disclosed. These discussions should give the employee information about how to improve in order to earn more.

When all employees receive an increase, typically it is either as a percentage of their present salary or as a set amount per hour or week. If you feel that some employees deserve a higher increase than others, you may add performance increases or bonuses as well. The basic difference between an increase and a bonus is that an increase is permanent and a bonus is a one-time payment that should not be expected to be repeated.

Be aware that if you give bonuses, employees can come to expect them to come automatically, particularly when they are given on some basis other than merit. Holiday bonuses are a good example of a monetary reward that may come to be seen as part of regular compensation. Employees do not necessarily understand that holiday bonuses are not mandatory but are given because of the employer's beneficence. Employers can become discouraged when no signs or gestures of gratitude are forthcoming from employees for a paid bonus. And if a holiday bonus is eliminated after employees have grown accustomed to it, this can cause financial pressures for employees who have come to rely on it for holiday expenses. Think about whether you want to set this precedent before offering employee bonuses.

Some managers may decide to pay bonuses based on a percentage of sales or another metric related to volume and generated fees as an incentive for those employees who sell certain products such as pet foods or insecticides. Of course, ethical considerations should dictate that nonveterinary employees should never be paid for recommending or inducing clients to purchase medical goods or services (Tannenbaum 1989).

Many other innovative ways to compensate employees for exemplary effort are suggested in the veterinary literature. Proceed with caution. Often, incentive programs are a Band-Aid solution for poor attitudes and inferior performance. If you are looking for solutions to these problems, consider whether they are symptoms of practice management problems that extend far beyond anything compensation can cure. Throwing money at such symptoms won't solve the problems; it will only prolong them.

Remember, many people are not motivated primarily by money. Employee surveys repeatedly show that compensation is not enough. In and of itself, a paycheck will not motivate many employees over the long run. Other workplace factors are just as important to employee satisfaction, including:

- Praise and recognition
- Promotions
- A pleasant work environment
- Well-maintained and modern equipment
- Job security
- Challenging and interesting work

If you focus on developing these intangible benefits, you may not have to worry about giving big bonuses or creating complicated incentive programs.

MANAGING CHANGE

One thing is certain in today's workplace: change. Some have called this era the "Age of Instability." So much change occurs every day that sometimes it feels like it is impossible to keep up. The fact is, all of the people in your practice will likely feel the same way, a bit off balance and forever trying to catch up with completing tasks, learning new information, and building skills.

It is hard not to be resistant to change in the workplace. Most people are trying to do a good job in the time they have available. The constant introduction of new information makes people feel nervous about managing time, conserving quality, and being up to speed with the knowledge they need.

A primary leadership duty will be to train and guide employee adaptability to change. Your goal is to create and maintain a team of employees who are excited to be successful in the face of change, rather than resistant to it. In the Age of Instability, managing change is part of everyone's job description (Pritchett and Pound 2008), not just yours as the manager. When managers make well-thought-out management decisions, employees are more likely to trust the changes that come.

Fortunately, good resources abound, because all companies are trying to stay relevant in the sea of change. Your practice leadership team must actively engage in initiating change, not to be troublesome to employees, but because the practice must change to be healthy and profitable. The more you can teach and lead the practice team through embracing change, the better.

Some talking points to remember:

- Change is a fact that is accelerating and will not go away.
- Resisting change is harmful to the practice and to those who are opposing it
- Resisting change takes more effort than working as part of the team to implement new methods of helping patients and clients
- Embracing change and figuring out how to adapt makes you more valuable to the practice

Here are some good resources for helping your team develop a mindset that leans toward working with change rather than against it:

- *Who Moved My Cheese? An Amazing Way to Deal with Change in Your Work and in Your Life*, by Spencer Johnson (1998)
- *Switch: How to Change Things When Change Is Hard*, by Chip and Dan Heath (2010)
- *The Employee Handbook for Organizational Change*, by Price Pritchett and Ron Pound (2008)

TERMINATION OF EMPLOYMENT

The one thing you hope you will never have to do is fire an employee. However, because firing may be necessary, you should understand a few things about employment law, among them, the changing definition of "at will" employment, how to avoid situations that might result in charges of wrongful discharge, and finally, how to fire an employee if the need arises.

At-Will Employment

In most states in the United States, employment is considered to be "at-will employment." This means that unless a specific provision in an employment contract states an agreed-upon duration of employment, employees may quit and employers may terminate employees "at will," according to their own preferences.

There are many exceptions to this general definition, and federal statutes, the efforts of organized labor, and labor contracts have significantly reduced the scope of the "at-will" definition of employment. Express exceptions to "at-will" employment include the following:

- Collective bargaining agreements (labor contracts between unionized workers and employing companies)
- Specific contracts that indicate a definite period of employment
- Dismissals based on race, sex, color, creed, or national origin, prohibited by the Civil Rights Act
- Dismissals based on age if over forty years old, prohibited by the Age Discrimination in Employment Act
- Dismissal because of pregnancy, prohibited by the Pregnancy Discrimination Act
- Dismissals that occur because employees refuse to work in a workplace that they consider unsafe or because they have exercised other rights under the Occupational Safety and Health Act
- Dismissal of an employee because he has filed for bankruptcy, prohibited by the Bankruptcy Reform Act
- Dismissal of an employee because of service on a federal jury, prohibited by federal law

The practice manager must be familiar with changing definitions of at-will employment. Understand that state, commonwealth, and provincial laws may differ from federal requirements. Whenever in doubt, confer with an attorney who is licensed to practice in the hospital's jurisdiction and able to apply employment law to your practice's particular circumstances.

Claims of Wrongful Discharge

Employers may be accused of wrongful discharge for several reasons. First, the claim may stem from reasons of public policy; the employee may allege that she was fired for refusing to comply with employer acts that were expressly prohibited by law. For example, the employee might claim she was discharged for refusing to commit perjury, refusing to fix prices, or being a "whistle blower" against the employer and bringing accusations of criminal or immoral activity against the practice. Wrongful-discharge suits might also claim that the employer broke implied contract rights, such as oral promises or a statement in an employee handbook implying a term of employment. Or an employer may be accused of breaking an implied "covenant of good faith and fair dealing" (London 1998).

The catalyst for a wrongful discharge claim is often an inappropriately handled notice of termination, that is, a notice that is poorly timed, poorly stated, or delivered too publicly. If a discharged employee feels publicly humiliated, a lawsuit is much more likely than if the discharge is made in a professional and appropriate way. In most instances, the decision to terminate employment may not be as important as how that decision is carried out.

Firing an Employee

Now that you have reviewed some circumstances under which you should not fire an employee, you may wonder when firing is necessary and appropriate. Firing an employee may be the best answer to several problems, including the following:

- Unsatisfactory performance of duties
- Excessive tardiness and absenteeism
- Dishonest or unethical behavior in the performance of duties
- Criminal activity within the hospital (such as stealing) or outside the hospital (such as drug abuse) that has been substantiated by a criminal investigation

In addition, if you have conducted a thorough review of the practice finances and organization and determined that one or more positions should be eliminated, some employees may need to be let go. In this case, they are being *laid off*, which refers to temporary suspension or permanent termination of workers due to business reasons such as an economic downturn, rather than *fired*, which applies to termination for cause, such as performance failure or gross misconduct. The method of employment separation matters because different unemployment laws will apply to them. In many states, a laid-off worker can receive unemployment benefits. Workers who separate from employment voluntarily are generally ineligible to collect unemployment benefits, as are those who are fired for cause.

If you have been keeping careful and complete personnel files, each and every reason leading to the termination of an employee should already be documented. Make it a habit to take the time to document problems and reprimands as they occur. Sign and date each written document as you prepare it. Where possible, ask the employee to sign and date the documents as well. The countersignature indicates that the employee was informed of problems and infractions and apprised of what would occur if there was no improvement. (See Figure 5.10.)

When you decide that an employee should be terminated, first be sure that the decision to fire was preceded by a series of clear, understood, and documented discussions with the employee. If you are firing an employee for unsatisfactory performance of duties, the employee should understand your complaints before the time of dismissal. Confer with the practice's engaged employment-law attorney to review the events leading up to the termination event. Follow his recommendations about additional steps to take prior to and at the point of carrying out the termination.

Don't fire an employee in haste, when you are angry, or immediately at the time of a transgression. When emotions are high, you are more likely to regret your words or actions later. Wait until tempers are cool and you have a chance to plan how you will handle the situation. Then you will be better able to be honest, control your emotions, and conduct the firing with dignity.

Once you have made a calm and studied decision to fire the employee, don't spend time and energy trying to avoid the event. Long delays between the employee's action and the

FIGURE 5.10 EMPLOYEE WARNING FORM

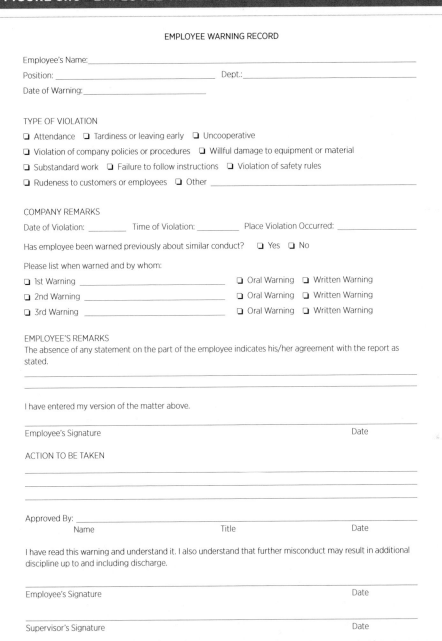

EMPLOYEE WARNING RECORD

Employee's Name:_____

Position: _____ Dept.:_____

Date of Warning:_____

TYPE OF VIOLATION

❏ Attendance ❏ Tardiness or leaving early ❏ Uncooperative

❏ Violation of company policies or procedures ❏ Willful damage to equipment or material

❏ Substandard work ❏ Failure to follow instructions ❏ Violation of safety rules

❏ Rudeness to customers or employees ❏ Other _____

COMPANY REMARKS

Date of Violation: _____ Time of Violation: _____ Place Violation Occurred: _____

Has employee been warned previously about similar conduct? ❏ Yes ❏ No

Please list when warned and by whom:

❏ 1st Warning _____ ❏ Oral Warning ❏ Written Warning

❏ 2nd Warning _____ ❏ Oral Warning ❏ Written Warning

❏ 3rd Warning _____ ❏ Oral Warning ❏ Written Warning

EMPLOYEE'S REMARKS
The absence of any statement on the part of the employee indicates his/her agreement with the report as
stated.
_____
_____

I have entered my version of the matter above.
_____

Employee's Signature   Date

ACTION TO BE TAKEN
_____
_____
_____

Approved By: _____
                   Name   Title   Date

I have read this warning and understand it. I also understand that further misconduct may result in additional
discipline up to and including discharge.
_____

Employee's Signature   Date
_____

Supervisor's Signature   Date discipline on your part might be viewed as indecisiveness by other employees, and this will threaten your ability to manage effectively.

Dismiss the employee in a private room, with the door shut, so other employees and clients cannot hear or interrupt. In most situations, it is advisable to include a witness, preferably one who is the same gender as the employee. This should be someone else in a supervisory or human resources position, not a peer of the employee being fired.

Discharge the employee at the end of the day, so that she will not have to encounter other employees when gathering personal effects and leaving the hospital.

At the time of the dismissal, have a final paycheck already prepared. Include hours worked through the current day, as well as earned vacation time and back salary. Ask the dismissed employee to sign a release forgoing her right to sue over the dismissal. Depending on the circumstances, and talking through options with the practice's attorney, you may want to provide severance pay as a means of obtaining this release.

If employee health care benefits are arranged through the practice, you should continue them at the employee's request and expense for the required period of time past the termination date. The Consolidated Omnibus Budget Reconciliation Act of 1986 (COBRA) allows for the extension of group insurance coverage to former employees and their dependents. COBRA requires employers to cover former employees whose medical conditions would prevent them from immediately getting coverage under a new employer plan. Many states have variations of the federal COBRA requirements called "mini-COBRA." These usually apply to businesses with much lower number of employees than the businesses affected by COBRA.

Require the fired employee to remove personal property from the hospital and to return keys or any other hospital property. Try to eliminate any reason the employee might have for returning to the hospital. In some cases, you may want to change the locks on the hospital doors, and if your hospital has a security system, to change security codes. Computer system passwords should be updated promptly.

Depending on the circumstances of the firing, you may or may not be willing to give the employee a reference for another job. You should decide this ahead of time and discuss your intentions with the employee at the time of the dismissal.

Document the firing, the circumstances preceding it, and the reaction of the fired employee in writing. Place the documentation in the employee's personnel file. If the practice is accused of wrongful discharge, proper and complete documentation of the entire process will be absolutely necessary. Whenever you suspect that litigation may result from a termination, call the practice's attorney and discuss the situation before firing the employee.

If the practice has insurance coverage related to employment practices (*employment practices liability insurance*, or EPLI), it is advisable to read the policy and contact the company for guidelines. Many companies provide hotlines to assist policy holders and offer Internet resources.

Do not allow the employee to continue to work after the dismissal, unless the dismissal resulted from reasons unrelated to work performance. Do not ask a fired employee to keep working because you need to get the job done until a replacement is found. Retaining an employee who is effectively fired can cause serious problems with other staff members as well as other risks and problems for the practice. Once an employee is terminated, do not allow him to do any additional work.

Your skills in firing an employee may be as important as your hiring skills. If you have competently coached and given corrective feedback to an employee who then continues to perform poorly or is the source of a serious problem, the sooner you remove that employee, the better off the veterinary hospital will be.

See Figure 5.11 for a sample Employee Termination Record. For more information about how to handle the termination meeting, see *The Changing Outplacement Process: New Methods and Opportunities for Transition Management*, by John L. Meyer and Carolyn C. Shadle (1994).

After the Termination: How to Handle Referral Calls

If you are contacted as a referral, remember the following:

- Under current law, it is still acceptable to give a "no comment" reference unless you have knowledge of an employee's propensity for violence. However, check with your attorney if you need help with a specific situation. It's advisable to have a game plan in place for future phone calls at the time a problem employee's work is terminated with your hospital for whatever reason. Case law and precedent rapidly change what is and is not appropriate for employers to do and say.
- To avoid defamation liability, only provide information, in good faith, that is true and can be proven true with written evidence. This means that to ensure that you can give accurate information later, you should document in the personnel file any pertinent events as they happen, such as episodes of violent behavior. Describe the event in the form of an opinion as opposed to a statement of fact (e.g., "in my opinion, Mr. Smith was acting erratically"). If the behavior warrants a police report, do call the police so that the incident will be documented.
- To avoid liability for claims of negligent referral, do not misrepresent the qualifications and character of a former employee if you have knowledge of that employee's propensity for violence or illegal behavior. Acts of violence and possession of weapons in the workplace are examples of the type of information that should be disclosed to prospective employers.

Practice Made Perfect

FIGURE 5.11 TERMINATION REPORT

TERMINATION REPORT

Employee Name:_____
(Last)   (First)   (MI)

Department _____ Position _____ Employee No. ____ Supervisor ____

Hire Date ____ Today's Date ____ Last day Worked ____ Termination Effective Date

Type of Separation (Check One)

❏ Resignation (attach letter of resignation) ❏ Dismissal ❏ Retirement ❏ Mutual Agreement ❏ Layoff
❏ Other_____

Reason for Termination
❏ Absenteeism/Tardiness ❏ Job Change ❏ Personal ❏ Reduction In Force ❏ Performance
❏ Violation of Policies/Procedures ❏ Company Shut Down
❏ Other_____

Employee Evaluation (check appropriate boxes)

Job Knowledge	❏ Poor	❏ Fair	❏ Average	❏ Very Good	❏ Excellent
Quantity of Work	❏ Poor	❏ Fair	❏ Average	❏ Very Good	❏ Excellent
Quality of Work	❏ Poor	❏ Fair	❏ Average	❏ Very Good	❏ Excellent
Initiative	❏ Poor	❏ Fair	❏ Average	❏ Very Good	❏ Excellent
Performance Under Pressure	❏ Poor	❏ Fair	❏ Average	❏ Very Good	❏ Excellent
Dependability	❏ Poor	❏ Fair	❏ Average	❏ Very Good	❏ Excellent
Attendance	❏ Poor	❏ Fair	❏ Average	❏ Very Good	❏ Excellent
Ingenuity	❏ Poor	❏ Fair	❏ Average	❏ Very Good	❏ Excellent
Policy Adherance	❏ Poor	❏ Fair	❏ Average	❏ Very Good	❏ Excellent

Recommendation: ❏ Without Reservation ❏ With Some Reservation ❏ Would Not Recommend
Rehire? ❏ Yes ❏ No If No, Reasons: _____

Additional Comments
_____
_____
_____
_____
_____

Signed _____ Date ____

For Office Use Only
❏ Cobra Notification   ❏ Insurance Company Notified   ❏ Direct Deposit Institution Notified
❏ Company Materials Returned   ❏ Dental   ❏ Vacation Due
❏ Retirement/Savings Distribution ❏ Health   Days ____
                               ❏ Life   Hours ____

HR Signature _____ Date ____

Adapted from materials by Amsterdam Printing and Litho Co.

160

In addition, if you are listed as a referral on future job application forms that a terminated employee submits elsewhere, you may be called by these potential employers. You must be prepared for this and know how you will respond to these calls. See the textbox entitled "After the Termination: How to Handle Referral Calls" for further information.

When Employees Resign

When employees decide to resign from employment, require that they provide notice of resignation in writing. The original notice must be kept in the personnel file. If you suspect that a critical feedback meeting is going to result in the employee quitting, have a resignation letter ready for the employee to sign.

Schedule an exit interview to allow a frank discussion of the employee's reasons for leaving and her job satisfaction. Listen carefully, and consider the employee's suggestions as you explore ways to improve the workplace environment so that you can continue to attract and retain qualified employees. The exit interview may be conducted thirty to sixty days after the employee's termination date. Many times, this delay will allow the individual to provide you with a more reasoned and open disclosure, particularly if personality conflicts with coworkers were part of the problem. Retain the exit interview documentation as a permanent part of the employee's file. (See Figure 5.12 for an example of an employee exit interview.)

Personnel Records

Human resource professionals and attorneys recommend that businesses have formal personnel file and record-keeping policies. Many employment-related laws include record-keeping provisions. Federal and state antidiscrimination laws require most employers to keep records of employee selection, promotion, demotion, reduction in force, and termination. Labor and immigration statutes require an employer to keep proof of an employee's eligibility for employment in the United States. Federal and state statutes require records of employee tax withholdings, payroll payments, salary and wage information, and tip income (Crook n.d.).

Principles of recordkeeping policy include: (1) protection of records from loss or damage; (2) physical design and policy that balances access with safeguarding confidentiality; (3) identification of records that must (or should) be stored separately; and (4) guidelines for retention and disposal. According to Attorney D. Scott Crook, employers should maintain five essentially separate record-keeping systems related to its employees. These include personnel files, medical record files, equal employment opportunity data, I-9 records, and payroll and benefits data.

Maintain a separate personnel file for each hospital employee that contains relevant materials related to the person's employment and excludes unnecessary personal information.

PAGE 1 SHOWN

˅

FULL FORM
INCLUDED ON
COMPANION
WEBSITE

FIGURE 5.12 EMPLOYEE EXIT INTERVIEW

EMPLOYEE EXIT INTERVIEW

Date:_____
Name:_____ Department:_____
Job Title:_____ Supervisor's Name:_____
Date Hired:_____ Date Terminated:_____

Type of Termination: ❏ Resignation ❏ Discharge ❏ Layoff ❏ Retirement

I. STATED REASON FOR TERMINATION
(Please check the reason that applies.)

RESIGNATION
❏ Returning to school
❏ Secured better position
❏ Going into business for self

Disliked:
  ❏ Hours
  ❏ Supervisor
  ❏ Type of work
  ❏ Wages
  ❏ Working conditions
  ❏ Other reason:_____
  _____
  _____
  _____

DISCHARGE
❏ Inadequate:
  ❏ Ability
  ❏ Suitability for position
  ❏ Drive
  ❏ Efficiency
  ❏ Cooperation
❏ Dishonesty
❏ Rules violation
❏ Absenteeism
❏ Tardiness
❏ Inadequate safety consciousness
❏ Other reason:_____
  _____
  _____

LAYOFF
❏ Temporary work
❏ Reduction of staff
❏ Other reason:_____
  _____
  _____
  _____
  _____

RETIREMENT
❏ Age
❏ Other reason:_____
  _____
  _____
  _____

Complete in DISCHARGE cases:
When was employee notified?_____ How was employee notified?_____

Complete in LAYOFF cases:
Was employee offered transfer? ❏ Yes ❏ No
To which department?_____ To which job?_____

II. PATTERNED INTERVIEW
This patterned interview has been designed to assist the interviewer to (1) evaluate the true reason for termination, and (2) make recommendations for rehire. The interviewer will ask these questions.

SELECTION
What kind of work have you been doing in our company?
_____
_____

These files should be kept in locked, secure cabinets that are accessible only to specific personnel that need to access them. If electronically stored, care should be taken to limit access to them, as well as backup files, however they are created. Employees should be able to see their own files, but only by request and in the presence of management.

A personnel record should contain the following:

- Original application, letter of qualification, records of contacts with references, résumé, if required, and any other application materials such as job-related tests related to hire (not medical tests).
- The various federal and state-mandated forms listed in the section earlier in this chapter entitled "The First Day," except for Form I-9, which should be managed through a separate filing regimen.
- An employee record form (see sample in Figure 5.13) showing the employee's date of hire, original salary, records of raises, promotions, demotions, and other details of employment history
- Performance evaluation forms
- Education and training records
- Awards and commendations
- Disciplinary records
- Attendance and vacation records
- Documentation of corrective-action feedback or other discussions related to performance of duties
- Lay-off or termination records, including a resignation letter from the employee and exit-interview documentation if the employee has resigned

Medical records should be segregated from other employee personnel records. Access must be carefully limited only to those who need to know the information, such as the employee's supervisor for purposes of identifying work limitations. Medical-record files contain information such as:

- Pre-employment drug screen results
- Post-employment physical exam results
- Family and Medical Leave Act Documentation
- Return-to-work releases
- Documentation of corrective-action feedback or other discussions related to performance of duties
- Documentation regarding disability and/or accommodation thereof
- Workers' compensation documentation
- Insurance claims documents
- Physician notes (Crook n.d.)

FIGURE 5.13 EMPLOYEE RECORD FORM/CONFIDENTIAL

CONFIDENTIAL EMPLOYEE HISTORY

Employee Name:_____

Employment Date:_____ Status: ❏ Regular ❏ Part Time ❏ Temporary

Years of Service:_____

PAYROLL DATA

Birthdate:_____ ❏ Male ❏ Female Social Security No.:_____

Marital Status:_____Name of Spouse:_____ No. of Children:_____

Federal Withholding: Exemptions Claimed_____ Additional Amount Withheld_____

Insurance	Date Eligible	Date Joined	Date Withdrawn
Life	_____	_____	_____
Medical – Self	_____	_____	_____
Dependent	_____	_____	_____
Major Medical – Self	_____	_____	_____
Dependent	_____	_____	_____

GENERAL INFORMATION

_____

Address	City	State	Zip	Phone

_____

Address	City	State	Zip	Phone

In Emergency Notify: _____ Relationship: _____

_____

Address	City	State	Zip	Phone

Relatives or Friends Employed by this co.

_____

Name	Relationship	Name	Relationship

Education Elem.:_____ JHS:_____ SHS:_____

College 1 2 3 4 Major:_____Other:_____

Special Skills or Training:_____

TERMINATION RECORD

❏ Resignation Date:_____ Reason:_____

❏ Dismissal Date:_____ Reason:_____

Recommended for Re-Employment

❏ Yes ❏ No Reason:_____

WAGE/SALARY HISTORY

Dates	Position and Classification	Rate of Pay	Reason for Change
From To		Amount	

Adapted from materials by Amsterdam Printing and Litho Co.

Federal I-9 records support federal law that require an employer to verify that an employee is eligible to work in the United States and to keep records of the verification process (see Chapter 6). These forms should be kept separate from other employee records for a number of reasons, including the fact the employers are not to use information on national origin in employment decisions in accord with nondiscrimination laws. Segregated record-keeping is one protection against the implication that nationality might have been a factor in any aspect of the employment cycle.

Because the Internal Revenue Code and Fair Labor Standards Act (FLSA) require employers to keep detailed payroll and benefits data, access should be limited. Keeping this information segregated from other personnel data is advised:

- Employee's full name and Social Security number
- Address, including zip code
- Birth date, if employee is a minor
- Work schedules
- Pay rates
- Earnings records
- Wage deductions
- Benefit records
- Hours worked daily and weekly
- Time records for each pay period, documenting the hours the employee has worked

It is important to keep time records because you may need to answer inquiries by government authorities and agencies. A time clock or computer program for recording employee work hours is the most efficient method of tracking employee time and creating time record documents. These also offer the benefit of being a controlled system. If your practice does not currently use a time clock or time-keeping software, install one or the other right away. Make its use mandatory for all employees. Time records maintained by hand on the "honor system" will not meet the management needs of a veterinary hospital. Increasingly, practices are installing biometric time clocks that use the employee's unique fingerprint to identify clocking in and out, reducing the opportunities for employee collusion in clocking in friends early or clocking them out late.

Statutes and regulations vary as to minimum requirements for personnel and payroll record retention after the final date of an employee's employment. Online search of regulatory agencies such as the Equal Employment Opportunity Commission (EEOC) will give you the most current required guidelines. Record policy is generally based on employer preference from some period of time that exceeds minimum guidelines, without maintaining them longer than is useful, and might be reviewed annually with the practice's attorney. With the foregoing caveats, a reasonable starting point for policy is a minimum of five years past the last date of employment. Workplace injury, medical examination records, and records of exposure to hazardous material may require much longer record retention time—even as long as thirty years.

If your practice has any employee benefits plans, such a pension and insurance plan, and any written seniority or merit system, keep records for the full period the plan or system is in effect and for at least one year after its termination.

Personnel management is perhaps one of the most complex areas of administrative expertise required in any business. Because you will be faced with many issues that are not discussed in this book, you should continue your study of personnel management in more specific areas, such as handling conflict resolution between team members or between management and practice employees, inspiring employee motivation, planning and taking disciplinary action, dealing with problem employees, and counseling employees with personal problems. Attendance and leave policies, benefit plans, and employee retention are just a few of the other areas that you should continue to learn about.

Legal issues also abound, and specific requirements change continually. Chapter 6 introduces some important general considerations. This book is intended to introduce you to the various aspects of employee management that are common in veterinary practice. For greater detail, keep adding to your practice management library. For suggestions, consult the "Additional Resources" section at the end of the book.

6

Employment Laws

With contributions by John B. McCarthy, DVM, MBA

Every aspect of personnel management is affected and controlled by some form of law. New laws are created frequently and old laws are continually clarified, both by case law and by regulations designed by enforcement agencies. Additionally, new agencies may be created from time to time that have some part to play in how you manage the practice's employees and administer your policies and procedures that pertain to their employment with you.

Clearly, managers must pay close attention to continually evolving guidelines and maintain excellent adviser relationships to mitigate risk of running afoul of regulations. Veterinary practices can be at risk for substantial liability, even for unintentional violations. In addition, practice owners and managers may be individually liable for noncompliance with certain laws and regulations.

This chapter reviews most of the federal laws of the United States that must be considered with regard to personnel management. Most states and provinces have companion laws that supplement and expand upon the federal laws, adding to the legal requirements for employers. Many states have distinct and more stringent laws, above and beyond federal law, that pertain to personnel management.

Canadian readers should check with their provincial registrar for applicable laws.

Immigration Control

The Immigration Reform and Control Act (IRCA) of 1986 affects all employers regardless of size. Intended to prevent illegal aliens from obtaining employment in the United States, the IRCA requires employers to take steps to verify that a newly hired employee is eligible for employment in the United States.

All employers must verify that every new hire is either a U.S. citizen or is authorized to work in this country. The IRCA applies to all employees: full-time, part-time, temporary, or seasonal. It does not apply to contract workers, so you do not need to obtain or verify information about independent contractors or their employees.

Verification of employee eligibility is documented on U.S. Citizenship and Immigration Services (USCIS) Form I-9, Employment Eligibility Verification (see Figure 5.7), which the act requires employers to complete for every new hire. By signing Form I-9, the employer attests that she has examined the required documents to ascertain that they reasonably appear to be genuine. Common sense is a useful guide. For instance, the documents should not look like someone has tampered with them, the typeface should be correct, there should be no misspellings, birthdates on separate documents must be the same, and so on. The employer is also attesting that the documents appear to relate to the individual presenting them. For example, the photo resembles the person; the name on the ID is the same as given, or, if different, can be explained (e.g., name change, national custom); and the identifying, nonchanging information, such as height and eye color, are accurate.

The employer is not responsible for detecting fraudulent documents. If the ID looks genuine and easily relates to the person, your obligations are met. In addition, if the documents reasonably appear on their face to be genuine and to relate to the person presenting them, you must accept them. To do otherwise could be an unfair immigration-related employment practice.

There are several documents that new hires can present to satisfy the requirements. Some documents are sufficient to establish both identity and eligibility to work (e.g., a U.S. passport or a Permanent Resident Card). Alternatively, the worker can produce a combination of documents, such as a driver's license to establish identity and a Social Security card to verify eligibility to work in the United States. The acceptable documents are listed on the instructions that accompany the I-9 form, which is available at the website of U.S. Citizenship and Immigration Services (www.uscis.gov). Be sure to use the most recent version of the I-9, as many earlier versions are no longer valid.

The employer can, but is not required to, photocopy any examined documents and keep the copies on file. If you choose to photocopy documents, you must follow this procedure for all new hires, and the document copies must be kept with the relevant Form I-9.

New hires must attest by signature on Form I-9 that they qualify for employment, and this must be done no later than the time of hire (the actual beginning of employment). The employer is responsible for ensuring that this attestation is properly completed by the time of hire, even though the proof-of-identity documents must be presented and examined up to three business days from the hire date.

All U.S. employers must retain the completed Form I-9 for each and every employee currently employed, citizens and noncitizens alike. This means that your practice files should also include completed Form I-9's for practice owners employed by the practice. In the event your practice is formed as a sole proprietorship, this is not necessary. The practice owner (the sole proprietor) is not required to have an I-9 on file for himself.

For additional information and to stay updated about any recent changes to forms and employer requirements, periodically visit the http://USCIS website. From here, you can access extensive instructions available in Form M-274, "Handbook for Employers."

Check your personnel files now. Time limits for compliance with the rules are stringent, and penalties for noncompliance with the rules are severe. For example, practices may be fined $100 to $1,000 for each employee whose identity and work authorization have not be properly verified.

The verification forms must be retained for three years from the date of hire or one year from the date of termination, whichever is longer. Most experts recommend that you maintain a secured filing location for all Form I-9's and any related photocopied employee documents that is separate and apart from other general employee personnel files.

The Fair Labor Standards Act

The Fair Labor Standards Act (FLSA), passed by Congress in 1938, sets basic minimum wage and overtime pay standards and record-keeping requirements and regulates the employment of minors. The FLSA can apply to employees in one of two ways: *enterprise coverage or individual coverage.*

In most cases, enterprise coverage applies to a business if it is engaged in *interstate commerce,* has at least two employees, and has annual sales or business volume of at least $500,000. Even if the business is not covered by the FLSA, some of its employees might be, if they are regularly involved in interstate commerce. Interstate commerce is defined very broadly by the statute and the courts, so the FLSA applies to many businesses and workers that one would not normally think are involved in interstate commerce. For example, processing credit-card transactions may constitute interstate commerce.

In all practicality, most veterinary practices are likely to be "covered" enterprises, thus bringing all of their employees under FLSA coverage. As a manager, you will frequently have issues that arise from questions about hours worked and exempt versus nonexempt status. Visit the U.S. Department of Labor website (www.dol.gov) regularly for easily searched questions and answers, and then progress to your practice's corresponding state website to determine what additional unique and special guidelines pertain to your practice.

MINIMUM WAGE REQUIREMENTS
The FLSA generally requires covered employers to pay their nonexempt employees at least the federal minimum wage and overtime premium pay of one-and-one-half times the normal rate

of pay for all hours in excess of 40 in a workweek, or, in some states, it is for all hours in excess of 8 in a work day. Each workweek stands alone.

Congress changes the minimum wage periodically, and some states set even higher minimum wage requirements. You should always know what the current minimum wage is in your state. You are also required to post, in a prominent location, the standard workplace poster displaying the federal minimum wage.

The FLSA makes reference to a workweek, the unit of time used for determining compliance with minimum wage requirements. A workweek is defined as 7 consecutive, regularly recurring, 24-hour periods totaling 168 hours. For the first 40 hours worked in any given workweek, each employee must be paid at least the minimum wage.

The overtime pay premium (1.5 times the regular rate) applies to all hours worked above 40 in a given workweek.

Here are some potential issues in determining what constitutes hours worked within a workweek as defined by the FLSA (U.S. Dept. of Labor, *Fair Labor Standards Act*, PowerPoint presentation, n.d.):

- *Hours "suffered" or permitted:* Even if the employer doesn't request the work, but knows the employee worked or permitted the employee to work, the work time must be compensated.
- *Waiting time:* This is counted as hours worked when the employee is unable to use the time effectively for his own purposes and the time is controlled by the employer. Waiting time is not counted as hours worked when the employee is completely relieved from duty and the time is long enough to enable the employee to use it effectively for his own purposes.
- *On-call time:* This is hours worked when the employee has to stay on the employer's premises or has to stay so close to the employer's premises that the employee cannot use that time effectively for her own purposes. On-call time is not hours worked when the employee is required to carry a pager or is required to leave word at home or with the employer about where she can be reached.
- *Meal and rest periods:* Meal periods are not hours worked when the employee is relieved of duties for the purpose of eating a meal. Rest periods of short duration (normally 5 to 20 minutes) are counted as hours worked and must be paid.
- *Training time:* This is the time employees spend in meetings, lectures, or training and is considered to be time worked and must be paid, unless
  » Attendance is outside regular working hours, and
  » Attendance is voluntary, and
  » The course, lecture, or meeting is not job related, and
  » The employee does not perform any productive work during attendance.

- *Travel time:* Ordinary home-to-work travel is not work time. Travel between jobsites during the normal workday is work time. Special rules apply to travel away from the employee's home community.
- *Sleep time:* Sleep time is broken down into two categories for purposes of compensation, based on the length of time the employee is on duty:
  - » If the employee is on duty for less than 24-hours and is allowed to sleep during that time or for a portion of that time and/or to engage in other personal pursuits, the employee is considered to be working for the entire period of time.
  - » If the employee is on duty for 24 hours or more, the employer and employee can agree to exclude bona fide sleep and meal periods.

The regular rate of pay is determined by dividing total earnings in the workweek by the total number of hours worked in the workweek, and may not be less than the applicable minimum wage. Certain employer payments to or on behalf of the employee are excluded from the determination of "regular rate of pay":

- Sums paid as gifts
- Payments for time not worked (paid time off)
- Reimbursement for expenses
- Discretionary bonuses
- Profit-sharing plan contributions
- Retirement and insurance plan payments
- Overtime premium payments
- Stock options

If an employee must wear a uniform, the financial burden of furnishing and maintaining the uniform (including laundry and repair) may not be imposed on the employee if the resulting wage would be below the minimum wage or overtime compensation required by the FLSA.

EXEMPTIONS

The FLSA provides for numerous exemptions from both the minimum-wage and overtime-pay provisions. For the first time in fifty years, the U.S. Department of Labor (DOL) made major revisions and clarifications of an employer's duty to pay overtime to certain employees under the FLSA. Final changes went into effect in August 2004. These changes primarily affect classification and salaries of "white-collar" workers, requiring employers to evaluate job classifications and payroll procedures for compliance under the new rules. The "541" or "white-collar" exemption is applicable to certain:

- Executive employees
- Administrative employees
- Professional employees

- Employees engaged in outside sales
- Employees doing computer-related work

To qualify for an exemption, the employee must meet the specific criteria for the exemption. In particular, the 2004 updates potentially affect practices with relatively low salary earners who have supervisory responsibilities or management-related responsibilities as well as workers with advanced education or specialized training (AICPA 2005, ch. 14). Exemptions are narrowly construed against the employer asserting them. Consequently, employers and employees should always closely check the exact terms and conditions of an exemption in light of the employee's actual duties before assuming that the exemption might apply to the employee. The ultimate burden of supporting the actual application of an exemption rests on the employer (U.S. Dept. of Labor, "ELaws," n.d.).

The three tests for exemption are related to salary level, salary basis, and job duties. Under the first test, the minimum requisite exempt salary level is $455 per week for most employees.

The second test for exemption resides in salary payment. The predetermined amount of compensation is paid weekly or on a less frequent basis, such as biweekly, semimonthly, or monthly. The compensation cannot be reduced because of variations in the quality or quantity of the work performed. The full salary must be paid for any week in which the employee performs any work, but need not be paid for any workweek when no work is performed. If the employee is ready, willing, and able to work, deductions may not be made for time when work is not available.

There are seven exceptions that permit salary deductions for an exempt employee:

1. Absence from work for one or more full days for personal reasons, other than sickness or disability
2. Absence from work for one or more full days due to sickness or disability if deductions are made under a bona fide plan, policy, or practice of providing wage replacement benefits for these types of absences
3. Offset of any amounts received as payment for jury fees, witness fees, or military pay
4. Penalties imposed in good faith for violating safety rules of "major significance"
5. Unpaid disciplinary suspension of one or more full days imposed in good faith for violations of written workplace conduct rules
6. Proportionate part of an employee's full salary may be paid for time actually worked in the first and last weeks of employment
7. Unpaid leave taken pursuant to the Family and Medical Leave Act

The third test for exemption relates to job duties. Here are the basics, but keep in mind that the details associated with each of these carve-outs are extensive. Consult with an employment-law attorney who is well versed in this area before drawing conclusions about how these factors apply to your practice:

1. *Executive duties:*
   A. Primary duty is management of the practice or of a customarily recognized department or subdivision of the practice.
   B. Customarily and regularly directs the work of two or more other employees.
   C. Has the authority to hire or fire other employees, or the practice gives particular weight to the recommendations of the exempt employee as to the hiring, firing, advancement, promotion, or other change of status of other employees.
   D. Includes employees with at least a bona fide 20 percent equity interest in the practice who are actively engaged in management of the practice. The salary level and salary basis requirements do not apply to exempt 20 percent equity owner executives.
2. *Administrative duties:*
   A. Primary duty is the performance of office or nonmanual work directly related to the management or general business operations of the employer or the employer's clients.
   B. Primary duty includes the exercise of discretion and independent judgment with respect to matters of significance.
   C. Examples of management or general business operations: tax, finance, accounting, budgeting, auditing, insurance, quality control, purchasing, procurement, advertising, marketing, research, safety and health, human resources, employee benefits, labor relations, public and government relations, legal and regulatory compliance, and computer network, Internet, and database administration; clerical duties do not count.
3. *Professional duties:*
   A. The employee's primary duty must be the performance of work requiring advanced knowledge, defined as work that is predominantly intellectual in character and that includes work requiring the consistent exercise of discretion and judgment.
   B. The advanced knowledge must be in a field of science or learning.
   C. The advanced knowledge must be customarily acquired by a prolonged course of specialized intellectual instruction.

Invariably, veterinarians engaged in the practice of veterinary medicine will fall under this exemption. (Many probably also meet the exemption for highly compensated employees.) However, the federal government issued a fact sheet that explains why veterinary technicians do not fall under the professional employee exemption (see U.S. Dept. of Labor, Fact Sheet #170, rev. 2008).

Other exceptions to the FLSA's minimum wage requirements include full-time students, student learners, and disabled workers.

The Wage and Hour Division of the U.S. Department of Labor issues certificates of exemption. The employer must apply for these in order to pay wages that are less than the minimum to these workers.

As for minimum wage requirements, some states do have overtime rules that are more rigorous than those of the FLSA. As a result, it is imperative for a practice manager to be familiar with state requirements as well as federal law.

RECORDS REQUIRED BY THE FLSA

Under the FLSA, employers are required to keep records on wages, hours, and other information for at least three years, but, as discussed in Chapter 5, record-keeping rules can vary depending on the applicable state and federal laws and regulations and the circumstances of the given practice. Retention of records for more than three years may be necessary. (For example, some lawsuits involving discriminatory pay practices may involve earlier records.) Records required for exempt employees differ from those for nonexempt employees, and special information is required about employees working under nonstandard pay arrangements. An accurate record of hours worked each day and total hours worked each week is critical to avoiding compliance problems.

Records need not be kept in any particular form. Time clocks are not required, although most practice managers are well aware that it is to their advantage to use them. (For more information, see U.S. Dept. of Labor, "Fact Sheet #21," rev. 2008).

FLSA-covered employers must post a notice explaining the act, as prescribed by the Wage and Hour Division, in a conspicuous place at each practice location. You can download free, up-to-date FLSA-compliant posters from the DOL website.

ENFORCEMENT

The Fair Labor Standards Act is enforced by the Wage and Hour Division of the U.S. Department of Labor. Compliance officers stationed across the United States carry out enforcement. Inspections may be initiated by the Department of Labor at random or after complaints are received from any source. Inspectors may inspect payroll records and may also interview employees. It is a violation of the FLSA to fire or in any way discriminate against an employee for filing a complaint or participating in a legal proceeding involving any of the provisions of the act.

The hospital manager should be aware of the many requirements of the FLSA. These include the minimum wage, overtime pay, and other requirements, such as regulations related to commission pay, bonuses, trainees, handicapped workers, part-time employees, and child labor. Additional information can be obtained from the U.S. Department of Labor website.

The FLSA does not require the following, but do keep in mind that some states do have laws covering some of these issues:

- Vacation, holiday, severance, or sick pay
- Meal or rest periods, holidays off, or vacations
- Premium pay for weekend or holiday work

- A discharge notice, reason for discharge, or immediate payment of final wages to terminated employees
- Any limit on the number of hours in a day or days in a week that an employee at least sixteen years old may be required or scheduled to work
- Pay raises or fringe benefits
  Here are some common errors to avoid:
- Confusing federal law and state law
- Assuming that all employees paid a salary are not due overtime
- Improperly applying an exemption
- Failing to pay for all hours an employee is "suffered or permitted" to work
- Limiting the number of hours employees are allowed to record
- Failing to include all pay required for calculating the regular rate of overtime
- Making improper deductions from wages that cut into the required minimum wage or overtime (e.g., shortages, drive-offs, damage, tools, uniforms)
- Treating an employee as an independent contractor

EMPLOYEES AND INDEPENDENT CONTRACTORS

Whether an individual is classified as an employee or an independent contractor is an important factor in determining the responsibilities of your practice under a variety of acts and regulations. These include:

- The FLSA
- The Federal Insurance Contribution Act (FICA)
- The Federal Unemployment Tax Act (FUTA)
- Internal Revenue Code (IRC) regulations determining income tax withholding responsibilities
- IRC regulations determining the requirement for providing benefits to an individual under evolving sections of the IRC
- IRC regulations determining the employer's responsibility regarding the many other laws related to "employees"

It is not always easy to determine whether someone who works for you is an employee or an independent contractor, especially since different regulatory bodies may have somewhat varying definitions or guidelines. There is no simple, black-and-white rule to provide guidance. Like so much of the law, situations depend heavily on specific "facts and circumstances" unique to your practice and on how case law has developed.

Employers should be aware that the IRS, the Department of Labor, and state-level regulatory bodies and tax authorities have an interest in classifying as many workers as possible as "employees" rather than as "independent contractors." The DOL and the IRS, working together to end the practice of employee misclassification, have published a Memorandum of Understanding regarding the independent contractor vs. employee issue.

In broad terms, an employee is an individual who performs services for your practice and who is subject to your control regarding what will be done and how it will be done.

The FLSA protects employees, but not independent contractors. The FLSA's definition of employee status is broader than the IRS common laws tests of such status. The determination of independent contractor versus employee standing considers the economic realities of the relationship rather than an agreement that purports to describe an individual as an independent contractor. The economic-realities test turns on whether the individual is economically dependent on the business for which he renders services (AICPA 2005, 17).

Six factors are generally considered by the courts in applying the economic-realities test under the FLSA:

1. The degree of control exercised by the practice over the individual's work performance (control over work hours, appointments and assignments, priority of work, hourly payment arrangement).
2. The extent of the relative investments by the practice and the individual in equipment and supplies used (for example, drugs and medical supplies).
3. The individual's opportunity for profit and loss through managerial skill (if the practice provides the opportunities and bears the risk of profit and loss, it is more likely that the individual is an employee).
4. The skill and initiative required by the work. Lower skill requirements weight toward employee status, but this does not necessarily mean that more skilled individuals, such as veterinarians, will qualify as independent contractors.
5. The permanence of the relationship. Longer work relationships imply employee status, especially when the nature of the work assignments does not vary much.
6. The extent to which the worker's services are an integral part of the practice.

The Internal Revenue Service (IRS) has traditionally used a more extensive set of twenty common-law factors to determine if an employer-employee relationship exists. They fall into three main categories: behavioral control, financial control, and relationship of the parties. These factors assess whether a business has the *right to direct and control* the actions of the worker. They are itemized in IRS Revenue Ruling 87-41 (see Table 6.1).

Under the twenty-factor common law test, an individual generally is considered an employee if the person for whom the individual performs the service has the right to control and direct that individual, specifically regarding the result to be accomplished by the work and the details and means by which that result is accomplished. The most important factor under the common law test is the employer's control, or rights of control, over the manner in which the work is to be performed and over the results of said work.

TABLE 6.1	DETERMINING EMPLOYEE OR INDEPENDENT CONTRACTOR STATUS
FACTOR	**EXPLANATION**
Instructions	An employee is required to comply with instructions concerning when, where, and how the work is to be done.
Training	An employee is provided with training to enable him or her to perform a job in a particular manner.
Integration	An employee's services are integrated into the operations of the business.
How services are rendered	An employee renders services personally.
Assistants	An employee works for a business that hires, supervises, and pays assistants to help the individual performing the services. An independent contractor hires, supervises, and pays his or her own assistants.
Employer-employee relationship	An employee has a continuing relationship with an employer and an employer-employee relationship exists.
Hours of work	An employee has set hours or work established by an employer.
Full-time work	An employee normally works full time or on a regular basis for an employer. An independent contractor works when and for whom he or she pleases.
Where work is done	An employee works on the premises of an employer or at a location designated by the employer.
Order and sequence	An employer directs the order and sequence in which the work must be done.
Reports	An employee submits regular oral or written reports to the employer.
Payments	An employee is paid hourly, weekly, or monthly. An independent contractor is paid by the job or by commission.
Expenses	An employee's business or travel expenses are reimbursed.
Tools and materials	An employee is furnished with tools and materials necessary for the provision of services.
Investment	An independent contractor has a significant investment in the facilities or equipment that he or she uses to provide services.
Profit and loss	An independent contractor can realize a profit or loss while providing services.
Number of clients	An independent contractor provides his or her services to multiple persons or firms at the same time.
Service offerings	An independent contractor offers his or her services to the general public.
Right to fire	An employee is subject to dismissal for reasons other than nonperformance of contract specifications.
Right to quit	An employee can terminate his or her relationship at any time without incurring liability for failure to complete a job. An independent contractor usually is responsible for the satisfactory completion of a job or project.

Source: Adapted from Internal Revenue Service, Revenue Ruling 87-41, 1987. For more information, see also U.S. Department of the Treasury, Internal Revenue Service, "Independent Contractor or Employee . . . " Publication 1779, revised August 2008, Catalog no. 16134L, available at www.irs.gov/pub/irs-pdf/p1779.pdf.

Not all of the factors are weighted equally. Indeed, not all of the factors need to be applied in every test. How the various factors are weighted in relation to the others depends on the facts and circumstances of each case.

In recent years, the IRS has grouped the more relevant factors into three main categories of evidence that show whether a worker is an employee or an independent contractor (U.S. Dept. of the Treasury, IRS, 2008). These are:

1. *Behavioral control:* Whether the practice has the right to direct and control the worker
   A. Instructions
      i. How, when, or where the work is done
      ii. What tools and equipment are used
      iii. What assistants are hired to help with the work
      iv. Where to purchase supplies and services
   B. Training:
      i. Whether the practice provides training about required procedures and methods
      ii. Whether the practice wants the work done in a certain way
2. *Financial control:* Whether the practice has the right to direct or control the business part of the work
   A. Whether the practice has a significant investment in the work
   B. Whether expenses are reimbursed, and if so, the proportion and amount of the reimbursement
   C. Who has the opportunity for profit or loss (the practice or the worker?)
3. *Relationship of the parties:* How benefits and contracts have been handled
   A. Existence of benefits such as insurance, a pension, or paid leave
   B. Existence of written contracts

If an individual in your employ has been treated as an independent contractor yet does not meet the standards imposed by the common law tests, you may still be able to consider that person as an independent contractor by utilizing a statutory safe harbor known as Section 530. Section 530 provides relief from federal employment tax obligations if certain requirements are met.

First, you must have a reasonable basis for classifying the employee as an independent contractor. The IRS provides the following examples of reasonable basis:
- You reasonably relied on a court case or an IRS ruling.
- You were previously audited by the IRS and were not told the contractor needed to be reclassified as an employee.
- You treated the worker as an independent contractor because you knew that was how a significant segment of the veterinary profession treated similar workers.
- You relied on competent legal advice.

Next, you need to be able to show that you have acted consistently in the way you have treated that worker and in the way you reported the worker's income. In other words, you should be able to show that: (1) You have always treated anyone doing that particular job as an independent contractor, and (2) you filed all required federal tax returns (including information returns, such as Form 1099-MISC) and the returns were consistent with your treatment of the worker as an independent contractor.

In all cases, great care should be taken before designating individuals as independent contractors. You classify an individual as an independent contractor at potentially significant risk to the practice.

Workers who believe they have been improperly classified as independent contractors can use a special reporting form to tell the IRS that they should only be responsible for their *employee* share of Social Security and Medicare taxes, in lieu of self-employment taxes. If an IRS audit were to categorize the individual as an employee, all back taxes would have to be paid by the employer. These taxes not only include the usual employer payroll taxes, such as Social Security and Medicare, but also the employee's portion of these taxes and mandatory federal income tax withholdings. The penalties and interest can be severe, especially when many payroll periods are examined and assessed.

Consider, too, that if the practice sponsors employee qualified benefit plans such as group health insurance, cafeteria plans, and retirement plans, the worker may have been eligible for them but did not receive the benefit while being treated as an independent contractor. When you add in the cost of legal defense and accounting fees for amending returns and refiling paperwork, the sum total of costs could literally bankrupt a veterinary practice.

Civil Rights

The historic passage of the Civil Rights Act of 1964 sought to bring about equal opportunity for all in the crucial area of employment rights. Under Title VII of the act, it is an "unlawful employment practice for an employer to fail or refuse to hire or to discharge any individual, or otherwise to discriminate against any individual with respect to his compensation, terms, conditions, or privileges of employment, because of such individual's race, color, religion, sex, or national origin."

The Equal Employment Opportunity Commission (EEOC) was created to enforce this antidiscrimination law. Although all businesses, regardless of size, are expected to avoid discrimination, the jurisdiction of the EEOC with regard to the Civil Rights Act only covers those employers with fifteen or more employees (meaning anyone with whom the business has an "employment relationship," including part-time workers). The U.S. Supreme Court has also ruled that former employees may sue their former employers under the Civil Rights Act.

This section will discuss several specific civil rights issues enforced by the EEOC: sexual harassment, pregnancy discrimination, disabled employees, and age discrimination. EEOC guidelines also cover discrimination related to religion, national origin, and affirmative action. As in all issues related to the law, consult your practice's attorney and current law for further details and up-to-date information. Many states and even local municipalities have regulations that overlap, are more rigorous, or change more frequently than the federal laws and should always be considered when addressing discrimination issues.

SEXUAL HARASSMENT

Title VII of the 1964 Civil Rights Act prohibits discrimination based on gender. There are three categories of sex discrimination: typical gender-based discrimination, sex discrimination based on pregnancy, and sexual harassment.

Sexual harassment claims were almost unheard of until the U.S. Supreme Court ruled in 1986 that sexual harassment is a form of sex discrimination prohibited by the act. Sexual harassment claims have risen dramatically since then. According to the EEOC, "unwelcome sexual advances, requests for sexual favors, and other verbal or physical conduct of a sexual nature constitutes sexual harassment when submission to or rejection of this conduct explicitly or implicitly affects an individual's employment, unreasonably interferes with an individual's work performance or creates an intimidating, hostile or offensive work environment" (EEOC 2002).

As this definition states, there are two types of sexual harassment: *quid pro quo sexual harassment* and *hostile environment sexual harassment* (sometimes called simply *environmental sexual harassment*). Quid pro quo sexual harassment occurs when submission to or rejection of unwelcome sexual conduct is used as the basis of employment decisions affecting the individual.

Environmental sexual harassment includes unwelcome conduct that is either sexual in nature or is directed at a person because of the person's gender, and that unreasonably interferes with the individual's job performance or creates an "intimidating, hostile, or offensive working environment," even if it leads to no tangible or economic job consequence. Sexist jokes, nude pictures in a magazine kept out in the open, touching an employee after being requested not to do so, or expressing criticism with sexist connotations could all be considered sexual harassment.

A hostile work environment can be created by particular conduct or a pattern of conduct. Factors that may suggest that a hostile work environment exists include: (1) the frequency of the conduct, (2) its severity, (3) whether the conduct is physically threatening or humiliating, and (4) whether the conduct unreasonably interferes with the employee's work performance (AICPA 2005, 33).

Be aware that virtually anyone can create a hostile work environment. The employer can be held responsible for the actions of employees, clients, and vendors. Supervisors, managers, and others in leadership positions, such as staff veterinarians, must be vigilant and keenly aware of conduct that may be leading to or causing a hostile work environment.

Whenever the employer knows or reasonably should know that another employee, vendor, or client is creating a hostile environment, the employer must take prompt, affirmative corrective action (ibid).

The core accusation in any sexual harassment claim is that the alleged sexual advances were unwelcome. In 1993, the Supreme Court further clarified the harassment standard by explaining that two requirements must be satisfied:

1. The conduct must "create an objectively hostile or abusive work environment"—in other words, an environment that a reasonable person would find hostile or abusive.
2. The victim must "subjectively perceive the environment to be abusive" in order for the conduct to have altered the conditions of the victim's employment. (London 1998)

A 1998 Supreme Court ruling found that employers are absolutely liable for sexual harassment by supervisors if the harassment has caused the plaintiff to experience a "tangible employment action," which is defined as hiring, firing, failing to promote, reassignment, or an alteration of benefits. This ruling also determined that it does not matter whether the harassment is understood by those involved as quid pro quo or as creating a hostile environment as long as "tangible employment action" occurred (ibid.).

As a result of this ruling, there is now greater pressure on employers to prevent harassment from occurring. Once it has occurred, an employer can do little or nothing to escape liability if the employee has suffered a "tangible job action" as a result of supervisor misconduct.

The EEOC encourages employers to "take all steps necessary to prevent sexual harassment from occurring, such as affirmatively raising the subject, expressing strong disapproval, developing appropriate sanctions, informing employees of their right to raise and how to raise the issue of harassment under the Civil Rights Act and developing methods to sensitize all concerned" (ibid.). The 1998 Supreme Court decision in fact would appear to require these steps to be taken.

OTHER PROTECTED CLASSES

Keep in mind that Title VII gives all employees the right of a workplace free of discriminatory intimidation, insult, and ridicule. Under federal law, workplace harassment can include a variety of conduct that can lead to environmental harassment (hostile work environment, including epithets; slurs; negative stereotyping; and threatening, intimidating, hostile, or demeaning acts that relate to race, color, religion, gender, citizenship, national origin, age, or disability [mental or physical]). Various states have enacted antidiscrimination laws that greatly expand federal-law restrictions, such as prohibiting discrimination relating to age for those between the ages of eighteen and thirty-nine, political affiliation, marital status, smoking, sexual orientation, appearance, and more (AICPA 2005, 29–33).

Note that harassment can include other forms of unwanted behavior directed at other protected classes, which include race, religion, national origin, age, reserve- or guard-duty status, and disability. Quid pro quo harassment applies to other protected classes as much as it does sex. Develop a clear practice policy prohibiting not only sexual harassment but also any other form of harassment. This policy should be well publicized at the practice, such as through posting with other legally mandated notification and prohibitions in the hospital policy manual, as well as on the practice intranet.

Regularly retrain employees about the policy, and document the training. A sample policy is included (see Figure 6.1).

Prompt management action is imperative with evidence of situations or employee comments suggesting quid pro quo or environmental sexual harassment. Your practice should maintain a clearly understood and publicized internal complaint mechanism. Because of the sensitive nature of harassment and the potential for employee fear of reprisal (especially in small businesses like veterinary practices), consider a back-up confidential reporting option, such as an outsourced hot-line service.

Employment practices liability insurance (EPLI) policies often include coverage for harassment claims in all categories of harassment as defined by the EEOC and claims related to hostile workplace issues. Insurance coverage has become increasingly important to practices because of the incidence of and expense associated with claim defense.

PREGNANCY DISCRIMINATION

The Pregnancy Discrimination Act of 1978 makes it clear that discrimination on the basis of pregnancy, childbirth, or related medical conditions constitutes unlawful sex discrimination under the Civil Rights Act. The basic principle of the act is that women affected by pregnancy and related conditions must be treated the same as other applicants and employees, on the basis of their ability or inability to work. The law applies to employers with fifteen or more employees.

This means an employer must treat a pregnant employee, with regard to performance of job functions, in the exact same manner that any other temporarily disabled employee would be treated. A pregnant employee must be allowed to work at all times during pregnancy as long as she is able to perform the functions of her position. An employer may not take fetal welfare into account when deciding whether to permit a pregnant employee to remain on the job (but the pregnant employee should be advised of any workplace hazards that could affect her pregnancy).

FIGURE 6.1 SAMPLE EMPLOYEE POLICY ON HARASSMENT

This is a suggested policy only—review this policy with legal counsel prior to implementation.

ANTIHARASSMENT POLICY

[Company name] promotes a harmonious, productive work environment in which no employee is subject to any form of harassment, discrimination, or intimidation. We strive to create a workplace where all employees are treated with respect and dignity.

All employees are covered under our antiharassment policy and are expected to comply with the policy provisions. Appropriate disciplinary action will be taken against any employee who violates this policy, which may include verbal or written reprimand, suspension, or termination of employment.

Harassment of any kind will not be tolerated and is prohibited. This includes verbal remarks that are derogatory regarding a person's nationality, origin, race, color, religion, gender, sexual orientation, age, body disability, or appearance; verbal taunting (including racial and ethnic slurs) or negative stereotyping; physical conduct designed to threaten, intimidate, or coerce; distribution, display, or discussion of any written or graphic material that ridicules, denigrates, insults, or shows hostility toward an individual or group because of national origin, race, color, religion, age, gender, sexual orientation, pregnancy, appearance, disability, marital status, or other protected status.

The practice strictly prohibits sexual harassment. Sexual harassment is defined as unwelcome sexual advances, requests for sexual favors, and other verbal or physical conduct of a sexual nature if:

- Submission to such conduct is explicitly or implicitly made a term or condition of an individual's employment.
- Submission to or rejection of such conduct by an individual is used as the basis for employment decisions affecting that individual.
- Such conduct unreasonably interferes with an individual's work performance or creates an intimidating, hostile, or offensive work environment.

Any harassment that is directed at a person because of that person's gender is also sexual harassment, regardless of whether it is sexual in nature. Conduct of this nature is prohibited by the practice, whether the person engaging in such conduct is a manager, supervisor, coworker, or third party (such as suppliers, customers, and service personnel).

An employee who thinks he or she has been subjected to any form of harassment or is aware of harassment in the workplace should immediately bring a complaint to the attention of the

CONTINUES >

> **FIGURE 6.1**

SAMPLE EMPLOYEE POLICY ON HARASSMENT, CONT.

owner or manager. If the complaint is directed against the owner, then it should be brought to the attention of the manager of the practice. All complaints will be promptly and impartially investigated, and the appropriate parties will be notified of the results. Investigations will be conducted as confidentially as practicable. Any employee found to have engaged in harassment will be subject to disciplinary action, up to and including termination.

The company will not retaliate against employees for making harassment complaints or bringing acts of possible harassment to the practice's attention.

Source: American Animal Hospital Association (AAHA), AAHA Guide to Creating an Employee Handbook, 3rd ed. (Lakewood, CO: AAHA Press, 2009), 16–17. Used with permission.

Congress made clear that the decision to become pregnant and to work while being pregnant is a decision for each individual woman to make for herself. Hospitals should have a "Pregnancy and Employment Policy" included in their hospital policy manual.

THE AMERICANS WITH DISABILITIES ACT

In 1990, Congress passed the Americans with Disabilities Act (ADA). Title I of the ADA prohibits employment discrimination against persons with disabilities. The ADA goes further than other employment discrimination laws by imposing on employers an affirmative duty to make reasonable accommodations for applicants and employees with disabilities. *Disability* means a physical or mental impairment that substantially limits one or more of the major life activities of an individual.

The law applies to employers who have 15 or more employees. The original law defined employees as individuals who had worked more than 20 hours per week for each working day in each of 20 or more calendar weeks in the current or preceding year. However, the Supreme Court has adopted a broader definition of employees under Title VII of the Civil Rights Act of 1964. Under this broadened definition, all workers who are on the payroll for at least twenty weeks during the year are counted in determining whether an employer meets the fifteen-employee definition. This definition is almost certain to apply to claims under the ADA (Kahn et al. 1999, 5–6).

Title I of the ADA prohibits employers covered under the act from discriminating against any qualified person with a disability with respect to practically every aspect of the employment relationship. This includes job application procedures, hiring, advancement, discipline, discharge, compensation, job training, leave, benefits, and all other terms, conditions, and privileges of employment.

The definition of "qualified person with a disability" is one of the key elements of the ADA statute. The EEOC regulations state that a "qualified" individual is one who "satisfies the requisite skill, experience, education, and other job-related requirements of the position such individual holds or desires, and who, with or without the assistance of a reasonable accommodation, can perform the essential functions of such position" (London 1998).

To ensure that your practice fulfills the requirements of the ADA, it is very important to prepare written job descriptions before you advertise and interview applicants. The regulations state that a written job description prepared before the job is filled will be considered as evidence of the essential functions of the job (Kahn et al. 1999). It should include not only the intellectual and skill functions but also the physical, time, and stress requirements. For example, if the job requires that the individual be able to lift a fifty-pound dog or bag of dog food, say so in the job description. Include any physical requirements that are part of the job, such as driving, sitting, lifting, and reaching.

If an applicant, except for limitations caused by a disability, is otherwise qualified to perform the essential functions of a job, the employer must consider whether or not the individual could perform these functions with the assistance of a reasonable accommodation. A reasonable accommodation is a modification or adjustment to a job or to the work environment that enables a qualified applicant or an employee with a disability to participate in the application process or to perform the essential functions of the job.

The employer is expected to make reasonable accommodations if, with that accommodation, the individual with the disability could perform the essential functions of the position. Employers are not required to lower quality standards in order to make an accommodation, nor are they required to provide personal use items such as eyeglasses or hearing aids.

Reasonable accommodations would include:

- Adjusting and modifying pre-employment exams and training programs
- Job restructuring (e.g., reallocation of nonessential job functions)
- Providing part-time or modified work schedules
- Reassigning disabled workers to vacant positions
- Making work and nonwork areas (restrooms, luncheon rooms, entrance space) accessible and usable
- Providing accommodation aids such as telephone headsets, electronic visual aids, magnifiers, and telephone amplifiers
- Providing adaptive computer equipment or software

- Lowering or raising desks
- Providing assistants such as interpreters
- Providing reserved parking places

A reasonable accommodation must be made unless the accommodation would impose an undue hardship on the operation of the business. The term *undue hardship* means significant difficulty, significant disruption of business, or significant expense. Undue hardship must be proven by the business on a case-by-case basis that takes into consideration the nature and cost of the accommodation as well as the size and the financial resources of the business.

Under the ADA, an employer may not ask employees about the existence, nature, or severity of a disability. An employer may not conduct medical examinations until after a conditional job offer is made, at which time medical examinations can be required, but only if an exam would be required of any candidate, with or without disabilities. Physicians performing the examinations should have a copy of the job description and can be asked if, in their opinion, each prospective employee is qualified.

Before a conditional offer of employment is made, employers may ask about an applicant's ability to perform specific job-related functions, that is, the essential functions as listed in the job description. An employer may also ask other questions that are not related to any disability (see Table 5.1) and may also require examinations that are not medical. Examinations given before the job is offered could include physical and intellectual-capacity examinations (spelling, typing, or grammar tests), but only if all applicants are given the same test and if a direct tie between the test and the essential functions of the job can be shown.

The ADA's protection extends to persons with mental disabilities. In 1997, the EEOC issued guidelines advising employers that they: (1) may not discriminate against qualified workers with a mental illness, (2) may not ask job applicants if they have a history of mental illness, and (3) must take reasonable steps to accommodate employees with psychiatric or emotional problems.

The ADA was amended in 2008, and several of the changes make it easier for individuals to demonstrate that they are covered by the ADA. For example, the amended statute expands the definition of "major life activities," which had been interpreted narrowly by several courts, including the U.S. Supreme Court. The amended statute also states that, except for ordinary eyeglasses and contacts, the effects of mitigating measures such as medications, prosthetics, cochlear implants, and oxygen therapy equipment are not to be considered when determining whether an individual is disabled. This change in the law is also a response to some Supreme Court decisions.

The Personnel Management section of "Additional Resources" at the end of the book contains a list of information sources pertaining to the ADA.

AGE DISCRIMINATION

In 1967, Congress passed the Age Discrimination in Employment Act (ADEA) to prohibit discrimination in employment because of age in such matters as hiring, job retention, compensation and other terms, conditions, and privileges of employment. The ADEA prohibits employers with twenty or more employees from discrimination against persons forty or older on the basis of their age. Employers must ensure that job announcements and employment application forms do not, in any way, attempt to discriminate against anyone on the basis of age.

The ADEA has special rules pertaining to pension and other benefit plans (AICPA 2005, 31). When designing a benefit plan for your practice, consult with an expert to assure compliance with the ADEA in addition to other complexities of employee benefit programs.

FAMILY AND MEDICAL LEAVE

Under the Family and Medical Leave Act (FMLA) of 1993, each eligible employee is entitled to a total of twelve workweeks of job-protected, unpaid leave during a twelve-month period. The FMLA covers employers with fifty or more employees for each working day during each of twenty or more calendar weeks in the current or previous year (weeks need not be consecutive workweeks). All employees (full time, part time, temporary, and permanent) must be counted as long as they were on the payroll at the beginning and end of each relevant workweek. To be eligible, an employee must have been employed for at least twelve months, although the months need not be consecutive. The employee must have worked at least 1,250 hours during the 12-month period immediately preceding the commencement of leave, and must work at a location where at least 50 employees are employed by the employer within a 75-mile radius. The leave must be for one of the purposes listed in the textboxes (see "FMLA: Reasons to Take Leave" and "FMLA: Qualifying Exigencies").

As for other federal laws, many states have their own family leave acts that may provide more generous benefits and have different eligibility requirements than the FMLA (AICPA 2005, 34). Carefully investigate your practice's obligations under state law at least annually. As laws change and/or as your practice grows in terms of its number of employees, additional requirements may apply to you.

Recent amendments to the FMLA provide for "military caregiver leave." Under this provision, a covered employee may request up to twenty-six weeks of unpaid leave to care for a covered service member with a serious injury or illness who is the spouse, child, parent, or next of kin to the employee.

Once an employer is covered by the FMLA, it is required to post a notice of FMLA rights in addition to following the guidelines for employer notice of FMLA designation requirements and employee notice of leave requirements. Information must be included in the employee policy

---

FMLA: Reasons to Take Leave

Under the FMLA, employees can request up to twelve weeks of unpaid leave for any of the following reasons:

- The birth of a child and to care for the newborn child within one year of birth
- Placement of a child with the employee for adoption or foster care, and to care for the child within one year of placement
- Care for a spouse, child, or parent of the employee who has a serious health condition
- Serious health condition that makes the employee unable to perform the functions of his position
- Any "qualifying exigency" arising out of the active duty or call to active duty of the employee's spouse, child, or parent (The qualifying exigencies are summarized in "Fact Sheet #28A: The Family and Medical Leave Act Military Leave Entitlements," which is available on the U.S. Department of Labor's website. The main points of Fact Sheet #28A appear in the accompanying textbox, "FMLA: Qualifying Exigencies.")

Source: Adapted from U.S. Department of Labor, Wage and Hour Division, "Family and Medical Leave Act," www.dol.gov/whd/fmla/.

manual, and if the practice does not have one, the employer must give the written guidance to employees of their rights and obligations under the FMLA (AICPA 2005, 38).

In June 2010, the Department of Labor issued an interpretation of the definition of "son or daughter" under the FMLA. That interpretation clarifies that a biological relationship is not required, and it gives some examples of parent-child relationships that would qualify under the FMLA. "Son or daughter" can include an adopted child, foster child, stepchild, legal ward, or child of any person in a position of "in loco parentis."

Under the FMLA, an employer must continue to provide the same health benefits, under the same terms and conditions, as the employer would have provided if the employee had been continuously employed during the entire leave period. In the event the employee fails to return to work after any unpaid leave has expired, the employer may recover the cost of any health benefit premiums paid during the unpaid leave, provided that the failure to return is not the result of a serious health condition or other circumstances beyond the employee's control (AICPA 2005, 37).

When an employee requests leave under the FMLA, employers may require medical certification. The Department of Labor has provided a medical certification form for health-care providers to complete.

FMLA: Qualifying Exigencies

The qualifying reasons for military personnel under the FMLA include the following:

- Issue arising from a covered military member's short-notice deployment (i.e., deployment on seven or less days of notice) for a period of seven days from the date of notification
- Military events and related activities, such as official ceremonies, programs, or events sponsored by the military or family support or assistance programs and informational briefings sponsored or promoted by the military, military service organizations, or the American Red Cross that are related to the active-duty or call to active-duty status of a covered military member
- Certain child-care and related activities arising from the active-duty or call to active-duty status of a covered military member, such as arranging for alternative child care, providing child care on a nonroutine, urgent, immediate-need basis, enrolling or transferring a child in a new school or day-care facility, and attending certain meetings at a school or a day-care facility if they are necessary due to circumstances arising from the active duty or call to active duty of the covered military member
- Making or updating financial and legal arrangements to address a covered military member's absence
- Attending counseling provided by someone other than a health-care provider for oneself, the covered military member, or the child of the covered military member, the need for which arises from the active-duty or call to active-duty status of the covered military member
- Taking up to five days of leave to spend time with a covered military member who is on short-term temporary rest-and-recuperation leave during deployment
- Attending to certain postdeployment activities, including attending arrival ceremonies, reintegration briefings and events, and other official ceremonies or programs sponsored by the military for a period of 90 days following the termination of the covered military member's active-duty status, and addressing issues arising from the death of a covered military member
- Any other event that the employee and employer agree is a qualifying exigency

Source: Adapted from U.S. Department of Labor, Wage and Hour Division, "Fact Sheet #28A: The Family and Medical Leave Act Military Family Leave Entitlements," revised February 2010, www.dol.gov/whd/regs/compliance/whdfs28a.pdf.

Except for highly compensated "key" employees, any employee who takes leave under the act will be entitled, on return from such leave, to be restored to the position held before the leave commenced, or to an equivalent position with equivalent pay, benefits, and working conditions. If a returning employee is no longer able to perform an essential function of the position upon return, the employee has no right to restoration to another position under the FMLA. However, if the employee is no longer able to perform the duties of the previous position because of a physical or mental condition, including the continuation of a serious health condition, the employer may be required to consider whether reasonable accommodations are possible under the ADA.

The FMLA expressly exempts "key" employees from the general reinstatement requirement. By definition, these individuals are the top 10 percent of the highest-paid employees who are employed by the employer within a 75-mile radius of the employee's worksite. A blanket restoration of such individuals to previously held or equivalent positions could result in substantial economic injury to employer's business operations. The employer must give written notice to "key" employees of their status and potential consequences when FMLA leave is requested (Kahn et al. 1999, 5.02).

Occupational Safety and Health

In 1970, Congress passed legislation establishing the Occupational Safety and Health Administration (OSHA) within the Department of Labor. OSHA requires that all employers, regardless of the number of employees, shall furnish a place of employment that is free from recognized hazards that cause or are likely to cause death or serious physical harm to their employees.

OSHA is authorized to issue workplace safety standards that are legally enforceable. Such standards include limitations on worker exposure to hazardous chemicals and maximum workplace noise levels. All employers covered by OSHA must comply with OSHA's Hazard Communication Standard, which requires employers to identify all hazardous chemicals to which employees might be exposed and communicate information about them to employees. Employers must develop and put into practice a written hazard communication program that describes the procedures by which they will comply with this requirement. OSHA also requires employee-training programs on hazardous materials and ergonomic risks in the workplace.

OSHA has the authority to conduct workplace inspections without notifying the employer ahead of time. Inspections are usually triggered by reports of injuries in the workplace or by employee complaints of unsafe working conditions or alleged violations of OSHA standards. OSHA is authorized to give citations and impose substantial penalties for workplace violations of OSHA regulations.

Few other federal laws or agencies bring as much concern to animal hospital administrators as does OSHA. Given the broad scope of the law and the fact that it requires employers to take proactive steps to educate and train workers, it is important that every employer become familiar with the basic requirements.

Managerial training programs focusing on these requirements must be among the hospital manager's tools. Resources include the DVDs *Be Safe: Veterinary Safety Training for the Whole Practice Team* and *Be Safe: Veterinary Safety Training for Medical and Technical Staff* as well as the book *Be Safe! Manager's Guide to Veterinary Workplace Safety* by Philip J. Seibert, all available from AAHA Press. Safetyvet.com is another helpful resource.

Workers' Compensation

Required by state statute, workers' compensation insurance protects the interests of employees involved in work-related injuries. For all accidental injuries, illnesses, or deaths arising out of employment and related to employment, employers are to provide compensation, both by replacing wages and by covering the cost of all reasonable and necessary hospital, surgical, and medical expenses.

A dog-bite injury inflicted on an employee by a patient is easily identified as an injury arising out of employment. Some injuries potentially causing a claim are more difficult to directly relate to employment. For example, a clinic employee who is injured while playing softball on a clinic-sponsored team after work hours might fall under workers' compensation jurisdiction.

Each of the fifty states has enacted its own workers' compensation laws, which cover virtually every employer. The state laws were enacted so that the employee does not have to go through the ordeal of a lawsuit to collect damages from the employer. Depending on the state, employers are required to obtain workers' compensation insurance or to prove financial ability to carry their own risk. Some states require employers to participate in a state fund, while others provide a competitive state insurance program as an alternative to commercial insurance plans. Hospital managers should be aware of the laws in their states.

Unemployment Insurance

The main objective of the national unemployment insurance program is to provide unemployed workers with modest financial support in the event of a temporary period of involuntary unemployment. Virtually all employers are covered by the program, which is financed almost entirely from employer taxes. The Federal Unemployment Tax Act (FUTA) provides funds that the states can use to administer unemployment benefits. Because of this joint administration, veterinary practice managers need to understand a double set of employer rules and send tax payments and tax returns to both the state and federal governments.

To qualify for unemployment benefits, all claimants must be able and available for suitable work. All states disqualify persons who voluntarily quit their jobs without good cause, are discharged for misconduct, or refuse an offer of suitable work. A relatively common occurrence is that an employee quits voluntarily and takes another job that doesn't work out, and then attempts to collect unemployment benefits from the first employer. When the former employee files for unemployment benefits with the state, a claim against the first employer results. This first employer may have had plenty of work available and may have preferred not to lose the trained employee in the first place.

Unfortunately, the burden is usually upon the employer to prove that a former employee quit without good cause or that there is another reason the employee should not be paid from the employer's employment reserve with the state. States follow a policy of reducing the employment tax on employers who show a history of stable employment. From the perspective of mitigating tax expense through elevated rates, which can stay high for many years, it is in an employer's interest to maintain low employee turnover.

Because practice managers are often responsible for refuting unjustified unemployment claims, it is important to have good records. Make sure all employees who quit voluntarily submit a written letter of resignation. Secure personnel files to prohibit tampering or loss.

Pensions and Employee Benefits

Employers may choose to provide their employees with some of a wide variety of employee benefit options that exist under law. Such legally prescribed benefits are generally known as "qualified benefits." The expense of qualified benefits can provide the practice with a tax deduction without the requirement to include the value of the benefit in the employee's income-taxable compensation.

Some qualified benefit program options include retirement income plans, stock purchase plans, group medical insurance, and prepaid legal services (Kahn et al. 1999, 1.05). Nearly every employee health and retirement benefit arrangement is governed by the Employee Retirement Income Security Act (ERISA) of 1974, which provides safeguards for employee interests in any employer-sponsored plan.

ERISA does not require that employers provide benefit plans, but it does impose requirements to protect the rights of participants. ERISA consists of three major sections. Title I prescribes reporting and disclosure obligations, minimum participation rules, vesting and funding requirements, fiduciary standards, and other rules. It is administered by the Department of Labor. Title II consists of amendments to the Internal Revenue Code and is enforced by the IRS. The last major section, Title IV, establishes a pension-plan benefit insurance program, administered through the Pension Benefit Guaranty Corporation (PBGC).

Both the IRC and ERISA impose substantial reporting and disclosure obligations on the plan's administrator. Annual reports of financial, actuarial, and other information must be filed with the DOL, the IRS, and the PBGC. The same information must be available to plan participants and beneficiaries. ERISA defines the fiduciary standards for covered employee benefit plans and rules of conduct for the plan trustee. Any employer who provides an employee benefit plan has a heavy duty of responsibility to be knowledgeable about ERISA provisions and about changes in the law affecting its administration (Kahn et al. 1999, 1.05).

Employee Health Plans

Health-care costs for employees and their dependents are a major source of concern, both for employees and employers. The law is still evolving because of the Patient Protection and Affordable Care Act (PPACA) of 2010 (as amended by the Health Care and Education Reconciliation Act of 2010), which is still undergoing challenges in the courts and in the political arena. Veterinary practice managers must stay abreast of these changes and be aware of how they apply to them. Some provisions of this law are described below. For updates, see www.healthcare.gov, a website managed by the U.S. Department of Health and Human Services. Other areas of health-insurance law that affect veterinary practice are the Consolidated Omnibus Budget Reconciliation Act (COBRA) of 1986, the Health Insurance Portability and Accountability Act (HIPAA) of 1996, and the Mental Health Parity Act (MHPA) of 1996.

COBRA, as amended in 1989, allows for limited continuation of group health benefits to covered employees who leave their employment under certain circumstances. The PPACA health-care reform legislation did not eliminate COBRA or change the COBRA rules (U.S. Dept. of Labor, EBSA "Health Care Reform and COBRA," n.d.).

COBRA's general requirement for temporary coverage extension applies to employers with twenty or more employees in the year prior to the coverage. Qualified individuals are allowed to extend their coverage (called *continuation coverage*) on a self-pay basis for a period up to eighteen months after termination of employment.

As for other federal laws, many states have their own versions of COBRA that can apply to employers. "State continuation" or "mini-COBRA" laws help workers in businesses with fewer than twenty workers continue health coverage after job loss. In some states, these laws mirror the federal COBRA law. In other states, continuation programs may differ in eligibility requirements, coverage duration, or benefits provided.

COBRA imposes numerous notice requirements on employers, plan administrators, and covered employees. Employers and administrators must provide timely notice in a number of events, and so must qualified beneficiaries, in order to avoid inadvertent waiver of their COBRA benefits (AICPA 2005, 57).

The Health Insurance Portability and Accountability Act protects workers' health-insurance coverage when they change jobs, limits exclusions for preexisting conditions, and prohibits discrimination against employees and dependents based on their health status.

The Mental Health Parity Act provides for parity between medical and surgical benefits and mental health benefits.

Beginning in 2014, the Patient Protection and Affordable Care Act, which became law in 2010, will require employers with more than fifty employees to provide group health insurance or pay a penalty of $2,000 per employee per year. For those with Health Savings Accounts, the statute increases the tax on nonqualified medical expenses from 10 percent to 20 percent. It caps the annual contribution to Flexible Spending Accounts at $2,500. As enacted at the time of this writing, the law requires everyone to have government-qualified health insurance or pay a tax (penalty). If your employees are not covered by a group policy, they will have to obtain insurance individually or pay the tax for being uninsured. This area of the law is under challenge in federal courts, so check for updates as mentioned above.

Polygraph Protection

The Employee Polygraph Protection Act (EPPA) of 1988 generally prohibits most private-sector employers from directly or indirectly requiring, suggesting, or otherwise causing any employee or prospective employee to take or submit to any lie-detector test. Furthermore, an employer may not discharge, discipline, discriminate against, deny employment or promotion to, or threaten to take any action against any employee or prospective employee who refuses, declines, or fails to take or submit to any lie-detector test; nor may such action be taken on the basis of any lie-detector test results.

The EPPA does permit polygraph testing of some job applicants by firms that provide security services (e.g., guards and armored car services) and companies that make, distribute, or dispense pharmaceuticals. The law also permits, under certain conditions, polygraph testing of employees who are reasonably suspected of a workplace crime resulting in specific economic loss to the employer (such as embezzlement or theft). However, any testing permitted by the EPPA is subject to stringent requirements designed to safeguard the employee's rights. Furthermore, any polygraph testing permitted by the EPPA is still subject to any applicable state and local laws and any collective bargaining agreement.

Required Notice Postings

Every employer, regardless of the number of employees, must post and maintain various Department of Labor posters in a conspicuous location frequented by employees. Required posters include information about the following:

- The Fair Labor Standards Act and Minimum Wage
- Equal opportunity provisions of the law
- The Family and Medical Leave Act
- OSHA Job Safety and Health Protection requirements
- The Employee Polygraph Protection Act
- The Uniformed Services Employment and Reemployment Rights Act
- Right to join/form unions and associations

The states also have workplace poster requirements, such as for posters advising employees of their rights under workers' compensation law and state minimum-wage and overtime requirements. The easiest solution may be to purchase a combination of federal and state posters from one of the many online companies that sell these at relatively low cost.

Every hospital manager must be aware of the practice's expansive responsibilities to its employees, the laws pertaining to personnel, and the related notice and posting requirements. Whenever questions arise regarding the applicability of these complex rules, which may span multiple jurisdictions and regulatory agencies, it is important to seek expert counsel sooner, rather than later.

This chapter has provided an introduction to some of the main areas of employment law pertaining to practice management. But we have really only scratched the surface. It should be a useful starting point as you make sure your practice is in compliance with state and federal law, but it is no substitute for good legal counsel. Be sure to ask your practice attorney about how these areas of law apply to your practice, and pursue further reading. Keeping abreast of the law will be a continual theme as you grow in practice management skills, knowledge, and expertise.

OPERATIONS AND MAINTENANCE

7

Reception and Front-Desk Procedures

When you ask a new employee, "What do you think is the number-one means by which our clients judge our performance?" the typical answer will be something like: "How well we take care of the patient."

Most experienced practice managers know that this answer is incorrect. Clients of veterinary practices judge competency on many levels. Quite frequently, the measuring stick is what the client first perceives through telephone conversations, the appearance of the front desk and the employees, and the general efficiency of the hospital team. The receptionist's demeanor and attitude may easily be the standard by which the veterinary service is first judged.

Most clients and potential clients are consumers who quickly assess competency based on immediate impressions. Reception area appearance, and the responsiveness and courtesy of the receptionist, play crucial roles. Reception is typically the first contact a new client has with the hospital once she has made a choice among the many veterinary service providers in convenient proximity. Written materials, such as brochures and handouts, as well as the practice website, also help to form and maintain client impressions. These elements can all create a seamless experience for the client.

Community reputation and referrals are clearly built over time through successful patient outcomes. Yet, clients equally judge competency on what they can see and smell, and especially how the hospital team makes them feel. Telephone etiquette, employee knowledge and communication skill, responsiveness, team-member appearance, facility aesthetics, and written materials are all critical parts of the hospital's success.

Being a "Walk-Around Manager"

Effective practice managers do not hide in the wings. Rather than sitting in a business office, preparing spreadsheet analyses and working on reports, a good manager will spend much of his time walking around the hospital ensuring that all aspects of the practice are as appealing to clients as possible, especially in areas of high client traffic. Watching and listening attentively to all aspects of people interactions are important parts of the fourth step of the management process: evaluating. If you have already planned, organized, and directed, the evaluation stage should go more smoothly than it otherwise would have, but this important step still should not be ignored.

As you walk around the hospital, be sensitive to mess, clutter, disrepair, and other signs of disorganization. Disorganization anywhere in the hospital is a symptom of organizational slippage. At the front desk, clutter and confusion can present blatant signs to clients of a poorly trained hospital staff and inefficient medical-care delivery. Disorganization can signal other potential problems, such as noncompliance with laws and regulations, theft and embezzlement, and poor practice profit resulting from excessive expenditures and lost revenues.

As the hospital nose, you should literally be sniffing out any bad odors that might give a poor impression to clients. Pay special attention to odors when you first come in each day; after you have been in the hospital for a while, you may no longer notice bad odors that are in fact offensively apparent to a client when first entering the reception area. Certain odors may be more apparent in some areas of the hospital facility depending on ventilation systems, construction, air movement, and patient population density.

As the eyes and ears of the practice, you will be watching and listening to team members as they communicate information. As you engage in "walk-around management," pay attention to the following:

- Do employees communicate information correctly and according to practice policy? For example, do clients receive correct, succinct information about animals that are hospitalized or have just had surgery? Or does it seem that employees are unclear about current patient status? When front-desk employees are not well informed, it erodes client confidence in the level of care and implies a lack of true concern.
- Do nonlicensed employees "play doctor" and make health-care recommendations, or do they encourage the client to make an appointment with the doctor?
- Do employees recognize potentially urgent situations and expedite appointments promptly and with assurance? Are these activities ever postponed or ignored?
- Are phone calls promptly made to clients to alert them to patient status changes or follow-up on client requests for information? Or are messages forgotten until the client instigates another call?
- Do reception-area employees exhibit confidence in the doctors and other team members? Can you hear pride about the hospital in their voices?
- Are employees courteous, respectful, and helpful? Do they exhibit the sort of attitude you expect from them?

- Do problems with angry clients, aggressive patients, and erroneous communications require extra front-desk assistance?

Building maintenance and phone-answering protocols will be discussed in greater depth later in the chapter, but try to keep the concept of being a walk-around manager in mind as you continue reading—and as you go about your day.

The Telephone: First Line of Communication

Unquestionably, the telephone is the most important instrument in your hospital. The telephone system is the communication source for nearly all of the hospital's business and the first mode of contact with most clients. It is a major client renewal source.

Uncontrolled, the telephone can be your worst enemy and the most significant single cause of client dissatisfaction. A priority for any hospital manager is to maintain an up-to-date telephone system and ensure efficient and courteous telephone use by staff. Telephone communication management includes investing in new equipment, maintaining the system currently in place, establishing guidelines for correct use by personnel, and training employees in two crucial areas: (1) courtesy and demeanor, and (2) efficient and knowledgeable response to client calls.

EQUIPMENT REQUIREMENTS

Technological advances in telecommunication devices, including business telephone systems, are progressing as rapidly as advances in computer software and hardware. Equipment choices are varied and complex. Upgrading the practice telephone system or installing a completely new system can be a significant expense.

Before making any substantial investment in practice communications equipment, take some time to research your options. Because telephone equipment technology changes so frequently, you'll want to be sure that people who give you recommendations are knowledgeable about the most current offerings. When talking with vendors, find out when they last attended a company training session. Find out if the company has experience equipping medical practices and offers training for them, including human hospitals, dental offices, and veterinary clinics. Ask for the names of other businesses that have purchased the recommended system. Check these references to determine their overall satisfaction with the equipment vendor, the equipment itself, and the company's service and maintenance programs (see the "System Maintenance" section later in this chapter).

Do not limit your research to information provided by the equipment company. If you network with other practice managers, now is the time to share notes. Conferring with your colleagues can help you design a phone system that allows the staff to handle incoming and outgoing calls efficiently while fully meeting client needs.

Another source of information is your own experience as a client. When you call other businesses, pay attention to how the phone calls are handled and critically analyze what might be potentially annoying to your own clients. For example, automated phone attendants are fairly commonplace as a replacement or substitute for a human receptionist or operator. Such an option can be modified to work well in the veterinary hospital setting, but you must be sensitive to client needs. The animal owner experiencing a possible emergency may not tolerate an electronic operator.

Equipment durability is another important factor in veterinary hospitals, where employees are notoriously hard on equipment. For example, sometimes employees have to count pills or control animals while they are on the phone, so handsets are frequently dropped. Look for handsets that lock firmly into the cradle of wall-mounted units. Make sure phones are tightly mounted to surfaces.

When damage does occur, the equipment will need to be repaired or replaced quickly and efficiently. When you are researching the phone equipment provider, be sure to find out how responsive the company has been with existing clients and how quickly equipment repair is accomplished (see also section below entitled "System Maintenance").

When planning your telephone system, define the specific options your hospital requires now and may require in future. For example, you do not want to buy a system that can handle only a limited number of telephone lines, because veterinary hospitals typically need to add additional lines as they grow. If your phone system restricts the number of lines to which incoming calls can roll, you may have to invest in a completely new system sooner than you would like. You certainly don't want clients in your growing practice to reach a busy signal!

When investigating new telephone equipment and installing new phone lines and Internet connections, think about how all of the telecommunication equipment within the practice will be integrated. Consider voice mail, after-hours answering messages, intercom messaging, and teleconferencing capabilities. Be aware that technological advances in veterinary medicine will also impact equipment-acquisition decisions. Videoconferencing capabilities and other forms of data transfers share many of the same networks that voice does, such as fiber-optic cable. In fact, it may be that much of your hospital's telephone communication will eventually be handled directly through the computer networked system, Internet connections, or wireless cell-phone technology.

Smartphone technology adds complexity in some ways that are important to consider, including human resources policy. Many veterinarians use various applications on smartphones to help with data research and also communicate with clients via voice mail, text messages, and e-mail. You may wish to consider policies limiting employee-to-client communication to practice-owned phone numbers, perhaps with practice-provided cell phones, and e-mail addresses provided by the practice, instead of allowing use of personally owned e-mail addresses

Planning the Phone System

The following is a recap of some areas that you should consider in designing the telephone system, planning for hardware purchases, and negotiating phone company services:

- Number of telephone lines required now
- Projection of number of lines required in the next three to five years
- Types of lines (e.g., plain old telephone (POT), digital, voice over Internet protocol (VOIP), dedicated, etc.)
- Best location for lines in the hospital (e.g., will you eventually need phone accessibility in each exam room?)
- Number of phone stations allowed by the system
- Integration with other equipment, such as computers, fax machines, scanners, message-taking devices, and digital recorders.
- Conferencing capabilities among various hospital stations
- Line privacy
- Hands-free options such as headsets and speakerphones
- Call-forwarding, call-waiting, caller I.D., and other service options
- On-hold messaging capability
- Voice-mail options

and phone numbers. It is a relatively simple matter to set up e-mail addresses that forward to a personal account, which can be redirected to forward to the manager's account in the event of employee termination.

Increasingly sophisticated and automated telephone instruments and services are available from telephone companies and other sources, many of which should be part of the telephone installation in most animal hospitals. But take care not to become so automated that personal telephone contact with the client is lost. Research what is available, determine the communication needs of the hospital, keep the hospital management philosophy in mind, and purchase only what is required. (For a checklist, see textbox, "Planning the Phone System.)

FINANCING THE PURCHASE

As with any equipment acquisition, there are several options for financing the purchase of a telephone system. The role of the practice manager in equipment acquisition varies from practice to practice; you may be called upon to research these options and give a recommendation to those who will make the decision, or you may have free rein in equipment acquisition.

Whatever your role in the decision, purchase financing has three basic options:

1. Pay for the equipment from existing available funds.
2. Obtain bank or private financing for the purchase.
3. Lease the equipment.

In most cases, outright purchase of needed equipment, including phone systems, is preferable to leasing. If you have any questions about the validity of a particular financing option, consult with the practice's accountant, who can give you specific figures and advice.

SYSTEM MAINTENANCE

As mentioned earlier, animal hospitals can be hard on telephone equipment, which is sensitive and expensive electronic hardware. Animal hair, dirt, blood, and moisture are sometimes difficult to avoid. Employees drop handsets and pull equipment off the counter when reaching for records or moving patients, and handset cords are often pulled to their limits. You will therefore have to give special attention to the servicing and replacement of your telephone equipment.

Ongoing service contracts should be strongly considered while equipment purchase is being negotiated. Review service agreements so that you know exactly what is covered and for how long. Remember, service calls, technician time, and replacement parts can be expensive for the practice if they are not covered under the terms of the agreement.

Lightning strikes, floods, and other catastrophes can also cause extensive damage to telephone equipment and other electronic hardware. Check warranties and service agreements as to what is covered in the event of such damage. Make sure that insurance policies pick up where warranties and service agreements leave off. Your insurance agent can help ensure that your valuable investment in equipment is adequately covered.

Interruption of the client communication network for an extended period can be more than an inconvenience—it can be financially devastating. Even if you have a good service agreement and full insurance coverage, consider integrating cell phones and/or an answering service into your system as an emergency backup. When the primary hospital line is down, incoming calls could be forwarded to these systems, providing a crucial stopgap during an emergency.

Also consider the fact that with many digital phone systems, the phones will not ring in the event of a power outage. Although the lines may remain operable, the ringers, which depend on electricity, will not ring. Check with your telephone equipment provider about the possibility of switching the system from a digital to analog basis during an electrical outage. Otherwise, emergency battery backup might provide a solution, similar to that used for computer system support.

Certainly, if your hospital is in a region where damage from severe weather, such as ice or snow storms or tropical storms, is possible, you may want to consider other options as well. Many practices choose to invest in diesel- or propane-powered generators to take over emergency provision of electrical services.

ADEQUATE ACCESS

Every hospital telephone system needs to have enough telephone lines for incoming calls. When first-time callers reach a busy signal, they may simply dial the next veterinarian found through their search engines or in the telephone book. Regular clients may be more patient, but they can also get discouraged with frequent or lengthy waiting. Also, when clients who have been kept waiting finally do get through to a receptionist, they may be more abrupt and less easy to please than those who did not have to wait, since they may feel the hospital has already been less than responsive.

Because client demand for veterinary hospital services can grow rapidly, it is extremely important that you constantly evaluate the capacity of your existing system to handle incoming calls. If it appears that the phones are busy most of the time or if you hear client complaints, ask the telephone company to survey the system for call attempts and completions. Teletraffic engineering measurements assess the level of line usage, the number of busy signals your clients experience, and the hours of peak use.

You can also evaluate your telephone usage with a survey of your own. Keep track of both incoming calls and outgoing calls for a test period, categorizing each call by type and time of day. From this you may be able to make better use of your phone lines by directing certain types of incoming calls to specific time periods. Once you have identified the least busy times of day, for example, you can instruct clients who will be calling for lab results, postsurgery instructions, and hospitalized patient status to call during those times.

Most practices have a single phone number listing but will subscribe to multiple phone lines. The system is then set up to enable each incoming call to be distributed to an available open line. The related telephone numbers are called a *hunt group*. If a large number of your clients are getting busy signals when they call, the most frequently implemented option is to add one or more incoming lines to the existing hunt group.

A second option is to add a private line or "back line" for outgoing calls. The number for this line is unpublished, so the line can be used exclusively for client callbacks, for follow-up medical consultations, for drug and supply order placement, for employee personal calls, and for all other necessary outgoing phone communications. Fax machines and credit-card authorization devices can be hooked into this line.

The telephone number for a back line is often given out to hospital contacts who need access, such as accountants, service providers, vendors, and sales representatives. Their calls can be routed outside the main hospital line, which keeps the main client-contact lines open, reducing the incidence of prolonged busy signals.

A third option is to add an electronic phone-answering capability (e.g., voice mail with automated phone attendant) to your phone system. Although many sophisticated, high-tech options exist, you must weigh the potential negatives before you choose. Some voice-mail systems result in complex tiers of caller options that may be difficult for a user to reverse navigate. Such a voice-mail system might produce nothing but client frustration. When evaluating possible automated-attendant voice trees, try to imagine how they would work for the client in an emergency situation. Might the client get "stuck" in one of these voice-mail mazes? Also, remember that many callers prefer personal contact to a recording. Besides, the personal touch of a friendly voice may give your practice a competitive edge.

If you conclude that a well-designed voice-mail system is a viable solution to the problem of busy signals, then you have several options to choose from. In systems using the hunt-group method described above, incoming phone calls roll over to any open and available line before the electronic operator kicks in. Only after all lines are in use will the client hear the voice-mail instructions.

With this system, some hospitals simply employ an explanatory message, such as: "Greetings. You have reached ABC Animal Hospital. All our lines are currently busy. A receptionist will be with you as soon as possible. Your wait should be no longer than a minute or two." Or the message can also give instructions for the caller to leave a message in a voice mailbox. A third option is to configure the system so that the client can request and receive immediate assistance in a perceived emergency situation.

In another voice-mail format, the automated attendant will answer first and give the caller a list of options from which to select. If you go this route, keep the option list short. Give the caller immediate access to an operator in case of an emergency situation. For example, "Hello. This is ABC Animal Hospital. If this is an emergency, please press 'one' now. If this is not an emergency, press 'two' to make an appointment, 'three' to check on the status of your hospitalized pet," and so on. When an emergency option is provided, the call can be routed to a line that is reserved for that purpose.

You may also contract with the phone company for it to host a voice mailbox that allows callers to record messages when all lines are in use. This is a good alternative when the phone system has exhausted its line capacity or if your practice owns an older system with no internally hosted voice mailbox options. A new replacement system may not be in the budget, so talk with your phone company to find what services they can offer that would supplement the practice's existing technology. Many times reception staff will resist the addition of more phone lines because they do not feel they can handle the current volume of telephone calls. However, if the practice is to grow, you must address both employee concerns and equipment and line needs. The practice's marketing efforts are going to waste if callers cannot get through.

A competent reception team may be truly unable to field additional lines in a timely manner, however. If you conduct a telephone survey, you will have a good idea when client calls and phone-line use peak. Use this knowledge to schedule additional employees for backup telephone duty. Consider segregating phone-answering duties from the reception desk during the busiest times of day. Commit to team training and retraining in client service, efficient routing of phone calls, and telephone courtesy.

EQUIPMENT LOCATION

The advice of an experienced telephone system consultant can be very helpful when you are deciding where to place telephone equipment. The key is to choose optimal locations for telephone stations, wiring, and jack access so that client appointment scheduling and other telephone activities can be carried out efficiently. The location of telephone equipment will depend in part on the current electronic sophistication of your system, but also consider how your system is likely to change in the future.

Plan for a telephone near every computer and every appointment book. If your practice has not yet moved to electronic appointment book use, strongly consider it. Otherwise, when using a paper-and-ink appointment book for scheduling, allow adequate desk space for the appointment book and any other essential books and reference materials that are needed when answering client calls, such as current fee schedules, typical service-bundle descriptions, emergency-procedure instructions, surgical admittance procedures, and important contact numbers, such as for emergency and specialty care providers. Some practices maintain several distinct appointment schedules. For example, there may be separate appointment schedules for outpatient care, inpatient care, surgical procedures, and grooming, boarding, and ambulatory services. More appointment books require more desktop space, in addition to computer and telephone space.

Large practice design should include a separate room or space, away from points of face-to-face client interaction, where telephone operators can handle incoming calls and appointment scheduling. (See also "Appointment Scheduling" later in this chapter.)

Be considerate of client privacy when planning telephone placement and employee training. Employees should be conscious of how easily conversations can be overheard, possibly breeching confidentiality of sensitive and personal information. Locate a number of telephones in areas where hospital staff can make calls without excessive noise or interruption and that allow for private, uninterrupted phone conversation.

You may decide to place telephones in exam and consultation rooms or near the surgery suite. Make telephones convenient to doctors so that client callbacks can be completed in a timely manner. A telephone in or adjacent to the surgery suite allows doctors to dictate patient histories to voice mail for later retrieval and medical-record transcription.

Cellular telephones and pagers provide a portable and convenient client communication option for key staff such as doctors and managers. Tax laws have changed to substantially reduce recordkeeping responsibility for personal use of such phones. In general, be aware of the potential for employee abuse of telephone-equipment privileges, especially for long-distance use or practice-provided cell phones. Part of a manager's responsibility is to track and control how telephones are being used.

MANAGING PERSONNEL AND TELEPHONES

To maintain the highest level of client service, your team needs telephone skill training. Knowing when to answer the telephone and what to say are as important as knowing when a companion animal is due for its first vaccines. Let's explore the basics.

Who Should Answer the Telephone?

Team members who routinely field incoming phone calls should be carefully chosen and trained. A pleasant, confident, and articulate voice on the other end of a telephone makes a big difference, especially to clients worried about patient health status. Your team's phone etiquette can help your practice gain new clients and keep existing clients satisfied.

When you choose receptionists, often referred to as client service representatives (CSRs) or client service associates (CSAs), consider their ability to project the desired hospital image. Many times other team members outside the reception department will need to handle the phones, either to fill in for or to back up your key operators. Make sure that all employees who do so have adequate training to competently answer the phone.

When Should the Phone Be Answered?

Whenever possible, the telephone should be answered by the third ring. Reception employees, including designated backup members of the practice team, should be so well-trained in client service that they jump to attention when the phone goes to the third ring. A frequent succession of three rings indicates that the primary receptionist is overloaded and needs a helping voice in serving clients promptly. Someone should be assigned to promptly answer phones whenever the receptionist needs assistance.

As practice manager, you are probably very aware of unanswered phone calls or extended ringing. When the hospital lines are extremely busy, it may be quite usual for you to jump to answer calls, even though there may be a "better" use of your time. You should be exceptionally sensitive to the prospect of losing potential clients by letting the telephone ring too long.

How Should the Phone Be Answered?

When people are in a hurry, they tend to start talking rapidly, before the mouthpiece is close enough to allow good transmission of sound waves. Instruct all team members to wait until the mouthpiece is close to the lips before speaking and to moderate the rapidity of their speech. Everyone who answers the phone should consciously slow down right from the start, when giving the name of the hospital and other prescribed information. No employee should be finishing a conversation with another person while picking up the handset to answer an incoming call.

Encourage employees to practice their answering technique and speech modulation. If you hear that an employee speaks particularly quickly on the phone, type a 180-word script and have the individual practice completing the script in one minute's time. A pace of 180 words per minute is ideal because it allows listeners to absorb information (Beaulieu 2009).

Be aware of the attitude your team members convey over the telephone. Voice carries emotion. Tone is also important. Some operators exude warmth and a friendly demeanor. Others sound cool and reserved. Others may seem professional and formal. Some have soft voices, perhaps difficult to hear, while others are much too loud. Some team members may come across as apathetic. The worst situation is the hospital employee whose telephone style is angry, hostile, argumentative, or abrupt, conveying a clear message: "Don't bother us. We don't want to waste time on your call. We don't care about your problems." Instruct all employees that they are to be enthusiastic and express caring in all that they say.

Every team member should be empathetic to clients, seeking to understand their feelings and the situations they are communicating. This empathy should be evident to the client over the telephone as well as in person.

A warm telephone presence can be learned through practice, even by those employees who are naturally more aloof. At a minimum, team members should engage in the practice of smiling while speaking on the telephone. Any employee who persists in abrasive and argumentative conversation should be removed from phone reception duty, no matter what.

What Should Be Said?

Simply saying "Hello" and nothing else when answering the practice phone will not convey the image of a professional, helpful team. Design a script that every employee should use to answer the phone. There are two rules: Identify the practice and identify yourself to the caller. For example:
- *"Thank you for calling Our Animal Hospital. This is Kimberly."*
- *"Good morning. Our Animal Hospital; Kimberly speaking."*

In some practices, the entire name of the practice will be recited, while others may prefer an abbreviated version, such as simply "Animal Hospital." There is no right or wrong way; decide what rolls off the tongue most pleasantly and presents the practice in accord with its marketing plan.

Every employee answering the phone should identify herself to the caller. Personal identification is perhaps the most important part of the initial greeting, but it is often the first phrase omitted when an operator is extremely busy. Don't let anyone on your team fail to include this introduction. Callers who are in a hurry or who are unhappy are much more likely to hassle a receptionist who has remained anonymous. Offering a name to put with the voice establishes personal rapport and responsibility. Remind all team members that this rule will save them grief while building positive relationships.

After the team member has given her name, it is time to stop and listen. The employee should get ready with pen and paper and let the caller speak. Nearly all callers will introduce themselves following the employee's greeting, if the employee says nothing else after giving her name. The team member should immediately write down the caller's name as a memory aid for the remainder of the call and for any follow up action that needs to occur (Friedman 2011).

If the caller identifies himself but it was difficult to hear the name, then the team member will need to get the proper name and spelling as soon as possible. A good way to do this is to say, for example, "I apologize. I know you said your name. I am Kimberly, and you are . . . ?" Once the team member knows the caller's name, she can personalize the conversation by looking up the client record.

When the phone is efficiently answered, an anxious caller is more likely to slow down and speak more calmly. Alternative scripts for taking client calls depend on the situation. One might say "How may I direct your call?" or "I am helping another caller. Are you able to hold for a few minutes?" If a caller must be put on hold temporarily, the receptionist should reintroduce herself when reconnecting to the call: "Hello. This is Kimberly. Thank you for holding. How may I help you?"

Every member of the team can easily master this classic phone-answering phraseology. In addition, a simple reminder can be posted at the reception desk: "Remember to CHARM our clients with each call!" CHARM is an acronym for the following keys to effective client service on the telephone:

- *Cheerful:* Smile when you answer the phone.
- *Hello:* Say "hello," the animal hospital name, and your name.
- *Actively Listen:* Write caller name. Identify the issue.
- *Respond:* "That's a good question," "I'll find out," or "Let's schedule a time."
- *Make:* Make the appointment (e.g., patient visit) or get call-back or other information.

Putting Callers on Hold

Be on the lookout for a hurried receptionist's tendency to put a caller on hold without politely asking if the caller has an emergency, or to ask the caller if he is able to please hold, but then not waiting for a response. In this situation, the receptionist goes through the motions, rattling off the prescribed phone-answering script, but the last phrase, "Can you hold?" becomes a demand, rather than the sincere question it was intended to be.

The hold button on the telephone can be the most dangerous tool in the office. Abused, the hold button can be a sure way to lose and dissatisfy clients. But there are times when the lines are exceptionally busy and callers have to wait for a few moments. It is the manager's job to implement reception guidelines that make this experience less irritating for everyone.

One solution is to ask a caller, "Do you have an emergency situation?" and then, if no emergency exists, to ask whether the caller can hold. Another very reasonable response is to say, "I have several calls waiting. Would you like to hold or would you like me to call you back in few minutes?" If your staff uses this technique, they must accurately collect the client name and telephone number and remember to call back promptly.

When your phone system has several lines that have hold buttons, your staff should follow three very simple and important rules:

- First, no caller should be put on hold before having a chance to give his name and the purpose of the call. Ideally, obtain a call-back number, too. If there is an emergency, a team member should deal with it promptly.
- Second, before a call is placed on hold, the team member should write down the name of the caller so that it can be repeated when the call is continued.
- Third, no caller should be placed on hold for longer than forty-five seconds. Most newer systems can be configured to emit an audible signal to alert the operator when a caller has been on hold for a predetermined and set length of time.

Ideally, your phone system should help you manage calls that have been placed on hold. Check with your telephone company and telephone equipment vendors about the availability of a telephone call sequencer, which will stack calls so that the person answering the telephone knows which one should be answered next.

Given that clients must be put on hold from time to time, consider whether they should sit there in silence. You do have options. Some phone systems are connected to a stereo radio receiver, so that the caller can hear the local radio station while on hold. This is probably the least attractive option, since the station might fade in and out if someone isn't constantly checking to assure that the fidelity is good. Also, consider the type of content being aired by the radio station. Talk shows, certain music, and advertising might be annoying to clients. In a worst-case scenario, one of your competitors might advertise on the station.

A second option is to play music selections chosen to fit the mood your practice is trying to create. Calming music is a good idea for clients who might be stressed or who dislike waiting. Various providers give access to fully licensed music programs for business environments so as to be in compliance with artist and recording-company legal rights.

A popular choice among veterinary practices is to use a professionally scripted and performed digital recording that mixes music with message voice-overs. A recorded voice names the practice, lists its hours of operation, describes available ancillary services such as grooming or boarding, introduces the doctors on staff, and provides other generic, medically oriented information. This alternative articulates and markets practice services such as brief messages about dental care or special senior patient health-care programs. Many companies provide these specialized recording services for veterinary practices; check the veterinary periodicals, print or online, for more information.

DOCUMENT TELEPHONE PROTOCOLS

Ensuring consistency in all hospital protocols is a continual management challenge. Team members come and go. New training and retraining are a certainty. Maintain telephone courtesy and protocol through a practice training manual, listing scripts and detailed guidelines about how to answer the telephone, what information to obtain and how to record it, and other necessary information.

To establish guidelines for the correct responses to client concerns, start by classifying the types of phone calls your practice receives:

- Caller wants to set up an appointment (see also "Appointment Scheduling" later in this chapter)
- Caller wants to talk with a doctor regarding a current patient
- Caller is inquiring about a hospitalized patient
- Caller has a specific patient-care question
- Caller wants to talk with a doctor but does not give a reason
- Caller has a question about a bill
- Caller has a nonspecific, general animal-care question
- Caller wants to know about hospital services and prices
- Caller doesn't have a provider and wants to know about your hospital
- Caller is responding to information received from hospital
- Caller is angry or abusive
- Caller is a cold-call salesperson
- Caller is current vendor or service provider to hospital
- Caller is family or friend of employee, and call is unrelated to hospital business.
- Other calls unrelated to veterinary practice

For each of these types of calls, decide what kind of response your receptionists should make. The response may be as simple as referring the call to a doctor's voice mail or to the billing department. The important thing is that the person answering the phone has guidelines for each situation that direct her in what to say or do.

Consider developing resource materials to help employees respond to frequently asked questions (FAQs). You can create a manual or develop an electronic database on the practice computer system. FAQ application software allows you to customize practice training materials with question-and-answer formatting. The resulting database may be able to do double

FIGURE 7.1 CALL-HANDLING WORKSHEET

GUIDELINES FOR CORRECT RESPONSES TO CLIENT CONCERNS

Type of Phone Call	Script – What to Say	Follow-up – Where to Transfer Call
Caller wants to schedule appointment.		
Caller wants to talk to the doctor about a current pet.		
Caller is inquiring about hospitalized pet.		
Caller has specific patient care question.		
Caller wants to talk to doctor but does not give a reason.		
Caller has a question about a bill.		
Caller wants to know about hospital services and prices.		
Caller does not have a provider and wants information about your hospital.		
Caller is abusive or angry.		

duty, since it will not only be a training tool but can also be adapted to provide a client self-help option on the practice website.

In the practice FAQ training resource, include guidelines for handling certain types of calls, such as emergency calls, personal calls, patient health questions, progress reports, and business calls. (See Figure 7.1 for a call-handling template.)

Develop another set of guidelines covering what to say and what not to say. Many times the same thing said in a different way will have a very different meaning to the caller. Avoid negativity and obstructive responses. Choose to be helpful and talk about what the practice team can do for callers. Nancy Friedman, a customer-service expert who is known as the "Telephone Doctor," discusses the "five forbidden phrases" and how to avoid them (Friedman 1987). These forbidden phrases are:

- "I don't know."
- "We don't do that."
- "You'll have to . . ."
- "Just a second."
- "No, we don't."

Friedman suggests that instead of these phrases, reception staff should say:

- *"Let's find out."*
- *"Here's what you do."*
- *"You'll need to . . ."*
- *"That may take a few minutes."*
- *"This is what we can do."*

Friedman's training materials are extensive. Here are a few selected recommendations that support excellent client communication:

- *Be a "double checker:"* Say, "I believe today's schedule is full, but I'd like to double check to see." This phrase tells the client the practice team cares enough about the value of the client's time to make sure it couldn't help the client out. Use it even if you are certain.
- *Don't multitask:* Give full focus to the client conversation so that no mistakes are made.
- *Listen and repeat what you think you heard:* Verify your understanding of the client concern.
- *Don't ever argue with a client:* When a client feels she is right but has incorrect information, you must delicately provide her with the correct information while allowing her to feel right along the way.
- *Apologize:* Use a sincere *"I apologize"* rather than an off-handed *"I'm sorry."*
- *Be positive:* Say *"It is my pleasure to help you"* or *"You are welcome,"* not *"No problem,"* which makes people feel like annoyances.
- *Be prepared:* Know your clients and your patients.

Communication Solutions for Veterinarians, a consulting firm, also offers telephone skills training for receptionists (see www.csvets.com). Another good resource, available through the AVMA, is *Telephone Courtesy & Client Service* by Lloyd C. Finch (1997). This book provides straightforward explanations and team training exercises for using the telephone effectively, with the goal of helping staff achieve quality client service through telephone etiquette. The four themes that Finch highlights throughout the book are:

- Understanding the basics of providing high-quality client service
- Learning proper telephone techniques
- Understanding the client and what the client wants
- Managing the client's perception by understanding the essential role client service plays in a veterinary hospital's success

AFTER-HOURS TELEPHONE SERVICE

Many practice telephone systems use automated answering systems after hours. Answering machines may be either stand-alone or electronically integrated with the telephone system. However, the system is only as reliable as the people who control its operation. If your hospital uses an answering machine, be sure that the message the client hears is clearly articulated and that there is no background static. It should contain helpful information and prompts. Few things are more annoying than having to call an answering machine more than once to try and understand a barely intelligible phone number or other information.

When using answering machines or after-hours voice mail systems, be sure that callers are offered the same options they have when the hospital staff is answering the call. If alternative phone numbers are provided, such as for an emergency-service provider or an on-call doctor's pager, make sure the number is repeated at least once in the course of the message so that callers can double-check it without having to call again.

Keep automated messages succinct, to the point, and free of extraneous or obvious information. For example, avoid the following:

- *"We are not here right now."*
- *"We are sorry we missed your call."*
- *"Your call is very important to us."*
- *"We will call you back as soon as possible."*

Here are some positive, useful, informational messages:

- *"We are open Monday through Saturday, 7 a.m. to . . ."*
- *"We will return your call on the next business day."*
- *"In case of emergency, call . . ."* (Friedman 2011)

Speak at a pace that will be easy for the listener to follow, and slow down a bit when stating a sequence of numbers so that the listener has time to write it down.

Some veterinary practices hire answering services for after-hours telephone answering by a live operator. Before contracting with such a service, obtain recommendations from other users. Once you engage an answering service, make sure the service personnel fully understand your practice's telephone-answering protocols.

To check on the service, periodically call the hospital number and listen to the typical responses clients are receiving, which may drift from practice standards. Answering-service contractors have the same problems with employee turnover and retraining that a veterinary hospital has. Although you should expect the service to provide the same telephone service and courtesy given by the practice team, you cannot always depend on consistency. Take corrective action as necessary.

Always place yourself in a worried client's situation. Think about how it would feel to have an emergency and not know who to call or how to get in touch with your trusted veterinary caregiver. Find practical solutions that will keep your clients well informed, and give them options that provide help rapidly in an emergency situation. Client trust and loyalty will reward veterinary practices that find ways to help their clients no matter what time of day or night.

CLIENT CONFIDENTIALITY

Telephone receptionists must take special care when responding to calls requesting information about clients or patients. State laws regarding the confidentiality of veterinary medical records vary. As the practice manager, you should be aware of applicable state laws. Many states prohibit the release of patient and client information unless a signed client authorization form is on file.

Requests for client or patient information are especially problematic when they are made by telephone because the caller's identity cannot be easily verified. Even if a signed authorization form is on file, it sometimes can be difficult to decide whether to give a caller the requested information. The caller may have no ownership relation to the patient or any right to information about the client or animal. Employees must know how to make a reasonable decision about how much information to reveal to a caller. Numerous types of situations can arise in which medical records are requested that the client may not wish to authorize (for example, in legal disputes involving animal bites or when the client is a breeder offering pets for sale).

If any practice employee receiving a request for patient or client information is unsure whether the caller has the authority to receive the information, she should refer the call to the manager or the attending doctor. In some cases, callers may be told that permission must be obtained from the listed owner before any information may be given to them. For more information on the confidentiality of veterinary patient records, refer to the American Veterinary Medical Association web page specifically addressing this topic (www.avma.org/advocacy /state/issues/sr_confidential_records.asp). See also "Consent and Release Forms" and "Legal Issues in Medical Record Management" in Chapter 8).

EVALUATING TELEPHONE POLICIES

As a manager, you have a right to expect hospital employees to follow rules and policies that the practice owners and managers have developed to ensure the consistent quality of functional operations. Because a client's first impressions of the hospital are so often made in that first phone contact, few management areas are as important as the telephone.

Once you have developed the hospital's telephone protocols and guidelines, formally published them in the hospital operations and procedures manual, and trained all employees in this important area, be sure to regularly evaluate their performance and update their training as needed (for example, through role-playing exercises, which are highly effective training tools).

To evaluate the hospital's client-facing presence via the telephone system, consider periodically monitoring their telephone conversations. You may wish to inform your employees that such quality-control methods are used regularly.

Some practices engage outside services to monitor phone-answering competency by calling as a client. You might engage friends or clients to call, too. Listen carefully from a client's point of view, critically assessing employee ability to field technical aspects of information dissemination as well as voice inflection, speech clarity, and overall courtesy and helpfulness. If you develop client satisfaction surveys, discussed later in this chapter, include questions about the hospital team's telephone etiquette and efficiency in meeting client needs.

The hospital can also contract with professional assessment services that provide regular, formal testing of receptionist skills and offer suggestions for improvement. You can also ask service providers who call the clinic to critique your staff. For example, you might request the practice's lawyer, accountant, and pharmacy company representatives to give you feedback after they speak with reception staff.

When employees are successfully handling client calls, do not hesitate to praise them for a job well done. These are employees you want to keep, and by rewarding them with compliments, you are adding to their job satisfaction.

Appointment Scheduling

Much of the difference between a controlled and efficient practice and a chaotic one lies in the execution of a smoothly functioning appointment system. The key to an effective appointment system is choosing the right density of appointment scheduling for your doctors and the practice.

Most practices now utilize practice management software for appointment scheduling. But the principles of a good scheduling system—efficiency, flexibility, and thoroughness—apply to computer scheduling and "paper" scheduling alike.

ELECTRONIC SCHEDULING: EQUIPMENT NEEDS

The right equipment selection supports the successful transition to electronic scheduling through the veterinary practice management software. Large flat-screen monitors are helpful for viewing patient and client information during the appointment-scheduling process. Receptionists, in particular, benefit from dual-monitor workstations that allow easy visibility of a full day's schedule on one screen and client and patient information on the other.

Flat-screen monitors of 22-inch diagonal measure or greater optimize reading ease, reduce eye strain and mistakes, and can be mounted vertically as well as the traditional landscape or horizontal orientation. Be creative about how paper clutter can be reduced and employee efficiency increased by using large monitors in various configurations and numbers per workstation, always with a telephone nearby. (See Chapter 8 for more information on practice management software systems.)

APPOINTMENT SCHEDULE CRITERIA

Every scheduling system should be based on the resources of the hospital and criteria specific to the practice, including the following:

- The number of doctors available during any particular period
- The relative efficiency of the doctors
- The time allotted to each appointment
- The number of patients presented by each client
- The types of cases seen
- The number of examination rooms (also called consultation rooms)
- The hours of hospital operations, including the hours available for scheduled and non-scheduled activities
- Favored client times for veterinary care

An effective appointment schedule should have two goals: (1) to eliminate client wait time, and (2) to maximize the efficiency of the doctors, the support staff, and the facility by minimizing downtime between clients or patient procedures. Realistically, the appointment schedule must have some built-in inefficiency because it must be flexible enough to allow for cases that require more time than expected as well as for unexpected emergencies. Even the best scheduling can be derailed from time to time by an unusual number of no-show clients or client emergencies.

An effective appointment system is able handle special requests or circumstances. Of course, as practice managers understand, what is truly an emergency situation and what the animal owner believes to be an emergency situation can be two quite different things. Without clear guidelines, it can be difficult for reception staff to know whether they should "work in" an unscheduled appointment when a client wants to see a doctor immediately. Ultimately, it is best in such cases to let client concern rule unless an emergency situation clearly does not exist.

If the perceived problem is not an emergency but the client believes it is, the reception staff should give the client options. For example, the receptionist might say, "The doctor is in surgery now. Could she call you at two o'clock? We also have an appointment time available at ten o'clock tomorrow morning. Or, you can bring Brandy now, and leave her for the technicians to tend to until the doctor is available. Or, we can direct you to the local emergency clinic immediately. Which would you prefer?"

The appointment schedule should list every doctor or other service provider who is available for appointments, clearly showing when each will be available. For example, in addition to veterinarians, your practice may include a licensed or registered technician or veterinary nurse who can handle dental procedures or patient treatment appointments. The appointment schedule must also be extensive enough to cover all hours of hospital operations during which formal client appointment times are scheduled. Because the arrangement of the appointment book is based on blocks of available time, the minimum time slots available will have to be defined. The most common minimum time blocks are ten and fifteen minutes, but some practices use five or twenty minutes as the basic appointment time units.

When planning an appointment schedule, also consider whether other activities—such as surgery, inpatient procedures, boarding, and grooming—are scheduled in specific blocks of time. For example, some practice managers will design a schedule that blocks all elective surgery procedures into two or three days a week to make the most efficient use of surgical staff. Each practice is different, and how various activities are scheduled depends on the number of doctors, facility size, hours of operation, client demand, types of procedures, and staff and equipment flexibility.

If a paper appointment book is maintained, it should be conveniently located in the reception area, close to both client check-in and the employee who schedules appointments. Oversized appointment books are popular, as they provide adequate writing area for all of the information that must be recorded.

As software advances, keep an ear to applications improving electronic appointment-scheduling efficiency for both clients and the practice team. For example, client and patient appointments can be synchronized through smartphone applications to request changes, send updates, and remind recipients of upcoming appointments. Doctors and technicians can also be automatically alerted to the clients and patient appointment changes to their schedules. Practice management programs will increasingly integrate appointment functions that enable real time contact with clients and employees through software.

RECORDING THE APPOINTMENT

As we have already seen, making a veterinary appointment is not as simple as merely filling an empty slot. To make an appointment accurately and efficiently, the reception employees need to obtain several key pieces of information, both from the client and from the appointment schedule. Additional information will be gathered from the client when he arrives with the pet at the time of the appointment (see "Collecting Client and Patient Information" in the "Reception" section later in this chapter).

Information to be noted on the appointment schedule at the time of the telephone call should include the following:

- Client's complete name, first and last
- Client's current telephone numbers, home, cell, and work
- Patient's name
- Presenting complaint (reason for the visit)
- Client status (new client or existing client, new patient or existing patient)
- Specific doctor request, if any

If the practice uses a computerized scheduling system that is integrated with the client database, most of the required information will already be entered for existing clients and patients. Additionally, many practices use Internet services that allow clients to securely access their veterinary records online to make amendments and corrections on their own. Such systems help speed appointment-making by decreasing record-keeping time, thus improving client service and enhancing patient care.

In all circumstances, it is important to check for any unrecorded changes in the client and patient information when making the appointment. Doing this consistently for clients who have not been seen recently keeps vital data up-to-date.

First, the receptionist will obtain the client's name and the patient's name and ascertain whether the animal is a current patient or a new patient. The client's telephone numbers will be next, unless they are already in the database. The receptionist should double-check any new spellings or numbers, updating the database as needed. It is important not to confuse two clients with similar names.

For clients who haven't been seen in more than four months, a good question to ask is, "Has any of your contact information changed since we last saw you?" The receptionist can also ask for any information that does not appear in the database already, such as cell-phone number or work number.

If time permits and the patient is new to the practice, the receptionist may wish to gather other information that is necessary for the preparation of a new medical record during this call. Otherwise, it will be collected in person when the client and patient arrive (see "Collecting Client and Patient Information" later in the chapter).

The next crucial step is to determine the primary client concern. Why did the client call for an appointment? The service requested by the client should always be written directly into the appointment book or included as part of the electronic appointment. This step may seem obvious, but surprisingly, it is often overlooked, especially when the hospital staff becomes very good at discerning additional services the animal should receive for good preventive care or when the hospital is very busy.

While identifying the client concern, the employee should estimate how much time will be required for the visit and determine which team member to assign the appointment. Is the appointment for a new puppy or kitten, or for a bird or exotic animal? These appointments may require more than the usual amount of time. Is this a potentially more complicated medical case than usual? Has the client requested a certain doctor? Is the appointment for a procedure that is usually performed by a technician? In addition, new patients will require extra time so that the doctor can get to know the client and patient.

The hospital procedures manual should include guidelines for determining the length of time necessary for various types of appointments. For example, ten minutes might be allotted for surgery follow-ups and medical progress rechecks, while twenty minutes (or two ten-minute slots) would be scheduled for annual wellness exams and vaccination boosters. Routine medical problems might receive twenty minutes. Three ten-minute slots, or thirty minutes, might be required for the first new puppy or kitten protocol, allowing time to communicate patient-care requirements to the client.

Standard appointment length is a matter of practice preference. Fifteen-minute appointments are also common, with times doubling to thirty minutes for extended issues.

Typically, practice management software programs can be customized to accommodate your preferences. When researching new software, determine the level of flexibility and automation the software allows in appointment schedule processing. Practice software can maximize scheduling accuracy and efficiency, and minimize the possibility of human error.

The number of examination rooms is an important parameter dictating the number of overlapped appointments that can be scheduled for a particular doctor or veterinary technician. Three examination rooms per experienced medical team of doctor, veterinary technician, and veterinary assistant are probably optimal because they allow for a technique called *dense scheduling* to be used.

Dense scheduling makes the best possible use of the facility space and the veterinary team. It involves overlapping appointments for optimal scheduling. For example, say that fifteen-minute appointments are scheduled for annual wellness care. In dense scheduling, an appointment could be scheduled every five minutes. After the client and patient are brought into the examination room, the technician would collect a basic history and patient physical parameters such as temperature, weight, and heart rate. The doctor comes in during the next five minutes to gather information, complete a physical exam, and discuss preventive-care options with the client. The doctor moves on to the next patient while blood, urine, and other patient samples are obtained to run laboratory tests. Or the technician may give vaccinations and parasite treatments at this time. Any prescriptions and instructions may be provided by the technician or doctor in the last third of the appointment.

You can read more about efficient appointment techniques in books such as *Zoned Systems and Schedules in Multi-Doctor Practices*, by Dr. Tom Catanzaro; *Receptionist Training Manual*, by Drs. Chris and Robb Heagle; *The Veterinary Receptionist's Training Manual*, by Drs. Wilson and McConnell; and *Client Satisfaction Pays*, by Dr. Carin Smith, among others.

To help your staff gather all of the information required to efficiently establish an appointment, use checklists and scripts of standard questions to ask. A script can be a helpful training tool for new employees and a continuing reference for those less experienced at handling appointment scheduling.

Part of the script may be the question, "How do you prefer we contact you for any reminders related to your appointment: cell phone, home phone, e-mail, or text message?" The client's answer then leads to identifying the correct e-mail address or phone number in the client record.

If the client is new, the receptionist should offer to send information (via e-mail or regular postal service) that will facilitate an on-time and well-orchestrated appointment, such as a medical history questionnaire or information about what the client should do if presenting the pet for labwork or a procedure requiring anesthesia. This is a good chance to showcase all of the practice's services, too, as a well-presented brochure may be sent to the client with the forms. Or, the client can be directed to the practice website or social-media page.

The receptionist should ask if the client is familiar with the hospital's location or needs directions. New clients can be asked to arrive ten to fifteen minutes in advance of the scheduled appointment in order to ensure that the new medical record is complete and that all necessary patient history data, such as information on prior vaccines and illnesses, can be gathered. You may wish to build this time into the appointment by simply giving the client an appointment time that allows for the extra ten minutes of record preparation. Otherwise, the client can print required forms from the practice website to complete at home or fill them out online, assuming the practice has invested in these client convenience features.

Before hanging up the phone or saying goodbye, the receptionist should repeat the appointment time and date back to the client. For instance, "Okay, Mrs. Smith, Fluffy has an appointment at ten o'clock a.m. on Thursday, June 22, for her annual checkup and vaccines. We'll see you then."

APPOINTMENT PROBLEMS

Even the most carefully planned appointment schedule will be thrown into disarray from time to time. Clients may simply not show up, or they might arrive late. Sometimes a client without an appointment will appear and ask to be seen by a veterinarian. With proper hospital protocols, some of these common problems can be avoided. In addition, effective possible solutions can be worked out in advance and become part of employee training sessions so that the practice staff is prepared to deal with them.

Giving clients advance reminders within twenty-four hours of appointments is a best practice for all client appointments. Options for reminding include personal phone calls, voice-mail or answering-machine messages, automated reminder call services, text messaging, and e-mail messages (which can be automated). Some of these services may be integrated with the practice management software or various web-based veterinary applications for client services. A wide variety of generic service options can be found via an Internet search for "reminder call service."

A "no-show" is a client who scheduled an appointment but subsequently broke it without notifying the hospital. No-shows can become habitual offenders. They may not understand or care that their failure to show up causes a problem with the schedule. If a client is a no-show on more than one occasion, make a notation in the client record. Practices develop different methods of dealing with tardy clients or no-shows. A common remedy is to call the known offender to confirm the appointment on the day before the appointment, or possibly on the morning of a late afternoon or evening appointment. Messaging by text or e-mail is a good supplementary action.

"Walk-in" refers to a client who comes to the hospital without a prescheduled appointment. Some hospitals do schedule open hours when clients know they can simply come in and wait their turn for time with the doctor. However, most hospitals do not have open hours because with scheduled visits it is easier to provide each client with adequate time and efficiently schedule doctors and staff. Also, for many clients time is at a premium and they do not like the inconvenience of waiting. Even so, some clients will choose to take their chances and simply show up with their animals.

Unless there is a dire emergency, a walk-in client should never be taken before a client who is waiting for a scheduled appointment. Taking a walk-in client may cause delays not only for clients already waiting but for clients with later appointments. The resulting subliminal message to punctual clients may be that their time is not valued and it is better to arrive late, since the doctor apparently runs behind schedule. Make no mistake: Clients become irritated quickly when their time is not honored, regardless of how caring and competent the medical team might be.

The practice team's challenge is to accommodate walk-in clients without upsetting the appointment schedule. Your appointment protocol should include several options. For example, the receptionist can let these clients know they will be seen as soon as possible but that there might be a wait of x minutes (the wait time can be estimated from the appointments that remain). Then the receptionist can offer to set up an appointment for the client at the end of the current day's schedule. That way, the client doesn't have to wait and can complete other errands and come back later at the appointed time.

Another option for a well-established client is to suggest leaving the pet so that it can be examined when a doctor is available. This option requires careful information gathering about the perceived issue being addressed, how the team can best reach the client, and preparation of any cost estimates and consent forms, as necessary.

If your hospital schedules clients by appointment only, courteously explain the policy to the walk-in client. Include this information in the hospital brochure and on its website, along with hours of operation. Politely ask the walk-in client to schedule future appointments, emphasizing the benefits of minimizing wait time and obtaining prompt and complete attention as each client deserves.

Some people arrive early for their scheduled appointments. Like clients who arrive late, "early birds" may have had to wait for their appointments on previous visits. They may believe if they come in early, they will be able to get in before the medical team is behind schedule. An unusual number of established clients showing up early or late for their appointments may be a sign of ongoing appointment-scheduling and time-management problems at your hospital.

Another potential scheduling problem presents when clients who are leaving or picking up patients need to speak with a doctor or veterinary technician but have no appointments to do so. Receptionists can try to predict when this will happen and provide for it when scheduling these clients. Otherwise, the practice may decide to simply provide some gaps in the appointment schedule to accommodate them.

Protocols for doctors and technicians and practice activity evolve over time, so continuously evaluate whether patient drop-off and pick-up scheduling provides for the effective client communication your hospital needs to accomplish. This same advice holds true for appointment scheduling in general and how the team coordinates its activities. For example, a common patient management practice uses technicians and veterinary nurses to meet with clients to discuss and identify concerns and to triage the patient. The doctor's time may then be used more efficiently for making diagnoses, establishing treatment plans, completing surgical procedures, and consulting with the client. You may need to set up specific appointment times for technicians and veterinary nurses who are working as triage specialists.

As the practice invests in laboratory technology, more procedures and tests may be completed while the client waits. In-house equipment expedites information gathering as well as diagnosis and treatment plans and also alleviates client anxiety in the case of an ill, elderly, or fragile patient. But keep in mind that as your practice incorporates more procedures into client visits, appointment times will have to be adjusted accordingly. The goal is to maintain a finely tuned workflow that minimizes bottlenecks and client wait time.

Be prepared. Review the appointment schedule at least daily so that you can anticipate and resolve problems before they arise. If you know the medical staff is running behind, direct the receptionist to call clients and give them the options of rescheduling or coming in later so that their wait time can be minimized. Most clients understand that emergency situations may disrupt the schedule and will greatly appreciate this small courtesy.

Reevaluate the scheduling format periodically. Make changes as they are required. If employees are standing around waiting for the next client, or if clients are often waiting for a long time, the system needs adjusting. Do not simply cope with a bad system. Your management goal is to redirect and reorganize appointment-scheduling protocol as needed to keep work flowing smoothly.

Reception

Practice success and employee livelihood depend on a thriving client base. New clients are gained and prior clients retained because they are treated with courtesy, respect, and professionalism. Their first experience of superb client service comes when they enter the door—in the reception area.

As we've seen, good reception begins even before a client arrives. The receptionist should check the appointment schedule for each client's name and organize patient charts and other paperwork that will be required during the visit. The client record should be checked, so that any missing information can be collected when the client arrives. With this done, the team is ready to greet the client.

GREETING CLIENTS

In most companion animal practices, the new client's first in-person contact with the practice will be with the receptionist when checking in for the first time at the front desk. The client will probably have "met" the practice already over the telephone, in what was hopefully a pleasant experience. Now the reception staff can reinforce that experience in person.

Clients will draw some preliminary conclusions about the practice within their first two to five minutes in the reception area (McCurnin 1988, 26). Therefore, it is crucial that a team member acknowledge clients in a friendly and welcoming manner as soon as possible after they enter. All team members must develop the habit of treating each person who enters the building as the single most important person they will meet that day.

If clients feel ignored, they are likely to have hard feelings. The longer a client has to wait before being noticed, the greater the effort needed later to regain goodwill.

The acknowledgment does not have to be verbal. If a receptionist is on the telephone or working with another client, simply making eye contact will suffice. A warm smile and nod will clearly signal, without words, that the client is welcomed. When finished with the first task, the receptionist should stand to greet the client.

Many times, a client will come in while the receptionist is busy with another team member. In this case, the client should be recognized promptly. The employee conversation should be truncated or interrupted as quickly as possible.

It is tempting to finish up a chore on the computer or complete other paperwork before dealing with a client who has just arrived. Train your team to warmly greet the client immediately even though it is an interruption of another important task. To avoid forgetting the task, employees can try marking their place in a document or writing themselves a brief reminder of where to pick up later. If the task is one that must be completed right away—for instance, logging important information in the appointment book or patient record—clients may be asked to wait a moment. But they should not have to wait too long.

Whenever possible, front-desk staff should greet clients and patients by name when they enter the hospital. This will go a long way toward creating a welcoming, friendly atmosphere. Front-desk staff can maximize their success in linking names with faces by using practice management software to store digital images of clients and patients linked with related records. The pictures are taken as part of the first appointment. These photos are easily retrieved, giving the hospital team a readily available resource for quickly identifying clients and patients on sight.

When a new client arrives, the receptionist may not know her name, but can still greet the client in a welcoming manner. If it can logically be concluded that the person walking in the door must be the next new client on the schedule (because of the type of animal accompanying the client), then the receptionist might say, for example, "You must be Mrs. Smith, and this must be Roxie. Isn't she a pretty girl." After the client confirms her name, the receptionist can say, "It is a pleasure to meet you Mrs. Smith. Welcome to ABC Veterinary Hospital."

If the first two to five minutes of the client visit are successful, it will be a measure of your managerial skills in choosing, training, and coaching the reception team.

EMPLOYEE PRESENTATION

The demeanor and appearance of hospital staff speak volumes to clients. A receptionist who is smiling, helpful, knowledgeable, neatly attired, and concerned is invaluable. Teach your employees to be well groomed and attentive to their appearance. Hospital policy may define acceptable jewelry, hairstyles, and clothing in an effort to enhance communication between staff and clients.

People remember through a variety of visual, auditory, and sensory inputs. Body language and facial expressions convey volumes about attitude and apparent sincere interest in others. A saying that is widely used in the medical profession is: "People don't care how much you know until they know how much you care." Body language and voice inflection convey an exceedingly large proportion of perceived information about how much you care.

Role playing with employees can increase awareness of how their voice inflections and body language affect client perceptions. Team role-playing sessions can be videotaped for employees so they can see how they appear to clients and learn how to communicate more effectively. Everyone on the practice team, including veterinarians, needs to receive training in communication skills and periodically refresh their skills through additional training in order to optimize the communication outcomes at the hospital.

Certain employee personal habits can detract from successful client communication. Employees who chew gum on the job, use chewing tobacco, or smoke may not be well accepted by many clients.

Employees should not smoke on the premises at veterinary hospitals. In this day of health consciousness, veterinary hospitals generally prohibit smoking. State laws vary in supporting practice efforts to provide a smoke-free environment for patients, clients, and employees. If local or state ordinances do not prohibit smoking in businesses, it may still be a perfectly acceptable policy for your practice to prohibit it. Your patients should not be exposed to second-hand smoke in a hospital environment. As a courtesy and to reduce littering on the premises, however, you might wish to provide an outdoor smoking area and trash receptacles.

The hospital hopes to create a lasting bond with the client, and the client's first impression is very important. If clients have a good first impression of the reception team, and they are satisfied with the overall care and service provided at your hospital, you will likely see them back with their companions for health care and related services.

For more information on communicating with clients, see "Effective Client Communication" later in this chapter and the textbox entitled "Recommendations for an Attentive Communication Style."

RECEPTION AREA APPEARANCE

By now you have seen that the reception area is not a "waiting room." The ideal reception-area team prepares each day's workflow by scheduling appointments in an efficient manner. It expeditiously manages client interactions. On-time arrivals are quickly greeted and escorted to consultation rooms, or their companions capably admitted for scheduled procedures, because as much as possible has been handled in advance of client and patient arrival.

Recommendations for an Attentive Communication Style

Here are a few basic guidelines for increasing effective and positive interaction:

- Stand and face the person to whom you are speaking.
- Point your feet toward the person, which will increase your energy and focus your attention.
- Use direct eye contact, without staring or looking intimidating.
- Shake hands when appropriate, but remember to be sensitive to those who may have arthritis and other types of hand pain by not gripping too firmly.
- Smile with your mouth and eyes.
- Raise your eyebrows to show openness and interest.
- Keep warmth and clarity in your voice; avoid monotone and mumbled responses.
- Address both the pet and the client by name.
- Maintain good posture, with your shoulders back and an open body position; convey relaxed confidence and availability to the client.
- Ask questions and repeat what you understand the other person to have said in order to ensure that they feel heard.
- Address all client concerns.

Although a well-organized and maintained appointment-scheduling system should ensure that most clients are promptly seen, on occasion a client will have to wait. For this and other reasons, the hospital reception area should be as pleasant as possible. Clients will be judging the rest of the hospital by what can be seen, smelled, and heard while they are waiting.

As mentioned earlier, hospital managers should walk through the reception area frequently to evaluate its appearance. The manager should organize and direct the team with daily checklists to ensure that employees are identifying and correcting deficiencies promptly. The reception area should be well lit, well ventilated, meticulously clean, and free of clutter.

Assign staff to keep waste containers emptied. Replace old magazines monthly with new editions. Discard dated copies that become worn and torn. Floors and safety mats must be clean. If old mats retain odors no matter how often they are cleaned, they should be replaced.

Inspect walls, door frames, and furniture legs for spatters of dirt, blood, saliva, feces, urine, and hair. These spills are normal daily occurrences in a hospital and so these inspections should be frequent and cleanup and sanitation prompt.

Watch that the area does not get too cluttered. Numerous vendors supply new pharmaceutical and preventive care information, and this literature is often posted on walls, doors, and windows or placed on tables and counters. Lots of information stacks up over time, but often very little is removed, resulting in a net gain. This can make the area look unkempt.

One way to solve the problem is to make tape and thumbtacks taboo. If an informational piece is worth posting, it is probably worth framing. Otherwise, maintain a neat, well-monitored bulletin board for interesting and timely postings. Date-stamp any posted item so that you can easily determine how long it has been there and remove it when it is no longer needed or begins to look worn.

Seating in the reception waiting area should be spacious enough to accommodate fractious animals without allowing contact between them. Clients must know to keep their pets securely leashed or restrained in carrying cases. Every client's safety, their pets' safety, as well as the safety of other clients, animals, and hospital employees, is of greatest concern.

Keep up with formal employee training to recognize animal behavior and posture signals that warn of fear or aggression. All employees should know what to do when a potentially dangerous situation may be developing. Predetermine the actions to take or not to take to avoid escalation of a problem. Quickly escort clients with animals that demonstrate aggressive postures to an isolated area, such as an available exam room. Employees should be well trained in bite prevention. They should also know how to calmly yet effectively intercede with clients who might be putting themselves and other people in danger.

Staff courtesy and attention to the waiting client is an important factor in client satisfaction. Depending on practice culture and likely client expectations, receptionists should communicate regularly with waiting clients. The receptionist should periodically re-acknowledge

Reception-Area Amenities

Here are some suggestions for maintaining an attractive reception area and keeping clients entertained (and possibly educated) while they wait:

- Play digital presentations of common problems relating to the health care of animals and preventive care recommendations. Flat-screen video displays can be mounted to walls. Showcase hospital images, personnel, services, and information through these or with digital photoframes.
- Provide a play corner or nook for children, being cognizant of keeping children out of harm's way.
- Provide a computer with Internet access for clients to use or provide free wireless Internet access.
- Install a fish tank (making sure it is regularly cleaned and tended).
- Put up bulletin boards for information on animal health care and community information pertaining to animals and patients, such as obedience training classes.
- Provide a bulletin board or album for informal pictures of hospital staff, clients, and patients with an open invitation for clients to add their own favorite pictures.
- Create an album or digital slide show of images and descriptions of areas of the hospital that clients cannot always readily visit, such as surgery, hospital wards, the radiography department, and patient treatment areas.
- Produce a professionally prepared video tour of the hospital, which could do dual duty through website marketing.
- If hospital design allows (e.g., glass reception walls), locate cat-boarding condos, patient adoption cages, or birds and other exotic animals, such as reptiles and amphibians, so that those in the reception area can see them.
- Provide a free coffee or other beverage service.

the client, perhaps every five to ten minutes or so, to provide a relatively accurate estimate of how much more wait time can be anticipated. If the wait will be long, give the client options such as rescheduling or keeping the animal while the client runs other errands. (For more tips on how to create an nice reception area, see textbox entitled "Reception-Area Amenities.")

COLLECTING CLIENT AND PATIENT INFORMATION

Each new client will be asked to provide the information required to complete hospital records. Earlier in this chapter, we discussed the information required to establish an appointment.

This information is usually obtained in the appointment-scheduling telephone call. When the client arrives at the hospital, the receptionist will need to gather additional information. The data required to complete the patient record at this time include:

- Name of client's spouse or significant-other companion and information on the extent of authority he may have over care of the patient
- Preferred method of payment
- Names of other owned animals that would typically be of the type seen by the practice (whether presented at first client visit or not)
- Patient information:
  » Species
  » Breed
  » Color/identifying marks
  » Sex and whether neutered
  » Age (birthday, if available)
  » Vaccination history (types and dates)
  » Previous medical history of significance

Depending on practice administration policy and goals, clients may be asked to provide additional optional information, such as:

- Children's names (if any)
- Birthdays of client and client's children
- Occupation of client and spouse/significant other
- Workplace address(es)
- Fax number (useful for practice communications to client)
- E-mail address (useful for practice communications to client)
- Driver's license number (for possible credit check or collection requirements)
- Name and contact information of patient insurance carrier (if any)
- Patient tattoo numbers or electronic identification

Many practices use a registration form or client check-in form to collect this information. The client can arrive early for the first appointment to complete it, or the form can be sent to the client ahead of time as a courtesy, by e-mail or postal mail. Alternatively, a link to the website version of the form can be sent by e-mail. The client can then complete the information in advance, rather than trying to remember the information at the time of the office visit while also struggling to control pets and/or children. (Sample Patient Information and Medical History forms are shown in Figures 7.2A and 7.2B.)

Having clients fill out the forms ahead of time helps to keep appointments on schedule, since clients have all the paperwork completed when they arrive. In addition, electronic forms

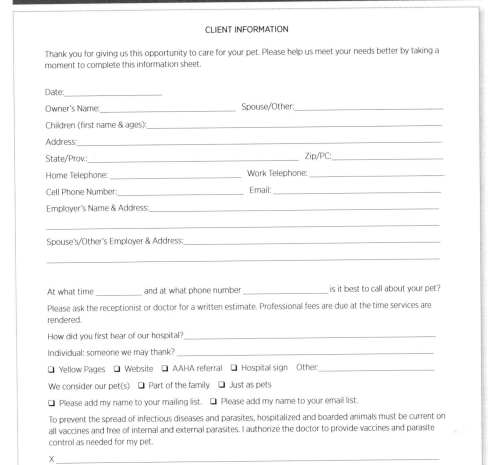

FIGURE 7.2A CLIENT INFORMATION FORM

CLIENT INFORMATION

Thank you for giving us this opportunity to care for your pet. Please help us meet your needs better by taking a moment to complete this information sheet.

Date:_____

Owner's Name:_____ Spouse/Other:_____

Children (first name & ages):_____

Address:_____

State/Prov.:_____ Zip/PC:_____

Home Telephone: _____ Work Telephone: _____

Cell Phone Number:_____ Email: _____

Employer's Name & Address:_____

Spouse's/Other's Employer & Address:_____

At what time _____ and at what phone number _____ is it best to call about your pet?

Please ask the receptionist or doctor for a written estimate. Professional fees are due at the time services are rendered.

How did you first hear of our hospital?_____

Individual: someone we may thank? _____

❑ Yellow Pages ❑ Website ❑ AAHA referral ❑ Hospital sign Other:_____

We consider our pet(s) ❑ Part of the family ❑ Just as pets

❑ Please add my name to your mailing list. ❑ Please add my name to your email list.

To prevent the spread of infectious diseases and parasites, hospitalized and boarded animals must be current on all vaccines and free of internal and external parasites. I authorize the doctor to provide vaccines and parasite control as needed for my pet.

X _____

COMMENTS:

_____

_____

INCLUDED ON
COMPANION
WEBSITE

prepared by the client are often more accurate and complete than those filled out in the office, as clients have time to track down all the information requested.

Admittance forms should always include the client's reason for scheduling the visit. Other patient needs, such as updating overdue vaccination boosters or completing deferred medical

FIGURE 7.2B ANIMAL MEDICAL HISTORY

ANIMAL MEDICAL HISTORY (Please complete all information for each pet.)

	PET 1	PET 2	PET 3
NAME			
Species (Cat, Dog, Other)			
Breed			
Description (Color)			
Sex/Castrated or Spayed			
Date of Birth or Age			
Current Medications			
Length of Time Owned			
Allergies			
Vitamins (Type)			
Diet (Kind of Pet Food)			
Type of Grooming Products			
Hours Spent Outside Each Day			
Dentistry			
Prior Illness			
Prior Surgery			

DATE OF LAST VACCINATIONS AND TESTS

CDV (Dog)			
CPV-2 (Dog)			
CAV-2 (Dog)			
FHV-1 (Cat)			
FPV (Cat)			
FCV (Cat)			
Rabies (Dog/Cat)			
Other Vaccines			
FeLV/FIV Test			
Heartworm Test/Result			
Heartworm Prevention			
Fecal Exam (Dog/Cat)			

PET ORIGIN

❑ Humane Society ❑ Pet Shop ❑ Breeder ❑ Advertisement ❑ Friend ❑ Stray
❑ Individual (Nonbreeder)

tests, can be identified from the patient history and from preexisting medical records. New patient protocols can also be applied in addition to the concern that the client has written on the form.

In their enthusiasm to do whatever is needed to support the patient's health, team members must remember to address the client's original concern. Although doctors and technicians may identify other patient health issues and recommended care requirements, the client will not be happy if his issue is not managed or questions are not answered, no matter how well the team members perform other parts of their jobs. Restating the concern on the registration form will support success.

The registration form may also be used to determine how the new client chose your practice. This important information guides management decisions about where marketing money will be budgeted to gain new clients. Finally, at this time you will need to communicate the practice's payment policies to the client (see Chapter 10 for more information).

Client registration forms can be a vital link in the initiation of the patient record. For new patients, previous vaccination history establishes the baseline data needed for the automated reminders. When clients cannot provide a previous vaccination history, receptionists should be able to create reasonable estimates based on practice guidelines and through training. A manager's responsibility is to establish practice systems that ensure team knowledge and compliance in maintaining complete and accurate client and patient records.

CONTINUING CLIENTS

Although much attention has been paid in this chapter to welcoming new patients and clients into the practice, the practice team must not forget to treat current clients with the same courtesy and concern. Not only do returning clients provide a steady and predictable part of the practice income, but they help attract new clients. Existing client satisfaction may be the most important factor in the growth of new client appointments. *The 1995 AAHA Report: A Study of the Companion Animal Veterinary Services Market* (AAHA 1995) concluded that nearly one-half (45 percent) of patient owners considered a recommendation by another person to be the most important factor in selecting a veterinarian.

Several other measurements of client-satisfaction are found in the 2007 AVMA Public Perception Survey. On a 10-point value-rating scale ranking the most recent visit to their primary veterinarians, 62 percent of pet owner respondents gave ratings of 8 to 10, indicating high value. On the question of "likelihood to recommend their veterinarian," 72 percent were "very likely" using the 10-point scale. Another 24 percent were in the midrange on the 10-point scale where 1 meant "very unlikely" to recommend the veterinarian. On the value scale, 34 percent rated the most recent visit at 4 to 7 out of 10, suggesting fair value for the money spent. On the value scale, only 4 percent of respondents were at a 3 rating or lower, correlating with poor value for the money spent. Similarly, 4 percent stated unlikeliness to recommend, with rankings of 1 through 3 out of 10.

Continuing clients return in part because of service satisfaction on previous visits. According to *The 1995 AAHA Report*, over one-half of patient owners have switched veterinary care at some point, although switching does not occur frequently. When a client does switch veterinarians, but has not moved from the area, the primary reason (25 percent) is having a bad experience. The 2007 AVMA survey shows that 11 percent of respondents were very likely to switch, higher than the 4 percent of respondents that saw low value and were very unlikely to recommend. Apparently enough respondents had a mediocre or below average experience, that caused them to consider changing primary veterinarians.

In the AVMA study, the key drivers of value derived from overall satisfaction with the veterinarian and the value of veterinary service were cited as:

- Confidence in medical skills
- Friendly
- Compassionate
- Informative
- Relaxing
- Veterinarians benefit society
- Inexpensive
- Veterinarians care for animals as well as or better than physicians care for humans
- Clean

Conversely, in the AAHA study, among clients who reported a bad experience, the following specifics were given:

- Poor attitude on the part of the veterinarian (38 percent)
- Poor care (31 percent)
- A dirty facility (12 percent)
- Nonprofessional behavior (8 percent)
- Inaccessibility (8 percent)

As you are walking around the reception area, evaluating procedures and acting as the eyes, ears, and nose of the hospital, keep these client complaints in mind. You do not want any clients to make their next visits their last visits.

Communicating with Clients in Print

Printed materials can be the backbone of the desired messages you want to convey to clients, from creating a uniform impression and decreasing mistakes to extending the brand image.

Successfully communicating hospital policies and procedures to clients in various written formats eliminates misunderstandings before they occur. To some extent, printed information relieves employees from repetitively answering common questions. Making information readily available in paper and electronic forms also serves to publicize many hospital services, which in turn may increase business.

Effective ways to communicate hospital policies and procedures include brochures, displays, and forms. Formal, written policies and procedures can help you, the manager, to better organize and direct team communications with clients. Websites, brochures, newsletters, computer-generated mass mailings, client surveys, and reminders will be discussed in more detail in Chapter 13, the chapter devoted to marketing.

Any type of practice-disseminated information can function as a communication tool of need-to-know hospital policies and procedures, while also performing dual duty in supporting the practice image and marketing efforts.

WALL DISPLAYS

All sorts of signs and informational pieces can be posted in the hospital for increasing client awareness and notification of important facts. Displays in the reception area or other client-visited areas might include the following:

- A roster of all doctors and team members, including their titles, degrees, and specialty status. (Be aware that your state may have specific guidelines and regulations regarding correct display of licenses.) This roster can be updated as necessary if you use a felt-covered changeable-letter board of the type designed for business and hotel lobbies.
- Photographs of the doctors and other veterinary team members on a wall display with their names and titles.
- Payment information (e.g., check policy, credit-card policy, or deposit requirements).
- Discount policies, if any.
- Hours and emergency procedures. (Hours and emergency telephone numbers should also be posted outside the front door or in a location that can be easily seen from outside the hospital's front door.)
- Boarding and grooming prices and other information, such as required vaccinations and parasite control.
- Framed photographs of pets and people (e.g., clients and/or employees with their pets).
- Artwork with animal themes.
- Medically oriented promotional information to advance client awareness of companion animal best care, such as dental care, nutrition, older pet needs, the importance of parasite management, and so on.

All practice materials, in hard-copy form or electronic, should uniformly reflect the hospital in a positive light, with accurate, up-to-date information presented in professional and appealing ways. Printed materials, website information, and wall displays should be reviewed at least once every six months. During your review, consider the following factors:

- *Content accuracy:* Does the information conveyed reflect current hospital policy and procedure? Are all named personnel still employees of the hospital? Are spellings correct?
- *Professional appearance:* Is the posting clean and dust-free? If the posting is covered with glass, is the glass clean? Is the lettering clear? Is the paper beginning to yellow?
- *Support the practice brand:* Is the most current practice logo consistently shown in all pieces? Are colors and font types consistent with the established practice marketing designs?
- *Tone:* Is the information neutral, or could it be misinterpreted as officious or overbearing? Is the information really necessary as a posting for all clients, or would the communication be better handled in a one-on-one conversation?

HOSPITAL FORMS

We will describe just a few of the many types of forms and other handouts here. Apply similar principles to the other forms your hospital uses. The client's understanding of the medical treatment plan, applicable fees, and other important information will depend on the accuracy and completeness of all forms. Through a consistent layout, font size and type, and logo, handouts can also support a uniform practice brand image.

Patient Care Plans

A patient care plan is a written estimate of services and related charges expected to be incurred from any patient medical or surgical procedure.

A written plan should be presented to the owner before care begins. It becomes a part of the written patient record and should support the axiom of providing for informed consent on the part of the client. Preparing and presenting the completed form to the animal owner or agent affords a golden opportunity to improve patient care and prevent misunderstandings.

When members of the practice team use a written plan to explain recommended care, the specific associated services, and related fees, the client has an opportunity to review the written plan and ask questions. To make an educated animal-care decision, the client may need clarification of any number of issues, such as the scope of the procedure and any alternatives to the suggested treatment. When medical, surgical, and diagnostic issues must be planned and questions addressed, the responsible doctor should personally speak with the client. These functions are the conduct of veterinary practice.

Presenting the case plan and fee estimate to the client includes arranging for payment of services. At this time, hospital staff typically request any deposit required by hospital policy.

Any prearranged financing agreements can be formalized and approved.

In most hospitals with computer systems, the treatment plan and related fee estimate is prepared using a template form on the computer. For frequently provided services, such as uncomplicated elective spays and neutering surgeries or prophylactic dental procedures, the estimate form can be standardized to include details about the component medical, diagnostic, and surgical services and medications included. A brief description of the procedure, including the reasons for performing it, and a review of predicted outcomes could be also included for client-education and informed-consent purposes.

An estimate form can also be a copy of the pre-prepared, itemized hospital invoice. A handwritten estimate is another alternative, although such an estimate will be more likely to contain computation errors. Of course, errors such as omitted services or medications can occur with any type of patient care plan and fee estimate form.

In some practices, the doctor in charge of the case discusses fee estimates with clients. Other hospitals allow technicians or practice managers to complete this communication. If the treatment plan and fee-estimate sheet is well designed and complete, any trained team member can discuss it with the client. However, if the conversation turns to making possible changes in the plan, the doctor must be involved.

Sometimes a client needs time to decide about the recommended care plan. Hesitancy does not necessarily indicate a rejection of the recommendation. When the plan and related fee estimate information is presented, the client should be given the opportunity to ask questions that have not yet been addressed. Some clients may need to have a few minutes alone to consider the options, especially when serious and expensive treatments are being recommended. The client may also need to discuss options with other responsible household partners.

Whoever discusses a fee estimate with the client should make clear that under certain circumstances, the estimate may change. Medical treatment and surgical procedures are both art and science. Different patients can respond differently to the same treatment, and sometimes unforeseen, but not unusual, changes in treatment protocol may be required. Assure clients that they will be notified and included in decisions when patient care requires changes or adaptations of the original care plan. Then follow through with communications, as promised.

The fee estimate and care plan is signed by the client and a copy is given to the client. Tablet computers and other interfacing devices allow clients to sign electronically in paper-light practices. The care plan and fee estimate is easily retrievable since it is part of the electronic patient record. Otherwise, a paper copy stays with the patient's paper file. In either case, the information in maintained even after the animal is discharged, especially if the owner was granted credit, in case of any later dispute over the charges. (See Figures 7.3A and 7.3B for an example of an estimate and admission form.)

INCLUDED ON
COMPANION
WEBSITE

FIGURE 7.3A ESTIMATE FORM

ABC ANIMAL HOSPITAL

Address: _____

Phone: _____ E-mail Address: _____

CASE TREATMENT PLAN

Client #: _____

Animal Name: _____

Date: _____

Notes: _____

Number: _____

Description of Services	Unit Price	Amount	Charges
_____	$ _____	$ _____	$ _____
_____	$ _____	$ _____	$ _____
_____	$ _____	$ _____	$ _____
_____	$ _____	$ _____	$ _____
_____	$ _____	$ _____	$ _____
_____	$ _____	$ _____	$ _____
		Estimated Total:	$ _____

Please Note:

This case treatment/surgical plan is only an estimate of service cost. We offer you the best possible care for your special companion. In order to give your pet good care and you the information you need to make informed decisions, we sometimes must run tests or do procedures that we did not anticipate when giving you this estimate. We will do our very best to inform you of any additional tests or procedures we believe necessary. Additional procedures authorized by you will cause an increase to this estimate figure.

PAYMENT POLICY

We accept cash, checks, Master Card, Visa, Discover Card, and Care Credit in payment of service. We cannot extend the privilege of charging services as this puts us in the position of becoming a lending institution.

DEPOSIT POLICY

Our hospital policy requires a minimum deposit of 50% of this estimate. Please leave this payment with the receptionist when your pet is admitted to the hospital.

Authorization to Treat: Amount: $_____

I fully understand the terms of this agreement and do authorize the hospital staff to perform the above-indicated services on my pet. I agreed that if I do not pay this account as agreed that any past due amounts are subject to costs of collection, including attorney's fees.

I am the owner or authorized agent of the owner of the pet presented for care.

By: _____   Date: _____

Received By: _____   Date/Time: _____

FIGURE 7.3B ESTIMATE AND ADMISSION FORM

ABC ANIMAL HOSPITAL

Address: _____

Phone: _____

CONSENT TO ADMISSION

Owner's Name: _____ Day In: _____
Pet's Name: _____ Day Out: _____

The undersigned hereby warrants that he/she is the owner or authorized agent for the owner of the above-named animal and does hereby request, consent, and authorize (hospital name), its veterinarians, personnel, and agents to board, care for, and treat said animal.

The undersigned acknowledges that other animals will be located on the premises and hereby authorizes the necessary care and treatment for any condition that may endanger said other animals and hereby agrees to pay the customary charges for such treatments. This includes, but is not limited to, parasites and infectious viruses.

The undersigned further acknowledges that no guarantees have been made except reasonable precautions against injury, escape, or illness with the understating that the undersigned will remain fully responsible for the cost of all services provided by (hospital name) and its authorized agents and professionals.

All animals admitted, must be current on their vaccinations and must be free of external parasites. Any animal found to have fleas or ticks will be treated at the owner's expense. We are not responsible for the loss of items left at the clinic such as leashes, toys, bedding, etc.

Emergency Phone Number: _____
Special Instructions: _____

ADDITIONAL AUTHORIZED WORK

1. Physical exam
2. Vacs: RV, DHLPP, CV, Bord, FVRCPC, FeLV
3. Fecal exam
4. Heartworm test
5. FeLV/FIV test
6. Nails/Anal sacs
7. Bath/dip
8. Other

Items left:
_____
_____
_____
_____

ESTIMATE OF FEES

Boarding fee _____ nights @_____ = $_____

Heartworm/Flea Rx _____ doses @_____ = $_____

Medication fee _____ doses @_____ = $_____

Prescription diet _____ meals @_____ = $_____

Other _____ times @_____ = $_____

Boarding fee $ _____
Additional work fee $ _____
Discount -$ _____
TOTAL ESTIMATED FEE $ _____

For office use only
1. ID card
2. Vcsc verified
3. Heartworm/flea tablets
4. Additional Work
5. Bath
6. Reserv. booked

No animal will be discharged without full payment. If I neglect to pick up pet within 5 days of the above date, you may assume that the pet is abandoned and you are authorized to dispose of the pet.

_____
Signature of Owner/Agent

Statement of release: I have examined my pet and have received it in good condition. It is free of fleas, ticks, and other problems.

_____
Signature of Owner/Agent

WE ARE NOT RESPONSIBLE FOR PROBLEMS AFTER THE PET LEAVES OUR OFFICE.

Special-Condition Handouts and General Animal-Care Information

The purpose of client handouts is to educate your clients about animal health care in general and their own animals' specific conditions. Sometimes this seems like an unceasing battle, but a successful practice will use all the resources it can to keep a position of authority when it comes to being a client's first choice for expert advice. Pet parents and animal owners are increasingly informed about animal care, receiving information (correct or not) from the Internet and other sources. You have little control over what your clients hear on television programs and from animal and pet supply stores, catalogs, nonveterinary press publications, and pharmacy advertising. However, you do control what they receive from your practice.

Your goal is to keep your clients informed about the facts and to dispel any misinformation they may have read or heard elsewhere. Printed materials can be valuable tools in explaining medical conditions, especially if a doctor or another team member takes the time to explain the handout and answer any questions. The information becomes even more valuable when it is made unique to the patient and client. By fully deploying practice management software and other programs to customize the information clients receive, you can ensure that clients know you are concerned about them and their pets.

One major benefit of computerization is the ability to create, store, edit, and customize practice forms, patient and client data, and other information. As data changes, electronically stored documents can readily be altered with word processing. Any document can be retrieved and printed, either for a particular client or for the entire client listing. For example, a letter outlining recommended prevention of heartworm disease can be updated as needed and printed for a general mailing, with each copy addressed to a different client, or disseminated by e-mail. Mailing lists and labels created from the client database streamline the distribution of timely and important animal-care information pieces, whether by newsletters, form letters, postcards, or e-mail messages.

A wide variety of glossy informational pamphlets can be obtained from animal food and pharmaceutical suppliers. Since these materials are developed as marketing tools for the companies in question, you will have to decide which ones provide information that agrees with your hospital's animal-care recommendations. Eliminate anything that does not agree with the practice mission and vision. You can also purchase noncorporate brochures from a variety of veterinary publishers, including AAHA Press and Lifelearn.

Not all online sources are suspect sources of information. Many companies developing veterinary website solutions, for example, have recognized the need for authoritative veterinary care and animal health information and designed valuable resources. These virtual libraries link with practice websites and often allow users to print selected information from them.

The Internet has permanently changed the nature of information research and dissemination. Veterinary practice managers must do their best to steer clients to reliable sources and to provide expert information endorsed by the practice doctors. Clients still will pay for expert advice, even with the ever-present probability of Dr. Google being searched to give an opinion, too. In your practice, guide the entire medical team to speak with a fairly uniform voice to minimize client and employee confusion. Teach clients to use information linked with the website, and hand them information that is in agreement with the medical team's opinions.

Checkup and Immunization Schedules

Every client should receive a schedule of future recommended veterinary checkups, vaccinations, tests, and preventive procedures. A life plan for wellness care, describing immunization schedules, parasite management, and follow-up appointments, is especially important for new puppies and kittens and other animals that have no previous history of veterinary health care.

Although patient-health pocket records are a nice touch, electronic versions are rapidly becoming preferred by clients. Whether the record is provided via a private log-in through the practice website or a paper version, however, the objective is the same: to fully involve the client in the health care plan for her companion animal. Both options allow the client to follow recommended practice schedules and keep track of completed appointments for immunizations, dewormings, diagnostic procedures, checkups, and surgical procedures for the life of the patient.

Commercially available client handouts can be customized with the hospital name, address, and telephone number. Vaccine manufacturers may provide your practice with patient health records when you purchase immunization supplies. Some hospitals design their own customized patient-health pocket records so that they can control the specific details, such as recommended regimens and preventive care suggestions. Publishers such as AAHA Press sell versions without pharmaceutical branding.

Effective Client Communication

As with any information that is important to patient care and support of client satisfaction, the reception team, and all team members, must communicate consistent information to clients in succinct, simple language.

As we've seen, veterinary practices cannot rely on verbal communication to relay important information and cannot depend on anyone's memory—the manager's, the employee's, or the client's. What is said in conversation is not necessarily heard, let alone understood.

And yet, written instructions must be accompanied by good oral communication. Many people do not read what you give them. If the practice team relies solely on written materials, you will still experience communication problems with clients. In client relations, as in staff relations, the hospital's greatest strength lies in a communication system that combines the best of written and verbal instructions.

EDUCATING CLIENTS

All team members have a role in client education, even, or perhaps especially, the receptionists. There are many resources available to you and your team that discuss the basics of client education. In *Educating Your Clients from A to Z: What to Say and How to Say It* (2011), Dr. Nan Boss discusses the basics of team-client communication for specific medical situations and educational opportunities with clients. Though veterinary technicians and veterinarians would more often engage in this kind of communication, receptionists may find the four-step process she describes to be useful in some situations. The steps are: engage, empathize, educate, and enlist.

Standardizing protocols, discussing protocols in team meetings, taking quizzes, and role-playing are all effective techniques for getting the whole team on board with medical recommendations. *Compliance* is a buzzword these days, but its importance is not diminished by its popularity in articles, books, and lectures. When the whole team supports the medical protocols laid out by the veterinarians, clients are much more likely to follow practice recommendations.

COMMUNICATING WITH DIFFICULT CLIENTS

Inevitably, the reception team, as the first and last defense, in any animal hospital will experience sensitive, emotionally charged situations. Clients can become angry, or they may be grieving and distraught over their pets' illness or injury. Dana Durrance and Laurel Lagoni go over both verbal and nonverbal communication basics in *Connecting with Clients: Practical Communication for 10 Common Situations* (2010). They offer a three-step process in which you lay the foundation, conduct the communication, and stay connected through follow-up care. Other communication skills that are helpful in the clinical setting include *normalizing, disclosure, paraphrasing,* and *active listening.*

Often, as hospital manager, you will be called upon to resolve potentially explosive situations. These challenging times can test the skills of even the most experienced and qualified managers.

Angry Clients

Angry, difficult clients will usually reach this stage gradually, not all at once. Most often, the cause is a communication breakdown that has created a misunderstanding. It is common for confusion to arise regarding financial matters.

Most often, timely and clear communication eliminates a client's anger and frustration. If problems with angry or unhappy clients are frequent in your hospital, one or more employees are probably not communicating with clients as well as they could. Listen to what is being said on the telephone, in the exam room, and at the reception desk. You will fairly quickly ascertain where and with whom the problem lies. You can then fine-tune procedures, document them, and train employees in how to carry them out effectively.

If a situation with an angry, complaining, or difficult client is escalating in the reception area or another public area of the clinic, move fast. Invite the client into a private room, such as an unused examination room, to discuss the situation. Public confrontation will make other clients feel uncomfortable. If there are new clients in the area, this can be a disastrous first impression. Furthermore, when a client is upset in front of an audience of other clients, emotions are more likely to become heightened and out of control. Take the audience away, and the client is much more likely to discuss matters in a calm and reasonable manner.

Whenever possible, if you are the practice manager, you should step into these situations to deal with upset clients. If that is not possible (for example, because you are not on the premises), someone else in a position of authority, such as a doctor, should take charge of the matter. A receptionist should never be left to deal with an angry client without assistance. A very arrogant and demanding person will often become much more reasonable when a doctor is involved, as doctors are often accorded a certain level of respect by members of the public simply because they are doctors. Make sure your team knows to whom clients should be referred in situations that are escalating.

When speaking with a difficult, complaining client, remember to listen. Try to understand the client's point of view and the reason for the complaint. Gather the information from the client in as quiet and friendly a manner as possible. Repeat what the client tells you, so that the client knows that you have heard him and that you understand what the issues are.

Immediately quoting policy or arguing the hospital's side will usually only aggravate the situation. Ask the client what could be done to resolve the situation to his satisfaction. Often, the client only wants a small concession. It is all right to break the rules from time to time. Letting an unreasonable client "win one" may well be worth far more than the aggravation involved in persisting in your own point of view (McCurnin 1988, 35).

The most important point to remember is that these situations are never resolved by confrontation and shouting matches. Stay calm and keep your cool. If you are too emotionally involved with the situation or are "taking it personally," it is time to ask another person to mediate.

Some clients are habitually upset and angry. If a client recurrently verbally abuses hospital staff, complains, or is unhappy no matter what you do, it might be best to refer that client to another veterinary clinic. This is always a matter to discuss with others in the hospital administration before making a decision.

The hospital might ask a client to choose a practice more suited to his needs for any of a number of reasons. The client is likely voicing discontent to other potential or existing clients. This could be costing the hospital clients over the long run. Having to deal with a chronic complainer is also very stressful and time consuming for hospital staff. Team loyalty increases dramatically when you fire a client that has been a continual problem. Finally, a client's abusive or dangerous behavior could result in an employee lawsuit against the hospital. You are responsible for keeping your employees safe on the job.

If the management team concludes that the hospital should no longer retain the client, send a letter to the client. Keep the message neutral, describing this as a no-fault situation. The letter should make the client feel that by mutual agreement, it has been decided that a switch to another hospital is in the client's and the patient's best interests. For example: "Mr. Smith, it seems that no matter what we do, we fail to meet your expectations. We no longer feel that we can do our best job for your pet or for you in this situation. Please provide the name of a hospital to which you would like us to send your pet's records. We assure you that this administrative task will be handled as soon as possible and at no charge to you."

Surprisingly, many difficult clients approached in such a manner turn over new leaves. They do not want to take their pets to another hospital. They really do like your hospital's services. These clients are just used to complaining and being difficult everywhere, and once a limit has been set, they may be able to change their behavior. But if they are truly abusive and dangerous, do not try to keep them.

The Client in Grief

Serious illness or injury to an animal or the death of a beloved animal companion are serious events in a pet owner's life and are often accompanied by a very real sense of grief. Grief affects every person differently. The emotion may be freely expressed or it may be internalized, but even clients who do not overtly reveal distress may be very affected by their worry or loss.

Whatever the client's demeanor, the situation should never be treated lightly. The entire team must be sensitive to the special needs of grieving clients, whether they are concerned over a sick pet, have lost a beloved pet, or face a difficult decision about a very sick pet. The human–companion animal bond and its implications for client communication and relations will be discussed in greater detail in Chapter 12.

Handling Abusive or Criminal Activity

Unfortunately, veterinary hospitals can be a target for criminal activity, especially since both drugs and money are on the premises. The well-being of your employees should always be a major consideration as you conduct employee training and plan and direct hospital policy.

If accosted or threatened, employees should not attempt to control the situation by themselves. Training should instruct them not to do anything that would endanger themselves in any way. Consider installing security cameras and an alarm device that employees can set off to contact the local police, especially if the hospital is located in a neighborhood at higher risk for crime.

Protecting employees against violence should be a primary goal of the hospital management. Ask local law-enforcement agencies to visit your practice to recommend changes in lighting, security systems, or building layout that will keep your staff as safe as possible. They can also often provide help with staff training to prepare team members to deal with dangerous situations. Do not wait until after an unfortunate event occurs to train employees. By making some simple changes now, you can keep your team and clients safer in the future.

Difficult situations like those described above are very rare, though it is necessary to be prepared for them. Most communications between the practice team and clients should be pleasant and rewarding—by emphasizing positive communication, you will be minimizing such problems. You will be keeping the focus where it belongs—on excellent patient care and service to the client.

Paying attention to the first impressions your clients receive of the practice will be an ongoing effort. Essentially, you are simply making sure that your clients feel welcome and that they have a positive experience, beginning with the first time they call or walk through the door for their visit. If you follow the front-desk procedures suggested in this chapter, you will be establishing good client relations and ensuring that clients return for many years to come.

8

Medical Records

A well-tended and carefully managed patient medical record system supports optimal patient care and enhances practice profitability. Astute practice managers pay close attention to how their practice teams use and maintain records. They also seek continual improvement to the medical record system to meet the ever-evolving expectations of the veterinary profession. A review of the patient medical record system is perhaps the best way to evaluate the practice team's ability to achieve its mission and objectives.

Medical record system structure and maintenance depends on the unique characteristics of each practice. Client and patient numbers, practice maturity, number of veterinarians on staff, and experience among staff professionals all factor into the choice of a medical record system and how it changes over time. Two different practices may use the same practice management software to manage patient and client records in very different ways. Even within a particular practice, individual medical records may display remarkable differences because of a variety of factors, including team-member depth of training and personal characteristics.

In addition, there may be both paper and electronic medical records (EMR) to maintain as well as various imaging results. Advances in computer hardware and software, often referred to as the veterinary practice information management system (VPIMS or PIMS), have caused some big changes to occur over the past decade in how veterinary medical records are stored. There is a learning curve taking place in many practices as they move from a paper system to a "paper-light" system.

Assimilating the variety of records into one meaningful way of tracking patient care and client communications, and ensuring that charges are captured, can be time consuming and sometimes frustrating. Misplaced and incomplete records irritate clients, employees, and the practice management team. The practice income stream relies on accurate invoices; any delays or inefficiencies in record completion can result in lost charges and invoicing errors, which increase the likelihood of client dissatisfaction and financial loss.

A significant management objective is continuous exploration, modification, and improvement of the practice's medical record system. The long-term goal for medical records includes the following characteristics:

- Are perfectly integrated
- Can be located instantaneously from any location
- Are secure and confidential
- Provide enough detail to prevent care gaps
- Still allow for team efficiency in completing them
- Meet any regulatory requirements
- Suffice to defend against malpractice claims

The more readily available, the easier to decipher, and the more complete the records are, the more likely it is that the practice objectives of excellent patient care, good client communication, and maximum revenue can be met.

Purposes of Medical Records

Medical records serve a variety of purposes. The Institute of Medicine has divided medical record uses into two large categories: primary and secondary.* The primary use relates directly to specific patient care. Secondary uses are not clinically based, but involve analysis of practice trends. Examples of secondary uses include studies of treatment costs, compilations of clinical trial data, determinations of how many patients had a specific disease, or counts of the numbers of dogs, cats, birds, horse breeds, or disciplines represented in the practice's patient base over specified periods of time.

PRIMARY USE: UNIQUE, INTIMATE PATIENT CARE

A patient medical record provides a logical organization of observations and conclusions about the patient's health. Patient medical records furnish documentary evidence of the patient's health status, incidents of illness or injury, preventive care, and medical treatment to date.

The record is also a forum for planning patient care based on observations and information collected from the client. This information is called the *medical history*. Patient history together with clinical examination allows the veterinarian to formulate possible diagnoses, determine testing procedures, and plan treatment. Doctors' notes about administered care and planned treatment constitute the treatment chart.

The medical record is like a story. The story recites what the client has observed in his animal and told the veterinary team. The story also tells what the team has observed about the patient. It describes the client's and team's care of the patient and the patient's response to that care.

* Portions of this chapter draw heavily on unpublished notes regarding evaluating information systems provided by Robert H. Featherston, DVM, MS, in 2000, and personal correspondence between Dr. Featherston and the author (Heinke) in 1999 and 2000, as well as the chapter on computer systems written by Dr. Featherston for previous editions.

In addition, the story recounts the relationship between the hospital team and the patient and client. Many team members will need to read and understand this story in order to competently perform their jobs.

The patient record includes tools and provides information for communicating with the client, both contemporaneously and in the future. The medical record sets a timeline for client contact and patient care, potentially over the lifetime of the patient. A comprehensive and detailed patient medical record documents past preventive health care and indicates when the patient is due for future medical services.

SECONDARY USE: BETTER MANAGEMENT THROUGH ANALYSIS

Medical records provide massive data, which is the basis for analysis, study, and evaluation of the medical care provided by the hospital and its team (AAHA 2000). A wealth of information can be gained by evaluating the medical records.

For instance, quality-of-care reviews to ensure compliance with practice medical care and prevention guidelines are an important secondary use of medical records. These uses are "secondary" not in the sense of being less important, but in the sense that they deal with larger, practice-wide issues and trends instead of dealing directly with individual patients and clients. As practice manager, for example, you can profile and compare the individual care providers (doctors, technicians, and veterinary assistants), measuring income production, number and types of cases seen, and success in treating cases. Routine peer review of medical records is the principal method of performing an objective quality assessment of patient care.

In 2003, the American Animal Hospital Association published an in-depth study called *The Path to High-Quality Care* to measure how well veterinary practices fulfilled their stated objectives of care as determined by practice team interviews and audits of patient records. The study quantified compliance in six areas:

1. Canine heartworm disease testing and prevention
2. Dental prophylaxis
3. Therapeutic diets
4. Senior screenings
5. Core vaccines
6. Preanesthetic testing

This study is an excellent example of the secondary use of patient records to concretely measure patient care in a few select areas against the predetermined practice guidelines. Practices exhibited large gaps between team *estimates* of completed care as compared to measured accomplishment through medical-record auditing. The record audits showed much less patient care in each tested area than practice teams and doctors had estimated. For example, auditing showed that 53 percent of the records for senior-aged dogs and cats showed no evidence of screening recommendations for screenings that had been defined in practice guidelines.

Auditing patient records to determine compliance with predetermined practice guidelines is an important adjunct to employee training, feedback, and coaching. Clients rely on the practice team to give consistent, concise, and reliable recommendations that allow them to make educated decisions about the health care they choose for their animals.

This secondary use of medical records deals with the practice's client education efforts, which translates into effective marketing strategies. If a veterinarian, for example, identifies a new medication or nutritional modality effective in controlling a breed- or species-specific condition, and relays this information to you, the practice manager, then you, in turn, can devise (or assign someone to devise) an e-mail broadcast to target clients narrowly defined with those patient types.

As practice manager you may also choose to analyze the client base from an activity standpoint. For example, you might look at the average number of patients, the average number of visits per year, where most clients live, how much clients spend in the course of a year, and/or how clients came to the hospital (referral, website, social-media venues, etc.). This information then aids your decisions about where to allocate practice funds intended to increase client-patient visits and referrals.

Record-keeping protocols to achieve both the primary and secondary purposes require a planned approach. In order to organize and direct your hospital's medical record system to its fullest potential, you first need to establish what the records will include and decide how they will be used. Defining a clear practice objective for medical records will help hospital staff maintain accuracy and clarity—two key characteristics of an effective medical record system.

Documents Included in the Medical Record

Although the patient's medical history and treatment chart are the primary components of an individual medical record, many other hospital and business documents are also considered medical records. Each hospital is different in the records it uses and maintains, and each patient case is unique in the records that are required and used in the professional judgment of the attending doctor of veterinary medicine.

Several levels of record keeping may occur in a single practice, involving both hard copy and soft (electronic) copy records. For instance, vaccination reminders and vaccination histories may be contemporaneously updated as part of the invoicing system through the practice management software, and the doctors' medical notes and patient treatment plans may entail a handwritten system with hard-copy filing. Radiographic films and laboratory results may be stored elsewhere in the practice. (See textbox, "What's in a Medical Record?")

What's in a Medical Record?

Here are some, but not necessarily all, of the documents that might be considered medical records:

- Client-patient registration forms
- Appointment books or electronic schedules
- Client consent forms
- Client release forms
- Patient history
- Patient identification records such as microchips and licenses
- Doctors' medical notes and problem lists
- Telephone consultation reports and telephone logs
- E-mail and text communications
- Exam-room report cards
- Routine hospital handouts for client education and instruction
- Radiographs, CT scans, and MRI scans
- Ultrasound images
- Electrocardiograms and other electrical examination results
- Photographs, videos, and electronically stored images
- Laboratory reports
- Reports from specialists and other veterinarians
- Necropsy reports
- Surgery logs
- Anesthesia logs
- Controlled-drug logs
- Adverse-reaction logs
- Radiography and imaging logs
- Ultrasound logs
- Laboratory logs
- Unexpected death logs
- Euthanasia logs
- Syringe and needle disposal and medical-waste logs
- Patient travel sheets, or circle sheets
- Patient care plans and estimate sheets
- Client financial records
- Patient discharge records and forms (adapted from Wilson 1988, 316–317)

Samples of some of these appear throughout this and other chapters; see also "What Should Be Included in a Patient Medical Record" later in this chapter for more information.

In essence, any electronic or paper-based information relevant to the care of patients and communication with clients may be considered a medical record. From the list shown in the textbox, you can appreciate that the hospital medical record system can become rather complex, voluminous, and challenging to manage in an efficient, cost-effective manner.

As mentioned, some of these records may be in electronic form and some may be in paper form, depending on how "paper-light" a practice is (Wilson 1988, 317; see also Slater 2007). More specific information about practice management software and EMRs appears later in this chapter.

As practice manager, you will need to work alongside the medical and technical team to come up with a list of items to be included as part of your practice's medical records. In devising a complete list of records to be retained, be sure to consider a variety of factors. Some of these factors are described below. You must consult with the practice doctors, and you must educate other team members about these requirements once the list is complete. You will also need to make sure all team members know how to follow record-keeping protocols. If the types of records kept are not consistent across all patients, both primary uses and secondary uses of the records will be hindered. Finally, plan to work alongside others to evaluate and modify record-keeping protocols on a regular basis in order to ensure the best possible patient care and reliable data management.

Balancing Record Cost with Record Benefit

Because the medical record system serves several purposes, the practice manager must balance the priorities of each objective when determining the types of records to be kept. For example, a medical record provides documentation that may protect against successful medical malpractice claims. If you viewed the medical record as a potential legal document, you might decide to retain a dated copy of each and every hospital handout given to a client.

Over a course of years, however, this method would require keeping an enormous amount of paper in the files. The paper retained might surpass the hospital's storage capacity, and the cost of printing and office supplies might become excessive. Misfiled records might be more common because of the volume of paper, resulting in increased staff frustration, time loss, and payroll cost.

Keep in mind that one major objective of the medical record system is to maintain the standard of patient care while obtaining revenue and realizing profit. A massive amount of detailed records might actually hinder rather than raise the quality of care (Wilson 1988, 316). In reality, private veterinary practices often have a bigger problem in the opposite extreme: records that are too brief and systems that are inadequate for maintaining compliance with fee capture policy or for enhancing the level or completeness of medical care provided.

Another challenge in private veterinary practice is the integration of financial management with patient care management. Practice managers have long yearned for record systems that would efficiently merge these two aspects of practice management. If drug inventory must be tracked for bill-paying and tax-reporting purposes, and medications dispensed should be recorded on the patient history, why shouldn't both occur simultaneously? Such a system would provide the best efficiency and the most detailed records.

Unfortunately, what satisfies the accounting and bookkeeping needs of the practice may not be suitable from a medical and surgical perspective. And, record-keeping protocols that suffice for managing patient care might not be adequate for effective client communication, or for assuring accurate invoicing and cash flow.

Most practice management software designed for veterinary hospital use starts with an income-centered perspective and related functions: invoicing clients, tracking accounts receivable, and recording dispensed inventory. Management of medical records and complex patient histories by these software programs developed more or less as an afterthought, deriving from the invoicing history for each particular client or patient.

Your management goal will be to sensibly monitor the effectiveness and efficiency of the existing record system in all its functions and formats in order to provide ever-improving outcomes in patient care and client service, while supporting the practice's profit motive. With the rapid advance of electronic applications, cloud computing, and equipment integration, you will need to stay current and modify patient data management as necessary, always balancing your options for new technology against the cost of reconfiguration and employee training.

Establishing a Medical Record System

Careful planning is the starting point for any effective and efficient medical record system. The existing medical record design is a mere starting point. Evaluate it from every perspective: appointment scheduling, client and patient data perpetuation, client notification of scheduled appointments and recommended patient care, invoicing completeness, internal controls and data security, compliance auditing, and more.

Your regular and recurring evaluations will lead to changes and adaptations of the existing system and team training about the hospital protocols to be followed. Parameters you will consider that lead to system modification include overall record design, format, recording methodologies, filing, data security, and storage.

Your decisions for system modification should be founded in the protocol for doctors' medical notes, the heart of the entire record. After all, practice clients are most interested in good patient outcomes for a reasonable price, and feeling that the practice team has their animals' best interests and their own at the center of all concern.

SYSTEM CRITERIA

Regardless of the type or format of the record system used in your hospital, the following criteria should apply to all examination and treatment records of veterinary services provided to animals:

- A separate record should exist for each patient examined. Typically, all patients belonging to a particular client are grouped together, with each patient having a separate file. Therefore, several different files (electronic or paper) could exist for a single client who owns several animals.

- Some paper-based filing systems create a separate file for each client but maintain all patient records for each client within a single folder. If a client has more than one animal, over the years these portfolios of patient files become rather bulky and difficult to efficiently use, especially during the course of an office visit involving one or two patients out of many.

- Multiple owners for a single animal often occur, giving another reason to have a single record for each patient. Practices with this situation must be especially attentive to careful identification of legal ownership, as confidentiality of patient and client information can be more challenging to manage. Employees must be attentive to possible ownership issues that can be associated with a single patient record.

- The record should provide readily retrievable information about the patient. The method of organization and filing should make sense and should be easy to use, as this helps ensure accurate record keeping by all staff members.

- The individual records should be well organized and should follow accepted standards for scientific writing, with the correct medical terminology and clear and objective language.

- The record must be composed as a legal document that will be admissible in a court of law. Keep in mind the prevailing legal viewpoint of "not recorded, not done." It is much easier to defend the practice against a malpractice suit when accurate, detailed records exist of the care provided. Incomplete records can increase legal liability exposure.

- The record must be accurate and legible. The value of medical records is in direct proportion to the thoroughness and accuracy with which they are compiled. Illegibility is a common problem in general practice and can compromise patient care. If a staff member cannot read what another person has penned, serious errors in medical treatment and client communication can easily occur, ultimately increasing liability exposure (AAHA, *Medical Records Manual*, n.d., 2.02).

WHAT SHOULD BE INCLUDED IN A PATIENT MEDICAL RECORD

Each medical record should include specific, permanently recorded information. The following list provides guidelines for recording information at the time of the first patient visit and updating it at each subsequent visit or hospital stay.

Client Identification

Record the full name (last name, first name, and middle initial), home address, home telephone number, cell-phone number, work address, work telephone number, and fax numbers of the client. Also obtain current e-mail addresses whenever possible.

Ask clients for their preferred modes of contact for reminders and important notifications regarding their pets' care. Establish a consistent way of capturing client communication preferences that will work well with your practice's record system. This step is essential, as not all clients regularly use text messaging or check for e-mail. Using these methods may work well for some clients, while for others it would mean that the message was not received in a timely way.

Patient Profile

Identify each patient by species, breed, sex, name, color, markings, and age (with date recorded) or date of birth. The patient's weight and body score should be recorded at each visit. If breed and/or age are not known, try to give reasonable estimates that are as specific as possible. For instance, "poodle cross" and "Lab mix" are more helpful descriptions than is "mixed breed."

Previous Medical History

A patient's medical history provides useful information for formulating a diagnosis and in planning and providing medical care, both from a preventive standpoint as well as for treating diagnosed abnormal conditions. Together with clinical examination and client interviews, the medical history enables a veterinarian to form a diagnosis and design a treatment plan.

Medical histories can be collected through a combination of forms, questionnaires, and interviews with the patient's owner. Generally, all interactions with a patient and discussions with the owner should result in updates of the medical history.

At the initial visit, interview the client to ask about and record information related to prior health problems. Include information from other veterinary care providers on the patient record. Other important data include prior medical treatments and surgeries, current medications, known allergies, and adverse reactions to prior treatments and medications. (See Figures 7.2A and 7.2B.)

Vaccination History

Record the dates of previous vaccines and boosters as accurately as possible. Ask the client for copies of vaccination certificates or other provider documentation for verification. Once the animal is a regular patient, review and update the vaccine history each time the patient visits or receives a vaccination. Identifying and recording the vaccination location on the patient's body is important for feline patients and is also a valid record-keeping protocol for all species of patients.

The Primary Complaint

Accurately summarize problems and information recited by the client. Discern what the client perceives to be the problem while listening for other details that could have a significant bearing on treatment. *Active listening* not only helps to ensure excellent patient care but also facilitates bonding between clients and the members of the veterinary team.

The veterinary team relies on owner observations of the patient a great deal in making diagnoses, determining medical treatment options, and identifying client-education needs because of the simple fact that animals cannot talk. Each team member who collects patient history, whether a doctor or not, must learn to be an expert listener. Listening is only the first step, however; what the team member hears must be clearly and concisely expressed on the medical record. As practice manager, your role includes providing training in this task, monitoring the team's consistency in completing records, and making needed modifications.

Physical Examination

At each patient visit, the veterinary care providers must contemporaneously compose brief reports of the results of the physical examination, listing any problems encountered. Although the physical-exam notes are brief, they should include observations of normal as well as abnormal findings. Typically, veterinarians will use abbreviations to describe physical exam findings so that they can be succinctly listed.

For example: "Oral cavity–NVL" means that "no visible lesions" were noted in the mouth. A trained reader of the exam notations understands that the oral cavity was indeed inspected and that no abnormal findings were observed. "Heart and lungs–WNL" indicates that the chest cavity was auscultated and that heart and lung rhythms and sounds were "within normal limits." Refer to AAHA's *Standard Abbreviations for Veterinary Medical Records* for more information.

Abbreviations can improve record accuracy, increase legibility, and reduce time spent writing or typing. Many hospitals derive their own special set of abbreviations, although many are common throughout the veterinary profession. Ideally, a veterinary practice should strive to use abbreviations that are universally accepted. In this way, new employees will be able to make sense of all notations. In addition, the notes will be easier to use in any litigation that might arise.

All hospital personnel must be able to understand what the abbreviations mean to be able to correctly interpret the records. Keep a master list or glossary of abbreviations for your hospital and periodically test staff members on their meanings. Misinterpreted abbreviations can be dangerous, even deadly.

Diagnosis or Possible Diagnoses

Veterinary care providers should make a record of both differential and definitive diagnoses. Medical diagnosis is the process of identification of a disease or disorder by analysis and examination. When the signs or symptoms of a health problem point to several possible causes, but a definitive diagnosis has not yet been established, the veterinarian should list all possible causes or potential diagnoses. These possible causes are called *differential diagnoses*. Additional tests and procedures will be needed to narrow the possibilities, usually leading to a definitive conclusion of cause. When a *definitive diagnosis* is made, it should be recorded as such.

For example, a dog may be hospitalized for bloody diarrhea, vomiting, and shock. On the medical record, the doctor will list possible causes, such as severe gastrointestinal parasite infestation or canine parvovirus. Once laboratory results show that this case is indeed related to parvovirus and not to massive hookworm infestation, it should be recorded as the definitive diagnosis, "canine parvoviral enteritis" (small bowel inflammation relating to the parvovirus strain infecting dogs). The patient record must include all the options considered and the steps taken in this process, not just the conclusion drawn at the end of the process.

Treatment Given or Prescribed

Team members must carefully list all drugs used in patient treatment as well as doses prescribed. State laws that regulate pharmacies may be applicable to veterinary hospital record maintenance and may govern how much information about particular prescriptions is included in the medical record. They may also regulate the labeling information required for all dispensed medication.

To enhance legibility, efficiency, and accuracy, veterinary practice management software enables printed pharmacy labels, including all requisite information, such as prescribing doctor, client, patient, and drug names; drug strength, dosage, and expiration date; and refill information. Software should also provide the option of including the same information in the electronically maintained patient record, resulting in a contemporaneous medical note as the label is prepared. In the event your practice uses paper medical records, consider printing two labels: one for the dispensed item and one to adhere on the paper medical record.

Laboratory Tests and Results

Technicians should record the results of all performed laboratory tests, including abnormal and normal findings, as a permanent part of the medical record. Even normal findings are important, as they provide a baseline reference point for future laboratory tests of the patient and can be evidence of a regular process for rule-out of possible disease conditions.

Laboratory tests are run on body fluid, tissues, and other specimens, covering a vast array of biochemical parameters and causative agent identification procedures. Sample testing investigates chemical abnormalities, cellular changes, and the presence of organisms or toxins, among other analyses. Lab tests include electrical activity or conduction studies, such as electrocardiograms (ECGs or EKGs) and electromyograms (EMGs).

Tests may be ordered from outside independent commercial laboratories (*reference labs*), or, if the hospital has the requisite equipment and capabilities, may be run in-house. In both cases, your hospital's record-keeping protocols should require staff to identify when a specific laboratory test was ordered; the laboratory used, if any; and the filing location of a report copy, if it is not included in the paper record or scanned as part of the EMR.

For EMR systems, hard-copy reports from specialists and laboratories might be scanned into the computer system and linked with the particular patient's record. Alternatively, the specialist or laboratory might transmit electronic documents via the Internet directly to the practice's computer system and patient medical database.

Most in-house laboratory equipment is driven by software that links with the practice management software. Equipment communication capability leads to accuracy, efficiency, and fee capture, as a lab test ordered from one human interface with equipment leads to processing and information in multiple locations. For example, invoicing a complete blood count to a specific patient could result in:

- An identification label printed for the blood collection tube and/or lab requisition paperwork
- An order sent to the in-house lab equipment and technician
- A notation made in the patient EMR
- An informational handout prepared for the client
- A reminder established to alert the practice that lab results are pending for inclusion in the record and discussion with the client

When the lab results are available, the lab equipment or reference lab might load the results to the patient record and electronically alert the attending veterinarian of their availability. See "Logs in Veterinary Practices" later in this chapter for more information.

Radiographic, Ultrasound, and Other Imaging Procedures

Practice medical records include diagnostic medical-imaging procedure results, which summarize findings from radiographic (X-ray) and ultrasound images, computerized tomography (CT) scans, and magnetic resonance imaging (MRI). Imaging technology is constantly advancing, and patient medical-imaging reports can include a wide variety of information sources, including interpretations of the images as well as the images themselves.

Some examples of other imaging-based diagnostic information include interpretations of videos that document behavior, lameness, and seizures; cytology and biopsy microscopic images; endoscopy studies; and digital images of skin, eye, ear, teeth, or other tissues; and surgical events.

As with laboratory reports, the medical record should include summaries of the findings, either as separate documents or as part of the doctor's notes. For example, a practice that uses traditional X-ray film development technology requires a system for filing the patient films, since they are too large to be bound into individual patient records.

For most lab results, the summary reports can also be bound into the patient paper medical record. In other cases, the reports are stored chronologically in a separate file system, either in paper form or as scanned versions for digital filing purposes. As practices evolve from paper patient records to EMRs, unique filing and medical record management systems evolve to manage and organize information. The overriding objective is to make archival and retrieval methods as flawless and easy to use as possible.

The medical record should inform the reader that the images exist and state where they can be found for review. This is particularly true in the case of digital images that are archived on a computer hard drive, on DVD, on CD, in a remote location via the Internet ("in the cloud"), or in some other electronic format, such as a USB flash drive. If the image cannot be directly linked to the electronic patient record for easy viewing, then the record should indicate the name of the image and where it can be found.

Managing and archiving digital patient medical images is a complex topic and is outside the scope of this book. Nevertheless, you should be aware of some basic concepts and standards. The global information-technology standard used to ensure interoperability of medical image systems is called Digital Imaging and Communications in Medicine (DICOM). The technology standard is required in integration with electronic health record systems and applies to image-related systems that are "used to produce, store, display, process, send, retrieve, query, or print medical images and derived structured documents as well as to manage related workflow" (Association of Electrical and Medical Imaging Equipment Manufacturers, DICOM brochure, n.d.).

Important objectives of DICOM include ensuring that all equipment is compatible with other current technology and will be compatible with future technology, regardless of vendor, and with health information systems and other developing standards. Another objective is ensuring that patient identification is imbedded with the image in a single data file, so that the two cannot be separated by mistake.

Consultation Reports

The record should include consultation reports, such as summaries of telephone consultations with the client by your hospital's doctors and any consultation reports from specialists to whom the patient has been referred. Specialist reports of referred patient treatment, results, and follow-up instructions should be bound into the paper record, scanned, or otherwise electronically filed as previously described.

For in-house doctor phone consultations, the veterinarian may make notes of what was discussed with the client on the patient medical record or type notes into the electronically maintained record, even while talking with the client. Doctor-client discussions by e-mail should be included in the medical record when they are pertinent to patient signs, diagnosis, and treatment recommendations. Your hospital will need policy guidelines for electronic communications, including handling patient images transmitted by clients when a doctor-client-patient relationship exists.

Prognosis

A prognosis is a medical prediction of the course and outcome of a disease. Once the diagnosis has been established, the attending doctor will usually make and communicate a prognosis to the client. The prognosis changes with time as the disease or medical condition takes its course, as treatment occurs, and as treatment is modified. The prognosis helps the client decide what level of treatment to engage for the patient (and pay for). Whenever possible, veterinarians should record the prognosis when it is first made and update it as the ill or injured animal is reevaluated over the course of care.

Surgical Record

Veterinary care providers must also make a comprehensive record of each surgical procedure undertaken for the patient. Each surgical record must include a variety of data, the specifics of which depend on the complexity of the procedure. In any patient case, the record should include the surgeon's name, the procedure name, and the anesthetic protocol. The anesthetic protocol includes type and dosage of each anesthetic agent used and the duration of anesthesia. Preoperative, intraoperative, and postoperative analgesics administered to control pain are listed by dose, type, and route of administration.

Description of the surgical procedure might be quite limited for a routine procedure, such as a feline castration. At the other extreme, a complicated orthopedic procedure might result in a quite detailed report, particularly where complications might be expected or results are uncertain. Details could include names of assistants, the length of time required to complete the surgery, the duration of the anesthesia and the recovery time, descriptions of bodily abnormalities noted during the procedure, and the types and sizes of surgical repair materials used, such as suture material, bone plates or pins, and surgical staples or glue. Even the method and antiseptics used for aseptically preparing the animal for surgery might be disclosed.

Dental Records

Team members should include information about the pet's dental history as reported by the client, such as evidence of pain, bad breath, drooling, loss of appetite, and weight loss, in addition to any observations made in the course of the dental examination. A dental chart is a permanent record of the dental history and should include examination and radiographic findings as well as a record of dental treatment. Findings that would be recorded include the condition of all teeth, identification of missing or broken teeth, and information about abnormal bites, periodontal diseases, and abnormal oral cavity lesions. Examples of comprehensive dental charts can be found on the American Veterinary Dental College website (AVDC n.d.)

Some practices consistently grade patients' overall gingival health through the use of a standardized scale. Images of the patient's mouth help to educate the client and provide an excellent record of oral health. Team members can make more consistent recommendations to clients in this important area of health care when good records are maintained.

The care provider should record any incidents of surgical management, such as extractions and other corrective procedures undertaken, and include any archive digital images taken before, during, and after such procedures. Treatments such as fluoride and enamel polishing, and recommended home therapy and routine preventive care, such as tooth brushing, should also be recorded.

Necropsy Reports

Necropsy is nearly synonymous with the more commonly recognized term applicable to humans, autopsy. A necropsy is an examination of an animal body after death to determine the cause of death. The doctor performing the exam describes normal and abnormal findings in the necropsy report. If possible, she determines a cause of death. Many times, the person performing the necropsy cannot determine a cause, even with very extensive and expensive laboratory testing. Laboratory tests could include microscopic tissue examination and tests for specific toxins. If laboratory tests are completed as part of the necropsy, the lab reports should be included in the necropsy report, which is filed with the patient record. If an outside pathologist performed the exam, that should be noted.

Care Plans, Estimates, and Consent Forms

A patient care plan lists the recommended procedures for the patient based on the patient history, the examination of the patient, lab findings, and differential or final diagnoses. The veterinarian may present this plan orally or in writing. It should include accurate documentation of hospital-proposed treatment and the client's acceptance or rejection of that treatment. A care plan includes an estimate of total fees for recommended services or a range of probable total fees. Fees are often presented in the form of a range because patients are unique. Their conditions and their responses to treatment will vary, and thus the final tally of costs will vary.

It is a good idea to create and update care plan templates that describe common procedures, including details of bundled services and expected total fee estimates or ranges. Team members can quickly update and customize template forms for the age, weight, condition, and other unique factors of the patient. Practice management software enables rapid creation of customized plans from templates and integration with patient records.

The care plan and any estimates given to the client, either oral or written, should be recorded in the medical record or filed with it in some way. All care providers should know that it is necessary to include doctors' notes and consent forms signed by the client. These forms provide documentation for the fact that all possible information concerning the risks, prognosis, fees, and alternatives of the procedure have been explained to the client in terms that the client can understand. (For more information, see the section entitled "Consent and Release Forms" later in this chapter.)

Organizing Medical-Record Data and Information

An individual patient's medical record eventually will contain a wealth of information, with the amount of data growing over time. The hospital manager, in consultation with the veterinarians, must determine how the information within each patient's files will typically be organized. Otherwise, it will be a haphazard pile of data that is virtually unusable. The better organized it is, the easier it will be to retrieve the information and use it to maximize patient care.

Typically, records have been organized in one of three ways: by source, by problem, or by some combination of the two. These three methods are described below. Whichever method is chosen, it should be applied consistently by all team members so that everyone can find the information they need as quickly as possible.

Neither the medical professions in general nor the veterinary profession in particular yet has a standardized method for organizing individual files. Widespread adaptation of electronically based medical records would likely cause rapid standardization of record organization, comparable to the previously described DICOM standards that led to compatibility in imaging protocols and technologies.

Electronic medical-record use by veterinarians and other medical professionals has lagged behind other automated data processes that have been quickly embraced. The lack of standardization is reflected in various practice management software programs that build in options and flexibility for the design of forms and data organization. Until the time of a standardization groundswell, you will need to know about the primary methods of organizing medical records and understand that practice-unique customization is common (Slater 2007).

SOURCE-ORIENTED MEDICAL RECORDS

In the 1950s, rapid advances in testing and treatment procedures resulted in physicians sorting records for individual patients by the source of information. Since then, source-oriented medical records (SOMR) have been widely used. In this method, data is entered on the record and grouped by the information source and then ordered chronologically within these categories. For example, possible information sources include the client oral history, physical exam findings, imaging studies, and blood tests. The chronological order is determined by date of office visit or period of hospitalization (*patient encounters*).

The information source types used in SOMRs include all of the documents listed in the previous section. The order in which each piece of information is recorded can be individualized to fit practice requirements and veterinarian preferences. For instance, using a free-form method, the doctor writes most entries as information from various sources that come to mind. As you might imagine, depending on the mental organizational skills of the doctor, the date-to-date history may be disjointed, or it may flow; it may be very detailed, or it may lack important details. Use of checklists can increase probability of doctors capturing all key information in a consistent manner.

SOMRs can be effective if they are well organized. As with any record type, legibility and completeness is crucial to a good record. Information from source documents should be easily retrievable. If your practice chooses this method, consider including a list in the front of the record summarizing the problems for which the patient has been treated. Practice management software can be configured to include diagnosis codes, which can be used in a computerized system as a convenient way to create these summary problem listings. This summary allows for powerful data sorting for patient histories of specific problems.

PROBLEM-ORIENTED MEDICAL RECORDS

In 1968, a physician named Dr. Lawrence Weed described a systematic approach for record organization based on identified health problems (Weed 1968; Salmon et al. 1996). Dr. Weed envisioned improved patient care through integration of problem-organized records through computer systems and medical information systems, including linkage to relevant medical research and knowledge (problem-knowledge coupling) (Shultz 1988; Clinical Informatics n.d.).

By the end of the 1970s, the problem-oriented medical record (POMR) was becoming the preferred mode of medical information management. It used a protocol of chronologically numbering identified patient health problems. The POMR links all diagnostic and therapeutic information to various patient health problems as they arise, are identified, and are resolved or managed.

Classically, POMR information is organized in four record sections:

1. The defined database, which includes the chief presenting complaint; the patient's profile, history, and physical examination findings; and laboratory and radiology reports.
2. The problem list, which is divided into three sections:
   A. the major problem list
   B. the minor problem list
   C. a medication table

A "problem" is anything that potentially threatens health and may require medical attention. Problems can be active, inactive, chronic, acute, ongoing, static, resolved, or in remission. The medication table documents the current various pharmaceuticals, supplements, and fluid therapies, as well as dosage information.

3. The plan section, which includes a written discussion of a planned course of action for the active problems at hand, including further diagnostic procedures, therapy, and client education.

4. The progress section, which includes doctor and technician notation of case observations, changes, and progress. Veterinarians write the progress notes in four consecutive parts, known as the "SOAP" format. The SOAP acronym stands for the following types of information:

S = Subjective information, including the presenting complaint and the patient's symptom history. The information is subjective, that is, it relates primarily to what the owner or caretakers have observed and interpreted and is more opinion than absolute fact.

O = Objective information, including the exam and laboratory findings. Objective information is based on scientific observation, as in a thorough physical examination. Objective information is more fact than opinion. A client's statement: "He has been crying all night. He is in horrible pain," contains both subjective and objective information. The fact that the pet has been vocalizing is objective information. The interpretation that the animal is in pain is an opinion, or subjective information. Since the animal cannot talk, it cannot verify the truth of the owner's opinion. Indeed, the animal might be suffering separation anxiety or some other distress unrelated to physical pain.

A = Assessment of subjective and objective information by the doctor. The doctor integrates all the information and comes to a tentative or final conclusion. A list of differential diagnoses or a final diagnosis would ordinarily be included as part of the assessment.

P = Plan that is based on the assessment. The plan can include rationale, suggestions, and recommendations for diagnostic studies; treatment protocol; surgical intervention; and client communication, including questions to ask. The plan can include doing nothing, taking a "wait and see" approach. Sequencing many be used, which describes subsequent steps to take after the first steps in the plan are taken and their results provide more information.

The POMR makes data efficient to retrieve and permits a rapid evaluation of the patient's condition at any given time. Information can be readily found in the record, since all of the entries are organized in the same way. For instance, if an employee wanted to find the most recent plan for client communication, he would simply look for the plan section (the "P" in "SOAP") in the latest record entry.

FIGURE 8.1 SAMPLE PROGRESS NOTES FORM

		PROGRESS NOTES

Owner's Name: _____

Patient Name: _____

DATE	SOAP	

One disadvantage of the POMR is the extensive time required to compose each complete entry. Even if there were no significant changes in patient status, the entire POMR format would be completed at each patient encounter, including a record of conversations with the client.

Oriented around apparently unconnected units of information organized by problem, the POMR challenges the medical team to look at the problem list holistically rather than in its natural format of *silos* of information (i.e., information systems that don't communicate with other systems, inhibiting knowledge flow and connectivity). In order to make a balanced recommendation of patient care, the medical team must consider complex interrelated body functions, priorities of treatment, and possible interactions (Clinical Informatics n.d.).

POMR methodology is commonly used in veterinary teaching hospitals. When it is used in for-profit, private veterinary hospitals, it often takes a much more abbreviated form than described here (Wilson 1988, 318; AAHA, *Medical Records Manual*, n.d., 2.02). (For a sample progress notes log, see Figure 8.1).

COMBINATION OF SOMR AND POMR

The third way to organize a medical record combines the source-oriented and problem-oriented methods. The combination approach is probably the most efficient way to organize the medical record from the private veterinary practice perspective.

In a combination method, the medical record includes a major problem list and a vaccination history and organizes the initial examination into the SOAP format. The major identified problems follow, with a source-oriented format, until the appearance of a new, significant issue. At that time, a complete and thorough SOAP write-up may occur.

FILING MEDICAL RECORDS

The hard-copy portions of medical records must be arranged systematically. Doctors' notes are maintained on cards or in folders. Options range from plain five-inch by eight-inch index cards to preformatted medical record pages for each part of the record, mounted in a file folder. The detailed records made on these sheets range from medical notes and surgical summaries to laboratory findings and ultrasound scans.

Several companies manufacture folder systems specifically designed for medical records in animal hospitals. These ready-made, professionally produced systems are easy to add to when more folders are needed. These companies have also devised sensible color-coded filing methods, which can make filing less time consuming and diminish the number of filing errors.

Cards and folders can be filed alphabetically, numerically, or with a combination of both. Since the alphabet is recognized and understood by everyone, alpha filing is the most commonly used filing system. With this system most employees can learn to file fairly easily because most people find it easiest to visualize information by name (client name, patient name, vendor name, etc.) in alphabetical order (Ancom 1999). The alphabetical method does not require a cross-reference file.

The main disadvantage of the alphabetical system is that the employee doing the filing must be able to spell accurately and recognize when files are out of alphabetic sequence. Unfortunately, misfiled records are common with the alphabetical system, especially when filing records of clients with the same or similar last names.

Numeric filing is more convenient when the records you are filing are identified with numbers, such as invoices, purchase orders, rabies tags, and health certificates, but it can also be applied to patient files. With the numerical system, each client is assigned a number, and records are filed from lowest to highest number. The numbers may simply be assigned in consecutive order, or they may be the client's telephone number. Clients' names and corresponding file numbers must be listed in a separate cross-reference file.

The numerical system's advantages are that numbers are easier to read and spelling is not a factor. Numerical systems are one of the most practical systems for large volumes of records because no file duplication occurs. Numerals can be put together in infinite combinations, so each number is unique (ibid.). The primary disadvantage is the need for an alphabetic cross-reference file. It can be more time consuming to use, because to find a client file, the employee must first look up the client's number. If telephone numbers are used, files need to be updated whenever a client gets a new phone number.

Implementation and ease of use in both numerical and alphabetical systems can be improved with *signaling devices*. Signaling devices can be colored metal or plastic tabs attached to the record or colored stickers attached to folders. Color-coded labels reduce file retrieval time, increase filing and sorting speed, and provide a way to quickly identify misfiled records.

Each combination of letters or each number has an assigned color. Signal tabs can also be used to designate specific groups of files. For example, patient files for animals that require vaccinations, dentistry, or other regular preventive services can be flagged at specified time intervals to indicate when reminders should be sent. Signals can also be used to flag clients who owe money. Colored tabs or stickers could be used to denote the number of days that the account is overdue or to indicate clients to whom estimates have previously been given.

Color-coded year tabs can also be used to show the last year of a patient or client encounter. Inactive files can be spotted at a glance using this system. Contact those clients who have not visited the hospital within a policy-defined period of time and purge the files according to the outcome of those communications.

The cost of misfiled records is hard to quantify (Stockner 1995, 179). Many employees dislike filing and will put the job off for as long as possible. Make your filing system as user-friendly as possible. Relying on employees' alphabetizing skill is not enough. If your practice uses a hard-copy medical record system, invest in a visual signal system. Otherwise, move the practice forward to electronic medical records through the veterinary practice information management system.

Logs in Veterinary Practices

A log is a continuous record, generally kept chronologically, for one particular veterinary service or service type. Logs serve multiple purposes, but three are paramount: (1) They are kept to comply with legal requirements, such as those mandating that records must be kept on the use of controlled substances; (2) they provide evidence in the event of a malpractice claim; and (3) they are convenient for quick data analysis and auditing.

Examples of the use of logs in data analysis abound. For example, the laboratory log could tell you the number of heartworm tests completed in the last month. As practice manager, you could compare this figure with the practice information management database to find out how many clients receiving a heartworm-test recommendation actually followed through with a screening test. You could see if sending a postcard reminder improved these rates. Or, you might use the surgery log to research average time requirements for various surgeries, which ultimately could enable you to make improvements in appointment-scheduling and workflow issues. Using the radiology log, doctors could compare various exposure techniques. In a pen-and-paper environment, each type of log is maintained as a separate record. Reference to the various logs can be made in each patient record where appropriate.

From a business management perspective, logs are also important for maintaining quality control. Logs, in conjunction with economic and financial data, help to justify certain procedures and the amount of work done in various service areas. Logs are also a useful resource for auditing the patient record system to ensure that test results were recorded in the patient record and that charges were captured for the work performed and documented in the log. For example, cross-checking the laboratory log of all tests run against the computer system for the same period of tests invoiced, can illustrate gaps where tests were not recorded.

The more commonly maintained logs are described below.

SURGERY LOG

The surgery log records every surgical procedure performed. The record includes:

- Patient name
- Patient weight
- Type of surgery
- Surgeon name
- Technician/veterinary nurse name
- Date and time of surgery
- Length of time to complete the procedure (start and stop times)
- Anesthetic induction and completion times
- Anesthetic monitoring systems used
- Any unusual occurrence

Veterinary technicians and nurses are most often responsible for maintaining surgery logs, although the surgeon may make special notations. The log entry can be completed as surgery progresses, with the surgeon narrating any details to be transcribed.

ANESTHESIA LOG

An anesthesia log can include:

- Patient name
- Patient weight
- Relative risk factor
- Types and dosages of anesthesia and other pharmacological agents used
- Type of surgery or other procedure
- Doctor name
- Anesthesiologist name
- Date and time of anesthetic procedure
- Length of time to complete the anesthetic procedure (start and stop times listed)
- Any unusual occurrence, including anesthetic deaths or serious complications

The anesthesia log may be maintained separately from the surgery log, since many anesthetic procedures are for purposes other than surgery, or it may be integrated with the surgery log to avoid redundancy.

Using an electronic spreadsheet such as Microsoft Excel to create a template anesthetic form can increase efficiency and accuracy in creating a patient's anesthetic plan. A form can provide for input of all requisite information, including dosages for anesthetic agents and pain medications, automatically calculated based on weight. It can also include an emergency plan. Once the electronically based form is completed, it can be printed in hard copy to keep with the patient during the hospital stay, added to the patient's file, added to the anesthetic log, and/ or saved as an electronic copy integrated with the patient record.

CONTROLLED DRUG LOG

Controlled substances are those drugs that are subject to abuse, the possession and use of which are regulated under the Controlled Substances Act. Under the act, the federal government classifies controlled substances according to their potential for addiction and abuse. Laws pertaining to doctors of veterinary medicine and their conduct as registered prescribers and dispensers of controlled substances are very specific and affect veterinary hospital use and control of these drugs.

Federal laws are enforced by the Drug Enforcement Administration (DEA), which requires strict records of controlled substances. State agencies may have even stricter standards. Whichever requirement is more stringent takes precedence.

By federal law, the hospital must keep a record of all controlled substances dispensed. Federal law states that a separate record, in addition to the patient record, is to be maintained for certain classes of drugs: "All inventories and records of controlled substances in Schedule II must be maintained separately from all other records. All inventories and records of controlled substances in Schedules III, IV, and V must be maintained separately or must be in such form that they are readily retrievable from the ordinary professional and business records" (U.S. Department of Justice 1990).

Federal law does not specifically require a separate log apart from the patient medical records and purchase documentation for any substance classified as less than Schedule II. However, maintaining such a log is strongly advised.

A separate log of controlled substances dispensed and administered provides significant benefits:
- The log provides a clear, concise, and contemporaneous record of all controlled substances administered and dispensed.
- The log provides an easy method of ensuring that all controlled substances are accounted for in the proper manner.
- The DEA will consider the log to be readily retrievable from the ordinary business records as defined by federal regulations. Thus, a separate log effectively keeps the DEA out of the practice's business records (Miller 1998).

Controlled-drug log requirements may vary according to state and provincial requirements. As a practice manager, you must be familiar with all areas of correct record and inventory maintenance of controlled substances. Noncompliance can result in extremely stiff fines, massive legal expenses, licensure loss, and bad publicity. Check with your federal, state, or provincial governments for the specific laws in your area. Every year, check for updates in the law, reread the requirements, and audit your hospital for compliance.

The need for strict attention to this area of practice management cannot be overemphasized. AAHA publishes a controlled-substance log that is reviewed by the DEA and specific to veterinary hospital use. The set is made up of six copies of the "Unopened and Opened Container Log" and two copies of the "Initial and Biennial Inventory Forms." Because the latter are stand-alone forms, you can easily store them separately from other drug logs, as required by law. Each copy of the "Unopened and Opened Container Log" features an initials entry log, an unopened container log, an opened container log, and a physical count log for added accountability. Using a separate log for each controlled substance is recommended for easy access to the pertinent information.

A sample of the AAHA log appears in Figure 8.2.

ADVERSE-EVENT LOG

Animals sometimes experience negative reactions to drugs and other therapeutic products intended to help them. An adverse-event log tracks any such incidents. If adverse events recur for the same product, it may be important to report the problem to outside parties.

Adverse drug reactions are unexpected side effects or unintended changes resulting from the administration of drugs. Adverse reactions can also occur in response to topically applied pesticides, commercially prepared food, and biologics such as vaccines.

As the MedWatch website of the Food and Drug Administration (FDA) states, the FDA has responsibility for ensuring the "safety and efficacy of all regulated, marketed medical products including drugs, biologics, and medical and radiation-emitting devices. Health professionals who monitor for and report serious adverse events and product problems to [the] FDA, either directly or via the manufacturer, are integral to this process."

MedWatch is the FDA safety information and adverse reporting service. The MedWatch program goal is to advance postmarketing surveillance of medical products used in clinical practice and to rapidly identify significant health hazards associated with these products.

The FDA arm for veterinary practitioners, the Center for Veterinary Medicine (CVM), maintains a separate adverse-reaction reporting site specifically for veterinarians (see www.fda.gov/AnimalVeterinary/SafetyHealth/default.htm). For FDA-approved drugs, veterinarians are encouraged to contact the drug company about any suspected adverse drug event (ADE). The company's technical services veterinarian will complete the FDA reporting forms.

FIGURE 8.2 CONTROLLED SUBSTANCE LOG SAMPLE PAGE

INCLUDED ON
COMPANION
WEBSITE

Drug Name _Diazepam_   Container Size_____ _5 ml_   Strength_____ _10 mg/ml_   Form _Injectable_

Date	Client, Patient	Client Address/ID (or bottle description/lot from unopened container log)	Unique Btl. #	Reason/ Notes	Amount Added	Amount Used	Balance	Initials	Initials When Physical Count Taken
1/18/20xx	STARTING BALANCE (from previous page)		5				2.6 ml		
1/18/20xx	Crandell, "Bubbles"	101 Oak Circle, Anywhere, USA 00111	5	Ear Flush		1.1 ml	1.5 ml	KLG	
1/19/20xx	Johnston, "Dudley"	202 Main St. Nowhere, USA 11000	5	Neuter		0.7 ml	0.8 ml	KLG	
1/19/20xx	Cranfield "Tess"	300 Grand Blvd. Someplace, USA 10011	5	Spay		0.8 ml	0.0 ml	RBA	
1/19/20xx	From unopened container log	AVRI1078 - exp. date Mar. 2015	6	new bottle	5.0 ml		5.0 ml	RBA	
1/19/20xx	Cranfield "Tess"	300 Grand Blvd. Someplace, USA 10011	6	Spay		0.6 ml	4.4 ml	RBA	KLG

Copyright 2011 American Animal Hospital Association

Non-FDA-approved drugs for animal administration can be reported directly to the FDA on a reporting form that is available through the FDA website (use Form FDA 1932a for voluntary reporting of veterinary adverse events and Form FDA 3500A for mandatory reporting of veterinary adverse events).

The FDA site includes information for reporting suspected adverse events involving animal biologics such as vaccines, bacterins, and diagnostic kits to the U.S. Department of Agriculture.

The Environmental Protection Agency (EPA) has regulatory jurisdiction over pesticides, including many popular veterinary products that are topically applied to the animal's skin or hair coat. Report suspected adverse reactions to EPA-regulated topically applied pesticides to the EPA. Information can be found through the websites of the FDA or the EPA, or through an Internet search for "Veterinary Pesticide Adverse Effects Reporting," which will guide you to a website for the National Pesticide Information Center. Veterinary professionals can fill out a form online.

The FDA site also provides instructions for reporting pet-food complaints electronically through a linked safety-reporting portal managed by the U.S. Department of Health and Human Services or by contacting the individual state's FDA Consumer Complaint Coordinators.

The diligence of veterinarians and their employees in reporting adverse reactions can help ensure that new safety information is rapidly communicated to the veterinary medical community. Fast reporting of adverse events can result in product labeling changes early in a new drug's life span, which is one reason for directly reporting to the manufacturer's technical veterinary team. Adverse-event logs are an important step in this process, in that they gather information that could ultimately affect the health of animal patients nationwide.

A commercial software product called the "Veterinary Pharmacy Reference" integrates with several popular veterinary management software programs, providing a searchable database of drug reactions.

IMAGING LOG

The imaging log records each and every radiographic image procedure and can be expanded to all forms of medical imaging technology used in the hospital, such as computerized tomography (CT) and magnetic resonance imaging (MRI). The log includes:

- Patient and client information
- The area of the body imaged
- The number and size of images obtained
- The machine settings used to obtain the correct exposure (technique used)
- The radiographic or other image findings (the veterinarian's interpretation of the image created)
- Initials of person taking radiograph
- Level of sedation (awake, sedated, anesthetized)

This log may be necessary to meet state or provincial government regulations regarding public health and radiation safety.

ULTRASOUND LOG

The ultrasound log records ultrasound procedures. Given the technology, logs may be automated to varying degrees within the system. Logged data should include:

- Patient and client information
- The area of the body scanned
- The location of stored images
- The ultrasound findings (the veterinarian's interpretation of the image created)

Many managers are incorporating telemedicine procedures into their practices, which involves transmitting images via the Internet to outside specialists for interpretation. In this situation, the log might also include the type of data and time of transmission, the number of images transmitted, and the name of the specialist receiving the images.

LABORATORY LOG

The laboratory log can be as extensive as needed. A hospital manager may implement a master log that records the laboratory work sent to outside reference labs and a second log for all procedures completed in-house. In-house logs can be maintained for microscopic studies, including fecal examinations, urinalyses, cytologies, and parasite smears; serum and whole blood work, including heartworm, leukemia, and similar "kit" tests, and complete blood counts and serum chemistries; or microbiology work, including microbacterial cultures and sensitivities as well as fungal cultures. These logs would include the following information:

- Outside reference lab log
  - » Client and patient name
  - » Date and time of sample collection
  - » Time of test
  - » Result of test
  - » Mode of shipment/carrier name
  - » Name of outside lab
  - » Type of sample sent
  - » Type of test
  - » Doctor name
  - » Date test results received
  - » Date client called
- In-house laboratory logs
  - » Client and patient name
  - » Date and time of sample collection
  - » Date client called
  - » Time of test
  - » Type of test
  - » Initials of test taker
  - » Result of test

As veterinary hospitals add high-end laboratory equipment beyond a microscope and centrifuge, separate logs may be established at each station. Expect computerized equipment to collect and store much of the data related to patient tests, so logs may be automated through use of such machines.

UNEXPECTED DEATH LOG

A hospital may maintain a log of deceased patients, including those who have died outside the hospital, also called a sentinel event log. If nothing else, this log provides hospital staff with a quick reference to identify patients that have died, thus improving client communication. Ideally, all employees know that a companion animal has died and are able to express condolences when next seeing or talking with the client, such as when the client comes to retrieve the cremation ashes or is calling to set up an appointment for another patient. It can be embarrassing when team members don't know that a patient with ten or fifteen years of history visiting the practice has passed on. Euthanasia procedures can be recorded either in this log or in a separate euthanasia log.

EUTHANASIA LOG

The euthanasia log records information related to patients who are humanely killed in accordance with professionally prescribed guidelines (for example, the "AVMA Guidelines on Euthanasia," available at www.avma.org/issues/animal_welfare/euthanasia.pdf). The log includes:

- Patient and client name
- Date and time of procedure
- Reason for elected euthanasia
- Method of humane euthanasia

If controlled drugs are used for euthanasia, this log not only provides retrieval information but also helps the practice meet legal requirements for recording controlled-substance administration.

SYRINGE/NEEDLE DISPOSAL AND MEDICAL WASTE LOG

In some states, logs that document medical waste generation are required. Even the disposal of deceased patients may be regulated. Many regulations promulgated by state environmental protection agencies may have application to veterinary hospitals. Every year, check with your attorney and state veterinary medical association to keep up with rapidly changing legislation in this area. Companies that provide assistance in maintaining OSHA compliance may offer ancillary support for meeting federal and state waste-disposal requirements.

CONSENT AND RELEASE FORMS

Many patient risks can be associated with medical treatment and surgery. Although quality veterinary services are commensurate with what is available in human medicine, they can be perceived as expensive by clients who do not understand the full scope of education, skill, equipment, facilities, pharmaceuticals, patient support systems, and other contributing costs involved.

To make informed decisions about veterinary health care for their animals, clients require clear and accurate information. Verbal communication alone may not be adequate. Many times, clients may not fully understand everything that has been said to them. Written information helps to clarify what might not be heard, understood, or remembered from conversation. Often, an essential aspect of client communication resides in written agreements between the client and the hospital about the level of patient care to be given.

In human medicine, the doctrine of *informed consent* requires that information be plainly conveyed so that a patient can decide on and approve a suggested course of care. In veterinary medicine, this legal doctrine is called owner consent, to differentiate the fact that animals are considered property (Rezendes and Kahler 2007).

The doctrine of owner consent is based on the need for clear communication with the legally and financially responsible owner of an animal to avoid misunderstanding about care and commensurate cost. The veterinary practice offers to provide certain services in exchange for the client's promise to pay. Owner consent helps each party to the agreement to understand the parameters of its obligations to the other party.

Information described in oral and written informed consent agreements includes known risks, alternatives, prognoses, possible complications, and an estimate of the fees to be charged. Discussion with the client, usually by the doctor when the condition or outcome is serious, and notes contemporaneously made in the medical record documenting the discussion, may fulfill the requirements of owner consent. Signed consent forms by traditional or electronic signature are part of the medical records and should be retained with them.

Written consent forms should be used wherever appropriate. Many times, the veterinarian or manager picks up a vibe that a particular client might end up being a problem. If difficulty or misunderstanding can be anticipated, obtain written consent.

Consider seeking written release from responsibility when the client is not following directions or recommendations about patient care. Another indication that written consent should be obtained is that an owner requests copies of information or documents pertaining to an animal currently under your hospital's care. In all cases where euthanasia is performed, a written consent form should first be obtained.

While the use of written consent forms can vary considerably, depending on the practice, practice location, perceived animal value, and type of medical problem, it may be simple, good practice policy to simply obtain written client authorization the majority of the time.

The AVMA has a position statement on owner consent (AVMA, "Owner Consent," 2007). You should be aware of it, as professional position statements help guide what veterinarians do in accord with professional ethical rules.

Possible types of practice consent and release forms to have available for client signature follow. These examples would apply when the client is giving the practice the authorization to proceed with a particular procedure while buffering the practice from certain liabilities:

- Consent for treatment
- Consent for anesthesia
- Consent to perform surgery (anesthesia consent could be combined with surgery consent)
- Consent for dentistry, including extractions
- Consent for euthanasia
- Consent to continue treatment for a terminally ill patient
- Release allowing the client to restrain an animal while it is being treated, although client restraint of the animal is against the advice of the veterinarian
- Request for release of medical records

- Release caused by refusal by the owner of specific tests or procedures recommended by the veterinarian

Many times, potential problems are easily resolved by simply asking a difficult client to sign a release form. The act of reading and signing a formal document defining the risks could convince the client to relent in her insistence to restrain a pet during treatment, for example.

Consent forms may be customized to meet the practice's particular needs. Frequently used forms should be available as computer templates or integrated with the practice management software, to be completed as needed. Electronic signing speeds the process and saves paper, although supplying a printed copy to the client may be a good protocol.

A useful source for sample forms is the book *Legal Consent Forms for Veterinary Practices* by James F. Wilson (2006), available through AAHA Press. The book includes samples of many different consent and release forms as well as a companion website with downloadable forms that can be customized.

Consent and release forms, like any agreement or contract, are legal documents. Before using any sample form, regardless of source, ask the practice's attorney to review it. Laws can change, and state laws vary. The reason for using legal documents is to mitigate potential problems later. If the document will not hold up in a dispute, you have wasted your time in using it and potentially increased the risk you intended to reduce.

Improving Practice Management through Medical Record Audit and Peer Review

Recall that a significant secondary purpose of medical records is to facilitate assessment of the overall quality of patient medical care provided by the hospital team. The regular, ongoing evaluation of medical records is integral to the overall practice management control system. The medical record standards you set and the monitoring processes you implement become control benchmarks for improving service quality and compliance.

Controls are aimed at minimizing lost fee charges, increasing doctor productivity and service provisions, and improving patient care. Patient record evaluation also seeks to find ways to provide services more efficiently, reducing wasted time, supplies, and other costs.

Although these secondary purposes concern practice-wide issues, often these issues can be identified through spot-checks of individual patient files. Medical record maintenance and compliance with standard practice guidelines, for example, can be tested with the following steps, using a single patient encounter:

1. Collect the patient travel or circle sheet, the hard-copy medical record (paper-file practice) or EMR (paper-light practice), the client check-in form, and the client transaction history from the practice management software system.

2. Compare records to test for understatements or discrepancies, that is, omissions of information from one record that appears in another.
3. Compare the records to the practice guidelines.

In this type of audit, you are comparing various documents that are unique to a single patient against one another to look for discrepancies and omissions. For example, the doctor's notes may refer to the fact that two liters of fluid were administered, but the invoice record might state that only a single liter was charged to the client.

This type of audit also tests for compliance of completed patient care against practice guidelines. For example, practice guidelines might state that when a pet receives a body score of seven, a member of the practice team should counsel the client about weight management and therapeutic nutrition options. Information on when the counseling took place should then appear in the records, along with any predefined follow-up exam dates for weight checks and estimated refill dates for the recommended dietary product. If the follow-up care is not being offered, opportunities to enhance animal health are being missed. Staff training in the corresponding areas can take place once the shortcoming is recognized.

REVIEWING FOR COMPLIANCE ACROSS JOB FUNCTIONS

When undertaking a compliance evaluation through an audit of medical records, begin with the receptionist. How competently does the receptionist capture the presenting complaint in the appointment register and the travel sheet? This information should carry through to the POMR and doctors' notes. Did the invoice capture all services and dispensed items, as proven through a cross-referencing analysis of all the information from the various source documents?

In these tests, you are checking the receptionist's ability to communicate with the client and capture all charges collected from doctors and technicians. The inpatient or outpatient travel sheet is cross-referenced to the invoice, as is the hard copy of the medical record or the EMR, which may have additional comments. The client check-in form may also isolate additional services that never made it to the examination room, or, if they did and were performed, never made it to the medical record and back to the invoice.

Cross-referencing the various information sources against each other elucidates how well the reception team is organized and trained and how attentive receptionists are to invoice detail. While receptionists are checked for compliance, the medical side of the practice can also be evaluated.

REVIEWING FOR MEDICAL SERVICES COMPLIANCE

When auditing records with the medical team in focus, you may find that the number of missed services can be remarkable. These omissions are costly to the practice. For example, a patient that was presented by the client with a medical problem might have been charged on the invoice for only a physical examination at the regular office visit fee. Missing commentary or doctors' notes in the medical record may reveal that additional services should have been offered, that recommendations could have been made, or that re-call and recheck reminders should have been scheduled. As the practice manager, your role is to meet with the various veterinarians and other team members, coach them in how to recommend all appropriate services, and train them in how to capture fees.

Medical personnel can also cause lost fees by handling discounts haphazardly. If several patients are seen in a single client visit, are the clinicians and receptionists making the right billing decisions about group discounts? It may be consistent with your practice philosophy to provide a nominal discount for multiple animals. However, arbitrary decisions to grant discounts can cause difficulties with clients on subsequent visits, not to mention the possibility of lost income. Make sure everyone agrees on how multiple patients will be handled, and then test subsequent records according to the resulting policy.

In evaluating a patient record from a medical perspective, look for thoroughness and appropriate follow-up care. Compare the record with whatever practice compliance guidelines have been put into effect. For example, if guidelines state that at every appointment, a patient is to be weighed and given a *body condition score* (BCS), do both a current weight and BCS appear for every appointment seen in the current week or month?

If guidelines do not exist or are in development, fall back to the question of known practice philosophy and values. Possibly revisit basic teaching hospital protocols for case management, particularly those involving record-keeping structures following the POMR and SOAP outline. Evidence of erratic record documentation supports the decision to implement and enforce standard record-keeping methods that will provide optimal documentation and the most organized approach to patient care and revenue capture.

REVIEWING FOR REMINDER AND CALL-BACK SYSTEM COMPLIANCE

When evaluating patient vaccination histories, audit the information-management reminder settings, including future notification dates and preset linkage with invoiced services. Are the requisite reminders for the various patient species in place, accurately reflecting practice care guidelines? If a client has several animals, does each have appropriate reminders in the system?

What will the reminders say, at the future date the system sends them to clients? Do reminders use client-friendly terminology, which will convey the importance of the services as well as their value?

When it comes to the reminder system, do not rely on hard-copy medical records if they are still in use. Practices in transition from manual systems to fully deployed electronic medical records that include doctors' notes may be missing essential reminders and re-call cues. Do not manage reminders through a manual system.

When migrating data from one type of practice management software to a different software program, be extraordinarily cautious. Maintain the old system in parallel with the new, and check client, patient, and reminder data meticulously for several months, if not for a full year. When transitioning from one system to another, the practice is at high risk for data-migration and data-linkage failures, potentially resulting in missed reminders, lost income, and increased costs through time expenditure and payroll.

When moving from a manual system to an automated one, incorporate the reminder system as rapidly as possible when adding clients and patients to the computer database. Reminder and re-call system automation has been shown to dramatically boost revenue realization through increased notification and client compliance.

Also audit the records for team call-back compliance in accord with practice guidelines. In multi-doctor practices, case follow-through might be made more difficult because of missed communications resulting from inadequate record detail. Review any medical-record commentary that suggests missed re-calls.

As an illustration, assume a patient presents with a client complaint of depression and diarrhea. A physical exam occurs, a fecal parasite screen comes up negative, and the veterinarian suggests additional laboratory tests that are not completed at the time of the first patient encounter. Does the medical record include the doctor's notes describing the plan, the specific tests to conduct, and a concrete time in which to accomplish the additional workup? Furthermore, was a re-call scheduled to find out how the patient was progressing, having been discharged with palliative therapy?

In the absence of such information, it is easy to assume that a clinician may have advised the client to call if further problems were observed, but the assumption could be wrong. Notations of client communications related to patient care should always be recorded in the medical record. In this example, an assigned team member should call the client, not rely on the client to call with a progress report. Complete doctors' notes should allow any other veterinarian to take over case management with little hesitation about next steps in the treatment plan or what to discuss with the client.

REVIEWING FOR COMPLETENESS OF PHYSICAL EXAM FINDINGS

Hospitals using paper medical records often make good use of rubber stamps or adhesive checklist templates, such as those for standard vital sign recording in accord with practice guidelines. Some practices integrate body-system examination templates as separate chart pages to encourage a systematic and complete approach to a thorough medical record. Templates and checklists both in the hard-copy and electronic medical records effectively cue the doctor to complete a systematic physical examination. The doctor can quickly check or make a notation by each body system designated on the template.

Templates can be based on body diagrams such as those illustrating body condition scores or allowing a rendition of the size and location of a corneal lesion. Diagrams allow the doctor to quickly indicate location and size of lesions or other findings. In some templates, the doctor makes a notation on the record about the status of the animal on the date of the examination by simply circling a "yes" or "no" answer. Templates like these are now widely available in electronic format for use with touch-pad technology.

One disadvantage to the template system is reliance on the doctor to include additional commentary regarding recommendations made to the client, plans for diagnostic workup, and a defined course of action for the current examination as well as for the future. The doctors must be dedicated to following through on these details.

Doctor efficiency in documenting physical examination findings and communication of care recommendations can be increased through dictation. Audio recordings made by the doctor can also be used, with a transcriptionist to key the information into the EMR. The narration can include patient history, presenting complaints, physical examination findings, plans for treatment, and care recommendations made to the client. Speech recognition software can also be used.

The resulting record should be legible and complete. It should provide a good roadmap of the patient's course of treatment, the patient's response to treatment, and plans for additional care.

HOW REVIEWS STRENGTHEN THE PRACTICE

Periodic medical record audits are a valuable practice management tool for evaluating doctor and technician competencies and compliance in treatment and charting as well as in other practice policies and systems.

An experienced team member can audit approximately ten patient records in thirty minutes. This includes making notations, assessing where tasks were not consistently completed, and planning follow-through in employee training or redefining care guidelines. A small investment of time in this key management process will yield a substantial profit.

Oversight of essential processes is a requirement that never expires. Recall that client adherence is primarily a function of solid and consistently delivered recommendations with adequate follow-through. Managers who consistently check records for completeness, consistency of recommendations, and follow-through via effective reminder systems can provide timely and pertinent feedback to the entire team while also bolstering practice profitability.

Whenever you are evaluating the medical record system, be open to rethinking organizational guidelines and the direction of employee development. Prioritize your activities, including the anticipated level of oversight needed to support accountability to defined guidelines and the practice's financial well-being.

Develop systems that promote good medicine and surgery. Make sure checklists, record-keeping forms, and templates are up-to-date. Reexamine the practice's time-honored systems for patient care and client communication. Do new technologies and work-flow processes suggest adaptation and change could enhance the quality of services and improve the income stream?

Thoroughly train and refresh receptionist client service skills as needed. Consider conducting cross-training and job rotations as well, so that team members develop ever-increasing knowledge about hospital procedures and protocols that helps them garner more income for the practice. Informal training sessions, such as *"lunch and learns,"* conducted periodically at less busy times can increase knowledge, revenues, client satisfaction, and patient care.

Leverage the expertise of your staff. For instance, use doctors with excellent record-keeping skills to regularly peer-review patient records prepared by veterinarians and technicians and to mentor case-management discussions. As an ancillary quality-management technique, have associate doctors review the patient records of the more experienced doctors and vice versa. Three-hundred-and-sixty-degree peer review allows the practice to optimize educational backgrounds, experiential knowledge, and different approaches to medical or surgical treatment.

Legal Issues in Medical Record Management

The patient record serves as a legal as well as a medical document. Medical records will be the most important and often the only documents introduced in a malpractice lawsuit. A complete, accurate, and legible medical record is a veterinarian's best defense against a client's allegations of professional negligence or malpractice (Allison n.d.).

By the same token, an incomplete, inaccurate, or illegible record can be considered as an admission of professional incompetence and a sign of service that is below the standard of acceptable care. Remember, "If it's not on the record, then it wasn't done," and if the record cannot be read, then the same conclusion may be made.

Here are some rules that will help to ensure complete and accurate medical records:

- Medical records must be handwritten legibly in black or blue ink, typed, or computer generated.
- Every person who has made an entry on a record should be identifiable, and by more than their handwriting. Each entry to the record should be dated and initialed, and for even more credibility, the time that the entry was made should also be noted.
- No record notation should ever be erased, covered with correction fluid, deleted, or in any way obliterated. If an error is made, it should be crossed out and the correct notation entered in the margin or in an addendum. Corrections must be dated and initialed and must contain an explanation for the change.
- Standard and approved abbreviations and notations should be used.

No matter how complete medical records are, many practices will eventually face questions that pertain to the ownership, possession, access, confidentiality, and retention of medical records, radiographs, and other supporting documents. From time to time, owners request patient records or other documents. Interested parties outside the hospital may request information on a particular animal. As an example, a pet-shop owner who wants to buy puppies from a breeder-client might inquire about inherited defects in an animal your hospital has treated. Governmental agencies, such as public health authorities, may request information and records pertaining to hospital patients. Veterinary medical records can also be subpoenaed.

Rights of veterinary medical record ownership, and access and questions of confidentiality and retention, vary by state or province. Only a few states currently have laws pertaining to confidentiality of veterinary medical records. The specific facts and circumstances of a situation involving requests for release of patient information will have a bearing on whether or not records are disclosed. Owner consent may or may not be required. It is commonly considered good practice not to disclose information in a patient medical record to another party without the client's consent (Hannah 1996, 570–571). Obtain the consent in writing if there is any doubt.

Generally, the original records made during the course of a patient's treatment are owned by the attending medical professionals or the hospital in which they are employed or are practicing. Records usually do not belong to the client. However, most states will hold that a client has the right to examine the records and a right to receive a copy of the records from the veterinarian, whether or not the client's bill for the treatment has been paid.

As with any situation that might involve litigation, the practice's retained attorney should be consulted when the hospital is confronted with demands for medical records or other documents by parties outside the hospital. An excellent resource on some of the legal intricacies and nuances of medical record ownership, confidentiality, and retention is Chapter 14 of *Law and Ethics of the Veterinary Profession* by James F. Wilson (1988). (See also "Client Confidentiality" in Chapter 7 of this book and the section on "Consent and Release Forms" that appears earlier in this chapter.)

Electronic Medical Records

Computer technology has evolved rapidly to provide efficient record storage and retrieval in veterinary practice and to increase data availability for improved patient care and analysis. The veterinary profession has benefited enormously from the advances of the past two decades in both computer equipment technology and software development. As equipment costs decreased, processor speeds accelerated, networking capabilities grew, data storage expanded, and speedy Internet access became a necessity, not a luxury.

And yet, no software programs are flawless. Some programs or program upgrades fail to do what they promise to do, and some can hinder productivity by introducing bugs and glitches. "Promise-ware" is the term given to software that is touted to do more than it is actually capable of doing (Sheridan and McCafferty 1993, 98). There is plenty of promise-ware out there, and it is wise to stay away from it by doing your homework.

It is important to find the right balance when incorporating computer technology into veterinary practice. Whereas some practice managers are too quick to adopt new technology, always wanting the latest thing, others resist new technology, causing their practices to lag behind. A savvy practice manager learns to balance the desire to jump ahead with a sense of caution—but not too much caution.

Investigate proposed system changes carefully, and dedicate plenty of time to planning before transitioning to a new system. Choose software that has been tested and reviewed positively by others, and purchase it from a practice-management software company that will provide adequate customer support and training.

MANAGEMENT SOFTWARE IS NOT QUITE PERFECT

Animal hospitals have varying capacities for maintaining electronic medical records. Often the ones that have not adapted computer technology have been limited more by employee resistance than by software capability. Practice-management software companies have developed highly integrated products, generally centering on the invoicing function, yet increasingly providing robust options for managing patient-care notes and medical records. These often effectively allow one data entry point to feed many purposes.

Most practice-management software programs attempt to provide the same benefits as paper records while adding new benefits that paper records cannot match. For example, paper records are very flexible because they allow the veterinary team to expand the patient chart to include whatever forms or information are deemed valuable. Veterinary practice-management software programs offer similar options through customizable word-processing templates. In the past, it was difficult to add a data field for a patient or a new client parameter. It is now common for practice managers to obtain help from program developers to write in a change or determine a work-around solution.

When investigating new software product, keep a must-have list and a wish list of the features you desire. Interview prospective providers and test-drive the software to see what each product is capable of doing without modification. Spend time at practices that use the software and interview their employees to gauge the level of software-company customer service. The software company should have a proven track record in supporting software operation, advancing changes, and providing training and other services (see also next section, "Choosing Practice Management Software").

As mentioned, many hospitals continue to use a combination of computerized and paper systems. Some hospitals use the electronic patient-medical-management portion of their computer software only to generate reminders and show which animal was treated on a particular sales invoice. To complete these baseline functions, the staff need only maintain the patient profile data (name, date of birth, breed, sex, color) on the computer. Even so, much more information can be compiled in the computerized patient record than the invoicing and reminder functions utilize.

Once the patient profile is established on the computer, the invoicing feature maintains a rudimentary patient and client history. Each time a service or product is charged to the client for that particular animal, an entry is saved in the patient record. The patient's computer history will therefore include key invoicing information: the invoice date (approximate treatment date); the services, products, or medicines that were invoiced; and the quantities invoiced. When vaccines are invoiced, the software should automatically update the reminder system to reflect the next date the patient is due for a booster immunization.

This automatic history function, based on the invoicing process, is in and of itself quite valuable. Even if a doctor has forgotten to write anything at all on the patient record, or if the hard copy of the record is lost, a record exists in the computer system that at least shows dates of treatment and what was done (assuming the doctor charged for everything).

Keep in mind, however, that this rudimentary listing of invoiced services and products on a specific date for a particular patient does not meet AAHA standards of medical record maintenance. If the "paperless" or "paper-light" hospital has no history of patient management and client communication in the electronic database other than the financial transaction history, then its medical record system will be sadly lacking.

CHOOSING PRACTICE MANAGEMENT SOFTWARE

When choosing practice management software, start by examining the training programs offered by specific software companies. Many offer trials of software, demonstrations, or even hands-on personal training during the implementation process. Depending on doctor and employee familiarity with the particular brand of practice management software, the available training can be a very important factor. Many practices invest heavily in an information management system but do not receive the full obtainable value because they simply do not know how to use all the available features.

Be sure to review the software product's medical-record features. Many of these programs provide for structured records with SOAP features, allow for rapid retrieval of historical patient data, and search records for treatments, diagnosis, and types of patients. Most top-shelf programs also provide integration with outside laboratories, allowing for quick access to easily searchable lab results, and include them in a patient's history. Full-featured programs can even directly interface with your own laboratory equipment. Also ensure that the system tracks all users who access and modify the record. (See "Record Alteration.")

However, medical records are not the only consideration when investing in practice management software. You will also need to find out how the software handles inventory tracking and reorder lists, for example. In addition, the software may offer a variety of reporting and analysis capabilities. You may be able to track financial measures such as revenues by profit center, or complete productivity reports and trend analysis. These capabilities can be very valuable. (For other features to consider, see the textbox, "Software Features.")

NOT QUITE PAPERLESS

Many practices are in transition, working from paper patient medical histories toward EMR systems. These systems should be based in strong quality controls and high medical-record standards commensurate with strong paper charting methodology. An otherwise well-organized veterinary office is the ideal candidate for implementing an EMR system. Starting with a good paper medical record system greatly helps in the transition to an electronic format. As Robert H. Featherstone put it, "Never computerize something for which you don't already have a good manual system." Transitioning poor medical record-keeping processes to an electronic format will not improve the quality of a medical practice or enhance a provider's ability to respond to a malpractice claim (Princeton Insurance 2008).

Generally, veterinary practice management software programs capture patient medical-record detail when a care plan with an estimate is created and at the point of invoicing. Additional information can be sent to the patient record through the invoice by including no-charge service codes. Examples of no-charge service codes are, "Your technician today was Jennifer, who is glad to answer additional questions you might have," or, "Thank you for your visit, Lisa, receptionist." These messages provide the client with helpful reference names and establish record data that aid in management of follow-up when questions arise about any issue related to the visit.

Other program options may include message codes that allow for client instructions to be added to the invoice. For example, several codes might produce the following messages at the bottom of the invoice: "Your pet has been diagnosed with a urinary bladder infection"; "Call us in 3 days if you do not notice any improvement"; "A repeat urinalysis and culture is scheduled in four weeks."

Many programs have incorporated templates that mimic traditional, successfully used forms, such as the patient examination report card. Standard exam observations can be preset to populate each health system field while also allowing for doctor overrides with customized

Software Features

Deciding which type of practice software to use is a big decision that will affect many different areas of management. The main issues are described in the accompanying text. Here are some additional questions to consider when choosing software for your practice:

- *Navigational ease:* How easy is it to get to various areas of the program from others?
- *Software intuitional ease:* How easy is it for employees to learn the program?
- *Screen organization:* How well are data fields organized in each part of the program?
- *User prompts:* Is it possible to customize alerts and pop-up screens that prompt the user to record important data before moving to the next task?
- *Scheduling interface:* Will you have the ability to view client no-shows, follow-ups, immunization compliance rates, and excessive downtime? Will you have the flexibility to modify the electronic appointment book for practice customization?
- *Boarding modules:* Does the program allow you to specify the needs of multiple pets in a single kennel, condominium, or suite (for example, detailed feeding and medication instructions, exercise needs, and the like)?
- *Whiteboard capability:* Are there large-screen displays of current patient treatment and surgery schedules in real time?
- *Reminder generators:* Does the program offer flexible linkage to a variety of services and products to generate follow-ups and repurchase recommendations, plus the ability to e-mail clients?
- *Invoicing:* Will you have the ability to easily spot a client's outstanding balance and last-payment information from an appointment screen or other commonly used part of the program?
- *Security features:* Are there multiple criteria for limiting employee access to nonessential areas of the user program interface?
- *Audits:* Are there comprehensive audit trails to evaluate the system for evidence of errors and fraud?
- *Patient record management:* Does the software allow for client access of basic patient information online so that clients can supply additions or corrections via the Internet? Such systems can decrease record-keeping time, improve client service, and enhance patient care.
- *Data backup:* Does the program have the capability to maintain complete and secure data backups? Is offsite data storage available to provide additional disaster support coverage?

descriptions of unique patient findings. The final report can be both printed as a client hand-out and included in the patient record as part of the history, assessment, and plan.

Lists of typical instructions and diagnostic comments may come preloaded with various software programs and can be customized with editing and additional information as desired by the practice. Coded comment and instruction lists can lead to inclusion of commonly used insertions on travel sheets. Doctors simply circle the codes associated with the instructions they would like to be added to the invoice and the electronic medical record for each patient.

Some hospitals maintain all doctors' notes on the computer and strive to eliminate hand-written records altogether. Hard copies of radiographs and laboratory reports may still need to be filed, and these can be referenced in the EMR. However, in most computerized practices, separate hard-copy medical records and logs are still maintained. Most doctors must still write comments on the records about subjective observations made by the client, physical-exam and test findings, differential diagnoses, and plans for treatment and communication (following the POMR and SOAP format). And many electronic documents, from invoices to paychecks to annual reports, are eventually printed out on paper. Thus, "paper-light" is a better term than "paperless." A truly "paperless" system is still something of a misnomer in today's veterinary practice.

DATA INPUT METHODS

Several methods may be used to electronically record doctors' notes to the computer. Here are a few:

Transcription. Doctors write notes longhand on the travel sheet, and a veterinary assistant, bookkeeper, or receptionist transcribes them later. Handwritten notes could be scanned and stored as is, but legibility must be good and hard-drive storage capacity adequate, with a reliable electronic filing system.

Typing. Doctors type notes directly into the EMR. When they are completed at the time of the patient visit, these notes may be more complete, since they are prepared contemporaneously with patient observation and client communication. The notes may be typed in at the end of the appointment hour, at the end of the day, or at the end of the week. As with manual record maintenance, the longer the wait, the less complete and accurate the information.

Templates. Doctors use EMR templates to speed data entry. For example, one template might be used to record a complete physical exam of a canine patient, while another is used for a feline patient. The doctor (or assistant) clicks the applicable check boxes for each body system describing normal or abnormal findings. Other templates could be used for laboratory results and findings, vital sign monitoring, SOAP notes, or just about any other need that can be created as an electronic form.

Advantages and Disadvantages of Computerized Medical Records

Advantages:

- Computers take up less space; no large filing cabinets are required.
- Information on the records may be more consistent, especially when more than one doctor is involved, allowing for quicker and more exact data retrieval.
- Client better perceives the quality of medical services provided because information regarding patient care is shared between team members and affiliate companies instantly and seamlessly. Complete and legible records are easily produced to provide to the client and other veterinary service providers, such as specialists.
- Depending on the method of input and the type of data, it takes less time to input information into the computer than to write the same information onto a record.
- Records will always be legible.
- Ease of accessing information from the patient medical history will make it much easier to target market for such services as senior patient workups, dental services, repeat visits, and vaccination reminders.
- It is easier to access medical records and other information from other locations. This is particularly necessary if the hospital has more than one outpatient location. It is also of interest if management and employees would like to be able to monitor records from another location.
- Referral case histories are more complete, resulting in better communication with the specialist and easier transfer of the case.
- It is easier to audit transactional activity and check for missing services or service opportunities, resulting in better revenue capture.
- Peer review is more efficient because records are easier to read and cross-reference with other medical information, invoices, and data logs.

Disadvantages:

- Computer downtime resulting from equipment and software problems can cause delays unless appropriate backup systems are in place.
- Records can be lost through electronic data corruption or if the computer system fails.
- Computerized records can be altered after the fact, unless safeguards are put in place.
- Computer records do not always accommodate detailed descriptions, templates, or special hospital forms and medical protocol recording.
- Storing medical records on the computer requires a much greater storage capacity than would otherwise be required, but hard disk space is becoming less expensive to purchase.

Assistant. Doctors dictate to team members partnered with them, such as veterinary assistants. Either by listening to the veterinarian describing exam findings and recommendations to the client, or from the veterinarian explicitly saying what to type, the assistant enters the visit details into the system. A computer terminal situated in each exam room allows an assistant to type information while the doctor interacts with the client and patient.

Dictation. Doctors dictate to a recording device. Handheld microcassette recorders work well, but they tend to get lost, dropped, and broken. Fortunately, low-end models are inexpensive. Another option is to record the information on voice mail through the telephone system. A medical transcriptionist retrieves the information later and types the medical notes into the database. Recordings can also be made into almost any cell phone.

Sound Files. Doctors speak directly into the computer's microphone. Dictation can be saved in an electronic file. However, keeping notes in electronic audio files requires a lot of hard disk space, and it could be tedious to find specific information, since the team member needing the information would have to listen to the entire file. Voice recognition software will transcribe narration directly to a text file and has evolved to the point of good accuracy.

Remember, maintaining doctors' medical notes and patient records on the computer results in more complete and more legible records than is possible on paper only if the data is entered accurately and promptly.

RECORD ALTERATION

One argument against computerized medical records has been that the EMR can be altered subsequent to the original input, leading to potential legal problems in the event of a claim. As noted earlier in this chapter, alteration of medical records at any time (whether paper or electronic) is a serious practice management issue, and strict policy and procedure guidelines must be in place to prevent it from occurring.

Recognize that electronic records create "behind the scenes" *metadata* that is attached to the records. Metadata is data about the data, and it creates an audit trail about file usage, such as when the file was created, processed, closed, reviewed, modified, opened by other users, and so on (Hansen and Brien 2011). With the rapidly increasing use of human EMRs, it appears that meeting certain parameters will satisfy the courts. In general, EMRs will be admissible as evidence if the court is satisfied that the information on the computer record is trustworthy, if the entries have been made at or near the time the event occurred, and if EMRs are recognized as standard operating protocol in the practice.

Prudence suggests checking with the practice's professional liability insurance carrier annually to determine appropriate policies to adapt or update, as well as other issues related to proper care and maintenance of medical records, whether paper or electronic.

The volume of data and records that must be maintained in a veterinary hospital is very large. Without a computer system, much of this information has to be duplicated. There may be multiple logs, locations, and records in which the same information appears. Eventually, computer systems will merge all these types of data so that one entry serves many purposes. Team members will be able to generate any needed report with only a few mouse clicks. The ideal veterinary medical record of the future will be entirely electronically based and maintained.

The possible advantages and disadvantages of computerized medical records are outlined in the preceding textbox, "Advantages and Disadvantages of Computerized Medical Records." The disadvantages are gradually disappearing as information technology becomes increasingly adept at overcoming obstacles with inexpensive solutions. Although the initial purchase of equipment and software is becoming less and less expensive, regular upgrades will continue to appear. Keep abreast of technological developments, and budget annually for hardware and software improvements.

9

Inventory Control and Management

I n all veterinary hospitals, the two greatest costs of operation are the cost of staffing and the cost of purchasing inventory for use in the practice or for sale to third parties. Inventory management is a critical component of practice profitability. A substantial part of practice resources may be invested in inventory at any given time, and lack of effective inventory systems is a common cause of poor cash flow.

Inventory has a variety of applications in a veterinary hospital. Drugs and medical supplies are a big component of inventory, but stocks of office and computer supplies, cleaning and janitorial supplies, and maintenance supplies are also necessary. Merchandise for resale is another major component. Inventory management concepts therefore apply to a wide variety of practice needs.

Simply put, the "stuff" your practice keeps on hand is the same as cash sitting on the shelves, whether those supplies might be vaccines or syringes, antiseptic or heartworm test kits, envelopes, or paper towels. The valuable stockpile of practice assets called "inventory and supplies" must be carefully acquired and controlled.

General Terms and Goals in Inventory Management

In accounting jargon, *inventory* is specifically defined as all goods owned and held for sale or use in the regular course of business (Meigs and Meigs 1987, 336). The inventory of products purchased for resale to clients is commonly called *merchandise inventory* (Fess and Warren 1987, 420). Items used in the course of providing veterinary medical and surgical services are called *professional inventory* or *medical supply inventory*. For this chapter's discussion of inventory management, the words "inventory" and "supplies" will be used interchangeably to include both merchandise and professional supplies. Please understand that the definitions for various tax-reporting and regulation purposes may be different.

Inventory control, for our purposes, is defined as the process whereby the need to maintain sufficient inventory to meet hospital operating demands is weighed against the monetary cost of carrying inventory (Tootelian and Gaedke 1984, 741). Optimal inventory control ensures that frequently used and needed items are always available and that return on investment for carrying and managing inventory is at the highest possible level.

As a hospital manager, you can contribute significantly to improvements in the hospital's profit margin through attentiveness to inventory control and management. Your practice-management goals include a tightly run purchasing department under the guidance of an astute inventory manager and a veterinary pharmacy that turns a profit. (For more information on the inventory manager position, see section on "Inventory Management Duties" later in this chapter.)

General goals of inventory control and management can be summarized by the following objectives:

- Clients can conveniently obtain refills and other items when requested and with the appropriate level of veterinary oversight through a valid doctor-client-patient relationship.
- Medications and supplies are available to treat patients when needed.
- Quantities of drugs and professional supplies are controlled to minimize hospital expenditures to the lowest practical level. Avoid large quantities that tie up cash unless discount savings can be shown to adequately offset the dollars tied up in idle inventory amounts on the practice shelves.
- Regular reevaluation of preferred pharmaceuticals and supplies occurs so as to minimize redundancy of products accomplishing similar purposes; streamline storage, ordering, and training protocols; and minimize employee confusion.
- Employees can efficiently order, stock, and dispense the needed items.
- Controlled drugs are properly monitored and secured.
- Appropriate security, systems, and safeguards exist to ensure that inventory and supplies will be used in the intended format.
- Employees are trained to know how to correctly handle supplies that represent potential health and safety hazards.
- Employees are well-versed in communicating the value of products dispensed through the practice and can respond appropriately to client questions about competing resources such as online pharmacies and big-box stores.
- Fees charged for pharmaceuticals and supplies are adjusted on a regular basis, and appropriate pricing is passed on to the clients of the practice.
- Sales achieve the planned level of profit.

To accomplish these goals, a workable hospital inventory system must be established, maintained, and adapted as needed. Like any other area of veterinary hospital operations, inventory management requires continual attention. Do not expect a one-time fix to solve inventory problems.

Practice owners and managers must be serious about maintaining adherence to inventory policies and procedures on a daily basis. Good inventory systems rely on good habits in handling and administering inventory and in billing for pharmacy and hospital supplies. As practice manager, you play a large role in ensuring this success.

It is important to remember that inventory is a revenue center as well as a cost center. These days, much of a manager's time in inventory management is devoted to instituting pricing strategies and improving client compliance with recommended preventive care guidelines. It is also devoted to team education about specific featured products, so that all team members will deliver consistent messages to clients about the products. To meet evolving client preferences, managers must be knowledgeable and proficient in advancing new pharmacy concepts, such as the use of the Internet for accepting client orders through a secure practice website.

Hidden Costs of Inventory

A common inventory control problem is running out of an item before a new supply is received to keep the item on hand. A simple but costly solution to this problem would be to purchase and maintain all items far in excess of expected use. For example, a hospital manager might purchase all of the anticipated supplies needed for the coming twelve months of patient activity.

The problem with this "simple" solution is that there are inventory costs extending far beyond the amount paid to the vendor. The annual cost of maintaining an inventory is much more than what you pay to suppliers.

The cost of the item begins with the *unit cost*. This is the amount paid to the vendor, including applicable sales taxes and shipping costs, divided by the quantity of the item ordered. But besides the unit cost, there are two other sources of inventory cost that are frequently overlooked: the *ordering cost* and the *holding cost*. Each time an item is ordered, ordering costs are incurred. Ordering costs include mostly labor-related expenses. The cost of labor includes an hourly wage paid to the employee performing the work, associated payroll taxes, and employee benefit programs. Employees must complete the following steps as part of inventory ordering, and the labor cost, and thus the ordering cost, increases with each step:

- Determine the amount needed
- Maintain vendor relationships (meet with sales representatives, shape synergistic relationship with them, secure the best pricing options)
- Obtain authorization for the purchase
- Fill out purchase orders
- Track backorders

- Receive and unpack items, compare items received with the shipping invoice, price items, and place items on the shelf
- Accumulate documents in a voucher packet; ready, approve, and transmit payment; post all transactions related to the acquisition in the practice financial records; and file, store, and manage purchase records, including those related to past years

The entire ordering process expends quite a bit of employee time. Not all purchases require each one of these steps to be completed; nevertheless, ordering costs can account for as much as 15 to 20 percent of the true total cost of the item.

Holding costs have to do with the costs of owning and keeping inventory on the premises in anticipation of their use. The largest holding cost is generally attributable to the capital tied up in inventory. Money paid to vendors to acquire inventory could have been alternatively invested to generate an income. Or, the money could have been used to reduce prior borrowings on which interest expense is being paid.

Other holding costs are as follows:
- Personal property taxes paid on the value of inventory as of a specific valuation date
- Insurance premiums paid on the average inventory value to protect against the risk of loss in event of a disaster, theft, or damage
- The utility and facility costs of protecting inventory against heat, cold, and humidity
- Loss due to obsolescence and spoilage if inventory is not used or sold before expiration dates
- Pharmacy licensing fees and regulatory compliance
- Per-square-foot facility costs associated with the space used to store inventory
- The cost of maintaining workplace safety programs (OSHA regulation compliance) that are attributable to inventory and supplies that are potentially dangerous to handle and store
- The cost of dusting items and maintaining them with an orderly appearance

The estimated holding cost for a veterinary practice ranges from 8 to 15 percent of the true total cost of an item.

Aggregated ordering and holding costs thus account for approximately 25 to 35 percent of the total true cost, depending on the amount of time the inventory is held. Cost also depends on management's success in safeguarding inventory from shrinkage as well as overall efficiency and effectiveness in purchasing the asset. For these many reasons, total inventory cost amounts to much more than what is paid to vendors.

Optimal inventory control must include astute purchasing policies so as to minimize ordering and holding costs, balanced with the opposing need to have required items on hand to operate the hospital. If the orders placed are too large, you have decreased the ordering cost but increased the holding cost. If the orders placed are too small, you have increased the ordering costs while decreasing the holding costs. Later in this chapter, we will discuss some optimal inventory ordering concepts and techniques.

What Should the Inventory System Do?

Essentially, the inventory system should ensure that all items used in the hospital are available when needed. Many important activities need to be accomplished to reach inventory objectives supporting this overarching goal. These objectives can be grouped into four basic functions—controlling, forecasting, purchasing, and selling:

1. *Control functions:* preparation and dissemination of written policies and procedures, establishment and maintenance of security and safety features, and regular monitoring and system adaptation through counting and accountability.
2. *Forecasting functions:* prediction of practice need through measurement of inventory in motion and determination of reorder points and quantities.
3. *Purchasing functions:* action taken on forecasts through analysis and negotiation of deals, vendor selection, and maintenance of time-efficient ordering and receiving strategies.
4. *Selling functions:* employee training, marketing, and strategic pricing, resulting in profit.

CONTROL FUNCTIONS

Although written policies and procedures underpin a strong inventory system, the system should be flexible. Products, treatments, and ways of supporting patient care continually evolve. An enthusiastic medical team will always be looking for new products and innovative and improved methods of enhancing animal health care. These new products and methods, in turn, drive inventory change.

Nevertheless, some inventory control functions will always be necessary. An efficiently controlled system should be able to provide a fairly accurate idea of inventory quantities and value at any given time. An inventory system that can provide accurate detail of inventory levels at any time is said to be a *perpetual* inventory system. When items are received, they are immediately added to the practice's inventory records. When they are sold or used, the invoicing procedure depletes them from the record of inventory count on hand. If inventory is accurately logged into the record-keeping system and invoiced as it is sold, the inventory levels reported by the system at any point should exactly match the *physical inventory* count at that time.

Taking a physical inventory means manually counting quantities on hand. A *periodic inventory* system uses records that rely on physical counts at the end of each financial period to determine the correct levels. Tax laws require an accurate inventory value annually, usually provided through a year-end physical count.

Counting inventory tests inventory system compliance. Every time an inventory count is completed, you, as practice manager, or with the assistance of the inventory manager, should figure out the variance from what the records indicate should be on hand. The evaluation proceeds as follows:

1. Add the beginning quantity for the selected item (the number at the beginning of the period) to the number of items ordered and received during the period (determined by means of either the inventory control card system or the electronic inventory management system, both of which are described later in this chapter).
2. From this sum, subtract the number of items sold during the same period of time (usually obtained from the practice's computer system).
3. Compare the resulting number to the physical inventory count at the end of the period. The numbers should agree.

For example, to test compliance for heartworm medication packs, the following computation would be done:

Beginning quantity on January 1, 20XX	500
Add number ordered and received, January 1 through December 31, 20XX	2,000
Subtract number sold January 1 through December 31, 20XX	<2,341>
Calculated quantity on hand on December 31, 20XX	159
Physical count of on-hand quantity on December 31, 20XX	150

In this example, the *variance* between the calculated number and the physical count is –9. Negative variances are expressed in the paperwork with brackets or parentheses. If there were 9 *more* heartworm packs on the shelf than the calculations say there should be, the variance would be +9.

More frequent physical counts reinforce the importance of good habits for safeguarding inventory, a valuable practice asset. Later in this chapter we will outline a method for designing your practice policy of completing cyclic counts, defining what, when, and how to count. When counting is done regularly, employees may be more aware of keeping good records in the inventory-management processes.

Accounting systems for veterinary hospital inventory management may be manual or computerized, but most often practices take a combination approach. Most veterinary practice management software includes integrated inventory-management modules. Even though these software programs include a number of helpful sophisticated control systems, hospital personnel must be trained in inventory management in order to make use of them.

Ideally, computer systems should provide perpetual inventory information, but usually they cannot in all situations. Computer inventory systems are very good at tracking merchandise quantities such as drugs, pet products, and similar items resold to clients. If negative or positive variances are occurring in these items, then as practice manager you must try to figure out why. User errors may be occurring during entry of inventory. Errors may be appearing on client invoices. In the case of negative variances, the practice may have a problem with theft of the products.

Medical and hospital supplies consumed in the course of patient care or completion of office work are much more difficult to track than merchandise. By emphasizing the importance of recording what is being taken out of inventory for these daily activities (e.g., through employee training), you may be able to reduce these discrepancies.

As in all hospital systems, *internal control* is a key concern in implementation of inventory management. Chapter 10 on revenue management covers the concept of internal control in relation to protecting revenue, but the concepts also apply to protecting inventory. Specifically, segregation of inventory duties will allow for adequate safeguarding of valuable practice assets. One person should not control all aspects of record maintenance and at the same time also control all ordering, stocking, and distribution of inventory. In such a system, there are no checks and balances to prevent theft, fraud, and error. At the very least, special attention must be given to reviewing and supervising that person's work.

Reviews can occur at several points in the inventory cycle. The most usual cross-check and verification occurs at the point that invoices are prepared for payment to vendors. In an ideal situation of duty segregation, the bookkeeper, who reconciles all vendor-related paperwork and pays bills, is not the inventory manager and does not make purchases.

The bookkeeper and, later, the owner (who signs checks), should critically assess the applicable documents and compare records of inventory on hand for reasonableness. Be aware that bookkeepers will not automatically complete a critical assessment without training of what to look for and how to look for it. An experienced veterinary practice bookkeeper will be familiar with drug and equipment names and uses, which is the baseline knowledge needed to be a skeptical critic of purchases coming through on invoices.

FORECASTING FUNCTIONS

The system should signal the manager when an item must be reordered to avoid an outage. The reorder timing should account for the estimated time delay between placing an order and receiving it. An item with a long lag time, or "lead time," requires a higher reorder level than an item the vendor can supply almost immediately.

Simultaneously with maintaining adequate inventory stocks, the system should mitigate supply quantities to levels that do not unnecessarily tie up capital. (For more information on the basics of reorder points, quantities, and timing, see the section "Using and Monitoring a Control-Card System" later in this chapter.)

As hospital manager you should stay familiar with routine estimated usage amounts, including those of seasonal items, and monitor the use of drugs and supplies. Order supplies at the proper time to ensure timely delivery in sufficient quantities and to take optimal advantage of discount and bargain purchase options.

PURCHASING FUNCTIONS

The inventory system should act as a contact management tool. It should readily provide information on how each item must be ordered, who to order it from, and how to avoid ancillary charges. The system should identify and track backorders and record when they are expected to arrive.

A good system makes cost-effective purchasing possible by identifying such factors as seasonal usage, which help you to determine optimal order times for larger quantities. An effective system also allows for identification of outdated items so they can be properly handled. In addition, an effective system ensures that vendor invoices match the contracted amounts and prices that were agreed upon when the orders were placed. Finally, the system should allow for immediate assessment of increased pricing to clients. When the vendor increases the price of an inventory item, the practice should pass the price increase on to the client.

SELLING FUNCTIONS

Ultimately, selling products of any kind through a veterinary practice should generate a profit. Selling functions include measuring the amount of profit realized as well as setting prices and supporting sales through a knowledgeable employee base. In a pure retail-selling environment, marketing is used extensively to drive sales. However, veterinary practice is primarily founded in animal-health-care services. Pharmaceutical and product sales are secondary to veterinary services, so the real practice selling function resides in promoting the value of expert opinion that supplements the product sale.

To track profit, management may look at items assigned to specific expense categories to create reports comparing inventory and supply expense with revenues generated from sales. *Gross profit* is the difference between the price of a product to the client (e.g., heartworm preventive) and the cost of the product to the practice. Some practice management software programs now attempt to represent the true cost of the products and services the practice offers in these calculations (e.g., by taking ordering costs, holding costs, and overhead considerations into account), so that managers can structure prices and fees accordingly.

Increasingly, however, there are competitive market forces at work that require managers to take other factors into consideration when it comes to price determinations. You are well advised to be mindful of alternative client sources for products and to regularly adapt your pricing strategies to coincide with larger practice objectives. More on pricing and profit appears later in this chapter (see "Break-Even Analysis as a Starting Point for Product Pricing").

Inventory Management Duties

By now you see that the entire cycle of supply acquisition and deployment, leading to veterinary practice revenue realization, is a big one. Most often, only one individual is assigned much of the responsibility for inventory management. However, the position requires competencies that include analyzing, negotiating, securing, accounting, and pricing.

A manager of a small practice may assume many of these responsibilities while leveraging her time by assigning tasks such as unpacking and counting to technicians and veterinary assistants, among others. In larger hospital operations, these duties may be split among several individuals to assure continuity and improve internal control functions. (See textbox, "Inventory Manager Duties.")

INVENTORY MANAGER CHARACTERISTICS

What qualities should you look for in an inventory manager? First and foremost, the inventory manager should be a good shopper and good at math and working with spreadsheets. Seek an employee who knows the value of working within a budget and the rewards found when staying within a budget's boundaries. She should be careful and not impulsive. Such a person will likely carry those frugal habits to careful hospital ordering. (See textbox, "Frugality in Inventory Management.")

The inventory manager often will need to prevent unnecessary duplication of similar medications that support the current service offerings. Sometimes, this means going back to the veterinarian who requested a purchase to point out the duplication. Thus, diplomacy and tact are also good skills for an inventory manager to have.

The inventory manager should have a basic understanding of the drugs and medical supplies used in a veterinary practice and their patient-care purposes. In large practices, the inventory manager may be working side by side with a veterinary pharmacist. The inventory manager may be responsible for regular updating of a practice-specific *formulary*.

A highly skilled and articulate inventory manager is an invaluable contributor to supporting pharmacy change in the practice. The inventory manager will likely need to participate in or even facilitate discussions with medical staff. In multi-doctor practices, veterinarians should regularly be debating care guidelines and the types of vaccines, biologics, medications, and other supplies that are appropriate to stock as care and services advance in accordance with veterinary medical knowledge.

Inventory Manager Duties

An inventory manager, who reports to the hospital manager, is typically responsible for the following tasks:

- Determining what amounts of specific supplies have been used in prior periods, being mindful of seasonal influences on usage.
- Computing and projecting quantities to order (*order quantity*) for the next period based on prior history and other factors.
- Determining the relative value of various inventory items to prioritize the level of control and amount of time to be spent managing those items.
- Counting and monitoring stock on a rotational basis.
- Assuring that stock outages are mitigated to the fullest extent possible.
- Accumulating inventory requests (requisition orders) from doctors and staff.
- Preparing purchase orders for submission to vendors.
- Meeting with pharmacy company representatives and supplier salespeople to learn about new products and pricing and to place orders. The inventory manager should know the schedules of the salespeople and company representatives who visit the hospital and must prepare accordingly in order to make efficient use of his own time and to show respect for the value of the reps' time. If the inventory manager is organized, he will be prepared to place orders that are large enough to take advantage of the best possible pricing from a company.
- Staying abreast of new developments so that products do not become obsolete.
- Being alert to manufacturing shortages that may result in serious impairment to patient care due to product unavailability. The inventory manager may need to stockpile some products at times or take other actions to alleviate the impact on the practice and its patients.
- Meeting with practice veterinarians to inform them of new products being introduced to clients.
- Keeping records of prior and current inventory-vendor pricing and price breaks.
- Staying aware of potential purchasing deals or discounts from different vendors.
- Accurately filing purchase orders for placed orders and tracking backorders.
- Overseeing shipment receipt and employee unpacking protocols.
- Ensuring that the information on shipment documents accurately matches what was actually received and unpacked.

CONTINUES >

- Ensuring that the information on shipment documents accurately matches what was included on the original purchase orders.
- Entering selected inventory data into the computer system.
- Updating sales prices of items to be resold to clients based on changes in cost, and updating the computerized inventory price lists accordingly.
- Routinely monitoring Internet-pricing of "shopped" items and prices published through other competing sources such as catalogs, and reporting findings to the practice manager, practice administrator, and/or practice owner.
- Securing inventory.
- Distributing inventory to the correct areas of the hospital.
- Rotating stock so that the oldest stock is sold first, by placing items on the shelves so that the newly received items are used after inventory already on hand has been depleted. Stock rotation is especially important with items that carry expiration dates. The inventory manager should be cautious about adding prices, codes, labels, or other information to received products that might damage the packaging. Such package alterations may prohibit the practice from returning the product at a later date.
- Periodically monitoring dated materials and removing close-dated items, or creating a plan for their quick use. One useful "at-a-glance" method uses colored stickers to identify the month in which the item will be outdated. Some suppliers will allow outdated materials to be returned for credit, but each vendor and supplier has different rules.
- Keeping track of items that come close to their expiration dates or that are not being used, and preparing plans to avoid this wastage in the future. Such a plan may involve adjusting purchasing quantities, consulting with other team members about the possibility of discontinuing the product, or contacting vendors to arrange for returns or exchanges. However, returns and exchanges may not be permitted.
- Watching for duplication of items through similar product lines and reducing such duplication.
- Ensuring that no outdated pharmaceuticals are available for use.
- Ensuring that all state and federal pharmacy and drug regulations are followed.
- Assisting the practice safety officer in maintaining required records for the Occupational Safety and Health Administration (OSHA) to ensure compliance with OSHA regulations.

CONTINUES >

> INVENTORY MANAGER DUTIES, CONT.

- Taking physical counts of inventory, comparing them to computer records for accuracy, and tracking and reporting variances.
- Identifying wastage and suggesting cost-savings ideas for waste elimination.
- Making sure the bookkeeper receives copies of all purchase orders and shipping documents, once they are reconciled.
- Providing the bookkeeper with records of items that have been returned to vendors.

Frugality in Inventory Management

The allure of new pharmaceuticals and products in bright and shiny packages is strong. New products are introduced regularly, with glitzy advertising and marketing to encourage purchase. Doctors, technicians, and purchasing agents are all susceptible campaign targets. Maintain practice protocols to reduce opportunities for impulse ordering of new products. Ordering a new item or line of products is not a problem per se, but ordering without prudent research and careful consideration is.

Procedures should be put in place to help those who make ordering decisions "stop and think." For example, when a veterinarian or other team member wishes to place an order, there might be a form to fill out with questions such as the following:

- What need does this product fill that we are not currently meeting?
- What are the advantages of this product over others that are designed for the same purpose? What are the disadvantages?
- If this item will be resold to clients:
  » What is the unit cost of this item, and what would the sales price be?
  » How much do competitors, including online sources, charge for this product?
  » How could the practice promote this product to clients?
- If this item is for use within the hospital:
  » How often will it be used?
  » Have veterinarians and other applicable staff members been consulted about whether it would be useful? What was their response?
- What is the shelf life of this product?
- Is the product subject to special federal or state laws that would require special attention by staff members?

This form could then be submitted to a practice owner for a second opinion.

The inventory manager must have in depth working knowledge of computer software use, inventory management software, and computer system integration with inventory management equipment. The manager should also possess good analytic skills in order to compare and interpret inventory-related reports. These skills improve the profitability of inventory as a practice revenue center that has high cost associated with it.

Inventory Benchmarks

You and your inventory manager should both have a working knowledge of the typical costs of inventory in private veterinary practice. Industry benchmarks are a starting point for analytic capabilities. It is then important to develop an understanding of the typical financial attributes of the unique type of veterinary practice in which you work. For example, small companion-animal practices will have different financial ratios from equine or large-animal or mixed-animal practices. Ambulatory practices tend to have different ratios from hospital-based practices. Emergency or specialty practices operate in a different way from daytime-only general practices.

Geographic location affects practices with a similar species mix. For example, practices located in arid climates often do not need to have as much flea or heartworm medication in stock as practices located in flea- and heartworm-endemic regions.

However, assess published financial benchmarks with a healthy dose of skepticism. Data is only as good as the quality of research behind it. Keep an eye out for benchmark data from a variety of different sources, and use your accumulated knowledge and experience when making comparisons with your practice, which is unique.

Your well-developed bookkeeping systems and chart-of-accounts coding accuracy should result in reliable expense categories that are related to inventory management, such as these:

- Drugs and pharmacy supply expense
- Heartworm, flea, tick, and parasite product expense
- Hospital supply expense
- Laboratory supply expense
- Radiology and imaging supply expense
- Anesthesia, dentistry, and surgical supply expense
- Therapeutic dietary product expense
- Premium and other dietary product supply expense
- Grooming supply expense
- Retail and pet product supply expense

One key statistic you will see frequently in the veterinary literature compares supply utilization against practice revenue realization. This information is gathered from the practice financial report called the profit and loss report (statement of revenues and expenses) and relies on the foregoing expense accounts. The benchmark calculation divides supply expense (the supplies used or dispensed in the financial period) by total practice revenue during the same period, typically twelve months.

Companion animal hospitals with good accounting systems will typically incur drug and professional supply expenses, including vaccines and parasite products, of about 12 percent of gross income. Hospital supplies, over-the-counter items, and ancillary supply expenses such as grooming supplies average 1.5 percent. Laboratory supply and reference laboratory expenses will run at about 3.75 percent of gross income. Anesthesia, dentistry, and surgery expenses amount to about 1 percent of gross income, and dietary product averages 2.5 percent of gross income.

Revenue centers will affect these financial ratios. For example, if the practice derives 15 percent of its total revenues from boarding services, this will cause the percentages for various supply categories to look much different (unusually lower, since boarding and grooming services generally average about 8 percent of total practice revenues).

One source for inventory and other financial benchmarks is AAHA's *Financial and Productivity Pulsepoints* study, published every two years. For comparison with the foregoing stats, the version published in 2011 (using data from 2010) reported drugs and medical supplies (not including laboratory, dietary products, and over-the counter items) at 14.6 percent of gross revenues. Food expenses (prescription and nonprescription) averaged 3.4 percent. Laboratory expenses came in at 3.7 percent, and over-the-counter expenses totaled 2.9 percent of gross income. This book also provides percentages detailed by practice size (total revenue ranges) and by full-time equivalency veterinarians.

Another good way to gain a better understanding of what your numbers mean is to compare them with those of other practices, ideally ones that are like yours but not in competition with your practice. To do this, consider taking membership in a business study group for veterinary practice managers and/or owners. Often, such groups meet regularly to discuss practice management issues such as improving inventory management (see the Veterinary Study Groups website at www.veterinarystudygroups.inc).

The bottom line regarding benchmark numbers is to know where to find them and the relative ranges, but not to rely on them as an indictment or as a validation of your own practice. Use them instead to inspire critical thinking about how your practice operates. Aim to show continual improvement over time in these ratios and other financial measures.

Balancing the Vendor Relationship

Often, the inventory manager is the primary person in the hospital who has contact with salespeople. Good and bad outcomes can result when one person has sole contact with salespeople. On the good side, having the inventory manager do this optimizes the way veterinarians spend their time, since veterinarians can spend their time with patients. The inventory manager can focus on how to obtain the best pricing, who the prime contact people are for different vendors, and the like. Less duplication and over-ordering problems result, and problem and fraudulent vendors more easily identified and remembered.

However, several potential downsides can also occur when one person is exclusively responsible for meeting with pharmacy and supply company representatives. The inventory manager may develop unfair biases for or against some vendors, for example. Vendors who could provide an excellent service to the practice might be excluded. In other instances, an inventory manager may have such an affinity for a particular salesperson that the practice pays premium pricing, when a better deal could have been negotiated with a competitor.

In some cases, there is little control or supervision of the relationship between the inventory manager and the salesperson. In extreme cases, this lack of oversight could result in fraud. A monopolistic relation with one vendor could occur in which the inventory manager receives kickbacks for placing all orders with one salesperson or vendor. No hospital manager wants to think that the practice inventory manager is capable of such things; however, these things do happen. Thus, the manner in which the inventory systems are set up should have built-in checks to prevent them.

In addition, when the inventory manager meets exclusively with the vendor representatives, practice veterinarians, including the owner, may lose the chance to nurture a valuable relationship with the vendors (Heinke 1998). The respect that managers try to foster in their clinics for clients and staff sometimes falls short when it comes to an integral practice resource, the suppliers.

Distributor and pharmaceutical-company representatives put forth extraordinary effort to serve their clientele well. They understand that their long-term success for serving veterinary hospitals is tied to the economic well-being of those hospitals. These individuals are highly educated and well trained by the companies that employ them. They provide some of the most cutting-edge information available as to new products in the pipeline, animal-owner concerns, upcoming potential backorders that may affect sales, and other issues. Their ideas can often help the practice serve its clients and grow.

Practice managers and owners who have nurtured relationships with their representatives know that they can rely on these partners in business to provide good feedback on how they are doing. If the representative likes the practitioner and the hospital staff, he will freely offer advice about how the hospital can be improved. He is seeing the hospital with fresh eyes and may be able to tell you how your clients likely perceive your services and the physical plant. At the same time, representatives have seen many other practices and may have come across ideas that will be good for your hospital.

Distributor reps are also well connected within the veterinary community. They may know where a practice is coming up for sale or looking for a merger. They may be able to help you find employees. They may be able to provide a wide variety of management support services, spanning inventory control, client service training, human resources and team development, marketing, and more. Be alert to these various offerings that may provide real benefit for overall practice improvements.

Practice management and financial success hinge on many little things done with care. A key factor is an interest in people and a respect for all members of your team. Distributor and pharmaceutical company representatives should not be treated as an afterthought. Instead, treat them with respect and reap the many benefits that they can provide.

Inventory Management Concepts and Techniques

Inventory control in veterinary practice can be handled manually or electronically. More and more practices have shifted to electronic inventory management. Even in these practices, however, the hospital manager and the inventory manager must understand the concepts of the manual system, as they still apply to electronic inventory management. All practices also need to have a purchase order system and a central supply system in place. The latter is best handled when it is ration-based.

MANUAL INVENTORY MANAGEMENT

Before electronic inventory management was possible, inventory management was handled by means of the inventory control card system. Inventory control cards are tried and true, and a thorough understanding of them is necessary in any inventory system. The same concepts are used in sophisticated electronic systems, but updated for the computer age. A sample of an inventory control card, aka product tracking form, appears in Figure 9.1. In this type of system, an inventory manager records information on a card for each item purchased. It can then be tracked, monitored, and reordered as needed.

What Is Tracked?

For each item purchased, the inventory manager records the following information on a card:

- *Item:* Size, color, strength, dispensing format (pill, liquid, paste, can, case, etc.), trade name or generic name, manufacturer and hospital code or SKU number (SKU stands for Stock Keeping Unit; see Glossary for more information)
- *Suppliers:* Company name, contact name, address, telephone number, fax number, website address, e-mail address, hospital account number, billing policy, and discount dates

FIGURE 9.1 SAMPLE PRODUCT TRACKING FORM

PRODUCT

Item: _____   Period Starting Quantity: _____

Product Type: _____   Minimum Quantity Required: _____

Category: _____   Period End Quantity: _____

Product Selling Price: _____

	DATE	QUANTITY	COST/UNIT	SOURCE	TOTAL COST
January					
February					
March					
April					
May					
June					

Total # Purchased _____

Total # Used _____

Total # Misplaced or Unaccounted For _____

Reviewed By: _____

Total Cost for Restocking/ Carrying/Ordering (# of staff hours X wages + payroll cost + cost for facility space) _____

Total # of Returned/Defective _____

TOTAL SIX MONTH COST _____

- *Quantity:* Number of each item ordered, quoted price, and date ordered; number of each item received, invoiced price, and date received
- *Reorder point:* Maximum and minimum level of stock at which reordering should occur
- *Invoice costs:* Price per item or unit, sales taxes, shipping, handling, and freight charges
- *Storage location:* Notation indicating whether the item is consumed in the hospital as part of patient care and/or is dispensed; number that should be readily available in each secondary supply area; how often items should be distributed from the central supply storage to restock secondary areas (treatment area, pharmacy, exam rooms, surgery suite, point-of-purchase display shelves, ambulatory vehicles, etc.)
- *Price to client:* Formula for determining price to be charged to client, including dispensing fees, minimum price, and mark-up over unit cost

Using and Monitoring a Control-Card System

Using the control card system, the inventory manager regularly and continually monitors supplies as to the amount on hand, the usage, and expiration dates. The manager creates and maintains an inventory control card on every item purchased and used in the hospital, distinguishing them by SKU. SKU records may be restricted to items used for the care and treatment of patients or may be expanded to include stationery, office forms, copier and computer supplies, janitorial and maintenance supplies, and other items. Equipment and furnishings are better segregated to a separate accounting journal or record-keeping system that is maintained specifically for long-lived assets with multiple years of use.

The inventory manager constantly monitors the system and regularly checks the inventory card records, requisition orders (requests from staff), and physical supply quantities throughout the hospital to determine which items have reached their reorder points.

After determining order needs, the inventory manager records all new information pertaining to each reordered item on the inventory card for that item. This should be done right away, generally at the same time the orders are placed, so that the task is not forgotten. If the card is not updated at this time, an order may be duplicated erroneously. By going back to the control card for an item, the inventory manager should be able to see immediately when it was reordered, how much was ordered, from whom it was ordered, estimated delivery date, and so on.

When the order is received, the manager makes note of all relevant information on the inventory card, including any price changes. Backorders are treated as not received. Prior to routing documentation to the bookkeeper, inventory manager should review the packing slip or invoice received with the shipment and make note of the following:

- Date and time of receipt
- Initials of person unpacking the shipment

- Initials of inventory manager
- Each item verified as to quantity, size, etc., and actual receipt
- Expiration date
- Any problems with the item, as well as the name of the person responsible for ensuring correction and resolution (for example, broken or missing items, wrong product, incorrect size or strength, short-dated expirations, and so on)

A "want list" may take the place of individual requisition orders from staff. Items that are in low supply are recorded on the "want list" by any team member. This requires careful attention by each employee to consciously note when she has depleted any supply stock, such taking the last package of suture out of a box or the last pills out of a bottle. When the last unit is taken, the employee must promptly write it on the want list.

A word of warning here: Want lists and requisition orders do not take the place of physical inspection of the shelves by the inventory manager. When physical inspection does not take place, problems can arise. For instance, if the inventory manager was not monitoring supplies, but was leaving everything up to the requisition orders and the want list, and a team member took the last item off the shelf of a certain product and never let anyone know, re-ordering might be delayed. The item would not be available when team members needed it. However, a want list and other creative systems can be used to prevent stock-outs and can act as helpful backups to physical inspection.

Using a Red-Tag System

A useful manual monitoring system is a *tagging* system. A tagging system can work with or without the inventory card system or its electronic alternative through the practice management software. For each item, the inventory manager creates a colorful tag that includes the name of the item and its size and strength or SKU. You can also place the name of the vendor you last ordered from, the reorder quantity, and the package price of the previous order on the tag, or this information can be recorded elsewhere. The tag is placed on a selected bottle or package that represents the point at which a reorder should occur.

For example, the inventory manager determines that amoxicillin drops should be reordered when five packages remain in inventory. The fifth from the last package is tagged. Team members dispense available packages in order. When they reach the tagged package, the tag is removed and placed in a box that the inventory manager routinely monitors. When tags appear in the box, the inventory manager knows it is time to order.

Like the want list, this system has its problems. Packages get out of order. Tags fall off. Employees put the tags in their pockets and forget about them. Even so, tagging does provide another valuable control to help ensure timely reordering.

ELECTRONIC INVENTORY MANAGEMENT

Inventory management software helps greatly in managing, tracking, and reordering hospital supplies and merchandise. When a hospital uses a computerized inventory system, the inventory manager's responsibilities are basically the same as described for the manual system. However, today's software programs provide a host of benefits.

They allow for detailed database information about vendors and stocked items. They record the transactional history with each vendor and the history of purchases for each item. Thus they take the place of the control card system by incorporating all of the information previously recorded by hand into a user-friendly database.

They also speed calculations and enhance cross-checks of controls. In the ideal electronically managed inventory system, one action by a computer operator should result in a whole series of coordinated computations and system updates.

These systems also allow for easy retrieval of information at multiple computer-terminal locations throughout the practice. Purchase orders, want lists, and requisition forms can be handled electronically, reducing the need for more paperwork. For example, forms can be completed via the computer and e-mailed internally to the inventory manager, who in turn can complete reorders electronically.

It's easy to see why most practice managers today do try to use an electronic database, although they can be frustrated by perceived deficiencies in electronic inventory management. Here are some of the other helpful features in electronic inventory management software programs:

- The computer can be preprogrammed with a reorder point for each SKU. The inventory program can then track usage and cue the inventory manager when it detects that merchandise quantities have dropped to the reorder point. Preestablished reorder points may rely on steady demand for SKUs that are not affected by seasonal fluctuations.

- Purchase orders can be prepared using the computer's integrated inventory coding system. Purchase orders can then be e-mailed to vendors or through direct connection to a vendor portal. The original copies are retained in the system.

- Once shipments are received, the electronic purchase order is updated to reflect receipt date, verification of quantities, and vendor prices. When the purchase order is updated to note shipment receipt, the computer updates account payable amounts and inventory-on-hand quantities.

- If the database has been set up to automatically calculate markup or margin pricing, the acquisition cost of the received SKU will be considered and a new selling price calculated. Any new client service invoice should immediately reflect the new inventory price. Pharmacy charges should be automatically calculated and added by the software in accord with preset parameters.

- As inventory is depleted through sales to the practice's clientele and as it is consumed in hospital use, the ideal system reduces the quantities in the computer's database. A *perpetual inventory* is thus maintained.
- The computer maintains an extensive history of each item purchased, including quantities, prices, and vendors. It thus provides a stronger, more robust control methodology and data analytics than the manual system.

Despite the obvious benefits, some practice managers and owners still have not fully embraced electronic inventory management. Some use some of its features but choose, for example, not to maintain perpetual inventory levels on the computer system. The labor time and cost for keying purchases to the system may be perceived as much greater than the inventory benefits gained by such tracking. Many SKUs constitute supplies that will be used up in the course of providing medical and surgical care. These "hospital consumables," such as disinfectants, gauze sponges, and needles and syringes, may indeed be difficult to track electronically. Resorting to manual strategies, such as tagging and physical inspection, may be necessary.

As much as possible, link items to specific invoicing codes that will also increase capture of expenses that should be passed on to the client. As an example, suture material can be charged by the pack with a specific SKU. Invoicing by the SKU and number of units supports detailed patient history about many aspects of the procedure, as well as enabling accurate inventory accounting.

After as many supply units as possible are linked to specific invoicing codes, there will still remain some supplies that are too difficult to track via a perpetual inventory system. One option is to calculate the expected monthly utilization rates of consumables based on practice history. This calculation should include analysis of the number of patients seen during each month sorted by departmental activity. For example, historical numbers of surgeries might drive predicted reordering points and quantities for surgical sponges, antiseptic solution, and anesthetic agents. This information can be maintained with a manual card system as an alternative to tracking with the practice management system, which can be too labor intensive and expensive if time must be expended keying in every supply order and arrival.

Despite the challenges of consumable supply management, electronic inventory monitoring should be embraced in significant portions of the total practice inventory and supply base. The more valuable the inventory item, the more important perpetual inventory management techniques become. Medications that are targets for drug abuse should be carefully monitored as well as secured. Controlled substances should be tracked on the computer system as a backup to manual logs of contemporaneous use and shipment receipt.

Expensive, dispensable SKUs that are easily tracked through individual unit sales recorded on the sales invoice should be electronically tracked. Relatively costly SKUs may be prone to internal theft. Safeguards should be instituted to reduce the temptation of theft, such as locking away the majority of available stock so only a week's worth is readily available (see later section about ration-based inventory methods).

As practice manager, you should know what inventory management software is capable of adding to your practice. In manual systems, control cards can be lost or misplaced. Data can be incomplete. The inventory manager may be spending a lot of time on tasks that could be automated and completed more accurately. Stay on top of how inventory management programs are changing, and incorporate new techniques that will improve efficiency in your practice.

PURCHASE ORDER SYSTEMS

A *purchase order* is a document issued by the practice to vendors to request the delivery of materials, including supplies, any other item to be placed in inventory, equipment, and the like. It specifies quantities and prices. Purchase orders can also be created when the hospital needs to purchase services, such as an equipment repair service call. A purchase order system traces every SKU from the time the practice determines that the item is needed to the point the purchase invoice is paid. Like other hospital forms, purchase orders are sequentially numbered for control purposes.

After preparing the purchase order, the employee responsible for placing the order may send a copy to the vendor, fax it to the vendor, send it electronically, or call in the order and refer to the purchase order while doing so. Sending a purchase order to a vendor is a legal offer to purchase, but no agreement exists with the vendor until it is accepted by the vendor.

A copy of the purchase order is retained in the practice files, whether it is in hard-copy form (and filed in numerical order) or in electronic form. The retained purchase order will be checked against the vendor's packing slip when the order is received. The purchase order and packing slip are sent to the bookkeeper to check against the purchase invoice before payment is made.

Many bookkeeping software programs integrate a purchase order system as part of inventory and accounts payable management (see Figure 9.2).

CENTRAL SUPPLY SYSTEMS: RATION-BASED INVENTORY

In very large hospitals, supplies and inventories, particularly drugs and pharmacy-related items, are stored in highly secured areas. Large quantities of supplies are stored in a limited-access central supply area and systematically rationed out to other areas of the hospital in smaller quantities. Limited access is often provided through electronic key fobs or other RFID (radio frequency identification) devices. Veterinary hospitals are increasingly using such devices to selectively control access of personnel to certain areas without the use of old-fashioned locksets and keys.

FIGURE 9.2 PURCHASE ORDER SYSTEM

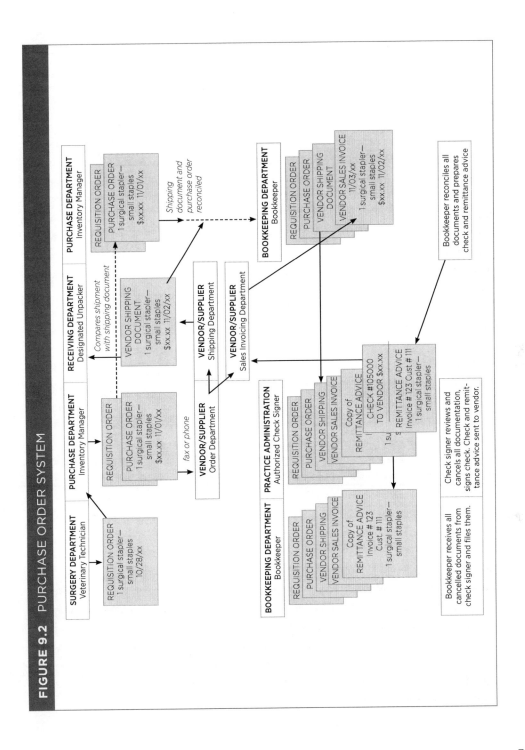

Ration-based inventory is based on a simple concept: When inventory is in publicly accessible and unsecured areas, such as treatment rooms, it is easier to control in smaller quantities than in larger quantities. SKUs that are almost depleted can be quickly identified while back-up quantities are still available in central supply. Wastage is reduced. Theft is easier to detect by walk-about management and visual scanning of the mini-storage area.

Theft in veterinary practice is a very real problem. People justify theft on the excuse that they think the practice will not be hurt by the theft or even notice it. When a veterinary practice purchases and stores large stockpiles of inventory, employees perceive that management is spending large sums of money on inventory and the practice is collecting even larger sums when the medications are sold. In these cases, an employee can easily rationalize that enough inventory exists that taking a few items will not do any harm.

If the loss goes unnoticed, incidents of theft will likely increase. Be aware: Any person in your practice with this mindset can and will steal from the practice. Age, position, gender, and economic status have no bearing on whether someone is capable of theft from the practice.

When large quantities of valuable product are sitting on the shelves and readily available to everyone in the practice, items become out of order. Products become outdated, and damage can easily occur. Staff members do not take care of what is available. Even if theft is not a problem (and it probably is, when inventory is in disarray), many other inventory management problems arise. A central supply under the control of one person alleviates disorganization and lost profit.

In a ration-based system, the practice manager and inventory manager purposely decrease the amount of inventory that is readily accessible. A clearly marked shelf where only one item remains is an excellent control feature. The objective is to ensure a reduced probability that an employee will take the inventory because of fear of being caught or suspected. A second goal is to ensure an orderly method for dealing with large amounts of inventory.

A ration-based inventory system results in "false" stock-outs, when limited and accessible inventory depletes during unexpected high-patient activity. A true stock-out would result in impaired veterinary care and sales. Indeed, true stock-outs are to be avoided, because if the practice does run out of an item, it must wait for a new shipment, borrow from another practice, or write a prescription for the client to obtain the medication elsewhere. Employee inefficiency, confusion, and irritation can increase, clients may be disappointed, and patient care may decline. Ration-based stock-outs are different because the item is readily available in central supply.

Ration-based stock-outs of common areas are a useful means to maintain inventory control without excessively irritating doctors and technicians. Back-up supplies can be requisitioned from the inventory manager who controls central supply. Timely reordering can occur, and meanwhile, the back-up cache provides immediate replenishment.

Facility Approach and Record Keeping

For an inventory rationing method program to work, the locations of primary and secondary inventory stocks must be designated. The central supply area must be secured and accessible to only one or two individuals. Keys to this area cannot be physically accessible to other people. Hiding keys will not work, because they can usually be found by a determined thief. If password control is used through an electronic keypad system, change the password regularly and safeguard them from others.

Consider implementation of other high-tech security measures as well, such as security cameras aimed on the entryways to central supply and RFID-controlled access areas. Limit the number of entry points: The more that are available, the more likely it is that security will be breached.

A practice may use the practice management software program's inventory module to assist in the change of inventory locations if it allows creation of electronic warehouses within the inventory module. Stand-alone inventory management software is another option. Otherwise, the inventory manager may simply use a paper-and-pencil system. The physical movement of inventory from central supply to the rationed secondary inventory areas should require sign-out reports detailing descriptions and quantities moved. In larger, busy practices, a designated employee may control the primary central supply and dispense requisitioned supplies from a pass-through window.

In unattended central supply rooms, the movement of supplies with concurrent sign-outs may occur once a day, once a week, or once every two weeks, and is contingent upon the need for inventory replenishment in outpatient pharmacy and treatment areas. The frequency of moving supplies will also depend on doctor tolerance for smaller quantities of at-hand supplies.

Dividing up responsibilities in a ration-based system is best because it provides for strong internal controls against theft, lax record-keeping, and the like. In short, it adds accountability. In a typical division of responsibilities, one person may be assigned the duty of determining when a reorder po int has occurred and requesting the item from central supply. Another person might be assigned the job of transporting it from long-term storage and delivering it to the short-term storage keeper. There might be a third person who would sign the item out to this person from central supply.

However the duties are segregated, there should not be one person who has control over both the asset and the record of the asset's movement. Of course, two people doing separate duties may collude to commit theft, but theft is less likely to occur when two people are involved because of the fear of being discovered.

Inventory Safeguards

One of the greatest safeguards against employee theft is a perpetual inventory system. In a perpetual inventory, the records maintained on the secondary supply common areas are easily compared on a weekly basis to the actual physical counts completed for each area.

The central inventory will be tallied much less frequently, with a physical inventory needed only once every six months to a year. (For more information on which supplies to count and how often in central and secondary supply areas, see the section later in this chapter entitled "Prioritizing Inventory.")

By maintaining a secure, rationed inventory system, you can minimize the cost of maintaining control. The inventory manager can compare and reconcile the computer-generated perpetual record of amounts held within the short-term cache to the physical count as performed on a short-term, periodic basis. Differences can then be addressed immediately.

Differences generally cannot be resolved when there are excessively long time spans between physical counts. If theft has actually occurred, the guilty party may have long departed from the practice before it is discovered. Other shrinkage issues, such as the incidence of damaged items, wastage, and missed charges for items consumed in the course of patient treatment, can also be reduced by using a ration-based approach.

Like theft, wastage is more prevalent when large supply quantities are available for use. The problem increases from lack of accountability. Without a ration-based approach and frequent inventories, inventory shortages due to wastage and cost overruns are not addressed as soon. Employees become slack about conserving supplies when questions are not asked. Invoicing accuracy may drop off, and dispensed medications may be omitted from the client bill. In management, what gets watched gets tended.

Implementing the Ration-Based Method

The methodology to enforce a ration-based inventory includes the following steps:

Understand the System. Management must understand how the system works and how it provides the practice with a valuable internal control structure. Management must support and enforce the system. If locks on the central supply are left unsecured because of owner laziness or some other reason, the system will be defeated.

Assess the Risks. Management must assess the probable risks involved to determine whether the risks are sufficient to justify the cost of maintaining control in a variety of situations. Some inventory items with a low-dollar value that are used on a frequent basis may be supplied to the rationed common areas on a much more plentiful basis than high-cost items would be. The cost of the unit has a direct bearing on the amount of inventory to be placed in the current cache. The desirability of the inventory item to various employees also affects the quantity rationed. A high likelihood of theft leads to low quantities readily available for use.

Evaluate the Labor Costs. Management must evaluate the labor cost of the perpetual inventory system and determine if physical inventory counts are worth the cost. For example, by placing minor amounts of inventory in a conspicuous location, the practice may be able to reconcile the current cache less frequently, perhaps once a month instead of once per week. Management might determine that the labor cost involved in having more frequent inventories will more than equal the benefit of maintaining tight control.

Inform Staff. Management must clearly communicate that tests are being conducted. All staff should understand that audits of inventory are performed on a periodic basis. The staff should see why inventory is held in such regard and understand that any attempt to take inventory will be met with consequences.

Ancillary Benefits of a Ration-Based System

A ration-based system has many other benefits. For example, because a ration-based system involves more constant tending, it diminishes the amount of obsolete items in inventory. Inventory stocks are logically ordered and located in a ration-based system, making items easier to find when needed.

Price changes can be accommodated more easily and in a more timely manner when they are considered in smaller units. If the at-hand cache is to be replenished on a more frequent basis, "just-in-time" pricing can be adjusted concurrently with the replenishment from the long-term stock based on the most current acquisition cost.

Duplication of drugs is also minimized. When two brands of the same drug are placed side by side, management has a greater opportunity to control duplicate ordering based on clinician preference. Finally, decisions in inventory are more evident at a glance when small numbers of units are used.

What, How, When, and How Much to Order

Learning how to manage inventory is best handled in small portions. Big-picture concepts will help you implement management and ordering systems that can be customized to fit the needs of your practice and to grow with it. First, you need to know how to prioritize the time you spend managing inventory by determining highest and lowest attributes of value and risk. Next, you need to know how to evaluate current stocks on hand and how to organize records to better manage them. You must effectively streamline inventory management processes, including perpetual inventory management, using inventory software.

Perpetual records require knowledge of terminology as well as application of the related concepts to inventory practices. This section introduces these inventory concepts, including safety stock, lead time, and inventory turnover ratios. Inventory management requires you to balance the costs of acquisition with the cost of holding inventory in storage until it is needed, which can be facilitated through use of multiple variables to mathematically determine the optimal order quantity.

PRIORITIZING INVENTORY

Selective inventory control is a profit-based management system that prioritizes inventory based on value and importance. Once the relative importance of inventory items is determined, you can develop suitable control systems and spend your time on what is most valuable to the practice.

The basic method uses Pareto's principle, or the "80/20 rule." The 80/20 rule, as applied to inventory, says that 20 percent of the items account for about 80 percent of the sales revenues. It also states that about 80 percent of the inventory cost exists in 20 percent of the inventory items. Third, 80 percent of profit can be predicted to come from 20 percent of products sold. These groups likely overlap, but they are not necessarily the same. It is helpful to know which items account for your practice's top 20 percent of total revenues, total cost, and total profit.

Because about 20 percent of the items carried in stock typically account for 80 percent of your inventory investment, you should plan to spend more of your time managing these items. Selective inventory control starts with *ABC analysis*, a method of sorting inventory into manageable components based on cost and relative value.

To carry out an ABC analysis, you will do the following:

- Use a spreadsheet software program.
- Manually input the hospital formulary or export the inventory lists from the practice management software to an electronic spreadsheet.
- For each item, determine volume consumed for the year.
- Calculate the *annual usage value* (AUV) by multiplying volume used in a year by the average cost.
- Place these results in a table like the one shown in Table 9.1.

Next, complete the following, while referring to the example shown in Table 9.2:

- Use the power of your spreadsheet tools to sort the SKUs in descending order by AUV.
- Calculate the cumulative AUV at each successive inventory SKU. The cumulative AUV for the second SKU in the series is its AUV plus the AUV of the first SKU. For the third SKU, add its AUV to the cumulative AUV total of the first two SKUs, and so forth.
- Calculate the cumulative percentage of AUV for each line of the table. Divide each successive cumulative AUV by the total inventory value to yield a percentage. For example, Table 9.2 shows that the ninth SKU is the Metronidazole 250 mg tablet with an AUV of $4,072.80 and contributing to a cumulative AUV of $137,022.08. The cumulative AUV divided by the total AUV of all purchases ($169,622.60) is 80.78 percent.

TABLE 9.1 SELECTIVE INVENTORY CONTROL: ABC ANALYSIS (EXAMPLE), PART 1

SKU	ITEM NAME	ANNUAL VOLUME	AVERAGE COST	ANNUAL USAGE VALUE (AUV)
#######	Amoxidrops 50 mg/ml (15 ml)	30	$ 14.27	$ 428.00
#######	Amoxidrops 50 mg/ml (30 ml)	120	$ 27.02	$ 3,242.40
#######	Clavamox 62.5 mg (1 tab)	2,943	$ 1.19	$ 3,503.57
#######	Clavamox 125 mg (1 tab)	982	$ 2.28	$ 2,238.96
#######	Clavamox 250 mg (1 tab)	561	$ 3.76	$ 2,109.36
#######	Clavamox 375 mg (1 tab)	722	$ 5.10	$ 3,683.64
#######	Clavamox Drops 15 ml	554	$ 32.54	$ 18,029.78
#######	Doxycycline 50 mg (1 capsule)	169	$ 0.41	$ 69.08
#######	Doxycycline 100 mg (1 tab)	6,402	$ 0.28	$ 1,765.55
#######	Metronidazole 250 mg (1 tab)	6,197	$ 0.66	$ 4,072.80
#######	Metronidazole 500 mg (1 tab)	6,410	$ 0.54	$ 3,445.07
#######	Metronidazole Susp 100 mg/ml	4,478	$ 2.06	$ 9,232.49
#######	Simplicef 100 mg (1 tab)	19,586	$ 2.27	$ 44,390.83
#######	Simplicef 200 mg (1 tab)	7,045	$ 4.41	$ 31,080.17
#######	Zeniquin 25 mg (1 tab)	1,412	$ 2.55	$ 3,607.31
#######	Zeniquin 50 mg (1 tab)	367	$ 4.69	$ 1,719.70
#######	Zeniquin 100 mg (1 tab)	778	$ 8.51	$ 6,619.37
#######	Cephalexin 500 mg (1 capsule)	16,902	$ 0.65	$ 11,012.30
#######	Clindamycin Oral Drops 20 ml	271	$ 25.34	$ 6,867.84
#######	Clintabs 150 mg (1 tab)	2,365	$ 2.42	$ 5,716.49
#######	Clintabs 75 mg (1 tab)	1,655	$ 1.44	$ 2,377.88
#######	Enalapril 2.5 mg (1 tab)	1,004	$ 0.24	$ 240.96
#######	Enalapril 5 mg (1 tab)	11,054	$ 0.12	$ 1,326.48
#######	Enalapril 10 mg (1 tab)	6,824	$ 0.24	$ 1,605.65
#######	Enalapril 20 mg (1 tab)	5,890	$ 0.21	$ 1,236.90

- Calculate the annual usage distribution. This is accomplished by computing the cumulative percentage of items (number of SKUs) for each line of the table. Again using the ninth SKU (Metronidazole 250 mg tablet) as an example, divide 9 the by the total number of SKUs (25) to yield 36 percent.
- Examine the annual usage distribution and group items into A, B, and C based on the percentage of AUV.
  » Class A = the 20 percent of SKUs that account for about 80 percent of the AUV. In Table 9.2, with a limited number of SKUs, the first 5 SKUs of the 25 listed (20 percent)

TABLE 9.2 SELECTIVE INVENTORY CONTROL: ABC ANALYSIS, PART 2

SKU	ITEM NAME	AUV	CUMULATIVE AUV	CUMULATIVE PERCENTAGE OF AUV	CUMULATIVE NUMBER OF SKUs	CUMULATIVE PERCENTAGE OF SKUs	CLASS
########	Simplicef 100 mg (1 tab)	$ 44,390.83	$ 44,390.83	26.17%	1	4.00%	A
########	Simplicef 200 mg (1 tab)	$ 31,080.17	$ 75,471.01	44.49%	2	8.00%	A
########	Clavamox Drops 15 ml	$ 18,029.78	$ 93,500.78	55.12%	3	12.00%	A
########	Cephalexin 500 mg (1 capsule)	$ 11,012.30	$ 104,513.09	61.62%	4	16.00%	A
########	Metronidazole Susp 100 mg/ml	$ 9,232.49	$ 113,745.58	67.06%	5	20.00%	A
########	Clindamycin Oral Drops 20 ml	$ 6,867.84	$ 120,613.42	71.11%	6	24.00%	B
########	Zeniquin 100 mg (1 tab)	$ 6,619.37	$ 127,232.79	75.01%	7	28.00%	B
########	Clintabs 150 mg (1 tab)	$ 5,716.49	$ 132,949.28	78.38%	8	32.00%	B
########	Metronidazole 250 mg (1 tab)	$ 4,072.80	$ 137,022.08	80.78%	9	36.00%	B
########	Clavamox 375 mg (1 tab)	$ 3,683.64	$ 140,705.72	82.95%	10	40.00%	B
########	Zeniquin 25 mg (1 tab)	$ 3,607.31	$ 144,313.03	85.08%	11	44.00%	B
########	Clavarrox 62.5 mg (1 tab)	$ 3,503.57	$ 147,816.60	87.14%	12	48.00%	B
########	Metronidazole 500 mg (1 tab)	$ 3,445.07	$ 151,261.68	89.18%	13	52.00%	C
########	Amoxidrops 50 mg/ml (30 ml)	$ 3,242.40	$ 154,504.08	91.09%	14	56.00%	C
########	Clintabs 75 mg (1 tab)	$ 2,377.88	$ 156,881.96	92.49%	15	60.00%	C
########	Clavamox 125 mg (1 tab)	$ 2,238.96	$ 159,120.92	93.81%	16	64.00%	C
########	Clavamox 250 mg (1 tab)	$ 2,109.36	$ 161,230.28	95.05%	17	68.00%	C
########	Doxycycline 100 mg (1 tab)	$ 1,765.55	$ 162,995.83	96.09%	18	72.00%	C
########	Zeniquin 50 mg (1 tab)	$ 1,719.70	$ 164,715.53	97.11%	19	76.00%	C
########	Enalapril 10 mg (1 tab)	$ 1,605.65	$ 166,321.18	98.05%	20	80.00%	C
########	Enalapril 5 mg (1 tab)	$ 1,326.48	$ 167,647.66	98.84%	21	84.00%	C
########	Enalapril 20 mg (1 tab)	$ 1,236.90	$ 168,884.56	99.56%	22	88.00%	C
########	Amoxidrops 50 mg/ml (15ml)	$ 428.00	$ 169,312.56	99.82%	23	92.00%	C
########	Enalapril 2.5 mg (1 tab)	$ 240.96	$ 169,553.52	99.96%	24	96.00%	C
########	Doxycycline 50 mg (1 capsule)	$ 69.08	$ 169,622.60	100.00%	25	100.00%	C

account for 67.06 percent of cumulative AUV. These SKUs have been marked "A" in the last column of the table.

» Class B = the next 30 percent of items that account for about the next 15 percent of the AUV.

» Class C = the remaining 50 percent of items that account for the remaining 5 percent of the AUV.

The result will be a table like the one shown in Table 9.2, but much longer for the actual number of SKUs in use in your practice.

The example shows only a small portion (25 items) of the entire practice inventory. In this example, the first 20 percent of the SKU items accounts for 67 percent (rather than 80 percent) of the AUV. Remember that Pareto's 80/20 rule is approximate, not exact.

The next 30 percent accounts for another 21 percent of the AUV. Class A plus Class B (52 percent of total SKUs) account for 89 percent of the AUV. In other words, nearly a full half of the SKU items (Class C) accounts for a mere 11 percent of the AUV.

When you complete an ABC analysis of your practice's supplies, you will likely find similar results. The 80/20 principle is an approximation of the distribution of items; the results of your analysis may produce numbers that fall into slightly different percentages. Nevertheless, the findings will enable you to prioritize the inventory items deserving more of your time and attention. In general, you will need to reduce the on-hand inventory of high-value items (though there may be exceptions for bulk purchases to benefit from discounts, and where excess high-value inventory will be kept under lock and key). Figure 9.3 illustrates the distribution of cumulative AUV (vertical axis) against the cumulative number of SKUs (horizontal axis) after cumulative AUV is ranked from highest to lowest value for each SKU listed in inventory.

Of course, you can have more than three classes if you so choose. For example, drugs listed as controlled substances by the U.S. Drug Enforcement Administration (DEA) present a level of risk that the AUV does not reflect. These medications should be set aside in their own Class "AA," but not included in the standard ABC analysis. Controlled substances require superior security, perpetual monitoring, and perfect record-keeping, no exceptions.

Here are some general guidelines for control use in the three classes determined by an ABC analysis:

- Class AA
  » Controlled substances
  » Highest risk / highest priority
  » Tightest controls
  » Frequent review and inspection (perhaps even daily) by a responsible doctor or chief of staff

FIGURE 9.3 ABC ANALYSIS GRAPH

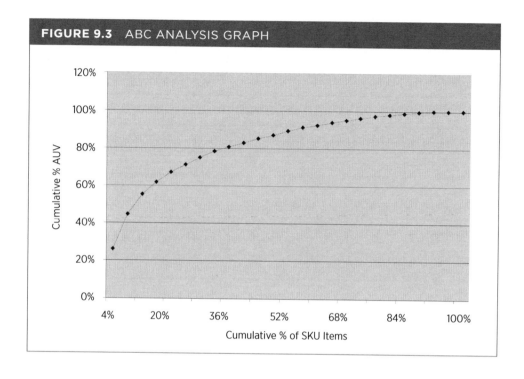

- Class A
  - » High value / high priority
  - » Tight controls
  - » Complete, accurate records
  - » Records updated in practice management system as stock is received
  - » Frequent and regular review by manager
  - » Frequent review and adjustment of demand forecasts
  - » Regular comparisons of physical stock to forecasts
  - » Minimize stocks on hand and reduce lead time
  - » Good security of surplus stock, when surplus is unavoidable
- Class B
  - » Medium priority
  - » Normal control
- Class C
  - » Lowest priority
  - » Simplest possible control

» Weigh cost-benefit relationship of micromanagement and stock savings

» Consider ordering larger quantities with bigger safety stock margins, if warranted

With Class C items, the carrying cost is low, so if you order less frequently you may be able to minimize the labor cost that happens with micromanagement. However, do not carelessly overstock and/or forget to manage these items. After all, Class C items make up about 50 percent of the SKUs moving through the practice.

Now that you have identified which items require more control time and attention, methodically plan your physical counting protocols. Good inventory controls require counting more than once or twice a year. Cyclical counting is the most palatable and effective way to manage stock. Below are some guidelines:

- Class AA (Controlled Substances)
  » Conduct weekly counts of the contents of drug safes accessed on a daily basis (secondary supply locations).
  » Conduct monthly counts of drugs secured in the central supply safe.
- Classes A and B
  » Divide into quarters.
  » Count one-quarter of the Class A and B stock each week. By the end of one month, you have rotated through the entire Class A and B stock.
- Class C
  » Divide into twenty-six sections.
  » Count one part per week. By the end of one calendar half, you have rotated through the entire Class C stock.

Be mindful of any Class A, B, or C items that seem subject to shrinkage as proven through repetitive variances in which the physical counts are persistently lower than the perpetual records indicate they should be. You may wish to throw them into the count more frequently until you see these variances clear up. If they do not, closer monitoring through daily spot checks, perhaps with video surveillance, may be required to identify the cause of the problem.

STREAMLINING THE OVERSTOCKED PRACTICE

You may be embarking on the overdue project of getting inventory back under control after it has run amok. A good place to start is an assessment of all of the products the practice has in stock. The ultimate project objective is to establish an electronic practice formulary that will be easy to keep up on a contemporaneous basis once it is set up.

To begin, print a list of the current products contained in the practice management database. This means all items that are invoiced to clients as part of services provided, including the drugs and supplies that are used and dispensed during the course of medical treatments and surgeries, as well as all items resold to clients, such as pet food for special diets. You may prefer to electronically export the list from the practice management database to a spreadsheet program such as Microsoft Excel.

You may subdivide the list into major categories, such as the following:

- Vaccines and biologics
- Antibiotics (orals and injectables)
- Otics
- Ophthalmics
- Antiparasitic medications
- Anesthetics
- Surgery
- Dentistry
- Hospital and treatment
- Laboratory
- Dietary products, therapeutic
- Dietary products, premium

After breaking the list down into parts, assign the pieces of the list to doctors to review and proofread. Ask them to check that the listed SKUs are in the correct category of usage. Complete this step if you previously used such categorized lists, as, over time, new SKUs will likely have been coded into incorrect categories as they were added to the database.

Complete a physical count of everything on hand, being sure to correctly account for the following:

- Name of item
- Number of items
- Volume
- Strength
- Expiration Dates
- Current locations

Your goal is to develop a detailed and complete SKU list that leaves no room for misunderstanding or error. To your spreadsheet listing, add any missing SKUs from what you've found on hand, and identify items that were exported from the practice management software that may need to be modified or corrected in some way. Take great care to ensure accuracy.

You will have to identify which items on the list are not correctly stated as unique SKUs, which, by definition are identifiable, minimum units consumed in a transaction. For example, injectable penicillin might be listed as 100 ml penicillin, with no clarity as to the dispensing volume (1 bottle, 1 ml, or 1/10 ml?) or the specific type of penicillin solution.

You should identify which items are no longer in use in the hospital, and which items were duplicated in the database. Eventually, you will have to correct the detail of each of these listed inventory items or move them to a "Do not use" category in the practice management system. A "Do not use" category is a work-around solution to allow an inventory item to remain unchanged in the database, and thus in the historic patient medical invoices, while moving it off the current SKU lists that team members have been trained to use on a go-forward basis.

Be mindful of the electronic patient medical records: Any item that has been previously invoiced carries a history into the medical record that must be preserved. You can modify your spreadsheet to your desired and envisioned SKU listing, but before making any changes to the original database you must talk with your software support team about how to proceed. You do not want the changes you make to the inventory control system to affect existing patient transactional histories.

SKUs are used in medical records, have fees attached to them, may be attached to services (such as an injection procedure), and may appear in the detail area of an invoice. Therefore, spend time getting familiar with all of the capabilities of the software your practice uses to track inventory. Look online for training and help from the software vendor. Read the inventory and invoicing modules of the software instruction manual.

Determine what the major profit centers will be and how to best organize drugs and supplies in the computer system in accord with the profit centers you decide are important to track. Start to group items according to treatment use and type on your master spreadsheet.

At this point, you may wish to reassess physical placement and storage of SKUs in locations most correlating with usage. One outcome of this project will be that each listed SKU will also have a physical location identified with it. Ultimately, the database and/or master spreadsheet will allow any employee to locate a product's location in the practice.

Team up with the doctors to debate product usage with an eye to streamlining and tightening inventory control through agreement about which products best fit with current practice care guidelines and which do not. Evaluate items that are sold infrequently and that expire before being completely used. Decide if you will continue to stock these products or only order when needed. If yes, consider charging out the entire purchased volume to the client even if all of it will not be used in the patient's care.

As an additional resource to controlling inventory, a practice-branded online pharmacy service may make sense and will still support use of a low-usage item while allowing clients to purchase them. Many veterinary distributors and independent supply-management companies provide online sales solutions for veterinary practices, and these can integrate rather seamlessly with the practice's website. Clients can order a selection of products and medications from the practice website even if the practice does not physically stock them. Purchases are sent from the supplier to practice clients after the order is verified by a practice employee.

The evolving inventory list that you will produce by taking all the steps described above will be the hospital formulary. It may include valuable information that cannot be managed through the practice management software alone. A formulary will include the following information: use/treatment regimen; species use; typical dosages; and contraindications. To supplement the practice management software, you will need to develop, in consultation with the veterinarians, an electronic document, likely in spreadsheet format, which serves as the ever-evolving practice formulary.

Once you have the spreadsheet well organized, correctly listing all the SKUs you wish to track going forward, you are ready to tackle the veterinary practice management database. Before proceeding, make sure you have done your homework, reading up on the software's inventory management applications. Call your software support team to clarify what is and is not possible and to learn how to avoid damaging any electronic patient medical histories. Carefully make a few changes and run test invoices on a fictional client-patient. Check the medical record that results.

With a careful stepwise process, you should be able to accomplish four goals:

1. Consolidation of existing inventory to a tight, manageable supply that will increase practice profitability and decrease SKUs on your shelves
2. Creation of a practice formulary
3. Creation of a physical inventory map
4. Reorganization of the practice management database to better manage inventory, including invoicing and integration to patient records

Although it is challenging project, ultimately the time you spend streamlining the inventory system will be well worth the effort.

DETERMINING QUANTITIES AND TIMING

The key to an efficient and effective ordering policy is the inventory manager's familiarity with the suppliers and knowledge of how the items are used in practice. This knowledge will make it possible to order the right amount of goods at the fairest prices. Here are some general suggestions of how and when to order inventory for an animal hospital:

- Know when suppliers' representatives will be visiting the hospital. Being prepared saves time.
- Keep a list of reorder items from each supplier. Prepare purchase orders if they are to be used. Try to order an entire month's requirement from each supplier.
- Deal with as few suppliers as possible. Working with a few vendors saves time in ordering, unpacking, handling, invoice checking, and bill paying. The hospital becomes a more

important customer account to the selected vendors, since it orders large quantities. In turn, the suppliers have more of an incentive to provide excellent service.

- Anticipate seasonal ordering (e.g., for heartworm preventives and flea products in the spring).
- Maximize use of vendor credit lines by timing order placement. Plan and make the most significant inventory orders the week after the day the vendor prepares monthly statements. Most companies "close their books" between the 25th and 30th of the month, so items ordered after that week will not be billed until the first of the following month. You can maximize use of practice money through order and payment timing and still take full advantage of purchase discounts from most vendors. Some vendors still allow a percentage discount if the statement is paid within a stipulated number of days of the invoice date. The statement includes all invoices for the month.
- Some companies have short purchase discount cycles, such as "2/10, net 30." This means that a specified percent discount is available if the bill is paid within ten days of invoice receipt (not of the statement date). If you wait until the statement date, you have probably missed the opportunity to take the discount. For these companies, promptly inform the bookkeeper when an order has been placed so that payment can be made from the shipping documents, if necessary. Know your vendor payment deals to maximize practice savings.
- Minimize emergency ordering, which can entail higher costs than routine orders (e.g., for overnight shipping) and are more prone to error, since inexperienced individuals are often placing such orders instead of the regular purchasing agent. When placing an emergency order, use a fax machine or electronic ordering system to be able to track what was ordered.
- Avoid ordering small quantities that may bear additional handling and shipping charges.

Figuring out how much to order of each item and when to order it can be a challenge. Too little of an item creates shortages, causes lost sales and services, and increases ordering costs. Too much of an item increases the expense of inventory holding. Not only do you need to know how much to order, you need to accurately estimate when to order and how much to have on hand while you are waiting for the order to arrive. (See "Determining When to Order.")

Forecasting is the measurement of inventory in motion. Correct measurement is a key to successful forecasting. Various measurement tools include:

- Historical sales and usage reports
- Purchase histories from your records
- Vendor reports of your practice's purchasing history
- Invoices from vendors
- Invoices to customers

- Inventory cards
- Customer input

To properly plan for effective inventory levels, the inventory manager should periodically analyze each item or class of items in order to do the following:

- Forecast demand for the next month, quarter, or year, including seasonal trends
- Determine acquisition lead time
- Plan usage during the lead time period
- Establish and monitor quantity on hand
- Determine reserve or safety stock requirements (Usry and Hammer 1991)

To meet these goals, it is helpful for an inventory manager to know these terms:

- *Operating level:* The inventory amount of an item that is expected to be used up between the point of order receipt and the time another order must be placed. The amount of an item should not drop below a predetermined amount (see "Safety stock" below), or stock outages may occur.
- *Lead time:* The time between the point of order and when shipment will be received. The lead-time quantity is the amount of inventory expected to be used up from the time the order is placed until the order is received. The lead time depends on vendor location and response time. The lead-time quantity should assure that at least one item will still be available when the new order is received.
- *Reorder point:* The time at which the purchasing manager should place a restock order with the vendor because supplies have fallen to a specified level. Reorder point is determined by the SKU quantity that will meet predicted normal operating needs until the restocking supplies arrive on the premises (lead time) plus the selected emergency stock quantity (safety stock). The reorder point quantity equals the safety stock plus the lead-time quantity.
- *Safety stock:* A desired inventory cushion, in excess of lead-time quantity, to help mitigate the event of a stock outage if shipment was delayed or if the item was placed on back order.
- *Inventory turnover:* A computation that relates the volume of merchandise sold to the inventory amount. For a veterinary practice inventory to be profitable, it must be held by the practice a relatively short period of time before it is sold or used. You can compute turnover to determine whether inventory items have the desired "shelf-life" or are sitting around too long and eating into profitability.

Inventory turnover can be calculated for the entire hospital drug and professional supply inventory, for selected segments (such as dietary products or laboratory supplies), or for individual items. Turnover calculations are useful for monitoring inventory-management decisions and for establishing purchase-order quantities and timing.

Calculating Inventory Turns

Every inventory and practice manager should know the basic formula for calculating an inventory turnover ratio. In its simplest form, the inventory turnover ratio is computed for all of the drug and medical supply purchases made in the course of a single year. The ratio equals the total annual purchases divided by the average inventory value on hand. The baseline data required to perform the calculation comes from the financial records:

- Value of drugs and medical supplies on hand at the beginning of the year, at cost (BI)
- Value of drugs and medical supplies on hand at the end of the year, at cost (EI)
- Sum total of drug and medical supply purchases (in dollars) made over the course of the year (DMSP)

Begin by calculating the *average inventory on-hand*. This is the sum of the beginning inventory (BI) and the ending inventory (EI) divided by 2. The result is the *average on-hand inventory* (AI) and is intended to approximate[1] the average cost of inventory on hand at any given time:

$$(BI + EI) \div 2 = AI$$

Now you can compute the inventory turnover ratio. Divide the total purchases during the year (DMSP) by the average on-hand inventory value, as calculated in the first step.

$$DMSP \div AI = \textit{Inventory Turnover Ratio}$$

The resulting inventory turnover ratio tells you how many times the entire inventory of drugs and medical supplies has been sold and replaced over a single year. Some items in the inventory may have turned more often (higher number per year) and some items may have turned over less often (lower number per year).

While this example is a basic computation for the entire inventory over one year, you can compute inventory turnover ratios for individual items or groups of inventory items. You can also compute the inventory ratio over different time frames, which might be helpful when considering the ebb and flow of operating activity, depending on the time of year.

In general, the higher the turnover ratio for a given period of time, the tighter the inventory control. There is no specific number that is correct in every situation, but the average turnover in companion animal hospitals tends to be around six times per year. Different experts will quote various ranges. For example, four to eight times a year has been commonly cited. Robert E. Froehlich (1987, 23) has written that eight to ten times per year (every thirty-five to forty-five days) is a good target range for veterinary hospitals. Higher turnover ratios are more attainable with a "just-in-time" inventory, where products can be obtained with minimal lead time from a vendor at appropriate quantities. However, the inventory manager must not be careless with spending too much time on frequent, repetitive ordering activities, which could defeat the benefits of faster turnover.

A very high turnover ratio, although appearing financially advantageous because it provides a faster return on inventory investment, has the danger of creating shortages. Ordering costs will also increase. The more orders required, the more labor involved in creating the order, unpacking the shipment, and accounting for the transaction.

Also, general economic factors can influence buying decisions, which in turn affect the resulting inventory turnover ratios. For example, during a period of rapidly escalating inflation, it may make sense to order large quantities before large price hikes go into effect, and therefore place orders less frequently.

Another common and useful calculation that follows from the inventory turnover ratio yields the average shelf life of inventory in days (ASLD). Compute ASLD by dividing the number of days in the period being measured by the inventory turnover ratio (ITR) for the correlating period. If the inventory turnover ratio measures the turns in a full year, divide 365 by annual ITR. If the inventory turnover ratio measures the turns in a calendar half, divide 182 by semiannual ITR.

365 ÷ annual ITR = ASLD

Figure 9.4 illustrates how the calculation of the inventory turnover ratio and the average shelf life in days works in practice for a veterinary hospital. Figure 9.5 shows how to apply these calculations to a single item, in this case 100 mg amoxicillin tablets, 200 per bottle.

Managers should track inventory turnover ratios and average shelf life in days over time because the resulting figures are useful indicators of inventory system function. The trends uncovered through this data highlight when and where additional attention should be spent in managing inventory.

Earlier in this chapter, we described a method of prioritizing inventory called *selective inventory management*. This process determines and ranks the inventory SKUs with the highest calculated annual value. Use the inventory turnover ratio computation to establish the turnover rates for the top 20 percent of SKUs, which comprise the practice's Class A inventory. The ITR for each of these high-ranking SKUs can be periodically spot-checked as a trend analysis for efficiency.

Evaluate whether turnover rates for other items should be determined as well. The resulting turnover numbers will give the inventory manager target turnover rates and therefore help in determinations of the maximum order quantity for each item. Remember, however, that turnover rates will not be constant over a year's time for seasonal items.

FIGURE 9.4 CALCULATION OF ANNUAL TURNOVER FOR A VETERINARY PRACTICE

Beginning inventory (1/1/XX)	$30,000
Ending inventory (12/31/XX)	$40,000
Average inventory ($30,000 + $40,000) ÷ 2 =	$35,000
Total purchases (1/1/XX through 12/31/XX)	$210,000
Inventory turnover ($210,000 ÷ $35,000) =	6 times per year
Average days on shelf (365 ÷ 6) =	60.83 days

FIGURE 9.5 CALCULATION OF ANNUAL TURNOVER FOR A SINGLE ITEM

Beginning inventory (1/1/XX)	150 tablets
Ending inventory (6/30/XX)	210 tablets
Average inventory for 6 months (150 + 210) ÷ 2 =	180 tablets
Total purchases (1/1/XX through 6/30/XX) – 4 bottles	800 tablets
Inventory turnover (800 ÷ 180) =	4.44 times per 6 months
	8.88 times per year
Average days on shelf (183 days ÷ 4.44) =	41.22 days

DETERMINING WHEN TO ORDER

Several factors influence the timing of orders:

1. The time needed for delivery
2. The rate of inventory usage
3. The safety stock level (Usry and Hammer 1991)
4. The effect of special manufacturer and vendor offerings

There are no generally accepted formulas for setting reorder points that apply in all situations. Scheduling a set reorder point would be relatively simple if usage rates were consistent. Lead time is also a variable factor. The more predictable the time between placing an order and receiving it, the closer the inventory manager can estimate the order date.

Typically, the reorder point is determined by normal, expected SKU consumption during the lead time plus the safety-stock quantity. The safety-stock quantity compensates for demand variability, which may not be predictable from forecasts based on prior use. If substitute products can be used in the event of a stock outage, then a safety-stock level may not be necessary.

The lead time quantity is determined by the average daily usage rate multiplied by the predicted lead time. If the practice does not use prior usage reports to determine average daily usage, the manager may reorder either too soon, and have too much product on hand, or too late, and run out before the new supply arrives. For example, if, on average, the practice uses 10 canine rabies vaccinations per day, and the lead time is 4 days, then the practice manager should reorder when 40 vaccines remain in the refrigerator, without consideration of safety-stock quantity. If, on the basis of experience or calculations, the practice keeps a safety stock of 20 rabies vaccines, then the reorder-point quantity is 60 vaccines.

Because perfect calculations of projected inventory usage and lead time are impossible, the inventory manager must assure a cushion to protect against stock-outs. Having the buffer provided by safety stock is usually the least costly method for protecting against a stock-out.

Safety-stock levels may be more important now than in the past in veterinary practice. Lead-time estimates are hampered by steadily increasing incidents of manufacturer drug shortages. This can become an obstacle to accurate predictions of reorder points. Manufacturing problems and regulatory issues are two leading causes of drug shortages (Stone 2011).

Working with the veterinary staff, the manager should identify which SKUs in the practice formulary are highly critical to patient care. Safety-stock estimates for critical SKUs should incorporate knowledge of predicted shortages. Shortage alerts may come from suppliers, and the manager may also obtain information from the FDA website, which attempts to list information about shortages that is voluntarily provided by manufacturers (see www.fda.gov/Drugs/DrugSafety/DrugShortages/ucm050792.htm).

Basic rules of inventory apply to safety stock. If the safety stock is greater than it needs to be, the carrying cost will be too high. If the safety-stock level is too low, frequent stock-outs will occur, resulting in inconvenience, disruption, and additional costs. The optimal safety-stock level is the quantity resulting in minimum total carrying cost and stock-out inconvenience (Usry and Hammer 1991, 247).

Most often in veterinary practices, inventory managers simply estimate safety-stock levels. Cost-accounting textbooks are useful resources for learning more about how the variables involved can be used to compute reorder points, as well as other aspects of inventory management. Much information can be found through Internet searches as well.

Most software programs with an inventory-management module include input areas for each criterion affecting when an item should be ordered. Data is required for:

1. The desired operating levels (maximum quantity to have on hand and estimated from inventory turnover calculations)
2. Lead-time quantities

3. Safety-stock amounts

When these parameters are entered, the computer system tracks inventory on hand. It cues the practice manager to order when the quantity falls to the total of lead-time quantity plus safety-stock amount.

A fourth factor influencing reorder timing relates to special manufacturer offerings. Most often these purchasing deals occur at the end of the calendar year. It is common for veterinary drug and biologic manufacturers to incentivize practices to place large orders for the coming year based on predicted product use and sales patterns. Incentives usually take the form of a combination of favorable pricing plus delayed payment plans.

On a per-SKU basis, supplier prices usually decrease with a veterinary practice's increasing volume commitment to a bulk purchase in advance of the new year. The manufacturer or supplier will also communicate expected annual price increases that will happen in the first quarter. The manufacturer may allow delayed payment that occurs months later, to coincide with practice revenue realization in the spring and early summer season when animal vaccinations and medication dispensing experience seasonal peaks.

All three factors will influence an inventory manager's buying strategies, which should be based on excellent knowledge of both practice product-use patterns and competing vendor offers. Delayed payment plans require the practice-management team to carefully plan cash-flow

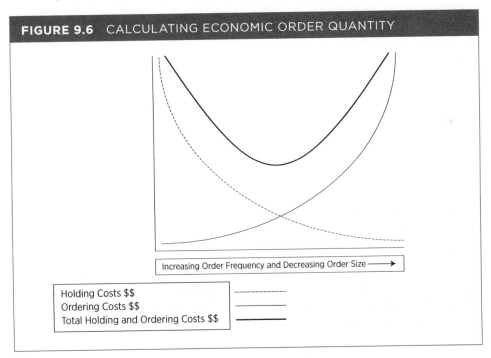

FIGURE 9.6 CALCULATING ECONOMIC ORDER QUANTITY

Increasing Order Frequency and Decreasing Order Size ⟶

Holding Costs $$
Ordering Costs $$
Total Holding and Ordering Costs $$

budgets. There is little that is more distressing than to be flush with client receipts in early spring, only to find the practice short of cash when large delayed pharmacy bills come due in May, June, July, and August. More follows in the section after next.

ECONOMIC ORDER QUANTITY

Managers should be familiar with the concepts encompassed by a mathematical model called *economic order quantity,* which finds the optimum order quantity by determining the point at which inventory ordering and holding costs are minimized. Recall that when the frequency of placing orders is high, the ordering costs are high and the holding costs are low. But when the frequency of placing orders is low, ordering costs are low and holding costs are high. These opposing factors are optimized using the economic order quantity formula. (See Figure 9.6.)

The *economic order quantity (EOQ) formula* is useful when both the demand and the purchase price for a SKU is constant over the course of a year and there are no discounts or delayed payment plans. It recognizes the three specific costs incurred in acquiring items for inventory that we discussed earlier: unit cost, ordering cost, and holding cost.

The formula determines the optimal quantity of any one item to be ordered each time an order is placed. Inventory management software may incorporate the computation, and you can explore further use of the concept through other sources. Managers should at least be acquainted with the formula, and for reference, it follows here:

$$EOQ = \sqrt{\frac{2 \times A \times F}{H \times UC}}$$

In this formula, the following definitions apply:

A = Annual demand in units
F = Fixed ordering costs incurred per order
H = Holding costs expressed on an annual basis as a percentage of unit cost
UC = Unit cost to purchase from vendor or supplier

OTHER MEANS OF INVENTORY CONTROL

There are numerous other ways to effect additional savings and profits from inventory. Every effort made has an additive effect, as small improvements add up to large gains.

As mentioned earlier, watch for deals that offer discounts for purchasing large quantities of an item. The discount must be sufficient to offset the costs of maintaining the inventory until it is sold (holding costs). Moreover, by timing orders and purchases to the vendor's billing cycle, you can delay receiving a bill for that item for at least thirty days, during which time you can sell or use the item.

Assume the practice's turnover number for a given item is 6 (meaning that on average, you can estimate that the full order will be sold in 60 days). If you have 30 days to sell the item before you need to pay for it, and the selling price of the item is twice the purchase price, then, from the sale of a 30-day supply of the item (one-half of the order), you have realized in revenues the amount of money due to the company for the 60-day supply. In essence, none of the hospital's current capital was used to stock the item in the hospital (if only unit cost is considered).

You may want to negotiate with drug and supply distributors to house the inventory for your hospital. If the hospital agrees to purchase a certain amount of an item solely from one distributor over a specified period of time, the distributor may agree to keep the product in its warehouse. It can then ship inventory on a "just-in-time" basis. The vendor can bill the hospital on a preset schedule or as your hospital requests. This agreement generally includes purchase discounts.

Using company credit cards to pay for supplies also allows for delayed payment while the practice has use of the asset. Make sure the credit card balances are paid off in a timely manner, however, to avoid high interest charges and/or late charges.

Here are some other tips for saving money on purchases:

- Comparison shop for supplies, especially sundries like toilet paper and towels or printed forms and stationery.
- Keep in mind that many products can be purchased for much less at certain times of the year, such as when the vendor is not as busy as other times or when salespeople are trying to meet end-of-year quotas.
- If your hospital uses large quantities of specially printed forms, consider bidding out the job. You may find that ordering greater than a three-month supply is advantageous.
- For equipment purchases, obtain bids from several vendors. Know exactly what equipment is needed to meet the practice's needs. Provide identical specifications to each vendor so that the bids will be comparable to one another.

One caveat on getting bids for large or expensive pieces of equipment: Keep in mind that sometimes a higher price reflects the extra attention a vendor pays to customer service and/or training in the use of the equipment. Or, it may reflect a better warranty, or better turn-around times when it comes to making repairs. Make sure you are comparing apples to apples. The extra support may be worth the additional cost.

RIGHTS OF INVENTORY OWNERSHIP

Inventory becomes an asset owned by the business as soon as title to it has passed from the vendor to the veterinary practice—in other words, the moment at which the sale is deemed to have occurred. The inventory may not necessarily be on practice premises when title passes. It could be at the point the inventory passes to the freight company engaged to deliver it.

You should be able to determine when title has passed (and practice liability for vendor payment has occurred) from the shipping documents. A *Freight on Board (FOB) shipping point* designation means that the sale occurs at the vendor's shipping dock, when the merchandise is loaded on the carrier. *FOB destination* means that title passes when the merchandise is delivered to the buyer (in this case, when the carrier unloads the shipment at the veterinary practice).

PRICING ISSUES

Inventory generally carries a high dollar value on the asset side of the balance sheet. Although inventory is an asset, it is nonproductive unless it is sold or used. Consequently, it costs money until it is sold or used.

In a veterinary practice, excessive inventory ties up funds, requires storage, and represents loss if it becomes outdated or cannot be sold. Part of the purpose of an effective and efficient inventory control program is to ensure that inventory generates a profit rather than draining practice resources. If there are items in inventory that are sapping practice resources, it is time to reevaluate having them take up space.

Regardless of how well you manage inventory, ordering, and payments for products, the system is doomed unless adequate charges are assessed and collected from clients.

Mark-up and Margin Pricing Methods

To maintain adequate revenues and profits, you must ensure adequate and timely product pricing. Two common methods of pricing include markup and margin pricing.

Markup pricing entails multiplying acquisition cost by a factor. Margin pricing determines the amount of profit desired for a given product line, and adding it to the cost of obtaining it from the supplier. Historically, the markup method is commonly used by veterinary practices and incorporated in practice inventory software modules; however, competitive market forces may be influencing changes toward a margin pricing strategy for some products.

With the markup method, a 100 percent markup on cost doubles the price for which the product was obtained from the vendor. A 200 percent markup triples the unit cost, and a 300 percent markup quadruples the unit cost to arrive at retail price. To determine the markup on an item, you must consider market competition and constraints as well as cost and practice philosophy. Product markups can easily range from a low of 40 percent to a high of 400 percent.

In veterinary practices, a 40 percent markup on product cost will result in a retail price that is very close to break-even point, when all costs of operations are considered. Being predominantly a service-based business, with a secondary reliance on inventory sales, veterinary practices appear to be relatively inefficient at managing inventory in a way that keeps sales profitable at markups of less than 35 percent.

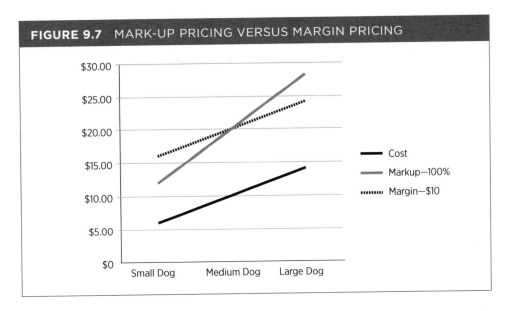

FIGURE 9.7 MARK-UP PRICING VERSUS MARGIN PRICING

Margin pricing differs from markup, in that a targeted dollar value is determined for profit. This amount is then added to the acquisition cost to establish the retail price charged to the client. In veterinary medicine, margin pricing may be an appropriate strategy when there are large differences in resulting price based solely on the size of the patient. With margin pricing, the price of a particular medication will increase much more gradually for the size of the patient as compared to a straight multiplier effect with the mark up method.

Figure 9.7 illustrates the difference between mark-up pricing and margin pricing.

Sometimes products serve as "loss leaders." In this case, the product is priced very low, below where a profit can be generated. It is a marketing technique to draw clients or potential clients to the practice in the hope that these clients will end up purchasing other products and services.

In most cases, the practice is better situated economically when it marks up products adequately. It is difficult to compete on merchandise retailing when big-box stores, catalog sale houses, and Internet outlets can sell the product for less than the amount for which your practice is able to purchase the products from a vendor.

Break-Even Analysis as a Starting Point for Product Pricing

Practice managers are reasonably concerned about how to price products of all sorts, ranging from a single prescription of antibiotics to medications repeatedly dispensed to treat long-term conditions. Without adequate pricing that recognizes all factors of product dispensing cost, pharmacy and related product sales can contribute to bottom-line losses, rather than supplementing profit.

In pricing discussions, it is important to understand the concept of *break-even analysis.* This relatively simple computation can affect the decisions you make about product markups. The break-even point (BEP) for any practice is the amount of revenue that covers all fixed and variable costs for the volume of the sales that have been made, without loss or profit. Another way to say this is that a practice's break-even sales revenue is the point at which sales revenues equal fixed costs plus variable costs, without generating either profit or loss.

A fixed cost tends to remain constant in monetary amount, regardless of variations in the volume of activity. A purely variable cost directly and proportionately fluctuates in amount in relation to the volume of activity.

When break-even analysis is applied to a single SKU, the break-even sales price (BESP) equals the SKU's fixed cost (FC) plus its related variable costs (VC). Purely variable costs are directly proportional to the SKU's sales price. This formula can help with many pricing dilemmas because it provides a baseline for a pricing decision.

From the most simplistic break-even aspect, we might only be interested in considering the actual costs of practice operations and product acquisition for pricing and prescribing. However, most astute practice managers understand that an incremental profit layer should be built into the price of every item invoiced or sold, to the extent possible and in light of many factors that affect client perception of price relative to value (refer to Chapter 13 on marketing for more on this subject).

The break-even sales price equation can be expanded to include the profit layer. Therefore, the expanded formula for pricing, including the profit factor, and where SP means sales price, appears like this:

$$SP = FC + VC + P$$
where:
SP = *sales price (of a SKU)*
FC = *fixed costs*
VC = *variable costs*
P = *profit*

Fixed costs are relatively straightforward when they are limited to a specific SKU held for resale without consideration of all other practice operational costs. For purposes of our calculation, fixed costs include attributed costs of obtaining the SKU to be sold, that is, the unit cost plus estimated ordering and holding costs. For example, if a box of heartworm preventive costs $10 (vendor's unit sales price), we can roughly estimate another 25 percent of unit cost for ordering and holding costs (as discussed earlier in this chapter, recall the range is about

15 percent to 35 percent). Therefore, the $10 box of heartworm preventive has a real, relative fixed cost of $12.50.

It is the variable costs, however, that are usually the key issue in ascertaining how much you will mark up a medication held for dispensing. Let's set aside profit for the moment, which is an important variable in and of itself when we use the mark-up method of pricing. Another significant variable component can relate to how hospital veterinarians are compensated. When the hospital pays doctors based directly on a proportion of overall revenue production, they may be eligible to receive a percentage of gross product sales.

In past years, doctors traditionally received 20 percent of gross collections attributable to them, which generally excluded boarding, grooming, and point-of-purchase sales. If a doctor's compensation is based on a 20 percent cut of any dispensed pharmacy sale, then that contracted commission becomes a significant variable component in determining sales price. Payroll taxes and benefits for that veterinarian must also be added to the 20 percent factor, for a grand total of approximately 25 percent. Thus, in this scenario, a practice could incur total compensation cost of approximately 25 percent of the sale of any given SKU assigned to the doctor's revenue production totals.

As mentioned above, the desired practice profit per dollar of sales revenue can likewise be computed as part of the variable cost. Assume, for example, that, like many small animal practices, your practice has a goal of maintaining a profit margin of at least 12 percent. Twelve percent of sales price then becomes the second variable factor.

Based on these figures, it is now possible to do the math and establish a price for the unit of heartworm prevention medication. The break-even analysis that follows is based *only* on the expenses directly associated with the specific product sale. Called *direct or variable costing*, this method does not consider all the other costs of managing the practice that must be supported by sales, such as overhead expenses for support staff labor costs, general and administrative expenses, and the bulk of facility and equipment costs. These overhead costs would be considered in an analysis that fully absorbs all identifiable costs (*full absorption cost accounting*).

Nevertheless, let's proceed with a simple out-of-pocket break-even analysis, where SP is sales price, and variable costs are expressed as a percentage of the sales price. Again, FC is for fixed cost, and VC is for variable cost. P stands for profit. To lay the groundwork:

$$P = 12\% \times SP$$
$$SP = FC + VC + P$$
$$SP = (unit\ price + holding\ cost + ordering\ cost) + ([DVM\ \% + desired\ profit\ \%] \times SP)$$

Now, to apply the math to our example:

$$SP = (\$10.00 + (\$10.00 \times 25\%)\,) + (25\% + 12\%)\,SP$$
$$SP = \$12.50 + 0.37\,SP$$
$$SP - 0.37\,SP = \$12.50$$
$$0.63\,SP = \$12.50$$
$$SP = \$19.84$$

The result shows that the sales price for a $10 box of heartworm medication must be $19.84 in order to obtain a 12 percent profit margin while also covering the unit cost (including related holding cost and ordering costs) and the veterinarian compensation cost. But remember: This computation does not include all the overhead costs that would be considered using a full absorption methodology. If they are not covered by the SKU pricing formula, these additional practice overhead costs would need to be subsidized by other departments. In essence, by using the foregoing direct costing methodology for pricing, pharmacy activities are subsidized by other revenue-generating segments of the practice.

For many medications used in long-term care of chronic conditions, questions arise about whether the doctor should be paid a percentage portion of the sale, which effectively becomes a commission. Even though a doctor signs for the prescription and authorizes its refill, some people believe commission-based pay is not appropriate in medical practices. There are a variety of reasons for this view. Such commissions should be minimal if calculated as a percentage of sales, or limited to a fixed fee, if not eliminated entirely. If we revise the calculation to omit the DVM's percentage of sales price, the result is as follows. Again, SP is for sales price, FC is for fixed cost, P is for profit, and we assume that P = 12% × SP:

$$SP = FC + P$$
$$SP = \$12.50 + 0.12\,SP$$
$$SP - 0.12\,SP = \$12.50$$
$$0.88\,SP = \$12.50$$
$$SP = \$14.20$$

With this pricing example, the $10 box of heartworm preventive is priced at $14.20. As in the prior example, this computation does not take all overhead expenses into account, as the full absorption methodology would.

As you might expect, use of the full absorption methodology has a significant impact on pricing regimens. Here is a simplified calculation illustrating how the full absorption method would apply to the same $10 box of heartworm medication. The computation excludes the doctor commission–based compensation percentage and adds a new variable factor of 45 percent of sales price, representing an estimate that every dollar of practice revenue must cover approximately $0.45 of overhead operating costs not previously recognized by holding and ordering cost assignments to the SKU. Here, OHC stands for overhead costs:

$$OHC = 0.45 \times SP$$
$$SP = FC + OHC + P$$
$$SP = \$12.50 + (0.45 \times SP) + (0.12 \times SP)$$
$$SP = \$12.50 + 0.57\ SP$$
$$SP - 0.57SP = \$12.50$$
$$0.43SP = \$12.50$$
$$SP = \$29.07$$

As this result shows, even a 1.4 times multiplier (40 percent markup applied to SKU cost, including the SKU's unit, ordering, and holding costs) may not be adequate to generate a return on medications, even when the doctor is not paid a percentage. With a 1.4 times multiplier, other segments of the practice operations must subsidize the fact of product sale throughout the veterinary hospital.

The expenses of running a capital-intensive business such as a veterinary practice demand that careful attention be given to pricing regimens for both service and product sales. Pricing strategies cause practice managers great concern in the face of a highly competitive marketplace when it comes to the products that used to be sold exclusively by bricks-and-mortar veterinary establishments, but are now sold by companies with less overhead, such as Internet firms. Client visits help sustain trusting relationships with the veterinary team, and managers must factor the potential loss of client visits related to pickup of medication refills and other products into their pricing strategies.

Sales and Use Taxes

States and local taxing agencies levy taxes on sales of merchandise and sometimes services. Many times, veterinary business owners erroneously believe that their practices are exempt from laws regulating such sales. They make this assumption because much of the human health-care industry is exempt (e.g., prescriptions of medications for people are usually sold without sales tax added) and because of exceptions for agriculturally based animal health care.

Most veterinary practices serving companion animals are, however, subject to sales-tax rules. Managers and owners should be aware that state agencies have significantly stepped up the number of audits of many types of businesses in an effort to improve sales-tax collection and remittance. Veterinarians have not been omitted from the fray. Despite these audits and well-publicized alerts, it is surprising that many hospitals still are not in compliance.

Sales-tax compliance applies to veterinary practice in two ways. First is whether tax needs to be paid to any vendor that sells the practice services, products, or supplies. Second is whether the practice is responsible for the collection of sales tax from its own clients when it sells services and/or products.

Unfortunately, no simple rule exists for veterinary hospitals. Each state and commonwealth has its own set of rules regarding sales tax, and they are often very complex. A good starting point is to contact your state veterinary medical association to find out whether it can offer any guidance through recent, up-to-date publications. In some jurisdictions, industry-wide audits of veterinary hospitals have been conducted and the results of those audits may have led to the publication of guidelines. In some situations, pharmaceuticals and other products are exempt from sales tax when the practice purchases them from the vendor, but the practice must charge a sales tax on the marked-up amount when selling the items to clients. The practice is then required to remit the sales taxes to the state.

In other situations, it is just the opposite: The practice must pay a sales tax on items and services purchased from a vendor or supplier, but there is no requirement to charge sales tax to the client. Be aware that the laws in this area are constantly being amended and clarified. Even if your practice was in perfect compliance a decade ago, it may no longer be.

Because of these complexities, properly accounting for sales tax can be very time-consuming. Check with your practice's accounting firm to find out if they are familiar with current sales-tax law as it pertains specifically to veterinary practice. The accountant may or may not have current information, and certainly you can engage the accountant to read the regulations and give you an opinion of how to best comply.

Next, check the website(s) of the state taxing authorities with jurisdiction over your practice. Practices now have easy access to state laws and rules via state government websites. Start with the state department of taxation website and find links to business and sales-tax information.

While you have the business taxation site in your browser, take a moment to sign up for automatic tax alerts. Most state tax websites provide them, and they are a useful back-up system to alert you to tax return due dates, tax rate changes, and changes in state law. Sales-tax laws and regulations change frequently, so receiving regular updates will help you fulfill your management duties for keeping the practice in compliance with rule changes.

Once you have found the sales-tax rules for your state, query for "veterinary" and "veterinarian." If you are fortunate, you may find an intelligible synopsis of the rules applying to private veterinary practices. Usually, however, the rules are not all together in one place and you will have to read through different documents to piece together applications to pet-food sales, boarding operations, pharmacy sales, pharmaceutical use in the course of patient treatment by the practice, nonprescription-type "over-the-counter" medication sales, and more.

If the veterinary practice serves clients in multiple states, it likely must abide by multiple sets of regulations that may or may not be coordinated between the various agencies.

Determine if different rules apply for dietary products, supplies consumed in-house, items resold to clients, or medicines administered to patients during the course of the office call. Each situation is different and may require special treatment. Don't forget that some or all services may also constitute taxable transactions. For example, boarding and grooming services might be taxable, but veterinary services might not be taxable.

For any one item purchased from a vendor, two different methods of accounting may be required for the same item based on how the item is being used. Dietary products are one example. In some cases, the practice may pay sales tax to the vendor for pet foods fed to a hospitalized or boarded pet, but the client pays the sales tax if the client is taking the same pet food home to feed to the pet.

Once you have determined the specific requirements of the state in which your practice is located, review the coding within the practice management software. The management program should allow you to determine and set the appropriate tax rate to use and to specify the items or services to which sales tax applies. Make sure that the coding is updated to properly reflect those items subject to tax and those that are not as changes occur.

When different sets of rules apply to the same items, such as in the pet-food example described above, sometimes an easy solution is to set up two accounts with a supplier, with one account being subject to sales tax, and the other maintained only for those purchases that are not subject to sales tax. You may need to set up dual accounts in this manner with each of the hospital's major suppliers.

Under this method, the practice's purchasing agent must make sure, when placing the order, that the order is assigned to the correct account with the distributor or vendor. Despite all due care, oversights and errors occur.

It is a good idea for another set of eyes to check the accuracy of these orders. For example, the bookkeeper can review invoices before making payment. The bookkeeper would thus notice whether a sales tax was or was not paid on a particular invoice and question any possible discrepancies. The bookkeeper would need to be familiar with the different requirements, and he would need to know how to determine whether invoices properly reflected the vendor account to which purchases were assigned.

The final requirement is to make sure that sales taxes are remitted on a timely basis. The timing depends on the volume of sales and on individual state requirements. The bookkeeper should keep a reminder system so that due dates are not forgotten. Penalties and interest can be substantial for delinquent filing.

Use tax is a relatively unfamiliar cousin to sales tax. Also known as a *compensating tax*, it compensates the state when sales tax should have been collected, but wasn't.

A common situation necessitating payment of the use tax is when out-of-state purchases are made. This includes purchases made through the Internet when the Internet company is in a different state from the company making the purchase. In veterinary medicine, for example, equipment purchased from an out-of-state vendor may require a use tax. This happens when the out-of-state vendor fails to collect sales tax for the state in which the practice resides. The practice owner or administrator often believes that she negotiated a wonderful deal because no sales tax had to be paid on what was a fairly significant purchase of equipment. In reality, the tax does have to be paid, but it is now called a use tax.

State laws require that if the vendor did not collect sales tax, it is the business's responsibility to cough up the difference. During state sales-tax audits, veterinary practices hardest hit are often those that made significant equipment purchases on which sales tax was not paid. States are quite attuned to these equipment invoices. The agencies will demand that the practice ante up after the fact. Penalty and interest costs, as well any cost of defense through an attorney or an accountant, can add quite a sting, not even considering the tax itself that is due.

Other out-of-state purchases commonly requiring use-tax computations include office supplies, computer reminder postcards, uniforms, and drug and hospital items. The practice bookkeeper should carefully review invoices, especially from rarely used vendors, to determine whether a sales tax should have been paid. If it should have been and was not, an ongoing tally must be kept of the total amount of purchases subject to use tax. At the end of the quarter or month, a calculation must be done and the use tax submitted.

Each state has its own use-tax remittance form. Some states have a separate form distinct from that used for sales tax. Other states and commonwealths combine both taxes onto one form.

Bookkeeping software programs ease the burden of doing the necessary computations. An astute bookkeeper will categorize purchases subject to use tax and assign them to a separate account as payment is made. At the designated date, he can then quickly create a report of the total purchases subject to use tax for the period. The grand total is multiplied by the applicable rate for preparation and submission of the tax return.

As you can see, inventory management is a complex topic—but for a manager who takes the time to understand it, it offers wonderful opportunities for cost savings and increased revenues. By reading this overview of the topic, you have taken a great first step toward understanding some of the issues involved. Perhaps you were aware of some of these issues already, whereas others may be new concepts for you. Take this information as your starting point and continue to learn from other sources about inventory, incorporating the new concepts over time, and your practice will be certain to benefit from your diligence.

IV

FINANCE AND ECONOMICS

10

Hospital Revenue
and Financial Control

A good practice manager persistently seeks ways to increase practice revenues and improve profitability. Financial matters and good patient care go hand in hand. Revenues and profits are essential to appropriate patient health care, and good patient-care outcomes lead to client satisfaction and a favorable revenue stream.

Clients expect reliable, responsive animal health care and will pay for these services, especially when they value the services provided and feel a sense of satisfaction about their experiences at the practice. Many factors that relate to client satisfaction and perceived value thus form a large portion of the manager's job description. As hospital manager, you must do all you can to ensure a continuum of service, value, and revenue.

The continuing financial health of the practice relies heavily on the practice health-care team's attention to prompt and courteous service. In exchange, the practice should expect prompt client payment and experience revenue growth.

How Fees Contribute to a Healthy Practice

Despite this logical sequence of exchange of money for services, there is a dilemma inherent in the caring image of the veterinary profession. Hospital employees, including doctors, want to help as many people and animals as possible, but are not necessarily willing to charge enough for their valuable time, knowledge, and expertise. And yet, the same staff expects to be paid well and to receive periodic raises, bonuses, ancillary benefits, and other incentives.

A practice manager must be fully aware of the high cost of operating and maintaining a veterinary practice. The breadth of hospital services and correlating fees are based on the costs of providing these services and the level of profit required to allow for future investment and growth. Costs of practice operations are always rising. Besides the cost of maintaining the practice's labor force, suppliers regularly increase their prices. The amounts expended on pharmaceuticals, reference laboratory fees, and the supplies necessary to support patient care increase every year.

The economic pressures include the cost of rapidly advancing medical technology. A veterinary practice manager must budget adequate monies for replacement and renewal of expensive medical, computer, and other equipment needs; for data security and software upgrades; and for the service contracts that are needed to support technology use.

Many hospitals for humans cover these costs in part with tax savings resulting from their advantageous nonprofit status. In veterinary medicine, taxes must be paid on profit before it can be reinvested back into the equipment and other high-tech needs of the practice.

As a service profession, veterinary practice has high labor costs. The expenditures required to maintain adequate inventories of all the items needed to provide the full gamut of veterinary services are high. Besides pharmaceuticals, the hospital must stock anesthetic agents, laboratory reagents, patient care supplies, personal protective equipment, and more. (For more on inventory control, see Chapter 9.)

Another fact of life in veterinary medicine is that hospital owners have a great deal of personal investment in the hospital—in real estate, equipment, personnel, and supplies. Owners often put their personal assets at risk by obtaining and guaranteeing significant loans, which in turn provide the capital needed to acquire hospital assets. The hospital therefore needs to cover more than current expenses; it needs to generate enough cash flow to repay outstanding loan principal balances and the interest expense on these loans. Owners expect to receive additional recompense for the investment risk they have assumed in the ownership of a veterinary practice, as well as for the hard work they have committed to doing in order to ensure the economic success of the practice.

Managers soon realize that small improvements result in big gains. For any given level of practice activity, a slightly higher fee or slightly lower cost of providing the service can add an additional profit dollar for each unit sale. That dollar is then available to improve the practice. Theoretically, if all *fixed expenses* and most *variable expenses* have already been covered, a slight fee hike results in pure profit return. If the practice gives away so much income in the form of discounts or free services that expenditures are not even covered by current income, then the manager will be trying to fill a deep hole before any profits can be measured.

The additional cash flows achieved by adequately charging for all services and quickly collecting on outstanding balances allow the practice to maintain the highest possible level of animal care. By charging appropriately and capturing and collecting all fees, the practice is able to add to the value of care by:

- Adding new medical equipment and technology to improve diagnosis and treatment of animal health needs.

- Acquiring a wide variety of pharmaceutical agents, diagnostic equipment, and other materials that allow the hospital to practice better veterinary medicine.
- Increasing the amounts budgeted for other areas of expenditure that help hospital employees, practice owners, and the hospital's clientele, including information resources about better care; a comprehensive practice website; fresh-looking uniforms; a well-maintained and clean hospital, with adequate repair and janitorial services, an attractive facade, and signage that makes the hospital easy to find in both routine and emergency situations; security and safety features such as surveillance systems; efficient management software systems; and detailed and well-maintained medical record systems.
- Providing adequate employee wages and salaries so that the practice can hire competent and personable employees, retain talented employees, encourage staff loyalty, and reward excellent performance.
- Investing in targeted, quality training and continuing education for every member of the practice team, and supporting career development opportunities leading to overall improvements in the level of health care provided.
- Ensuring the fiscal stability of the practice and consistent performance in excess of practice break-even targets, so that it will continue to be a healthy community presence to meet the demands of the current and potential clientele.
- Advancing consistent veterinary care in accord with the practice mission and core values, which will lead to perpetual employee pride in the organization.

Your management approach to sustaining revenue growth will be multifaceted. The veterinary team's consistent performance in client communication and service is one aspect, but employees do come and go. Individual motivation and attentiveness to the details of income collection may vary quite a bit. Think about the skills you will need to direct team members and to boost their confidence and abilities to articulate services and value to clients. Your competent oversight, leadership, and mentoring aptitude will be a constant requirement. No one-shot fix achieves results; constant vigilance and resourcefulness characterize the hospital manager.

A manager's attentiveness to ensuring profitability creates many benefits for the practice and all of its stakeholders. Over the course of years, the benefits compound. The hospital, its owners, the patients and clients, and the employees all reap the rewards of an adequate fee schedule, fairly charged and prudently collected.

As practice manager, you must carefully design and organize your practice's specific systems for managing the revenue stream. You must then monitor and adapt that system as needed throughout the years. In short, you must constantly tend and refine the practice systems in order to maintain the highest possible level of efficiency, so that the practice will collect adequate amounts of money to provide excellent care, to support the practice team, and to continually improve.

The fee-income and revenue system includes these components:

- Appointment scheduling
- The reminder system
- Client discount policies
- Employee discounts
- Client credit policies
- Care plan and estimate preparation and presentation
- Payment-option adaptation and management
- Receptionist and cashier accuracy in recording and collecting charges
- Team training in invoicing accuracy when invoicing for services provided or products dispensed
- Accounts receivable management
- Collection policies
- Regular fee schedule increases
- Strategic fee modification
- New service and revenue center development, deployment, and marketing
- Patient medical chart maintenance and concurrent invoicing of patient services as they are provided
- Patient care guideline development, team education, training, and competency in client communication
- Medical record audit and compliance assessment
- Target goal determination and communication
- Team feedback and coaching

Every service transaction depleting hospital resources should result in collected revenues. This will not happen without team-member and managerial compliance with many of functions just listed.

Revenue collection policies are at the heart of hospital income realization, since the practice manager and team members are responsible for ensuring that payment occurs. In this regard, essential duties include proper recording of transactions, effective client communication underscoring the value of veterinary services, confident presentation of estimates and invoices, safeguarding of hospital records that document amounts charged, and timely, safe banking of all revenues collected.

Basic Recording Methodology

A key step in ensuring revenue maximization is creating and evaluating a system for tracking and recording services provided, inventory sold, and revenues collected. A wide variety of practice management software systems are available to help you run your practice as efficiently as possible.

Programs customized for veterinary practice use are probably a best bet, as the database structure incorporates features that are possible but challenging to retrofit to a small business accounting solution such as QuickBooks. Consider that the practice not only needs to invoice a client for services and products; it also needs to allocate services and prescriptions to a specific patient owned by the specific client.

When invoicing occurs, the system needs to deplete inventory from the perpetually maintained database. Invoicing for services may need to automatically result in specific reminders for future services, such as phone calls or other client communications. The services also need to be attributed to the care-giving professional assigned to the patient.

The program should automatically track invoices that have not yet been paid (client accounts receivable). As time passes, and clients pay their bills, the system should accept payment input and show that the aging balance has been satisfied. If clients do not pay outstanding invoices in a timely manner, the system should track the balances and add finance charges to the extent allowed by state law. The result will be updated reports showing each client in arrears, the length of time for which payments are overdue, and the last payment amount and the date the payment was made.

The system should also allow for inclusion of doctor and team notes, which can be linked to the patient records to create a useful history for future reference. (See Chapter 8.)

Finally, the invoicing system must provide security: a means to ensure that audit trails are captured and essential areas of the program and database are protected by passwords. Client and patient confidentiality are additional concerns to manage.

Strong internal accounting controls are also an important function of veterinary practice management. This is especially true in the age of technology. Computer use has increased, rather than controlled, the frequency and magnitude of fraud and theft incidents. "Trust but verify" is a good warning to any practice manager or owner overseeing practice financial systems, whether the practice tracks revenue and invoicing by computer or manually. (See Chapter 11 for more information on accounting and bookkeeping.)

Although some practices still use manual systems, most now use electronic methods because of their many benefits. Those who still are using a manual method should seriously consider upgrading to an appropriate computerized method.

MANUAL SYSTEMS

In manual methods of recording financial transactions, the handwritten charge slip serves as an itemized record of charges for both the client and the hospital. The total daily charges are recorded by the hospital in a daybook, otherwise called a "sales journal."

The charge slip is generally completed in duplicate, with one copy retained by the hospital and the other given to the client. This method has the advantage of simplicity and is less costly to implement than a computer invoicing system. However, the charge slips provide little, if any, easily accessible information other than the total amount charged and the client name. This was especially the case in past decades.

Although charge slips could include other important detailed information, because the slips are handwritten, compiled data would be tedious to collect. Much potentially valuable practice information is never gathered. Theoretically, one could sort through the slips to look for broader trends, such as total annual income from ovariohysterectomies, preanesthesia lab screens, or feline vaccinations for the entire year. But this would take a great deal of time so normally is not done. A computer system, however, can compile and summarize this kind of information automatically.

Another disadvantage to a manual invoicing system is that it is vulnerable to internal theft. Safeguards are tedious to maintain by hand. A computer system can guard against theft in ways that a manual system cannot, but also requires risk-management oversights in other ways.

One of the largest disadvantages to a manual system is override of standardized fee schedules and how services and products are invoiced. Large variations can occur among several doctors in the same practice. Even the invoices created by a single veterinarian for similar patient presentations can be quite different. Ultimately, the practice revenue stream suffers from human override and error.

Practices still using manual systems often purchase commercially available *one-write systems*, that is, systems utilizing overlapping carbonless paper records to memorialize the same transaction to several records simultaneously. This allows the recorder to transfer information from the charge slip to the practice's summary journal of sales. From a single written entry, two records are created, an invoice for the client and a duplicate history for the hospital financial record.

If your practice uses a manual system, even if it is well designed and relatively efficient, you may want to consider integrating it with the practice management software to boost client communication frequency, patient record detail, and revenue capture.

ELECTRONIC METHODOLOGY

Manual recording systems are increasingly unusual in North American practices. Typically, the entire receipting process is accomplished through a computer system. Computers have replaced both one-write systems and electronic cash registers in most veterinary practices.

Well-designed computer systems, along with effective recording processes, maintain consistency in fees charged, automate estimate preparation, keep track of amounts collected, and provide contemporaneous tracking of medical cases as they progress through the hospital. Sophisticated software programs designed for the veterinary hospital can summarize data in a variety of formats and reports from a single entry.

Data from an itemized invoice can be used to record fee income, to generate patient health messages and reminders about future appointment dates, to adjust accounts receivable, to provide income-generation data, and to adjust on-hand inventory levels.

Recording the Transaction

The saying "Garbage in, garbage out" applies to practice management software systems as much as it does to any other computerized collection of data—or manual methods, for that matter. The veterinary practice information management system (VPIMS) is only a tool. Your practice must keep proper standards and protocols in place for it to work properly and yield information that may be valuable in assessments of practice operating results. When used to maximum effect, the software can aid you in executing many different types of management decisions.

Table 10.1 summarizes the normal sequence of events that occurs in capturing revenues from veterinary services.

In no particular order of importance, here are some of the issues. First, the most current fee schedule must be precoded and preloaded into the database. You may need to list multiple variations of a common service to distinguish minor differences. For example, for well pets receiving health checkups, you could use categories such as annual wellness examination, examination with vaccinations, second puppy examination, third kitten examination, or semi-annual senior examination. When designating types of examinations involving ill animals, you could use variations such as medical examination—complicated, progress examination, brief progress examination, complicated lameness examination, recheck infected ear examination, courtesy examination, and so on.

Any particular service can evolve into variations on a theme, which will likely be confusing to employees until they are trained in understanding the codes and associated procedures. Long-term medical problems, such as an ongoing troublesome ear infection, may require explicit definition as to what procedures are included in repeat examinations and at what point patient examination constitutes a completely fresh office call and physical examination to be invoiced. Employees must know how to communicate this information to clients. An added complexity is for employees to know how to use the computer codes corectly for these different types of examinations and their corresponding charges. Adequate training and then regular record audits are essential.

Once employees understand these matters, they need to know how to determine the specific patient-care services to be invoiced for each type of event. They also need to know how to

TASK	HOW TO CAPTURE REVENUE
TABLE 10.1 CAPTURING REVENUE IN ELECTRONIC HEALTH RECORDS	
Discussing fees with clients and providing estimates	The estimate is generated from the invoicing function within the computer system and printed for the client. Some practices format generic estimate bundles that are based on prior experience with particular hospital, medical, or surgical cases. These can then be customized, printed, and reviewed with the client.
Providing patient services	A patient tracking sheet, listing computer codes and associated services, is used to highlight the various services provided. Medical personnel need to contemporaneously update the tracking sheet or invoice with each service or inventory item as it occurs or is dispensed. They should not rely on memory to capture patient care at a later time.
Preparing invoices	The receptionist or other team member transfers the computerized estimate onto an invoice and adds any additional services that were required. Whether or not an estimate has been used, tracking sheets for inpatient or outpatient care are checked and coded into the computer invoice. Careful notation of quantities and amounts should be made. For example, if an animal has been hospitalized for three days, a quantity of three days of hospitalization for a pet of that size should be keyed into the computer system. A major cause of error in invoicing is keying in the wrong service code or inputting the wrong quantity. Some practices use bar-code scanners to reduce these errors. In this type of system, each service item and product SKU is given a unique bar code.
Presenting invoices to clients for payment	An invoice is presented to the client, usually at the end of the visit, although some situations may result in invoicing in advance of the service, such as in the case of euthanasia procedures. Receptionists and other personnel involved in invoice presentation must be well trained in communicating information on the invoice in a confident manner that supports the value of the veterinary care provided.
Collecting and recording fees	Payment is recorded into the computer system at the invoicing menu, using the correct code for the method of payment: cash, check, credit card, medical credit card, or charge on account. A printed invoice that shows a zero balance or balance due is given to the client.
Monitoring accounts	The computer automatically posts to the client's account the amount owed and the payment method and amount. In the event an invoice is not paid when closed, it will be included in the entire accounts receivable listing of all open accounts. A billing for any open account can be generated as needed.
Billing	The computer will automatically generate a billing statement at the close of the month when cued for unpaid invoices. The practice manager should also check for any open invoices in the system to ensure that all are appropriate, such as when an animal is still hospitalized or the client has not yet picked up and paid for medications that have been invoiced. The computer automatically ages the accounts into the next month and assesses billing and finance charges in accord with preestablished rates and unique practice database criteria selections.

explain these services beforehand to clients in order to receive client authorization for services to be performed.

The service provider, with the help of the computer system, will need to itemize the services and products for each transaction. This is usually done on a tracking sheet. There are many different names for the *tracking sheet*. Sometimes it is called a *patient service tracker* (PST) or a *data collection sheet*. Other names are *circle sheet* (because applicable coded items are circled) or *travel sheet*. The service provider could be a doctor, veterinary technician, veterinary assistant, receptionist, or other team member.

Ideally, two team members will cross-check each other's itemized invoice drafts to make sure all patient care and services are captured correctly and the right computer service codes used. When the itemized services and products are keyed, or bar codes scanned into the computer, pricing is calculated automatically based on fees previously entered into the computer database.

Several sample tracking sheets are presented in Figure 10.1. Tracking sheets include service and medication descriptions and the corresponding computer codes or bar codes. Different tracking sheets may exist within the same practice, with each one customized for use in a certain type of case. For example, there might be different versions of the sheet for outpatient and inpatient medical procedures; surgical and dental procedures; and boarding, grooming, and ancillary services procedures.

Some software programs allow customized forms to be printed or incorporate patient-processing features that function in conjunction with the record-keeping system. These types of programs decrease redundancy in information collection and reduce opportunities for errors.

Tracking Sheet Protocols

When a client presents a patient to the hospital, the receptionist or client coordinator initiates a patient tracking sheet. The client's name, patient's name, the date, and other details are completed on the top of the sheet. The receptionist may then mark the specific services requested by the client or needed by the patient. Needed services are dictated by predetermined practice guidelines for routine wellness, such as annual exam and visit, vaccination booster, fecal analysis, urinalysis, and other laboratory tests. Other services and needs may be identified as well, such as nail trim, flea and heartworm preventive refills, and nutritional consultation.

With a paper tracking sheet, use a brightly colored highlighter to mark the requested services. Highlighted codes increase visibility, reducing the risk that a task won't be completed or invoiced. Colors can be assigned uniquely to personnel to increase record-keeping efficiency and assist in communication when questions arise.

The tracking sheet accompanies the patient medical record and any other necessary documents to the doctor or technician attending the client and patient. The medical team is

FIGURE 10.1 SAMPLE PATIENT SERVICE TRACKER

Date	Pet	Description	Charges	Payment Credits	Adj.	Current Balance	Previous Balance	Name

1. Professional Evaluation
❑ Initial Examination _____
❑ Regular Examination _____
❑ Comprehensive Examination _____
❑ Re-examination _____
❑ Presurgical _____
❑ Health Certificate _____
❑ 2nd opinion _____

2. Emergency Fee

3. Vaccinations
❑ Puppy
❑ Kitten
❑ DA$_2$PP—Canine Distemper, Adenovirus, Parvo, Parainfluenza
❑ DA$_2$PP _____
❑ FVRCP—Feline Rhino, Calici, Panleukopenia _____
❑ Feline Leukemia Vaccination (FeLV) _____
❑ FIV _____
❑ Leptopirosis _____
❑ Lyme _____
❑ Rabies 1 yr _____
❑ Rabies 3 yr _____
Other: _____

4. Parasite Control   S   M   L
❑ Hookworms   1   2   3 _____
❑ Roundworms   1   2   3 _____
❑ Tapeworms   1   2   3 _____
❑ Whipworms   1   2   3 _____
Other: _____

5. Dental Care
❑ Dental Radiographs _____
❑ Ultrasonic Scale & Polish
❑ Extractions _____ @ $ _____ ea.
❑ Oral Hygiene (Dispensed) _____

6. Laboratory
❑ Fecal Flotation   Pos   Neg _____
❑ Fecal (Direct)   Pos   Neg _____
❑ Urinalysis   Norm   Abnorm _____
❑ Culture & Sensitivity _____
❑ Fungal Culture _____
❑ Gram Stain _____
❑ Heartworm (test)   Pos   Neg _____
❑ Blood Count   (CBC)   (HCT) _____
❑ Thyroid Profile _____
❑ Chemistry Profile   1   2   3   4 _____
❑ Glucose _____
❑ Needle Aspirate _____
❑ Ear Cytology _____
❑ Allergy Testing _____
❑ FeLV/FIV Test _____
❑ Skin Scraping   Pos   Neg _____

❑ Schirmer Tear Test   Norm   Abnorm _____
❑ Fluorescein Stain   Pos   Neg _____
❑ Vaginal Smear _____
❑ Histopathology (Biopsy) _____
❑ Cytology _____
Other: _____

7. Injections
❑ Antibiotics _____
❑ Allergy Shots _____
❑ Anti-inflammatory _____
❑ Analgesic _____
❑ Heartworm treatment _____
❑ Vitamins _____
Other: _____

8. Outpatient Procedures
❑ Ear Flush _____
❑ Anal Sac Expression _____
❑ Wound Preparation _____
❑ Bandages/Wrap/Dressing Change _____
❑ Nail Trim _____
❑ Wing Clip/Beak Trim _____
❑ Euthanasia _____
Other: _____

9. Electrocardiogram
❑ Stat

10. Radiology
❑ Survey Films & Interpretation
    Number of Views _____
❑ Special Studies & Interpretation
    Organ System
    Number of Views _____
❑ Certified Rad Interpretation _____
❑ Ultrasound _____

11. Anesthesia
❑ Premedication _____
❑ General (Injections) _____
❑ General (Injections and Inhalations) _____
❑ Local _____
❑ Sedative _____

12. Surgery
❑ Operating Room _____
❑ Surgical Packs _____
❑ Electrosurgery _____
❑ Cryosurgery _____
❑ Soft Tissue _____

_____
_____
❑ Orthopedic _____
_____

CONTINUES >

> **FIGURE 10.1**

SAMPLE PATIENT SERVICE TRACKER, CONT.

12. Surgery (cont.)

Other:_____

13. Fluid Therapy

❑ I.V. Catheters & Infusion Sets _____

❑ I.V. Fluids_____Liters _____

❑ S.Q. Fluids _____

❑ Blood Transfusions_____ _____

❑ Respiratory Therapy _____

14. Hospitalization

❑ Dr. Supervision

_____ days @ $_____ day _____

_____ days @ $_____ day _____

❑ Nursing Care

_____ days @ $_____ day _____

❑ Ward Occupancy

_____ days @ $_____ day _____

15. Boarding S M L

❑ Canine

_____ days @ $_____ day _____

❑ Feline

_____ days @ $_____ day _____

16. Medication (Pharmacy Rx)

❑ Prescriptions _____ _____

_____ _____

_____ _____

_____ _____

❑ Prescription Diet (_____) _____

❑ Heartworm Preventive _____

❑ Multiple Vitamins _____

❑ Flea/Tick Control Products _____

Other:_____

17. Baths   S   M   L

❑ Regular Bath   C   F _____

❑ Medicated Bath   C   F _____

❑ Bath/Dip (Flea & Tick) C   F _____

❑ Bath/Dip (Mites)   C   F _____

Other:_____

Total Charges _____

Deposit _____

Balance Due _____

Cash	CK	MC	VISA	Initial:

Payment is due when service is rendered.
Deposit is required on all inpatient services.

Home-care Instructions:

Please call nurse to report progress in _____ days

Heartworm/Urine/Fecal test requested in
_____ days

Revaccination recommended _____

Internal/External parasite control _____

Reworming Recommended _____

Suture Removal in _____ days (please schedule appt.)

Reexamine required in_____

Follow-up blood work   ECG, X-ray _____

Additional comments: _____

_____

_____

_____

_____

_____

_____

_____

_____

_____

_____

_____

responsible for completing the scheduled services that are highlighted on the sheet. They will also record on the tracking sheet any additional services performed and medications dispensed.

If the doctor highlights any additional services, the technician should check the sheet to make sure it is complete. If the technician prepares the tracking sheet, then the doctor should scan it for completeness. The goal is to ensure accuracy through cross-checking by involved personnel.

The finalized tracking sheet serves as the basis for capturing all completed service and dispensed item codes for each transaction into the computer system. Determine who has this responsibility and keep the process consistent to maximize quality control.

Often, a cashier or receptionist will key the information from the tracking sheet into the computerized invoice form at the conclusion of the visit. A doctor or technician may initiate the invoice from a computer terminal in the treatment or exam room, and perhaps even complete it. Regardless of process responsibility, accuracy of data entry is of prime importance. The correct code and quantity of any items used must be selected. If, for example, a cashier erroneously entered the code for a medical progress exam every time a doctor provided a complete physical exam, substantial practice dollars could be lost over the course of the year, assuming a progress exam is coded at a fraction of a complete medical examination service charge.

Coding errors can also lead to erroneous patient histories, as invoiced services are included in the electronic medical record. Incorrect coding of dispensed medication could have disastrous consequences. For example, a prescription refill could be made on the basis of the medication that was incorrectly listed in the electronic medical record carried over from the tracking sheet to the invoice.

Invoicing systems that incorporate bar-code technology can help to ensure accuracy. In these systems, each service and product are given a distinct bar code. The bar codes appear on the tracking sheet, and the cashier uses a handheld scanner to capture the correct services and quantities into the computer system.

Whatever entry method your practice uses, it is important to cross-check the invoicing system with a periodic review of procedure and accuracy. In this review, you will randomly select tracking sheets from the past week or month and compare them against the invoices stored in the computer system. Check for discrepancies between the services listed on the invoices and those highlighted on the tracking sheet. Check for incorrect quantities as well as for erroneous service or product coding. If you find errors in these spot-checks, then it might be time to schedule a staff retraining session in which you can review coding and fee-capture protocols.

Tracking sheets are generally kept for a year and then disposed of. The computer software retains invoice histories until the system is purged. Generally, invoices should be kept a minimum of three to five years, though most computerized practices keep them longer because hard-disk storage is relatively inexpensive.

Using the Tracking Sheet for Inpatient Services

Inpatient tracking sheets are unique in that the service coding usually covers a series of days when the patient was hospitalized. The tracking sheet may have columns that allow services to be marked off day by day; alternatively, a new tracking sheet might be started for each new day of hospitalization.

As with other tracking sheets, inpatient tracking sheets are most accurate when they are reviewed by several sets of eyes and when each item or service is entered in a timely manner. A common problem with inpatient cases is that medical care providers may procrastinate about marking down the specific services completed during the course of each day. As a general rule, the services should be highlighted and quantified on the tracking sheet as they are completed. Otherwise, staff may rush through a last-minute reconstruction of all the services that occurred during an animal's stay, trying to create an invoice and discharge the patient at the same time. If tracking-sheet preparation is tardy and invoice preparation is hurried, charges and services are much more likely to be missed (or mistakenly added when they were not provided), resulting in lost revenues for the hospital (or overcharges for the client).

Many practice managers insist that, at the least, the prior day's tracking-sheet information be entered into the computer system at the start of a new day of hospitalization. This method ensures that charges are up-to-date. This protocol also makes it easy to retrieve information on the services provided and the patient's medical status when the client calls. The total current charges to date, calculated by the computer, can be checked against the estimate. This information can help the hospital team anticipate financial questions and make sure that the client is informed if the cost of care is approaching the estimate.

During a patient stay, several doctors or care providers may be responsible for different services (e.g., diagnostic, supportive, or surgical roles). Many practices track the income production of individual doctors. When this is the case, staff completing data-entry tasks must take care to ensure accuracy when assigning the care providers to the services provided. Each hospital has a different system for assigning services or dispensed items to the responsible providers.

Transaction Recording Accuracy

The importance of accuracy in recording transactions cannot be overstated. A recording error can have widespread implications, since financial-transaction recording has several purposes, including:

- Providing the client with a detailed and informative breakdown of services provided and products purchased.
- Providing the client with a statement of the total charges to be paid.
- Providing the hospital bookkeeping department with the data needed to record the transaction in the hospital's financial records.
- Providing the bookkeeping department with income information required by law.
- Providing medical staff with a history of completed services that become part of the medical record.

The accuracy of transactional recording ultimately determines the success of the hospital's financial control system, and more attentiveness to accurate recording can actually increase hospital revenue. Veterinary practice management software programs can generate an almost unlimited number of reports, sorted by different parameters. But these management reports are only as good as the accuracy with which the data are originally recorded. If your staff accurately records transactions, you can confidently evaluate how the practice is doing this year compared to the same time last year in different areas.

For example, you may want to find out how many preventive care examination or *wellness visits* were completed in the first quarter of several consecutive years. Or you might want to know how many radiographic procedures were billed by Dr. Smith as compared to Dr. Jones. You might be interested in assessing how many new clients were seen this year and whether the number is on track with your projections. All of this data depends on accurate transaction records.

Your job as practice manager is to direct and evaluate your team's attention to all phases of transaction recording. The reliable data that results will assist you in making crucial decisions about future practice activity and goals for veterinary service.

Payment Methods

Revenue is defined as "the price of goods sold and services rendered during a given period of time" (Meigs and Meigs 1986, 78). Another way of saying this is that revenue is the income a practice realizes from its normal activities, otherwise called practice operations.

Revenues equal the value of services rendered and inventory sold, even if actual collection has not yet occurred. Hospital revenues include services and products charged on client accounts as well as those paid by various means during a specific period. (See discussion of cash versus accrual accounting in Chapter 11.)

When a client agrees to purchase services and products and the hospital has provided those services and products, revenues are said to be realized, whether or not actual collection in the form of money has occurred. Revenue realization can take many forms: cash, check, money order, credit-card payment, charge on account, promissory note, dedicated health-care credit card transaction, or insurance reimbursement.

Each of these payment forms has some inherent risks for the practice. In accepting any form of payment, management is responsible for reducing the associated risks, as much as possible, through systems, protocols, and monitoring. Each payment type requires the practice to set up safeguards against theft and loss. Following is a review of the forms of revenue realization and the risks and concerns involved with each.

CURRENCY
Although still common, cash payment is diminishing as consumers increasingly use credit cards, debit cards, and other forms of payment. Cash generally accounts for 15 percent or less of total practice receipts in many veterinary practices. Even so, a practice that generates several thousand dollars in daily revenues could have substantial cash receipts on hand at any time.

There are two primary risks in accepting cash payment for veterinary services. The first is that the cash may be counterfeit and of no value to the practice. Consult your bank for tips on how to spot counterfeit bills. You can also find information on the Secret Service website (www.secretservice.gov). Keep in contact with your bank and police department so you are alerted if counterfeit money is currently being passed in your area.

The second risk is that cash is hard to trace and is highly susceptible to internal theft. Once cash is stolen from the cashier's drawer, it may be impossible to determine who took the cash and when. Similarly, once cash has entered the drawer, it may be impossible to tell where it came from, making the source of counterfeit currency difficult to trace.

To safeguard against these risks, keep cash reserves at low levels. Don't retain cash receipts over several days running; instead, make deposits on a daily basis. If you are too busy to make deposits daily, consider engaging a courier service to pick up deposits at the hospital and deliver them to the bank. If your practice collects a significant amount of cash during a day's activity, consider making two daily deposits rather than one.

Do not keep large amounts of cash within view or reach of clients or employees. Deposit excess cash and checks into a secure slotted safe on the premises. Review the security of the cash drawers in the reception area. You might be amazed to see how easy it is to reach over a counter to relieve the cashier's drawer of $100 or $1,000. Such a split-second act can be made by a person off the street, a client, or an employee. Once the theft has occurred, tracing the crime to a person or time may be impossible.

An important safeguard against such theft is cashier drawers that lock the moment they are closed. Cashiers can open them only with a key or computer invoicing software. Cashiers should never leave drawers unattended, especially when no automatic locking device exists. One quick moment of inattention can result in hundreds of dollars of loss.

In busy practices with more than one cashier on a shift, configure the payment area with two or more secure cash drawers. Pair exclusive use of each drawer with a single cashier. At shift changes, require any cash drawer to be reconciled with invoice records for that shift, and receipts secured in the business office safe, before a new cashier starts with a new opening drawer. Otherwise the shift-change protocol must require the departing cashier and starting cashier to both sign off on the reconciliation at the shift change when the drawer changes hands without being cleared back to its opening balance. More information about managing cash drawers appears later in this chapter (see "Collection Guidelines").

MANUFACTURER COUPONS

Many pet food manufacturers and pharmaceutical companies provide coupons for consumer purchase of products sold through veterinary practices. When accepted by the practice, manufacturer coupons should be treated like cash.

Cashiers must be trained to know which products the practice carries and which corresponding coupons will be accepted. Determine if the practice management software needs to be configured to recognize and use a specific coupon as a payment type. After checking the validity of the coupon expiration date, the cashier will apply the coupon as payment to the open invoice, followed by other forms of client payment.

At the end of each shift, collected coupons should be reconciled with invoice totals for the shift and secured for timely submission to the related manufacturer(s). The bookkeeping system must be adapted to record submitted coupons as an account receivable, or amount due from the manufacturer. The receivable can be cleared with subsequent receipt of a manufacturer check that is deposited to the practice checking account.

PRACTICE GIFT CERTIFICATES

Gift certificates must be secured and treated like cash. The practice needs a procedure for selling gift certificates, and another procedure for accepting gift certificates as a payment for services.

Gift certificates should be numerically sequenced so that each sales record can be easily reconciled to a specific transaction that resulted in a client's purchase of a gift certificate.

The computer system will require a payment code correlating with the receipt of a gift certificate in payment of services. Once a gift certificate is added to the cash drawer, it must be reconciled with payment records at the end of the shift, just as any other monetary instrument is.

PERSONAL CHECKS

As a contractual obligation to pay for services, a personal check is a *negotiable instrument,* that is, a paper document that can move freely in financial transactions as a substitute for money (Corley and Shedd 1990, 655). There are two types of negotiable instruments, notes and drafts; a check is a draft. By signing a draft, the signer, in this case a client, orders a bank to pay money to the payee, in this case, the veterinary hospital.

By signing a personal check, the client vouches that funds exist in the account on which the check is drawn. Second, the resulting signed check requires that the stated amount will be transferred to the hospital's checking account on demand. When the client check is deposited to the hospital's bank account, the hospital's bank acts to demand funds from the client's bank and checking account.

Writing and signing a check for payment when funds are inadequate to pay the specified amount can constitute a felony. Despite the legal obligations and ramifications, many people write checks from accounts that are not adequately funded to cover the payment promised. Very often, inadequate funds represent an oversight or miscalculation by the client. The client mistakenly believes the account funds are adequate to cover the check written.

Your hospital should maintain a check-acceptance policy. The specifics of the policy will depend on the history of "bad"-check receipts in the practice. Typically, such policies require that checks meet the following criteria:

- *Adequate identification:* The check should be preprinted with the payer's name, address, and phone number. It is also helpful if the check includes the date the checking account was opened at the bank. Many times, the month and year the account was opened will be listed adjacent to the payer's name. This bit of information may give you more confidence in accepting a check from a new client who does not have a history with the practice.
- *In-state account:* An out-of-state account may signal that the client will disappear in short order, leaving the practice with a bounced check and little recourse in collecting it.
- *Payer's account:* Avoid third-party checks, that is, checks written to the client from a third party, endorsed by the client, and signed over to the veterinary clinic by the client for payment.
- *Written for the amount owed:* Do not accept checks written for more than the amount owed, which require the hospital to accept the check and give change back to the client in the form of cash. The obvious worst-case scenario is that the check bounces. The hospital is out not only the amount of the services charged to the client but also the amount of cash that was given as change.
- *Written from an established account:* Check numbers greater than #300 might indicate that the client has used the checking account for some time. Checks having no number or very low numbers, such as #102 or #110, may suggest an inadequate client history with the account. Reviewing check numbers is not a foolproof screening technique. Many companies will print personal checks starting with any number a person desires. The account may have never had a check written from it even if the check number is #30352.
- *Preauthorization by a check-verification service:* For a nominal fee, you can engage a check-verification service to help you determine the risk of accepting a client's check. These services validate the checking account and check-writer's history or provide a statistical analysis predicting the level of risk that any particular check represents. Check-verification services may also offer a more expensive service option of guaranteed payment of checks from payers who don't show evidence of outstanding bad checks at the point of processing.

Any check-acceptance policy should be communicated to new clients. General disclosure can be made in printed material, such as the practice brochure, new client registration forms, and in account payment information provided on the practice website. Hospital policy should specify the forms of required identification, such as a driver's license. Disclose any ancillary charges that will be assessed to the client in the event a check does not clear and is charged back against the hospital's account. Hospital policy should also include the collection and charge assessment procedures for a "bounced" check.

Because banks assess very high returned-check fees, both to the payer and to the payee, veterinary practice payment policies should clearly state that any client who passes a bad check will not only pay the amount owed but will also pay any fees that were assessed to the veterinary hospital by the bank. If it is legal in your state, you may also wish to add an additional service fee for returned checks, since tracking down clients and arranging their payment on bad checks costs the practice employee time and trouble.

Cashier training should include these two points: First, always make sure that the check is signed before accepting it and closing the invoice, and that the amount is correct in both locations on the check (numerals and spelled-out version). Second, before closing the invoice, make sure the check is in the till and not still in the client's checkbook! Once received, each check should be endorsed with a stamp on the back that includes the hospital name, a "For Deposit Only" qualification, the name of the depository bank, and the business checking account number.

ELECTRONIC CHECK PROCESSING

Halfway between check and debit-card payments is electronic check swiping and processing equipment. Handwritten checks are scanned and transmitted for deposit as they are received. The cashier will know quickly if the bank will accept the check as valid, and the transmission eliminates the time needed for compiling deposits and the risks incurred by having to transport them to the bank.

CASHIER'S CHECKS, TRAVELER'S CHECKS, CERTIFIED CHECKS

A cashier's check is a demand draft drawn on the bank itself, rather than the client's account. After a cashier's check has been given to the hospital in payment, the client cannot stop payment on the check.

Traveler's checks are similar to cashier's checks in that the draft is drawn on the institution issuing the check. Traveler's checks are negotiable instruments only when they have been completed with the identifying signature. Cashiers should understand that traveler's checks must be countersigned on acceptance, and the signature must match the signature already on the face.

A certified check is a draft that has been pre-accepted by the payer's bank. By certifying the check, the bank assumes responsibility for payment and sets aside funds from the client's account to cover the check (Corley and Shedd 1990, 658).

Although they are less common than personal checks, cashier's, traveler's, and certified checks are less risky modes of payment.

CREDIT CARDS

Credit cards are the most popular way of paying for veterinary services. In most cases, not being able to accept credit cards can substantially reduce a practice's cash-flow potential. It is not necessary to accept every type of credit card. Cost and client preferences will be among the factors you consider when deciding which types of cards will be accepted at your hospital.

In order to accept payments by credit card, the veterinary hospital will contract with a merchant bank or a financial company that will handle credit-card transactions for the practice. The merchant bank may or may not be the same bank that handles regular business checking for the practice. The contract specifies when and how credit-card transactions will be submitted to the merchant bank and what sorts of charges will be assessed by the merchant bank and paid by the veterinary hospital.

Every year, the amount of revenues a typical practice receives through client credit-card payment increases, with the total fees assessed amounting to 1.5 percent to 2 percent of total practice gross revenues or more. Practice managers must regularly reread contracts and compare offers from different banks and other financial institutions. In addition, there is not just one type of fee, but many, so make sure you understand all the fees that are involved. Typically, the fees include a percentage of each transaction, and the percentages vary depending on card origination and other factors. There may also be a flat fee per transaction, a transaction authorization fee, and various surcharges and/or account maintenance fees.

The fees can add up to a substantial amount taken by the bank in exchange for processing client payments by credit card. Some banks and companies assess the fees once per month, usually as an automatic draft from the practice business checking account. Other contracts stipulate that fees will be immediately withheld from the day's gross total of client credit-card payments. In this case, the net credit-card collection available for immediate deposit into the hospital's account is the amount charged by the clients less the various bank fees.

A practice manager cuts expenses where possible, and this is one of the most challenging areas in which to conduct cost comparisons because of the processors' complex and convoluted ways of assessing fees. Ideally, you should periodically compare merchant bank alternatives every twelve to thirty-six months. Check with veterinary organizations such as AAHA for affinity programs that negotiate favorable merchant fees on behalf of members. Compare rates and ancillary fees. Check monthly merchant statements to ensure that additional charges have not been added or that rates have not changed without your knowledge.

Another cost savings can be found in reducing bookkeeping time required to reconcile credit-card related deposits at month end. Cashiers should close out all credit-card transmittals at the same time the hospital's computer invoicing system is closed out. For many practices, this is at the end of the day, but some practices choose to close transactions at midday so that the majority of deposits are posted to the account that same day and not held overnight. The best arrangement allows the credit-card bank's transaction-batch totals to match the daily deposit totals from your veterinary practice management software system. If your merchant bank combines several transaction batches into a single checking-account deposit, sorting out these deposits and reconciling the practice's bank statement at the end of the month can be extremely time consuming and expensive when considering the fully loaded cost of a competent bookkeeper.

A third savings can be found in making sure that the assessed merchant charges for monthly transactions are accumulated and assessed as one lump fee to the checking account at month's end. Some processors assess fees with each batch, which is more costly for two reasons. The first reason is that you do not have use of the full credit-card depository amounts for the entire month. Fees are assessed with each batch, rather than with a monthly grand total applied a full thirty days after the earliest transactions have occurred. The second reason is that, when processing fees are assessed based on each batch, reconciliation of the bank statement then becomes a time-consuming challenge, and bookkeeping labor cost again increases. If credit-card batch totals are minus ("net of") the merchant bank charges, the true gross amount of client payments received will exceed the monthly bank statement detail of deposits. To match credit-card charge transactions reported net of merchant fees with the total of client payments, bookkeeping adjustments must be made so that operating revenues are correctly reported and so that financial statements are accurate. (See textbox, "Negotiating Credit-Card Processor Contracts.")

Although credit-card fees will take a hefty chunk out of client gross receipts, practice managers should understand the advantages of accepting credit cards in payment for veterinary services. Clients using credit cards may be more likely to accept the complete array of recommended animal health-care services. Charging accepted services to a credit card may seem less expensive than paying by cash or writing a check.

More services might be used by the client, coupled with creative monthly payment plans using credit cards or other payment alternatives. A complete annual wellness program can be structured for unique species, breeds, and ages. With life-long wellness programs, the practice team can use guidelines to customize a comprehensive annual program for each pet. Annual program price can be satisfied by manageable monthly payments ranging from three months to a full year. When offering a payment program, the practice must assure the security of client credit-card information, which might be best managed through the credit-card or other payment processor. PayPal is a good example of a provider that offers secure management of recurring payments.

Another advantage of allowing invoice payment by credit cards is that transactions are electronically transmitted for immediate bank authorization, potentially improving cash flow.

Negotiating Credit-Card Processor Contracts

When reviewing merchant bank options and the equipment they supply for processing client charge transactions, consider these additional factors:

- If you purchase rather than rent the card swipe terminal, what happens if it breaks?
- Does the processor you are renting or purchasing also print a tape or copy for the client? If not, is an add-on printer available? What will it cost?
- Are any special hookups required for the electronic equipment? If there is an equipment warranty, how long will it cover the equipment parts? Is labor covered? Will it provide replacement equipment?
- Can you negotiate a discount if you rent or purchase the processor and printer together, rather than separately?
- How many days does it take for credit-card transactions to be deposited into the practice's checking account?
- When you sign the merchant bank contract, are you locked in for a number of years, or can you change immediately should the relationship go sour or you find a better deal?
- Are there any hidden fees or expenses about which you have not been informed? Ask for written verification of all contractual details and a copy of the agreement to read carefully in advance of signing.
- Is the proposed merchant fee rate only temporary, with a massive increase within six months or at a year?

When clients charge veterinary services on personal practice accounts for later payment, cash flow is delayed, and the practice incurs the labor cost of creating invoices, sending statements, and collecting, recording, and applying payments to open accounts. Through credit cards, the practice avoids the expense of the collection procedures that may be encountered with unpaid accounts and bounced checks.

Finally, veterinary hospitals are better positioned to minimize accounts receivable and maintain high average transaction charges when credit-card payments are permitted because the client can pay the full amount of a large invoice immediately. Thus the practice receives payment promptly for comprehensive services such as intensive medical cases, advanced dental procedures, and orthopedic surgery. Practice cash flow is maintained. This advantage often outweighs the cost exacted at month's end when the merchant bank fee hits the bank statement.

Following are some other guidelines for accepting client credit cards for payment of veterinary services:

- Cashiers should confirm that the signature on the receipt is the same as the signature on the card. If the credit card is not signed and you do not know the client, ask for alternative identification, such as a driver's license.
- Be careful to return the credit card to the client once processing is finished.
- The credit-card swipe terminal should be updated with the most current software to ensure maximum security. Receipts should show only the last four digits of the card number. No full credit-card numbers should be stored anywhere in the practice, including in the client computer record.
- Credit-card numbers can be easily stolen and are used in identity theft schemes. Due to the increasing risk of identity theft, Congress passed the Fair and Accurate Credit Transactions (FACT) Act of 2003. With several other federal agencies, the Federal Trade Commission jointly issued regulations called the "Red Flag Rule" in 2007 that require certain creditors to develop and institute a written identity-theft prevention program. Because of confusion as to their application, mandatory compliance with the rules was delayed multiple times.

While the Red Flag Rules do not pertain to most veterinary practices, it is advisable to take adequate steps to prevent identity theft so that your clients or employees do not become victims. (See textbox, "Safeguarding Client Information," for more information.)

Credit cards rejected by the processing bank or other financing institution usually indicate the client is a poor credit risk. In cases when a large bill is anticipated, such as with a lengthy hospitalization or complicated surgery, obtain the client's credit-card number at the time of admission and complete the authorization check immediately. Many practices charge deposits to the credit card before the services are rendered, with the client's permission, and after a client consent form is signed. If the credit card does not clear, you will have time to contact the client and arrange for an alternative form of payment.

DEBIT CARDS

The debit card essentially replaces personal checks drawn on personal bank accounts. Like a credit card, the debit card is swiped through an electronic processing and authorization machine. If adequate funds are in the client's account, the amount of purchase is drawn from the account and transferred to the hospital's bank for deposit.

As with credit-card use, debit-card use requires the practice to have an agreement with the bank stipulating any charges and discounts that will be assessed. Clients may or may not be charged fees by their banks for using debit cards. The veterinary practice accepting debit-card payment always pays a fee.

Debit cards save on the labor required to compile deposits. Since a transaction is electronic, it eliminates the risk associated with losing or misplacing a client check, and the funds

Safeguarding Client Information

As in so many areas of policy and procedure, safeguarding clients' personal information can be accomplished through a combination of both technology and employee education. Good resources are available through the Federal Trade Commission. Five key principles guide security of information:

- *Take stock:* Know the extent of client and employee personal information contained in the practice files, including computer data.
- *Scale down:* Only retain information essential to running the veterinary practice. Eliminate any credit-card numbers and related information from client and patient records.
- *Lock it:* Protect all information in the care of the practice.
- *Pitch it:* Properly dispose of information that is no longer needed. (Shredding services are a good option.)
- *Plan ahead:* Have a written plan of what to do in the event of a security breach and possible information loss or theft (Federal Trade Commission 2011).

transfer nearly immediately. If the client's account is inadequately funded to cover the transaction, you will know immediately, rather than having to collect on a bounced check.

DEDICATED HEALTH-CARE CREDIT CARDS

A dedicated health-care credit card works like a Visa card or MasterCard but can only be used for certain kinds of services. Like regular credit cards, a dedicated health-care card for veterinary services can only be used at veterinary practices that choose to accept the card. Among companies providing this client payment option, a common vendor in the industry is CareCredit. Other providers with comparable services include Butler-Schein Financial Services.

As with accepting regular credit cards for invoice payment, the veterinary practice contracts with the health-card provider company. An enrollment fee may be applicable. When a veterinary client uses a dedicated health-care card to charge veterinary services, the card provider assesses a contracted percentage of the total amount charged. The percentage is usually higher than the fees associated with regular credit cards.

Clients can easily apply for a dedicated card, often right at the veterinary practice's check-out desk. Applications are submitted by phone or Internet. A new client's creditworthiness can be rapidly verified through the card company, which grants a line of credit if the client's credit history is satisfactory. The client can then immediately charge any veterinary services to the card, even the very same day the application was submitted and approved.

The veterinary practice is paid in a manner similar to method used with regular credit cards. Generally, the fee charged to the dedicated card is electronically deposited to the practice checking account within a few days, less the contracted merchant fee amount.

Dedicated health-care cards provide another payment option to your clients. A client may be short on cash, or other credit cards might be at their limits. A dedicated card provides a separate line of credit, allowing the client to accept and follow through on treatment recommendations rather than defer them. The dedicated cards often offer attractive payment plans and interest rates to the user as compared to other modes of credit. Dedicated cards benefit the hospital in that they allow clients to accept higher priced veterinary procedures while passing the risk of collecting money to an outside party. Essentially, the veterinary practice chooses to accept a slightly lower payment for services in order to avoid the hassles of collecting from clients on amounts owed.

To make an educated decision about accepting this mode of payment, the practice manager must weigh the benefits against the fee amount assessed by the dedicated-card provider. Animal health-care financing companies often provide attractive marketing materials to help inform clients about financing and payment options, thereby increasing client acceptance of treatment recommendations.

PET HEALTH INSURANCE

Pet health insurance was first offered in Sweden in 1924. In various European countries, policy purchase now extends to up to 48 percent of pet owners. Insurance coverage continues to be used at low levels in North America, at about 1 percent of pets (Trupanion n.d.). New companies and products continue to be launched, and growth in the pet health-insurance industry can reasonably be expected.

Pet health insurance is not like human health insurance. Because by law animals are considered property, pet health insurance works in much the same way that casualty insurance for property like cars or homes traditionally works.

An insurance policy of any kind is a contract or agreement between the insurance company (insurer) and the person buying the policy (the insured). The insured party—in this case, the veterinary client—pays a premium to the insurance company so that the insurer will take on the risk of monetary outlay for veterinary care if the pet becomes ill or injured. In the event of injury or disease, the insurer agrees to pay for medical services in accord with the contract (the terms stipulated in the insurance policy).

As with any insurance policy, pet health-insurance policies vary. The insured party must decide how much of a premium she is willing to pay in order to mitigate risks. If the client opts for a policy with a low premium, the policy may provide very limited coverage and/or have a high deductible. If the client purchases a policy with a higher premium, the policy should provide coverage for more services and/or have a lower deductible.

When a client has pet health insurance, the veterinarian should be outside the process of collecting on the insurance claim. The veterinarian is not a party to the insurance contract, but merely provides the needed veterinary services when and if injury or disease occurs or in accord with covered wellness plans. The privity of contract, or legal relationship, exists between the insurance company and the insured party, the animal owner. The client, in accord with customary hospital fee-collection policies, should pay the veterinary clinic and then seek reimbursement from the insurance company. Unlike human medical practice, veterinary practices do not handle the insurance claims process for the client.

At this point in the development of the industry, veterinary practices do not enter into contracts with pet health-insurance companies to accept the prices they specify for different services. Whether or not that will be the case only the future can tell. The benefit that many veterinarians see in the growth of the pet health-insurance industry is that it may allow for more complete treatment for animals. Euthanasia might not be elected as early or as often. The downside is that the companies may attempt to control or regulate the prices charged for veterinary care.

One difficulty with insuring pets is that there are wide variances in the life expectancies of different breeds and species. Different disease predilections and inheritable conditions occur. The insurer may err in determining the level of risk, by underestimating the going rate of treatment in the region, or when factoring in other conditions that could affect how much has to be paid out to policyholders. In such situations, total premium collection may not be adequate to satisfy state insurance regulators and the needs of insured animal owners.

If insurance providers find they are underestimating the actual cost of pet medical care and insured party claims, premiums will increase. Fewer diseases and injury incidences will be covered, and pressure may be put on veterinary practices to manage their fees for services and restrict the care or diagnostics recommended to clients. In order to grow and develop successfully, the pet health-insurance industry will need to accurately assess risks and costs, and then design the contractual relationship between the insurer and the insured accordingly.

BARTER TRANSACTIONS

In a bartering arrangement, a person agrees to trade goods or services with another party without monetary exchange. For example, a veterinary practice owner may agree to provide veterinary services to a client who, in exchange, agrees to reroof the hospital building. Sometimes, veterinary services are freely given in exchange for something of personal value. An example would be when a veterinarian-owner accepts a hunting dog as payment from a client in exchange for providing veterinary care for the client's horse. The bartered property can be anything that the practitioner would otherwise be required to purchase with personal funds.

Although casual trade arrangements are more common in small businesses, more formal transactions occur through *barter exchanges*. Businesses that are members of barter exchanges swap services and products with other businesses that are members.

Income taxes cannot be avoided by entering into barter transactions. Barter exchanges are required to report transactions in accordance with IRS rules. In casual trades as well as more formal barter exchanges, the value of the bartered goods and services represents revenue realization. The practice is required by the IRS to record such transactions in its records, and the value of the bartered goods and services must be included in the gross income of the practice. Think of a barter arrangement as just another sales transaction of practice goods or services in which a form of payment was received, but with a different form of tax reporting that must be followed. The service or the item received by the practice (in the examples above, what the roof or the hunting dog otherwise would have cost) must be included as practice income at the time received. Accurate accounting and record keeping can help the practice manage barter transactions.

Because of the added complexities of tracking bartered services, many practice managers prefer to avoid them. Bartering veterinary services for personal goods can set a bad precedent for practice operations and for maintaining staff morale and honesty.

Transactions occurring through a barter exchange must be reported to the IRS on Form 1099-B. This includes the value of cash, property, services, and credits or barter (trade) dollars added to your account by the barter club. If a barter is made outside of a formal barter exchange, and if the goods or services the practice has received from the other party have a value of $600 or more, the practice must send a Form 1099-MISC to the service provider as well as to the IRS. This form reports the value of veterinary services received by that person in exchange for other goods or services.

For example, if the person re-roofing the hospital receives veterinary services worth $1,000 in exchange for his work and supplies, the value of the roofing job approximates $1,000. You issue a Form 1099-MISC to the client to report the $1,000 of income constructively received by him. By law, the practice must also have a Form W-9 (Request for Taxpayer Identification and Certification) on file for that individual, which includes legal name, address, and Social Security number. The only exception would be if the person was incorporated as a business and the goods and services were provided through his business, as the law currently stands at the writing of this book. Congress continues to look at tightening the rules to expand reporting requirements, which will massively increase the record-keeping and reporting responsibilities of veterinary practices.

In addition to sending a Form 1099-MISC to the person, $1,000 of veterinary service income must be reported as revenue. Ultimately, then, the people or businesses on both sides of the barter arrangement are reporting the fair-market value of the services and products they have received as income and paying the required tax (see samples of forms in Figures 10.2, 10.3, and 10.4).

ACCOUNTS RECEIVABLE OR CHARGES

Accounts receivable are the client debts owed to the veterinary practice, usually resulting from services provided on credit, although they can result from any sales made on credit. Essentially, a receivable results when the client and the practice agree to keep an open account for the client subject to a specified payment plan.

An outstanding client account balance represents the hospital's right to payment for veterinary services rendered or goods sold, but this right is not evidenced by a promissory note or other written documentation. When evidenced in a written agreement for payment, the client account receivable becomes a client *note receivable*.

The monetary balance in the accounts receivable ledger represents past revenues earned by the hospital but not yet paid with currency or another form of payment such as a credit card or personal check. Charging on account has historically been very common in the medical professions, including the veterinary profession. A veterinary hospital is not obligated to provide services and sell products on a charge basis, however. Many practices selectively do, but to a much lesser extent than in the past. Such agreements are increasingly rare in small animal practices.

The attitude toward credit leniency varies with economic circumstances, market forces, client creditworthiness, and practice owner philosophy. Time spent in collecting accounts receivable can be expensive and frustrating. Credit cards have made instant borrowing from an alternative source possible, making it less necessary for clients to need credit extension from the veterinary practice. Hospital managers typically require clients to pay as they go and to borrow money from another party, if necessary, rather than having the hospital carry and manage accounts receivable.

Still, there are good reasons to allow client charges on account. Many clients have long, dependable payment histories with the practice. These trustworthy clients may be used to charging, or the patient may get into an emergency situation that results in higher than usual expenses all at one time. Some clients represent excellent credit risks. The hospital manager, knowing that payment will occur in short order, extends credit to maintain client goodwill.

Moreover, medical, diagnostic, and surgical care service fees can add up quickly in a complicated case. An owner may want all of the offered services recommended in the best interest of the animal but may not be able to pay for them all at once. Extending credit to a client with a good credit history may allow the practice to provide services that might otherwise be declined. An excessively restrictive credit policy may result in honorable clients delaying or declining recommended veterinary care.

PAGE 1 SHOWN

⌄

FULL FORM
INCLUDED ON
COMPANION
WEBSITE

FIGURE 10.2 1099-B

☐ CORRECTED (if checked)

PAYER'S name, street address, city, state, ZIP code, and telephone no.	**1a** Date of sale or exchange	OMB No. 1545-0715	**Proceeds From Broker and Barter Exchange Transactions**
	1b Date of acquisition	2011 Form **1099-B**	
	2 Sales price of stocks, bonds, etc. $	Reported } ☐ Sales price to IRS } ☐ Sales price less commissions and option premiums	
PAYER'S federal identification number RECIPIENT'S identification number	**3** Cost or other basis $	**4** Federal income tax withheld $	**Copy B** **For Recipient**
RECIPIENT'S name	**5** Wash sale loss disallowed $	**6** If this box is checked, boxes 1b, 3, 5, and 8 may be blank ☐	This is important tax information and is being furnished to the Internal Revenue Service. If you are required to file a return, a negligence penalty or other sanction may be imposed on you if this income is taxable and the IRS determines that it has not been reported.
Street address (including apt. no.)	**7**	**8** Type of gain or loss Short-term ☐ Long-term ☐	
City, state, and ZIP code	**9** Description		
Account number (see instructions)	**10** Profit or (loss) realized in 2011 on closed contracts $	**11** Unrealized profit or (loss) on open contracts—12/31/2010 $	**14** Bartering $
CUSIP number	**12** Unrealized profit or (loss) on open contracts—12/31/2011 $	**13** Aggregate profit or (loss) on contracts $	**15** If box checked, loss based on amount in box 2 is not allowed ☐

Form **1099-B**   (keep for your records)   Department of the Treasury - Internal Revenue Service

Department of the Treasury, Internal Revenue Service

PAGE 1 SHOWN

⌄

FULL FORM
INCLUDED ON
COMPANION
WEBSITE

FIGURE 10.3 1099-MISC

☐ VOID   ☐ CORRECTED

PAYER'S name, street address, city, state, ZIP code, and telephone no.	**1** Rents $	OMB No. 1545-0115	**Miscellaneous Income**
	2 Royalties $	2011 Form **1099-MISC**	
	3 Other income $	**4** Federal income tax withheld $	
PAYER'S federal identification number RECIPIENT'S identification number	**5** Fishing boat proceeds $	**6** Medical and health care payments $	**Copy 1** **For State Tax Department**
RECIPIENT'S name	**7** Nonemployee compensation $	**8** Substitute payments in lieu of dividends or interest $	
Street address (including apt. no.)	**9** Payer made direct sales of $5,000 or more of consumer products to a buyer (recipient) for resale ▶ ☐	**10** Crop insurance proceeds $	
City, state, and ZIP code	**11**	**12**	
Account number (see instructions)	**13** Excess golden parachute payments $	**14** Gross proceeds paid to an attorney $	
15a Section 409A deferrals $ **15b** Section 409A income $	**16** State tax withheld $ $	**17** State/Payer's state no.	**18** State income $ $

Form **1099-MISC**   Department of the Treasury - Internal Revenue Service

Department of the Treasury, Internal Revenue Service

FIGURE 10.4 W-9

Form **W-9**
(Rev. December 2011)
Department of the Treasury
Internal Revenue Service

**Request for Taxpayer
Identification Number and Certification**

Give Form to the
requester. Do not
send to the IRS.

Name (as shown on your income tax return)

Business name/disregarded entity name, if different from above

Check appropriate box for federal tax classification:

☐ Individual/sole proprietor ☐ C Corporation ☐ S Corporation ☐ Partnership ☐ Trust/estate

☐ Limited liability company. Enter the tax classification (C=C corporation, S=S corporation, P=partnership) ▶ _____

☐ Other (see instructions) ▶

☐ Exempt payee

Address (number, street, and apt. or suite no.)

Requester's name and address (optional)

City, state, and ZIP code

List account number(s) here (optional)

Print or type
See Specific Instructions on page 2.

Part I Taxpayer Identification Number (TIN)

Enter your TIN in the appropriate box. The TIN provided must match the name given on the "Name" line to avoid backup withholding. For individuals, this is your social security number (SSN). However, for a resident alien, sole proprietor, or disregarded entity, see the Part I instructions on page 3. For other entities, it is your employer identification number (EIN). If you do not have a number, see *How to get a TIN* on page 3.

Note. If the account is in more than one name, see the chart on page 4 for guidelines on whose number to enter.

Social security number

Employer identification number

Part II Certification

Under penalties of perjury, I certify that:

1. The number shown on this form is my correct taxpayer identification number (or I am waiting for a number to be issued to me), and

2. I am not subject to backup withholding because: (a) I am exempt from backup withholding, or (b) I have not been notified by the Internal Revenue Service (IRS) that I am subject to backup withholding as a result of a failure to report all interest or dividends, or (c) the IRS has notified me that I am no longer subject to backup withholding, and

3. I am a U.S. citizen or other U.S. person (defined below).

Certification instructions. You must cross out item 2 above if you have been notified by the IRS that you are currently subject to backup withholding because you have failed to report all interest and dividends on your tax return. For real estate transactions, item 2 does not apply. For mortgage interest paid, acquisition or abandonment of secured property, cancellation of debt, contributions to an individual retirement arrangement (IRA), and generally, payments other than interest and dividends, you are not required to sign the certification, but you must provide your correct TIN. See the instructions on page 4.

Sign Here
Signature of
U.S. person ▶

Date ▶

General Instructions

Section references are to the Internal Revenue Code unless otherwise noted.

Purpose of Form

A person who is required to file an information return with the IRS must obtain your correct taxpayer identification number (TIN) to report, for example, income paid to you, real estate transactions, mortgage interest you paid, acquisition or abandonment of secured property, cancellation of debt, or contributions you made to an IRA.

Use Form W-9 only if you are a U.S. person (including a resident alien), to provide your correct TIN to the person requesting it (the requester) and, when applicable, to:

1. Certify that the TIN you are giving is correct (or you are waiting for a number to be issued),

2. Certify that you are not subject to backup withholding, or

3. Claim exemption from backup withholding if you are a U.S. exempt payee. If applicable, you are also certifying that as a U.S. person, your allocable share of any partnership income from a U.S. trade or business is not subject to the withholding tax on foreign partners' share of effectively connected income.

Note. If a requester gives you a form other than Form W-9 to request your TIN, you must use the requester's form if it is substantially similar to this Form W-9.

Definition of a U.S. person. For federal tax purposes, you are considered a U.S. person if you are:

- An individual who is a U.S. citizen or U.S. resident alien,

- A partnership, corporation, company, or association created or organized in the United States or under the laws of the United States,

- An estate (other than a foreign estate), or

- A domestic trust (as defined in Regulations section 301.7701-7).

Special rules for partnerships. Partnerships that conduct a trade or business in the United States are generally required to pay a withholding tax on any foreign partners' share of income from such business. Further, in certain cases where a Form W-9 has not been received, a partnership is required to presume that a partner is a foreign person, and pay the withholding tax. Therefore, if you are a U.S. person that is a partner in a partnership conducting a trade or business in the United States, provide Form W-9 to the partnership to establish your U.S. status and avoid withholding on your share of partnership income.

Cat. No. 10231X

Form **W-9** (Rev. 12-2011)

Department of the Treasury, Internal Revenue Service

Practice owners must guide other policy regarding credit. Emergency cases might be presented by a good Samaritan or an infrequent user of veterinary services with little prior transactional history at the hospital. Or perhaps it is a long-standing client who presents his own animal in dire circumstances, but who also has a history of passing bad checks. When an animal's life is in the balance, the health-care team will need to know what to communicate and how to proceed quickly in accord with practice owner wishes. Clearly stated policies and employee training should occur in advance of such instances.

Even with good clients, long outstanding credit balances can create communication problems and ill will. The client who owes the hospital money may resent the bills that come every month. The client may feel guilty about owing money and may hesitate to bring the animal in for additional services until the balance is cleared. A client that has a long-standing balance may even take the animal to another hospital, rather than face the hospital to which money is owed.

Allowing the client to charge a bill is the same as loaning the client that amount of money. Because of the individual circumstances, the hospital may be willing to assume the risks of a lender. And yet, to mitigate the risk of holding the money, the practice should take reasonable precautions to ensure that the "loan" is repaid.

To start, the hospital administration must decide whether and under which circumstances it will agree to accept a charge on an open client account. If your hospital will not provide services on a charge basis, communicate the policy to clients before performing any services: "ABC Animal Hospital does not carry client accounts. Clients are responsible for paying in full at the time of service. We accept cash, personal checks, debit cards, credit cards (state which ones), PayPal, and health-care credit cards (state which ones)." This information can be included in the registration materials given to the client at the first visit.

If the hospital does wish to permit clients to open charge accounts, then two policy components must be planned and implemented: client credit policy and charge account policy. The client credit policy establishes the prequalification criteria by which a particular client is permitted to open an account. A hospital may require a client to have a minimum of two years of pristine payment history without problem (i.e., invoice payment in full at time of service with no bounced checks, credit cards that clear consistently, and no requests for the practice to hold checks until a later date).

The charge account policy should establish credit limits, payment due dates, payment methods, and invoicing procedures. For example, the hospital may require full payment before the twentieth day of the month. It may require payment by check or cash and not by credit card to minimize the cost of credit-card merchant fees. The policy should also specify when billing and interest charges would apply and should be in compliance with federal and state laws pertaining to "truth in lending." The practice's attorney should be able to explain the laws and supply the necessary information you will require for compliance.

When opening an account for a qualified client, a charge account information form should be used. The form specifies the terms of the agreement, including finance and billing charges that will be assessed. A sample credit information form is presented in Figure 10.5.

Complete the charge account information forms in duplicate. Retain one copy in a secured hospital file. Give the other copy to the client. The form should request adequately detailed information to allow collection pursuit, should the client default on the promise to pay. The mere act of written formalization of the charge arrangement often entices the client to simply pay the bill by check or credit card and not open a charge account.

Practice credit and charge-account policies should specify:

- Standard prequalification procedures for a client of unknown credit standing
- The process for identification of clients prequalified to charge and how they are flagged in the record system
- The total invoice amount that the client can charge without approval by either a doctor, the manager, or an owner
- The maximum permissible amount that a particular client may charge
- The percentage of a bill that must be paid at time of patient discharge and the resulting percentage that can be charged by the client
- The procedures for managing aging accounts and collecting overdue accounts receivable (see Stockner 1983, ch. 10)

Employee training is required to ensure appropriate communication of practice revenue collection, credit, and payment policy. The following methods of client communication and collection-related activities can bridge from and to employee training materials:

- Disclosing practice policy in a brochure or handout that is suitable for discussion with the new client (for example, *"Payment is required when services are rendered, unless prior arrangements have been approved. Our practice accepts payment by cash, check, or credit card"*)
- Displaying a sign at the reception desk that uses similar policy wording
- Providing guidelines in practice printed information and possibly by posting information in select locations such as examination rooms (for example, *"We provide written patient care plans so that clients are fully informed of recommended care and associated costs. Please freely discuss any questions or concerns with your pet health-care team before your pet receives veterinary services"*)
- Asking the client, *"How will you be paying today?"* before the patient receives services (remember, once the client is with the doctor, all may be lost)
- Communicating a brief synopsis of payment options when establishing an appointment with a new client
- Using a credit or check verification service
- Preauthorizing a deposit on a credit card

FIGURE 10.5 SAMPLE CREDIT INFORMATION FORM

CREDIT AGREEMENT

Name of Client: _____

Address: _____

Employer: _____

Work Phone: _____ Home Phone: _____

1. Amount of Unpaid Professional Fees: $ _____
2. Credit Service Fee: $ _____
3. Total Amount Financed: $ _____

TERMS:

Each of the below monthly payments is due as expected by the _____ of the month. If payment is not received at our office in 15 days, a _____ LATE PAYMENT CHARGE will be added to the account.

INTEREST:

18% per year (1 ½% per month) of the unpaid balance of the amount financed and late charges that may apply For the first 90 days, this is included in the Credit Service Fee. After 90 days, interest (at the rate of 1 ½% per month) will be added to the account.

AGREEMENT:

Monthly Payment $ _____

Final Payment $ _____

Late Charges or Interest $ _____

I agree to make the first monthly payment the _____ of _____, 20_____, and subsequent payments each month until paid in full. I have read the above, agree to the terms and interest rate, and have received a copy of the agreement.

_____   _____

Date   Signature of Client

- Asking the client to complete a credit application form before extending credit (a point system can be applied to the questions asked on the credit application to establish a scoring system for credit approval and the level of credit approved; Wilson 1995, 61)
- Reviewing the client's prior credit and payment history with the practice (check under other possible names if there has been a change in marital status or partners)

The practice may also wish to follow these two simple and commonsense prequalification procedures:

1. Call the client's listed home telephone and/or cell-phone numbers. Make sure they are in service and are correct. If the lines have been disconnected, consider offering only minimal credit extension, if any.

2. Call the client's employer to verify employment and length of employment. Check the company website. If the employer's business appears to be closed, check the secretary of state online information regarding businesses in good standing or identified as possibly impaired (Wilson 1995, 58).

Chapter 11 briefly discusses accounts receivable as part of an overview of accounting and bookkeeping in practice management. Below, you will learn more about how to collect accounts receivables.

Collecting Current and Overdue Payments

Four basic processes make up the accounts receivable function. Two of these, credit prequalification and charge-account policy management, are discussed above. The other two are remittance processing and collections. Remittance processing systems are collection processes and include methods of tracking and billing client receivables.

ACCOUNTS RECEIVABLE

When a practice allows clients to pay for services on credit, it must maintain a record system that does the following:

- Identifies which clients owe the hospital money
- Accurately tracks the amounts owed
- Adds a billing charge or an interest charge to an account as determined by the hospital policy (if allowed by state laws)
- Adequately discloses finance rates and other charges in accord with local and state laws
- "Ages" accounts receivable by the number of days since the account was charged
- Generates a statement for billing purposes on at least a monthly basis
- Records those accounts that are paid and enters that information into cash receipts for the day payment is received
- Produces reports of current and overdue amounts owed to the hospital

Like so many other management duties in veterinary practice, these tasks can be carried out manually or electronically.

Manual Accounts Receivable Management

If the hospital employs a manual system of revenue recording and control, you can begin by separating those transaction forms that are not paid at the time of discharge from those that are paid. The records of unpaid transactions initiate the accounts receivable subledger. A manual system requires careful monitoring and meticulous computations by the employees who are responsible for maintaining it. As described below, usually there are at least two employees involved, in a system with strong checks and balances.

All the details of each account—statements, billing charges, interest, account aging, and payments—when recorded manually, are usually recorded onto individual client ledger cards. The use of colored "flags" on the ledger cards assists billing personnel in monitoring and managing aging accounts. One color might signify 30-day accounts, another 60-day accounts, and so on. Each month, flags are changed to update the ledger-card status.

Because theft is easier to hide when records can be altered and manipulated, good accounting systems separate payment-handling tasks from record-keeping tasks. The person responsible for aging accounts, billing clients, and computing amounts outstanding should not handle payments received from clients. Neither should this person handle mail that includes payments from clients.

When the practice receives a client payment, the receipt should be included in the current day's deposits by the cashier. A copy of the check or client receipt is given to the accounts receivable clerk, who then updates the client's ledger card and the accounts receivable ledger to the correct balance. Thus record keeping is separated from payment handling.

Computerized Accounts Receivable Management

One significant advantage of computerization is that it automates computations and management of accounts receivable. When the invoice is completed and the client has not paid in full, the balance is automatically posted to the client's account. If the client's record in the computer database has been flagged for assessment of billing charges or interest, the computer will automatically calculate these in accord with the rates recorded in the computer system.

All open accounts are automatically aged when a billing period (usually one month) closes. When a payment is received, it is entered as a payment in the computer system applied to the correct client account name or number. The computer computes and adjusts the balance. If the balance is paid in full, the computer removes the account from the receivable listing. When the client makes partial payment, the receivables report usually lists the last date of payment and amount. A comprehensive computer-generated accounts receivable aging report provides an immediate, detailed picture of the unpaid accounts of the hospital.

RAPID COLLECTION

Hospital collection policies and procedures should be formalized in writing (Cottle 2011, 33). Make sure the entire staff is aware of them. Policies should cover the following invoicing and collection issues:

- Interest charge assessment
- Discounts, including when, who, why and how authorized
- Account balance write-offs
- Use of outside collection services
- Procedure for deciding and taking legal action
- Discontinued client relationship, including what circumstances and the authority for final decision and communication of same

- Shifting of collection responsibility to a doctor, an owner, or other specified personnel

Collection is simply an extension of billing. If fees were clearly explained to the client in anticipation of the work, quality veterinary services were provided, and the client made a concrete commitment to pay, then collection should not be difficult or controversial.

Management's primary concern is that collection of accounts occurs in a timely manner. As a general rule, the longer a balance goes unpaid, the harder it is to make full collection. The key to full collection on accounts receivable lies in prompt and accurate billing. Clients are usually much more willing to pay when patient treatment is still in process or the results are still fresh in their minds. A planned system of collection enables your hospital to follow up on outstanding accounts on a regular basis.

COLLECTION TIPS

Hospital procedures can help expedite the collection process. At the point of patient discharge, when the charge is made, a client who is prequalified for credit should receive a complete and detailed invoice. An invoice lists all services provided to the client at a specific time and may include multiple patients.

Sometimes credit is unexpectedly extended, such as when a new veterinarian or other poorly trained employee fails to complete prequalification procedures before emergency patient care is given. At patient discharge, talk with the client and solidify agreement as to when the account balance will be remitted. Often the agreement is formalized through a written payment plan.

Some practices will adopt policy wherein employees request clients to remit payment as soon as possible at the time of providing clients with their detailed invoices. If your hospital provides ambulatory services where clients may not be present when the animals are treated, such as in a food-animal or equine practice, the practice should send out invoices immediately, or, at the latest, on the day after the services were posted to the client account. The goal is to speed up the payment cycle, understanding that if the practice waits to bill clients at month end, timely client payment receipt could end up occurring as much as 60 days after the date of veterinary care.

A statement is different from an invoice. A statement summarizes the client's charge-account activity, including each outstanding invoice, aged totals, and assessed finance charges. Statements are generated once a month, usually only for accounts carrying a balance. If an invoice occurred in the most recent 30 days, a detailed copy of it should be included with the statement. Statements and invoices should completely communicate all terms of the hospital's policy on the account, such as billing charges and interest on overdue accounts.

To encourage timely payment, the practice might include a billing charge on the statement, if legally permissible. If the practice uses a billing charge, the statement could include a message such as, "Billing charge does not apply if balance is paid within 10 days of receipt." Including a payment envelope with the statement may also help expedite payment.

The first billing statement should be sent no later than 30 days after an unpaid invoice is generated. Statements are generally sent at month's end, but the practice may gain an advantage by timing the hospital's statements to arrive on a different date, perhaps just in advance of the majority of bills sent by other creditors.

Statements should be sent at the same time each month. They must not be delinquent. Statements should be neat, accurate, and complete, giving the client an itemized accounting of the amount owed. The employee who prepares them should double-check the client name and address, make sure adequate postage is attached, and include the payment envelope for the client's convenience.

Complete return address information and hospital phone numbers should be clearly listed on the statement. If the first statement is paid within 30 days after being sent, it is considered to have been *paid currently*. Although a billing charge may be added if it is practice policy, interest is usually not charged on an account paid currently.

Any account that remains unpaid more than 30 days after the first statement was sent should be considered overdue. For this reason, the aging of accounts is generally categorized into 30-day periods: 30 days, 60 days, 90 days, and more than 90 days since the first monthly statement was sent.

Maintain a hospital policy defining consistent collection protocol of overdue accounts receivable. Concentrate collection time on receivables in the 30- to 60-day range, because these are relatively recent and have a higher probability of collection.

30-Day Accounts

Each client with an account at a 30-day level has received at least the original invoice and one mailed billing statement. The second billing statement is now required. The statement should include the interest charge allowed by law, as well as a new billing charge, in accord with hospital policy.

Generally, 30-day accounts are not major causes for concern, because a high percentage will be paid. But once an account is nearing the second statement date and into the 60-day category, you should follow up with the client. This can best be accomplished by a phone call to the client to ascertain if there are any concerns that have caused the delay. Your goal is to promptly address issues and resolve them with the client. (For more information on what to say, see the later section entitled "Calling Clients with Delinquent Accounts.")

Consider adding a handwritten note on the second statement, such as, "Your account is now overdue. Please remit payment promptly. If your payment is in the mail, thank you!" If the practice is computerized, standard collection messages can be cued to automatically print on all 30-day and 60-day statements.

60-Day Accounts

Accounts aging to the 60-day category are due for their third monthly statements as they near 60 days from the first statement date and as much as 90 days from the point of original service. Interest and billing charges continue to accrue. At this point, nonpayment should be considered a potential problem, especially if your phone calls have not been returned or if the client has not paid in accord with any agreed-upon arrangements made through prior discussions.

Include a stronger message on the statement. A personal note from the doctor may have more weight and success than a message from the manager or bookkeeper. Better yet, call the client as soon as possible to determine the problem and to regain commitment for payment. You may be able to obtain credit-card information and authority to pay the invoice immediately when talking with the client.

If you cannot talk with the client, a computer-generated collection letter can be enclosed with the statement. Two sample collection letters (also called "dunning" letters) are shown in Figure 10.6. Note that both of these letters follow the basic rule of a good collection letter: brevity. Long, rambling letters that insult the client for not paying or that recite all the hardships nonpayment has caused are much more likely to be ignored. Ask the practice attorney to review your proposed dunning letters to assure they follow collection law regulations.

Collection letters should be sent discriminatingly, since better collection results can often be attained with personal phone calls or a meeting with the client. The hospital policy for overdue account collection should include telephone calls to all clients whose accounts have not been paid by 60 days. Do not leave messages on the answering machine. Persist until you have talked with the responsible party. If you are not able to obtain and process a credit-card payment, ask the client to give you a specific date on which payment will be made. (See "Calling Clients with Delinquent Accounts.")

90-Day Accounts

After 90 days, the practice will be sending the fourth monthly bill. A 90-day account is in serious risk of default. Collection probability is now down to somewhere between 65 and 80 percent. On the 90-day statement, give the client a specified number of days to pay, after which the account will be turned over to a third party for collection. Name a contact person at the hospital and instruct the client to call immediately if payment by that date is not possible.

Another phone call to the client is also in order. The person handling 90-day and over-90-day accounts should confidently ask for payment, reminding the client that animal-care

FIGURE 10.6A SAMPLE COLLECTION LETTER

ABC ANIMAL HOSPITAL

[Ms. Jane Smith]
[123 Main Street]
[Anywhere, Any State 00000]

November 6, 2XXX

Re: [$1,206.46]
[#12345]

Dear [Ms. Smith]:
We note that your account of $1,206.46 was overdue as of _____, _____. Please pay this account promptly. For your convenience, we accept major credit cards. Simply call or E-mail your credit card number and expiration date, and we will credit your account.

If you have already sent the check in the mail, we apologize for the inconvenience and thank you for your payment.

Sincerely,

FIGURE 10.6B SAMPLE COLLECTION LETTER

ABC ANIMAL HOSPITAL

[Ms. Jane Smith]
[123 Main Street]
[Anywhere, Any State 00000]

November 6, 2XXX

Re: [$1,206.46]
[#1234]

Dear [Ms. Smith]:
This is your second reminder that you owe us $1,206.46. Please pay this balance promptly. We appreciate your patronage, and wish to continue providing veterinary care to your pets, but we need your cooperation and payment to do so.

We accept major credit cards. Simply call or E-mail your credit card number and expiration date and we will credit your account.

Thank you for your prompt attention to this matter.

Sincerely,

services were undertaken with the understanding that all fees would be paid without undue delay. The telephone call should project a stronger message than the 60-day call. (See "Calling Clients with Delinquent Accounts," below.)

The client record should be flagged to eliminate future credit eligibility.

Over 90-Day Accounts

Unless the client has made some attempt to contact the hospital and make payment arrangements by this time, most over-90-day accounts should be turned over to a collection agency without further delay. In some circumstances, you may decide to extend the in-house collection efforts beyond 120 days, depending on factors such as the size of the bill and the relationship with the client.

Waiting any longer than 120 days to try to continue your own collection efforts will probably only make the account less collectible. If you decide not to pursue third-party collection, remember that continuing to send statements is a costly procedure. A better choice may be to simply write off small accounts as bad debt.

Flag the client record of any account that you write off or turn over to a collection agency. Some people who have not paid bills will return to the hospital at some point in the future, sometimes years later. It is sad to say, but an occasional villain banks on the fact that no one will remember the theft and will try to use your practice's services again. Sometimes they do pay the next time around, but sometimes they do not. Flagging the file of such poor-risk clients will give your team a shot at disqualifying them if they attempt to pass prequalification screens at later dates. You can even request that this person pay the old account before engaging any new services.

Calling Clients with Delinquent Accounts

Any employee who calls clients about overdue accounts should be well trained in the task, whether she is the practice manager, a doctor, or a bookkeeper. In general, the person calling should have authority to make decisions as well as the correct demeanor. Courtesy, tactfulness, and firmness are good qualities. Each employee making collection calls should also be current in knowledge of collection laws, such as when calls can be made, what can and cannot be said, and the necessity of using care in knowing with whom they are speaking.

If the practice team has done a good job of establishing and following credit qualification policy, telephone calls to clients about payment matters should be infrequent. Most clients who have prequalified for credit and are fully informed of credit policies will pay their account balances accordingly.

The objective of a collection call is to courteously resolve any problems that the client perceives, leading to payment of the outstanding account. If a client is not making payment because of dissatisfaction with veterinary services, it is certainly in the practice's best interests for you to know about the problem and resolve it rather than have bad feelings lead to a client speaking poorly of the practice.

Other problems that have led to the nonpayment may also be identified and quickly resolved. For instance, a client may be overwhelmed by other bills, and a reconfigured payment plan with your practice might result in regular payments, albeit over a longer period of time than was originally planned.

When there is no valid complaint about veterinary care, the employee making the collection call should be persistent about getting a firm commitment for payment. Without being judgmental, a collection caller should demand that the client fulfill the obligation to pay for services and products already provided.

Throughout the conversation, the caller should pay attention to what is said and take notes, so that the correct actions can be taken when payment does not occur as originally promised. Sometimes, it appears that a client may be looking for any excuse not to pay the bill. In general, when it has already been determined that the client is not dissatisfied with services, stay focused on gaining commitment for payment and avoid lengthy discussion of the animal whose care generated the outstanding invoice. Practice policy should guide collection-call protocol for specific issues in other cases—such as when a patient has died or been euthanized—resulting in an outstanding account balance that has gone unpaid.

When talking with slow-paying clients, keep the conversation on point and repetitive: When and how is the account going to be paid? Here are additional suggestions for making collection calls.

- You will be more likely to be successful with both client satisfaction and telephone collections if the first call is made before the bill is long overdue.
- Have at hand a copy of the original invoice, estimate, and other records that substantiate the charges the client agreed to pay.
- Make sure that your facts are correct.
- At the first call, inquire if the client has some previously unstated concern about the veterinary services. If so, obtain the client's recitation of pertinent information. When the client expresses concern about veterinary care, tell the client that you will discuss the situation with the attending doctor and then call the client back. You may also offer the client to have the veterinarian call. Get a specific time to call the client so that you do not play "phone tag." Practice policy should clarify the responsibility of doctors to promptly return

calls to clients in any situation where some expression of dissatisfaction with patient care has become apparent.

- When calling, be aware of the client's rights under the laws of fair credit. Check with the hospital's attorney for information and guidance about maintaining legal practice collection procedures.
- Do not let the client assume you have lost interest in collection. Be firm, proactive and assertive, and make repeated calls (Cottle 2011, 33).
- Endeavor to obtain commitment from the client. If you have received a definitive promise of payment by a certain date and payment does not occur, follow up immediately.
- Note reminders of scheduled follow-up calls where you won't miss them—on a wall calendar, in an electronic scheduler, or on the aging accounts lists that you use to record the results of your contacts.
- Do not make downward account adjustments to encourage payment when collection is difficult or lengthy. A downward adjustment may create an impression that services were originally overbilled or there was some deficiency in them. The implication of service deficiency could be extremely detrimental if it is perceived that professional negligence or malpractice was involved (ibid., 34).
- Be prepared to give the client some options, such as smaller payments deferred over a longer time. If you arrange an extension of time, remind the client that the interest and billing charges will continue to accrue, and explain the consequences of defaulting on the agreement.
- As a last resort, you can reduce the account balance and accept a lower remittance, as it is better to receive some payment than none at all. Send written acknowledgement of any reasons for the adjustment—for example, the client's financial condition or communication lapses that led to misunderstanding the amount of patient care the client authorized. Also, make clear that the compromise does not represent a diminution in the value of professional services. The adjustment is a one-time occurrence and a deviation from the hospital's standard policy. You may also consider discontinuing service to the client after payment is made (ibid.).

Proper administration of accounts receivable and collections can be time-consuming and sometimes problematic. Many of these potential problems can be mitigated through effective prequalification procedures that reduce the risk of extending credit to clients who are not creditworthy. Evaluating accounts-receivable aging reports regularly will allow you to adjust practice policies when necessary, thereby preventing significant cash flow troubles due to poorly executed collection activities.

Collection Agencies and Legal Action

Whether you use collection agencies to collect on an overdue account depends primarily on the amount of the bill and your relationship with the client. Most collection agencies limit the account total they will accept. Collection services keep anywhere from 35 to 50 percent of any amounts collected on the account. Collection agencies generally collect this percentage when the account is paid by the client, but some will collect up-front fees on all accounts turned over to them by the practice.

Keep this cost in mind when you're deciding whether it's worth it to contract with a collection agency. Another issue to consider is that once the practice turns a client account over to an agency, the hospital may very well lose the client for future veterinary services. Although you probably don't want this person as a client any longer, under some circumstances you may not want to risk losing the client. (See Table 10.2 for collection tactics to avoid.)

Many agencies only write harsh collection letters that generally get more aggressive as they proceed. Be sure to read the standard form letters the agency uses, and try to ensure that they follow prevailing legal standards and pass muster with the practice's owners, since they do, to a certain extent, reflect the practice's image.

Some people who owe money will pay as a result of collection letters, particularly if they come from a credit bureau's collection division. Clients receiving such letters from a credit bureau may be concerned about the adverse impact on their credit history and may decide to pay the bill. Whatever collection services are contracted, request a statement documenting the agency's collection success before contracting with it. Make sure their tactics don't conflict with your practice's code of conduct and overall policy of client service.

If the agency you use is not successful in collecting the bill, the next step is legal action. Some states allow you to pursue collection attempts in small-claims courts, which do not re-

TABLE 10.2 COLLECTION TACTICS THAT MAY CONFLICT WITH FAIR CREDIT LAWS	
UNLAWFUL ACT	**TACTICS TO AVOID**
Libelous statement	Never make a statement reflecting negatively on the client's character or reputation.
Extortion	Never threaten to distribute bad credit information about the client.
Invasion of privacy	Do not contact anyone (e.g., an employer) about the debt other than the client or an immediate family member.
Assault and battery	Never threaten any physical action if the bill remains unpaid.
Harassment	Do not call the client at unreasonable times or at work. Do not make threatening statements about the action you might take that might be considered harassment.

Source: Adapted from Priscilla K. Stockner, A Practice Management Manual for Veterinarians (Ocean Shores, WA: Stockner and Associates, 1983), Chapter 10.

quire that an attorney be involved in the collection process. Even if the process does not result in the collection of the overdue bill, the court may serve judgment against the client. This action may prevent the client from selling any property before the judgment is cleared. If you win the case, the client's wages may be garnished until the payment is completed.

Before entering into any legal process for the collection of overdue accounts, weigh the costs and time involved against the chances of recovering the owed money. Managers who contemplate suing a client for fees should consider the following:

- The possibility that the client may file a counterclaim for malpractice, whether or not valid (even if you believe that no malpractice was involved, remember that the litigation costs and time involved in such cases may surpass any recoverable outstanding fee, plus foregone revenue from not being available for other work)
- The potential detrimental effects of litigation on insurance premiums
- The effect of possible negative publicity on the potential and current client base
- The possibility that even if a suit for fees is successful, the client may have no recoverable funds
- The possibility that recovery of funds may take several years, even with a judgment in favor of the practice (Cottle 2011, 35)

It is important to identify potential bad debts early so that they can be kept to a minimum. A well-managed veterinary practice will have sound financial controls that will help protect against granting credit to poor credit risks. Keep all personnel informed, and remind staff frequently of the credit and collection policies so that they will be applied consistently and in a professional manner. Establish strong oversight systems to ensure that doctors and other employees adhere to the agreed-upon policies.

Review all practice credit and collection policies annually. Keep up with changing standards and market conditions when it comes to practice rules and procedures, as well as employee training, in these areas. Remember, the more you can avoid unpaid fees and write-offs of delinquent accounts, the more capital your practice will realize for investing in and advancing improved animal-care services (ibid., 36). Besides, most veterinary personnel would rather focus time and energy on patient care rather than hounding clients for payment.

PROBLEMS WITH REVENUE COLLECTION AND BILLING POLICIES

As manager, be alert to the following danger signs that indicate problems with billing and collection policies.

- Declining profits
- Difficulty paying bills as they come due
- Final invoices for cases frequently higher than care plan estimates costs, resulting in more service write-offs

- Increase in the number of bad accounts written off and the monetary value of write-offs
- Lower average transaction charges
- More client "controversy"
- Employee unhappiness or resistance to fees, and dissatisfaction or discomfort with the billing process
- Accounts receivable balances aging longer
- More client invoices going into accounts receivable, rather than being paid at time of service
- More discussion at management meetings about fees, billing and collection issues
- Less owner compensation and stagnant wages for all employees (Cottle 2011, 35)

These problems can quickly lead to serious financial trouble, so act quickly to resolve them.

Safeguarding Hospital Revenue

When revenues are collected, they must be protected from loss, theft, and mishandling. As manager, you are charged with a huge responsibility: You must plan, organize, direct, evaluate, and adapt procedures and systems to ensure that revenue losses are minimized as much as possible.

Revenues represent a substantial practice asset, whatever form they take. Even collections that are realized through credit-card payment and checks are readily converted to cash. The vast majority of accounts receivable will be converted to cash within a relatively short period of time. All realized revenues allow the business to pay its vendors, pay employee wages, buy new equipment, maintain and repair existing equipment, expand and improve facilities, and invest in advertising and marketing.

The process of safeguarding revenue is multifaceted and complex. A successful system relies on physical protections, well-trained employees, and exemplary record-keeping systems. Checklists of issues to be considered in safeguarding revenues are presented in the accompanying textboxes. Please note, these are not comprehensive lists of all the extensive management details that contribute to maximizing and safeguarding practice revenue.

If services are provided and products are dispensed to clients, but revenues are lost, records are misplaced, or records are altered to disguise theft, the hospital may be irreparably harmed. Your reputation as a practice manager could be damaged as well. Following proper collection guidelines helps to ensure that this does not happen.

COLLECTION GUIDELINES

Cash and checks should be kept in a secure place as they are collected throughout the day. Typically a cashier's drawer is used. Electronic cash registers serve the purpose well, as the

Fee Schedules

In order for any veterinary practice to maintain profitability in the face of the increasing costs of patient care, the management team must regularly adjust the practice fee schedule. All employees must be able to explain fees to clients so that they can make educated, well-informed choices among health-care options for their companion animals. The following guidelines can help you establish practice procedures on setting, applying, and collecting fees. Conduct periodic reviews of fee-schedule compliance at your practice using this checklist, and regularly execute changes as needed.

SETTING FEES

- Fee increases should reflect inflationary effects and costs of doing business in your practice's area.
- Leverage the Internet to investigate cost-of-living statistics and trends in the practice area. The Bureau of Labor Statistics, the Consumer Price Index, the Quarterly Census of Employment and Wages, and other statistical sources can help you keep a pulse on the practice's market area.
- Evaluate competition via the Internet, especially for vendors competing in product sales (for example, for prescription pharmaceuticals sold via both virtual and paper catalogs).
- Acquire the AAHA veterinary fee guide to benchmark commonly invoiced services by region.
- Plan fee updates a year in advance as part of the practice budgeting routine.
- Consider applying regular, periodic fee increases across all services (for example, raising all fees by an incremental percentage once per year, half-year, or quarter) so as not to fall behind. Many practice administrative teams keep waiting to raise fees because they intend to evaluate each fee on a line-by-line basis. When the reviews do not take place, and therefore the increases are not implemented, these practices quickly fall behind. Meanwhile, costs continue to increase.

APPLYING FEES

- Once the new fees are established, they should be accepted by all staff members as an appropriate reflection of the skills and care provided. To implement the fee updates, they will need to be communicated to clients.
- All members of the practice team must be confident about the value of veterinary care so that they do not hesitate to talk about fees with clients.

CONTINUES >

- The fees should be clearly explained to clients in a way that supports the value of patient services. Regular staff training and role playing is an important factor in excellent communication with clients—and excellent communication with clients builds client loyalty to the practice. It reinforces the team's expertise in providing excellent care for a fair price.
- Medical personnel should recommend treatment in the best interest of the patient without second-guessing the client's desires or ability to pay. The client will make a decision about treatment options based on sound, solid information and recommendations by hospital staff.
- Care plans and associated fee estimates should be prepared and clearly communicated to clients to avoid problems with uncollectible accounts.
- Discounts should be minimized to the extent possible.

COLLECTING FEES

- All team members should contribute to contemporaneous completion of patient service tracking forms and, in paper-light practices, to inputting service and care transactions as they occur so that charges are not missed.
- Employees must be diligent and careful in invoicing and writing patient records, so that accurate and comprehensive records result with all services and products charged to the client.
- Employees should keep clients aware of the total amount of accumulated charges as care progresses.
- The team must follow clear guidelines as to when total invoice amounts require client payment, keeping abreast of the cost of care for a complicated patient case. Client payments should be collected to keep below ceiling guidelines.
- Maintain current and well-communicated guidelines of client payment expectations and credit policies.
- When all team members follow the practice policies, payment problems are minimized.
- Regularly train team members about fee communication, invoice presentation, payment collection, and patient discharge coordination to maximize the probability of full payment at the time of service.

Revenue Realization Controls

A practice manager's job description usually includes careful attention to assuring collection and banking of all revenues charged to and collected from clients. Many steps in systematic and timely revenue collection require monitoring. The following can serve as checklists for your practice in these areas.

PREVENTING LOSS
- Management hires honest employees and carefully cross-checks references during the hiring process. The practice uses drug and background checks as standard hiring procedure.
- Cashiers exercise attentive care and caution while collecting the various types of monetary equivalents from clients: cash, checks, credit cards, charges on account, manufacturer coupons, gift certificates, barter credits, etc.
- Cashiers pay careful attention when making change for cash transactions.
- Checks accepted for payment are scrutinized for flaws, and immediately endorsed or scanned for electronic deposit.
- The hospital facility is well lit and well maintained, discouraging grand theft and robbery and enhancing employee security.
- Secure systems and equipment are in place for storing collections awaiting transfer to the bank or other financial institution.
- Periodically, practice management reevaluates the means of depository transport, to see if better, safer and more cost effective methods are available.
- Cashiers' drawers are locked so that they cannot be readily accessed by unauthorized personnel or outside parties.
- Cashiers' drawers are hard to see and access from across the reception counter.
- Each cash drawer is imprest (consistently starting with a given amount of cash for change) and assigned to a single cashier. All cashiers have total responsibility for protecting and balancing their drawers for the duration of the shift.
- Cashiers' drawers are reconciled with collection records at least once per day, and more often in busy practices and those with multiple shifts
- Cashiers are responsible for the reconciliation of their personally assigned drawers.

CONTINUES >

- Cashiers immediately investigate and resolve cash shortages and overages.
- Refunds from the cash drawer are limited to a set amount, such as $10. Beyond the preauthorized refund limit, responsible management personnel must authorize refunds before a refund check can be written to the client.
- Employee check-cashing through the cashier's drawer is prohibited.
- Petty cash for miscellaneous practice cash expenditures are not obtained from the cashier's drawer but from a separate dedicated fund for this purpose.
- Fee collection, invoice, client credit, and deposit records are cross-checked by employees who do not handle collected cash, checks, or credit cards.
- Practice management assures deposits are made to the bank or other financial institution once per business day, at the minimum.

ENSURING PROMPT COLLECTION

- Strict procedures are established that define what payment methods are allowed and how client payment will be accepted.
- Credit-card payments are authorized and processed immediately.
- All employees consistently comply with accounts receivable charging policies.
- Collection policies are aggressively maintained and delinquent accounts are pursued promptly.
- Procedures are in place for resubmitting nonsufficient fund (NSF) checks to the bank after contacting the client and accessing processing fees.
- NSF checks are safeguarded for future deposit or prosecution.
- Client challenges to credit-card charges are promptly investigated, and communication is made with the merchant processing bank and client to resolve them.
- Practice owners and managers regularly read the aging accounts receivable report and personally make calls to slow-paying clients to resolve any issues and obtain agreements for payment.

drawers can sometimes be electronically linked to the practice computer system that prints client invoices. A simple drawer, built in under a counter, can also suffice, as long as it can be locked securely in the event the cashier must leave the post and the drawer is unattended.

This storage place should be as inaccessible as possible to clients and all employees other than those responsible for revenue collection and custody. If there is concern about possible armed robbery, receipts may be deposited directly into a locked slotted safe as they are

Record Maintenance Controls and Procedures

Practice managers are responsible for data management and record control. This aspect of management has become increasingly important as veterinary hospitals have moved toward electronic environments. Whether in hard-copy or electronic form, records must be handled to prevent information loss, mitigate practice risk, and improve employee efficiency. Management controls are centered in policies that require good organization, accuracy, and completeness and procedures that specify exactly how to obtain those objectives.

PREVENTING LOSS OR ALTERATION OF RECORDS

- Define and enforce procedures for computer backup media rotation and offsite storage to prevent data loss and/or outsource backups through the Internet to a reliable "cloud-based" solution.
- Close out charge-card batches with the merchant processor or bank on a daily basis.
- Number invoices sequentially (in manual systems).
- Account for all invoices and cross-check them with appointment records.
- Close out computer databases on a daily basis and print activity reports for audit purposes.
- Bank statements should be received unopened and then reviewed by the owner for irregularities before going to the bookkeeper for reconciliation of the bank account. Only designated owners should have Internet access to practice bank accounts, and they should regularly check recorded deposit and expense activity and print activity reports to provide to the bookkeeper for account reconciliation purposes.
- Persons with responsibility for the maintenance of accounts receivable and collection procedures should not be the same as those physically handling payments and preparing deposits.
- Persons opening and logging mail content, including client payments by check, should not be the same as those controlling accounts receivable ledgers and making adjustments to client account balances.
- If large mail payments occur on a frequent basis, contract with an outside service to receive the payments and immediately post them to the practice's bank accounts, rather than having clients send payments directly to the practice.

REVIEWING DATA FOR INACCURACY

- Review audit trail reports to spot irregularities and odd account adjustments.
- Compare computer reports or manual one-write ledgers of revenue collected with

CONTINUES >

the daily bank deposit slip for accuracy and evidence of any irregularities, including possible delays in bank deposit occurrence.

- Reconcile bank statements in a timely manner to spot discrepancies between the time monies were collected and prepared for deposit and when deposits were actually made.
- Look for discrepancies between deposit amounts that clear on the bank statement and deposit amounts reported on the daily reports.
- Ask questions when records don't jibe.
- Periodically review computer settings to assure correct sales tax rates, finance charges, billing fees, and preferred-client discount rates (e.g., senior citizen or employee discounts).
- Frequently review bad-check listings and aging accounts receivable reports to ensure ongoing employee attentiveness to collection and billing protocols.
- Regularly review inventory quantity adjustment reports, perhaps weekly or monthly. Frequent adjustments and especially downward adjustment of inventory amounts on hand may indicate that charges are being missed when products are dispensed to clients or that product has gone missing for other reasons such as internal theft.
- Conduct periodic medical-record audits to compare doctors' notes with estimates and invoices. Check records for services that were estimated and provided but not invoiced.
- Measure incidents of specifically targeted patient services and product use and compare them to the veterinary practice's care guidelines and goals to evaluate compliance gaps. Compliance gaps show that although clients were seen and patients treated, the sum total of defined services and/or product sales fell short of targets set for optimum patient welfare in accord with practice guidelines for early detection and wellness enhancement.

collected, so that only a manager or outside party with the combination can gain access to the collected receipts. This security method is used at many all night gas stations and convenience stores. A visible sign stating that cashiers do not have access to cash receipts may also discourage robbery attempts.

For each cashier's drawer, establish a set amount of funds that will be in the drawer at the beginning of each shift. Usually this is $50 to $150. Include small bills and coins in this amount, since this beginning amount, called imprest, represents what is available to make change for transactions during the coming hours of business activity. Ideally, each cashier is assigned custody of a single cash drawer and is responsible for the funds collected and deposited to it during his shift as a cashier.

The daily drawer closeout procedure compares the counted revenues with the receipt records. The type of receipt record used depends on the practice's sales invoicing system. In all cases, the cashier must verify totals with an adding machine, print the tape, and bundle it with the receipts. The total on the tape provides evidence of reconciliation for each revenue type: cash, credit card, checks, and coupons.

In computerized practices using practice management software, the cashier should print the daily receipt report for his shift. The report tallies check, credit-card, and cash transactions, with each client transaction listed. With some software, the report is configured as a deposit report that can be efficiently used as a substitute bank deposit slip, eliminating the cashier's manual preparation of one that includes details of client names, check numbers, and amounts.

In the case of a manual invoicing system, the cashier will compare the receipt counts with the total of the amounts listed on the one-write system register, the total of the duplicate sales slips, or the total from the cash register tape. Where electronic transmission of credit-card payments occurs, the cashier will use the card swipe terminal to tally the batch total when it is closed out at the end of a shift.

At the end of his shift, the cashier counts the total collections in the drawer and is responsible for balancing the drawer. When the beginning imprest amount is subtracted from the total amount counted, the remaining balance should agree with the total receipt records for the shift. A bank deposit can be prepared at this time to summarize the collected amounts, and these shift receipts are safely secured in the slotted safe away from the reception area or other designated repository. The cashier's drawer is left with only the starting imprest amount to begin the next shift. The new shift cashier counts the imprest amount with the prior shift cashier in attendance, with each cashier as a witness to the correct amount in the drawer.

Alternatively, at the end of the shift, the cashier will count and balance the drawer and bundle the receipts with the adding machine tape, as before. The cashier then submits the entire drawer to a designated person in the practice business office. The new shift cashier obtains a fresh cash drawer, containing the correct imprest amount, from the business office.

For smaller practices, the drawer may only be opened once at the beginning of the day's activities and closed once, after the last transaction of the day's activities is processed. In the event the cash drawer stays open the entire day, a necessary safeguard is for the cashier leaving and the cashier taking over the next shift to jointly reconcile the interim closeout. If a bank deposit is not made at the close of the shift, the interim checkout is not a final process but is meant to identify receipt shortages and overages while all responsible employees are still available.

When receipt overages or shortages are discovered, the responsible cashiers should review the appointment book, receipt copies, computer audit trails, and their memories to resolve the differences. The sooner cashiers recognize and address discrepancies, the more likely it is that they will be resolved. Through this reconciliation process, unresolved errors are promptly brought to management's attention by the next step in the internal control process: the bookkeeper's review of the reports that have been prepared each day and submitted for posting in the overall practice accounting system.

Make cashiers accountable for addressing out-of-balance reconciliations that result from their shifts' activities. If you do not, the practice will likely suffer from many more out-of-balance problems in the future. Employees are much more attentive to exact change making and careful collection techniques when they know their time and credibility are at stake. In most cases, regular spot checks of the cashier's reconciliations and asking questions about differences are effective tools for gaining compliance. In no case, however, should a cashier be balancing the drawer by using his own funds.

When deposits are prepared, cashiers should inspect each check that has been collected, making sure each one has the current date, signature, payee, and correct amounts, even though this should have already been done at the time of payment. As mentioned earlier, as checks are received throughout the day they should be endorsed with a stamp on the back. The stamp should include the hospital name, a "For Deposit Only" qualification, the name of the depository bank, and the business checking account number. The person doing the final inspection of the checks should look for these stamps as well.

After final closeout, the cashier remits all collected revenue, less the established imprest amount, to the manager or another responsible person for safe storage. The cashier drawer and its imprest amount also will go into a safe for overnight storage. Supporting reports and adding machine slips may be included with the bundle or relayed directly to the bookkeeper for verification.

Make or arrange for a deposit of collected funds to the depository bank at least once daily. In some areas, it might be appropriate to make a night deposit rather than leaving the daily receipts in the hospital overnight. Some practice managers prefer that employees not be responsible for transporting deposits, especially in locations posing personal threats. In this situation, arrange for an armored car to pick up deposits on a daily basis, or the practice owner or manager may take responsibility for transporting the deposit.

Many banks now offer remote online deposits. This service enables you to scan paper checks and have the scanned images of the checks electronically transmitted to your bank for deposit directly into your checking account without leaving your office. Although you still need to go to the bank to deposit cash, you may be able to reduce the frequency of the trips.

In all possible methods of receipt processing and reconciliation, managers and owners must periodically review and make careful assessment of internal control functions. These reviews are necessary to mitigate the risk inherent in any one person accumulating a concentration of responsibilities for physical management of receipts and/or records pertaining to receipts that could lead to embezzlement or theft.

METHODS OF INTERNAL CONTROL

Practice managers must be concerned about minimizing the risk of internal losses. A practice manager cannot be everywhere at all times, so systems must be devised to help reduce the chance of loss and theft. The accounting profession has a term for these systems and methods: internal control.

Internal control includes "all measures used by a business to ensure against errors, waste, and fraud; to assure the reliability of accounting data; and to promote compliance with all company policies" (Meigs and Meigs 1986, 27). These measures are generally implemented to prevent loss of revenue due to the actions of an employee or employees. These actions could be accidental or deliberate. Revenue loss can be in the form of money, supplies, time, equipment, or other valuable practice assets.

One basic internal control principle is that no one person should handle all phases of a transaction from beginning to end. If, for example, one person enters the invoice, collects the revenue, handles the drawer closeout, records the daily receipts, makes the bank deposit, and reconciles the bank statements, significant problems can result (ibid., 11). Errors and omissions would not be found unless there were detailed audits of the transaction, and even then, loss could be successfully disguised through destruction of records.

This important internal control principle results in a concept embracing the division of duties. Wherever possible, record-keeping duties should be kept separate from asset custody duties. The person comparing and maintaining records should not tend or safeguard the assets. The person who reconciles the bank statement should not control the deposit or take it to the bank or process client credit cards. The person who reviews the daily records and cross-checks deposit amounts with invoices and computer-system reports should not make the collections or prepare the deposit. The person who adjusts client accounts receivables for write-offs should not handle payments made on account by the client.

Be aware that no matter how well you divide duties, you cannot easily detect fraud committed through collusion. If two employees with different areas of responsibility work together to hide their actions, they may be able to thwart the best system of internal controls, at least for as long as they remain on friendly terms with one another!

Remember, your most effective tool for detecting internal theft and fraud is a good system of cross-checks in a well-thought-out internal control system. Management, including owners, should regularly review systems to evaluate them for weaknesses, since job duties and responsibilities can shift. The practice's accountant rarely discovers embezzlement or theft. Most frequently, detection occurs when another employee complains about the perpetrator or management makes the discovery through monitoring and oversight activities.

Your goal is to establish administrative systems that reduce the opportunity for theft, embezzlement, and waste of valuable practice assets without unreasonably impeding your staff's ability to effectively and efficiently care for patients and respond to client needs. Doing this requires that you think and act first like a business owner. Veterinary practice professionals tend to be kind, trusting, and forgiving individuals, and often they do not demand an appropriate level of accountability from staff members. Do not fall into this trap. You have a fiduciary responsibility to your practice, your employees, your partners, and your family. Strong practices mandate strong leadership. (See textbox, "Managing Risk of Internal Theft," for additional methods.)

DETECTING AND HANDLING EMPLOYEE EMBEZZLEMENT

Embezzlement is a risk that no one likes to consider. However, for the sake of the practice, be vigilant. Implement the guidelines suggested above. Watch for signs of potential trouble. Pay as much attention as you can to what is going on in your employees' personal lives. Embezzlement problems might be signaled by certain employee behavior. Keep an eye on any staff member who does any of the following:

- Evidences sudden, unexplained wealth—for example, new expensive clothes, car, home, hobbies, horses, jewelry, plastic surgery, and the like.
- Constantly talks of money problems or asks for advances.
- Receives calls at work from creditors.
- Refuses to take vacations or share job responsibility.
- Frequently complains about bookkeeping entries and errors made by others.
- Is under significant economic stress because of family illness, divorce, or loss of income
- Has known gambling tendencies.
- Is disorganized and cannot produce financial information or records promptly when requested to do so.

Be attuned to incidents of missing records, an increasing number of client complaints about billing errors, and daily closings that always balance to the penny. Typically, daily closings will sometimes be a little off due to unintended human error; if an employee is cheating, the numbers may be a little too perfect, especially if there are other warning signs (see textbox, "When Losses Are Evident").

If guilt is determined, terminate the employee immediately. Do not think that you can trust this employee again, no matter what the reason for the embezzlement. Send a clear mes-

Managing Risk of Internal Theft

In addition to segregating responsibilities, consider implementing the following internal policies and systems:

- All staff members handling money and accounting processes should be bonded. Talk with your insurance agent about including employee theft coverage (also called employee dishonesty coverage) in the business insurance policy. Your accountant and insurance agent can help you decide what level of theft coverage to carry, and limits should be reassessed annually for possible adjustment. Often, insured businesses do not carry employee theft insurance amounts sufficient to cover actual losses when they occur. The veterinary profession has had many incidents where embezzlement schemes greatly exceeded $250,000, as best as could be measured after the fact of discovery.
- Staff members who handle money, process transactions, and manage accounting records should be carefully selected. Including background checks as part of your practice's standard hiring procedure is likely cost-effective in the long run.
- Install security cameras to monitor areas where employees handle cash and transactions as well as other practice areas representing higher risk for loss, such as inventory storage and valuable equipment locations.
- Require employees who handle money and manage accounting records to take vacation days consecutively, ideally for a minimum of one week and optimally for two weeks. Assign another staff member to take over these duties while the employee is away. This policy helps uncover any embezzlement schemes, which tend to unravel when the perpetrator cannot be present to control records and activities.
- Cross-train staff to share and rotate duties. Cross-training keeps practice procedures moving without too much disruption when a key position becomes vacant, keeps employees more challenged with new learning experiences, and makes it less likely that any employee will gain absolute power and control over any segment of practice activity.
- Periodically take an active part in the check-out and other transactional procedures yourself.
- Charge slips, manual invoices, or computer data forms should be serially numbered. Staff should be well aware that forms are checked for missing numbers. Voided forms of any type should be retained, not thrown away.

CONTINUES >

- If your practice is computerized, do not keep manual invoices on hand. Insist that all transactions be invoiced through the computer system.
- Change invoicing software passwords frequently. Every employee should be logged into the system under her own unique password so that audit trails clearly identify each employee originating a transaction.
- Limit employee function in the practice management software to only those necessary in order for the employee to efficiently perform his job functions.
- Many software programs include training modules that enable employees to practice using the software using fictitious clients and patients, including the generation of practice invoices. Once employee training is complete, eliminate employee access to training modules through password management or deactivation of these parts of the software program.
- Regularly audit computer reports to look for evidence of unexpected voided or reversed transactions, changes to client accounts, and client refunds.
- All expense payments should be paid by business check or from a petty-cash fund. Do not allow funds to be dispersed directly from daily receipts.
- When balances do not tally, ask questions. The employees with duty responsibility should be expected to promptly explain any discrepancies.
- A doctor with authority or the hospital manager must approve all discounts, refunds, or account write-offs exceeding predetermined amounts. Require this person to add a dated signature to every discount, refund request, or write-off he approves.
- Place a sign at the cashier's station that reads, "Please request a receipt for all transactions." Cash theft is often disguised by a cashier not invoicing transactions, including deleting prepared invoices without posting them when clients pay with cash. Alternatively, place a sign on the exit door that reads, "Did you receive a receipt for your pet's care today? If not, please ask for the practice manager."
- Regularly inform employees through clear policy communication that theft of any kind is cause for immediate dismissal and possible prosecution.
- Do not set bad examples. Owners and managers should follow the same rules as other employees.
- Create a work environment that encourages honesty. The practice should set and maintain high standards for moral and ethical conduct. Standards cannot be arbitrarily applied; they must apply equally to all personnel.

sage to all other employees: Theft will not be tolerated. If you do not pursue prosecution of blatant theft, other employees will not be deterred by practice rules.

Employee theft can be very pervasive and costly. As small businesses, animal hospitals can be particularly vulnerable because financial control systems often are relaxed to reduce cost. Because veterinary practices tend to have a small number of employees, it is often difficult for them to segregate duties at all times according to the recommendations listed above.

Do not consider any employee wholly incapable of theft. Given the right combination of external pressures, psychological reasons, and lax internal controls, even employees who seem very loyal can make bad choices. Most employees who steal have rationalized their actions and do not consider them to constitute theft. Whenever possible, always have two staff members handling the money. Take an active part in all revenue-handling activities, and do not take anything for granted. (For more information on internal controls, see Chapter 11.)

When Losses Are Evident

If you suspect embezzlement, proceed with caution and a careful plan of action. When an employee is stealing, the fact usually becomes fairly clear eventually and practice managers are pretty certain who is responsible. However, suspicions may be hard to confirm and often are proven false, sometimes years later when the real perpetrator confesses. Accusing someone of theft without concrete evidence to support your allegations could result in a lawsuit. If you find your practice in this situation, consider the following steps:

- Notify the hospital owners and/or any others who share managerial responsibility with you; do not try to handle the situation alone.
- Secure important and relevant hospital records. Make sure you have working backup copies of computer data. These backups should be stored with an owner and possibly another responsible person or trusted party, such as the practice attorney.
- Inform the bonding or insurance company as soon as possible, as theft coverage provisions will likely require it. The company will likely have helpful resources available to assist you as you determine what action to take.
- Contact the hospital accountant and attorney for advice and enlist their aid in conducting a review of the hospital records and internal control procedures.
- Reassign duties so that money-handling and record-keeping or bookkeeping tasks are shared or reallocated.
- On the attorney's or insurance company's advice, contact the police. Make no accusations.
- Do not talk about specific dollar amounts involved.

Managing all the varied aspects of practice revenue is a significant part of your role as practice manager. Making day-to-day decisions about the financial health and safety of the practice will require you to balance directive and participative leadership, as you must determine and enforce policies and protocol and while also guiding and encouraging your employees to observe them. Whether you are resolving issues of internal control, determining credit policies, overseeing collections, or managing accounts receivable, you will need your full repertoire of manager's skills: planning, organizing, directing, and evaluating.

11

Accounting and Bookkeeping

Accounting is "the art of measuring, communicating, and interpreting financial activity" (Meigs and Meigs 1986, 1). In a veterinary practice, the purpose of accounting is to provide sound and reliable financial information to a variety of decision makers who plan and control the activities of the business. Practice owners and managers rely on accurate financial data to make informed judgments and decisions. Dependable accounting information is vital in setting organizational goals and tracking progress toward those goals.

Other important decision makers who rely on accurate financial information about veterinary practice operations include outside parties such as creditors, potential investors or purchasers, banks, and state and federal governments. Bankers and suppliers are concerned about a practice's stability, and they want to assess its financial soundness before making loans or extending credit. Investors, such as new veterinarians buying into the practice, are interested in its current financial health and future prospects. Government agencies require information for taxation and regulation purposes.

When veterinary practices are consolidated into larger corporate entities, they may become publicly owned. The Securities and Exchange Commission (SEC) demands stringent reporting before stock in a corporation can be publicly traded on a stock exchange. Then shareholders require regular financial reporting, and the law mandates it. Larger incorporated veterinary practices may also offer employee stock ownership plans (ESOPs). Employees who own stock in the practice become vitally interested in its stability and profitability.

Accounting and Practice Management

The individuals who depend most heavily on accounting are those charged with the responsibility for the daily direction of veterinary hospital operations. This is you, the practice manager.

Consider the wide variety of data available from accounting records and the many ways that you can utilize this data in practice management. Here is a partial list of the information that you might obtain from the practice's accounting system:

- Practice profitability, based on operating income less operating expenses
- Total operating income collected over any selected period of time
- Revenue or income sources by profit center, by service provider, and by location
- Amount owed to each vendor and creditor of the hospital (trade accounts payable and loans payable), and time outstanding (aging of balances)
- Amounts owed to the hospital by its clients (trade accounts receivable), aging of balances, amounts in collections, and accounts written off as uncollectible
- The number of animals that have received treatment and the average charge per patient
- The number of reminders to be sent in coming months for vaccines and other services, the number of past due or delinquent reminders, and the predicted revenue that can be projected from reminders
- The total employee hours worked in any particular time frame, in addition to hours of paid time off and overtime hours worked
- Amounts of taxes withheld from employee wages and amounts of taxes owed to the various taxing agencies
- Projected employee hours of paid time, hourly rates of pay, and total payroll burden the practice must pay
- Qualified benefit cost, such as health insurance and employer retirement contributions, and predictions of how cost will integrate with a total payroll budget
- Records of hospital-owned equipment, when each item was acquired, and purchase prices
- Inventory counts and value of veterinary pharmaceuticals, hospital supplies, and other supplies on hand
- Inventory that has been sold and the profit it generated
- Sales taxes collected and due to the state

As this list demonstrates, accounting plays a crucial role in all aspects of veterinary practice operations, including even patient record maintenance and treatment documentation. Inventory and supplies consumed during treatment administration, surgeon and anesthesiologist time involved in complex orthopedic procedures, and coordination of estimates and invoices with actual services are all examples of data traced by accounting.

The veterinary practice accounting system is the sum total of methods used to keep records of practice financial activities and to summarize these activities in periodic reports. Accounting information is primarily, but not exclusively, composed of financial data about business transactions, expressed in terms of money. Because mere transaction records are of little use in making informed judgments and decisions, this recorded data must also be sorted and summarized, then presented in significant reports (Fess and Warren 1987, 9). A good accounting system results in timely production of the reports that management deems necessary to evaluate, plan, and execute, incorporating the principles of cost versus benefit.

Despite the importance of accounting to every area of veterinary practice management, many practice managers lack accounting and finance knowledge. It is quite common for hospital employees to grow into a management position because of competencies in other areas, such as excellent client and staff communication skills. Technicians, veterinarians, kennel workers, and receptionists may all find themselves in management positions with no formal training in finance, bookkeeping, or accounting systems.

In fact, a key skill that many practice owners seek when hiring a practice manager is basic veterinary hospital financial and bookkeeping aptitude. You will need to coordinate with the practice accountant to determine how information gathered can be used to control operations efficiently and economically. But you also owe it to yourself and your practice to be familiar with the basics of accounting systems, bookkeeping, and terminology.

Like the medical professions, accounting has a special jargon all its own. Until you are acquainted with basic words, meanings, and concepts, you will have a difficult time understanding accounting, which is often called "the language of business." This chapter will introduce some elementary accounting terms and principles; you might also consider taking college courses or seminars that teach bookkeeping basics, financial reporting concepts, and accounting software use.

Accounting and Bookkeeping

Accounting and bookkeeping are closely associated activities, with the accounting process depending on the information produced by the bookkeeping process. However, they are two very distinct undertakings, requiring different degrees of education, training, and professional competency.

Bookkeeping is the process of recording business data in a prescribed manner. Writing checks to vendors and summarizing the bills that have been paid is an example of a bookkeeping function. General principles guide financial data collection and recording, but individual veterinary hospitals often develop their own variations, depending on personnel competency, computer system investment, and other factors.

For example, a practice bookkeeper might be responsible for all the financial records of the hospital, or may only keep records on one segment, such as amounts owed by clients (accounts receivable clerk). Bookkeeping duties may be divided among several different employees. One person may have primary responsibility for accounts receivable while another handles accounts payable.

Bookkeeping work is primarily clerical, and computers now play a significant role in handling the bookkeeping segment of veterinary practice income and receipts. Information that was once logged by hand in ledger books and summated with a *ten key* can now be gathered, sorted, and summarized by robust software programs, which simultaneously create invoices and amend patient records.

In most animal hospitals, a bookkeeper or manager keeps the income and expense journals on a regular basis through computers and software. Sometimes, a practice owner or family member of the owner will handle significant portions of bookkeeping duties because of confidentiality and risk issues related to the potential for financial record manipulation. (See Chapter 10 for more information on the risk of revenue loss and implementation of internal controls.)

Accounting activities are different from bookkeeping functions. Accounting requires the use of transactional data gathered by bookkeeping to identify, measure, and report financial information to practice owners, managers, and other parties interested in economic measurements of a business's activity results. Accounting also involves the design of the hospital's accounting system and resulting records. Besides preparing reports from bookkeeping data, accounting encompasses interpretation of what the reports mean. After all, financial reports are of little use if they cannot be deciphered (Fess and Warren 1987, 9).

Interpretation leads to planning. As mentioned in Chapter 3 on strategic planning, goals should be set in measurable terms. Many goals become incorporated into budgets, which are a natural evolution of financial reports. Budgets link historical results accumulated by bookkeepers, summarized in financial reports, and interpreted with the help of the accountant to the future and to the entrepreneurial vision established by the practice's leadership team.

BOOKKEEPING DUTIES

The bookkeeper's duties basically involve recording the transactions into the journals and ledgers. While the bookkeeping function is relatively repetitive and straightforward, it takes time and skill. Bookkeepers do not require degrees or licenses, but most will have taken business and accounting courses in a college or trade school. Important bookkeeper attributes are attentiveness to detail, neatness, consistency, accuracy, and organization.

Do not assign bookkeeping tasks to just anyone with time available. Various bookkeeping responsibilities are best handled by as few people as possible to achieve conformity and continuity in record-keeping processes. At the same time, the practice manager must make sure that the bookkeeping system itself allows for continuity and conformity, no matter which employee is assigned the job. The system design should be clear and consistent so that another trained person could step in and take over bookkeeping duties should the current bookkeeper leave the practice's employment.

While minimizing the number of people involved in the bookkeeping processes is important, it is also important to ensure that appropriate internal controls are in place. The bookkeeper is in a unique position of record creation and control that can easily enable embezzlement, particularly if duties expand beyond recording transactions and cross-checking other employees' prepared documentation, such as cashier records of fee income deposits. If the bookkeeper has access to and handles bank deposits, then a significant principle of strong internal control function, segregation of duties, has been violated. (See textbox, "The Basics of Internal Control Systems.")

The bookkeeper must have basic knowledge of and familiarity with computer operation and Internet use. Look for competent use of bookkeeping- and accounting-related software programs, including a spreadsheet program such as Microsoft Excel and a checkwriting program like Intuit's Quicken, or deeper capability in a small business accounting package such as QuickBooks. Bookkeepers should be comfortable using cloud-based software applications, which are increasingly used for practice bookkeeping to aid in communication with the practice's accountant, for ease of access and oversight by owners, and for reliable data backup.

The American Institute of Professional Bookkeepers (AIPB) provides excellent resources, education, and credentialing of bookkeepers as well as a free weekly bookkeeping tip e-letter

---

The Basics of Internal Control Systems

As you recall from Chapter 10, proper segregation of duties entails making sure no single person is in charge of or controls more than one of the following functions:

- Authorization
- Recording
- Custody

Authorization duties entail the ability to approve transactions. For example, approval of supply orders, approval of client refunds and discounts, and approval of offering client services on credit all relate to the authorization function.

Recording refers to the actual data entry process, typical duties of a bookkeeping position. For example, entering bills and payments into the bookkeeping software, entering deposits into the bookkeeping software, and preparing bank and credit-card reconciliations are all recording function duties.

Custody duties involve the physical handling of assets. For example, receiving incoming supply orders, receiving cash and check payments from clients, and accessing the practice's bank account and having possession of signed checks for vendor or employee payment are duties of the custody function.

The chief objective of establishing and maintaining appropriate segregation of employee duties is to ensure that no employee has the opportunity to both commit a fraudulent activity and also conceal that fraud (see Chapter 10 for more information).

(see aipb.org). The website also provides access to a bookkeeper's hiring test. (See Figure 11.1 for a sample test to give bookkeeper job applicants.)

A check-writing software program will generally suffice very well for bookkeeping in veterinary practices with up to $1 million or $1.5 million in annual gross receipts. With higher annual revenues, the practice's accountant may recommend a more sophisticated software program, such as Intuit's QuickBooks or Sage's Peachtree.

For very large practices, professional accounting software might be used after analysis and consultation with the engaged accountant. The bookkeeper will most likely need special training to proficiently use any of these high-end programs. One common practice management error is to buy software that exceeds the abilities of key bookkeeping personnel, which can include the practice owner.

In most animal hospitals, many duties beyond simple check writing and transaction recording are assigned to the practice bookkeeper. The following sections discuss possible bookkeeping tasks and can be used as a model for creating a job description and developing training opportunities for an animal hospital bookkeeper.

MAINTAINING PAYROLL RECORDS AND PREPARING PAYROLL

Payroll represents an extensive and high-risk responsibility that extends well beyond the preparation of individual employee paychecks. Although time-keeping software solutions may supplant some of the following, typically duties have included properly recording employee hours worked by summarizing time cards or time-clock reports. The bookkeeper must be proficient in converting minutes into fractions of an hour to correctly compute hourly wages, then applying the correct hourly rate to the time worked, considering overtime requirements. She must track accrued (earned, but not paid) vacation hours, sick time, and other paid time off for each eligible employee and accurately subtract it as it is used.

The bookkeeper may also be required to evaluate employee scheduling, including hours worked in comparison with the schedule, and report variances to practice administration. Since labor cost is by far and away the single most significant cost of running a veterinary practice, payroll controls and recording through the bookkeeper and management team are crucial to preserving adequate practice profitability.

The bookkeeper must stay current with laws regulating tax withholding. Often this is done with the help of an outside payroll company. Withholding laws and payroll tax return preparation have become an increasingly complex aspect of small business management. Even payroll companies make mistakes, so practice managers should develop and monitor procedures that include careful administrative review of final payroll reports of hours worked, employee names, paid time off, and withholding.

FIGURE 11.1 BOOKKEEPER EXAMINATION

PAGE 1 SHOWN

˅

FULL FORM INCLUDED ON COMPANION WEBSITE

PART I. PAYROLL

1. If an individual works 54 hours in a week and is paid $10.00 per hour, what is his gross pay for the week? Assume that he receives time and a half for over 40 hours of work per week.

2. An individual earns $2,300 of gross pay for the week. His payroll deductions are as follows:

OASDI Tax – 6.2% of his pay, up to a maximum of $117,000.
Medicare Tax – 1.45% of pay
State Income Tax Withholding $75.00
Federal Income Tax Withholding $205.00
City Income Tax Withholding $40.00

His cumulative earnings for the year (not including this week's pay) were $120,500. What is the amount of his net pay for the week?

3. Bill Murray receives a 5% commission on merchandise he sells in excess of $1,000 per week. Bill sold $10,000.00 worth of merchandise during the week. What will be his gross pay for the week?

4. Please give the correct Internal Revenue Form number for each item.

A. Wage and Tax Statement
B. Employer's Withholding Allowance Certificate
C. Federal Unemployment Tax Return
D. Quarterly Employment Taxes (Social Security and Federal Withholding)
E. Used for reporting interest and dividend payments

5. The employees' earning records for the calendar year of ABC Animal Hospital are presented below:

Employee	Cumulative Earnings
Assad, Ann	$30,600
Bauman, Lee	$45,000
Medford, Phillip	$5,000
Miller, Pat	$10,100
Sawyer, Jan	$80,500
Timmons, Bill	$187,000

The OASDI component of FICA Tax during the year was 6.2% on an individual's first $117,000 of annual earnings, and the Medicare component of FICA Tax was 1.45% on all earnings. The unemployment rate for the year was 0.8% for the federal portion of up to $7,000 and 2.3% on the state portion for the first $8,000 of earnings. Compute:

A. Total company earnings subject to FICA.
B. Total subject to unemployment compensation taxes.
C. Employees' share of taxes assuming that employee does not pay unemployment insurance.
D. Employer's share of payroll taxes.

PART II. BANK RECONCILIATION

PROBLEM #1
The bank statement for the ABC Animal Clinic indicates a balance of $2,109.50 as of January 31. In addition, the following information is also provided:

The bookkeeper with payroll processing responsibility must make the correct calculations regarding withheld amounts for taxes, garnishments, voluntary employee contributions to retirement plans, repayment of advances, copayment for insurance coverage, and any other withholdings that might be required. She must correctly record payroll checks in the clinic accounting system to reflect gross wages and the various withholding amounts and remittances. (See Figure 11.2 for an example of gross pay, tax withholdings, and net pay.)

MAINTAINING PERSONNEL FILES

The bookkeeper may be responsible for maintaining each employee file, recording vacation and sick days, and determining employee benefits as directed by hospital policy. Making sure that Forms W-4 and other necessary personnel-file documents, as completed by each employee, are up-to-date may be an additional responsibility.

DEDUCTING PAYROLL TAXES AND COMPILING TAX REPORTS

The bookkeeper may be responsible for ensuring that the various taxes withheld from employee wages, called trust funds, as well as taxes that are the responsibility of the employer, are deposited on time with the appropriate tax-collection agencies according to the correct procedures. Payment of trust funds to the federal and state governments is one of the largest responsibilities any employee might bear. If funds are not paid, the bookkeeper may be held liable for that money even though he has no ownership or financial interest in the veterinary business. If the bookkeeper does not have personal responsibility for actually making the deposits, he may at least be accountable for ensuring that deadlines are met by informing the responsible personnel of deposit amounts and deadlines.

At designated times throughout the year, the bookkeeper with payroll duties will prepare the required city, state, and federal reports pertaining to payroll. These reports inform the involved agencies of the various taxes due to federal, state, and local governments. In nearly all cases, late submission of reports or delinquent tax payments will result in penalties, which may be substantial. Interest may be assessed for each day of tardiness. Massive penalties and interest can accumulate when subsequent deposits or reports are also tardy.

Each type of tax has different reporting and deposit requirements. As a veterinary practice grows and as payroll gets bigger, tax deposits usually have to be made more frequently and contemporaneously with the actual paycheck issuance. The bookkeeper must work hard to stay current with these requirements, as the number of reports, the information reported on each form, and the due dates for reports and filing are subject to change.

Laws also stipulate what reports and forms must be maintained on file in the hospital. A payroll bookkeeper's best friends are a current copy of the IRS publication entitled "Circular E," an information bulletin that comes with the quarterly payroll report form (Form 941), and

FIGURE 11.2 SUMMARY OF WITHHOLDING TAXES

Please note that each state varies in regard to the specific taxes that must be withheld from an employee's gross wages. Periodic reconfirmation with the practice's certified public accountant, chartered accountant, or payroll company is recommended. Types of taxes and tax rates change with new legislation, and different laws may apply to your practice as circumstances change. The following example does not include all the various taxes that might have to be withheld from the employee's wages.

Gross Wages	$1,000.00
Less:	
Federal Income Tax Rate depends on employee, claimed dependents, and other factors. See form W-4.	(250.00)
Federal Social Security Taxes OASDI (Old-Age, Survivors, and Disability Insurance) – 6.2% on a base wage that is adjusted annually by the IRS.	(62.00)
Medicare (Hospital Insurance) – 1.45% of all wages.	(14.50)
State Income Tax Rate depends on employee factors stipulated by the state. Employee may be subject to tax withholding by more than one state. Some states do not have an income tax.	(50.00)
Regional Income Tax Rate and occurrence depend on locale.	(10.00)
City Income Tax Rate and occurrence depend on locale.	(18.00)
School District Tax Rate and occurrence depend on locale.	(6.00)
State Disability Insurance Tax Some states may access a tax to the employee over and above what the employer pays.	(1.00)
Net Wages ("Take-Home Pay")	$588.50

bulletins from state and local payroll tax agencies. With Internet connectivity come options for e-mail notification. The bookkeeper should regularly check all pertinent tax filing sites and enroll for automatic e-mail notification of deadlines and tax changes.

Given all the details and duties of payroll bookkeeping, not to mention the legal ramifications of making an error, it's no wonder that many practice administrators engage the services of a professional payroll preparer. The staff hours required in proper payroll preparation may very well exceed the cost of outsourcing payroll services. Some CPA firms will handle payroll preparation in addition to the income tax preparation, but the best option for keeping costs low and minimizing errors is often to use a payroll-specific professional organization. The practice accountant may be able to direct you to a reputable outsourcing organization. See later in this chapter for more information regarding selection of a payroll processing company. (See Figures 11.3 and 11.4 for sample forms 940 and 941, and 11.5 for internal controls.)

MANAGING EMPLOYEE BENEFIT PLANS AND EXPENSE REIMBURSEMENT

Employees may be eligible for a variety of qualified, pretax fringe benefits. Such fringe benefits can include health insurance, group term-life insurance, cafeteria plan participation, profit or pension plan participation, or qualified medical expense reimbursement. Some others are educational assistance, transportation benefits, achievement awards, and moving expenses. Since the rules are very specific, the hospital manager should talk with the practice accountant to clarify issues and read up on these subjects on the IRS website (irs.gov). Look for the most recent edition of Publication 15-B, "Employer's Tax Guide to Fringe Benefits." The bookkeeper will be responsible for verifying benefit invoice accuracy, correctly accounting for payments that constitute fringe benefits, and maintaining good records.

The bookkeeper may also need to assist the practice manager in establishing practice policy that fixes employee eligibility for the various benefit programs the practice chooses to offer. The nuances of part-time versus full-time eligibility must be understood in terms of federal and state laws that might identify cutoffs for each type of employee. Each employee's average hours of work per week over time may need to be carefully tracked in order to ascertain when that employee's class might change from part-time to full-time worker, or vice versa.

New employees may be ineligible for certain benefits until they have worked an adequate number of weeks as established by practice policy within the confines of any laws that may apply. The bookkeeper would likely be responsible for keeping tabulations of deadlines as to when an employee is eligible to apply for group health insurance or some other benefit program, and also to help the employee complete and submit the requisite paperwork.

Many practices also reimburse some employees for documented, out-of-pocket, business-related expenditures. The bookkeeper may be responsible for ensuring the correct computation of these benefits and expenditures, verifying documents and receipts substantiating the amounts to be paid, and preparing payment for authorized signature and reimbursement in a timely manner.

DOCUMENTING SPECIAL PAYROLL ISSUES AND TAX REPORTING DETAILS

Tax regulations require that a business be reimbursed for any employee personal use of equipment that is owned or leased by the hospital, such as vehicles and laptop computers. Throughout the year, the bookkeeper may be responsible for checking records such as mileage logs to ensure that personal use is contemporaneously documented as required by federal tax law.

FIGURE 11.3 FORM 940

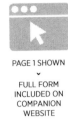

PAGE 1 SHOWN

˅

FULL FORM
INCLUDED ON
COMPANION
WEBSITE

Form **940 for 2010:** Employer's Annual Federal Unemployment (FUTA) Tax Return

850110

Department of the Treasury — Internal Revenue Service

OMB No. 1545-0028

(EIN)
Employer identification number ☐☐ – ☐☐☐☐☐☐☐

Name *(not your trade name)*

Trade name *(if any)*

Address

Number   Street   Suite or room number

City   State   ZIP code

Type of Return
(Check all that apply.)

☐ **a.** Amended

☐ **b.** Successor employer

☐ **c.** No payments to employees in 2010

☐ **d.** Final: Business closed or stopped paying wages

Read the separate instructions before you fill out this form. Please type or print within the boxes.

Part 1: Tell us about your return. If any line does NOT apply, leave it blank.

1 If you were required to pay your state unemployment tax in ...

1a One state only, write the state abbreviation . . . . **1a** ☐☐
- OR -

1b More than one state (You are a multi-state employer) . . . . **1b** ☐ Check here. Fill out Schedule A.

2 If you paid wages in a state that is subject to CREDIT REDUCTION . . . . **2** ☐ Check here. Fill out Schedule A (Form 940), Part 2.

Part 2: Determine your FUTA tax before adjustments for 2010. If any line does NOT apply, leave it blank.

3 Total payments to all employees . . . . **3** ☐ .

4 Payments exempt from FUTA tax . . . . **4** ☐ .

Check all that apply: **4a** ☐ Fringe benefits   **4c** ☐ Retirement/Pension   **4e** ☐ Other
4b ☐ Group-term life insurance   **4d** ☐ Dependent care

5 Total of payments made to each employee in excess of $7,000 . . . . **5** ☐ .

6 Subtotal (line 4 + line 5 = line 6) . . . . **6** ☐ .

7 Total taxable FUTA wages (line 3 – line 6 = line 7) . . . . **7** ☐ .

8 FUTA tax before adjustments (line 7 × .008 = line 8) . . . . **8** ☐ .

Part 3: Determine your adjustments. If any line does NOT apply, leave it blank.

9 If ALL of the taxable FUTA wages you paid were excluded from state unemployment tax, multiply line 7 by .054 (line 7 × .054 = line 9). Then go to line 12 . . . . . . **9** ☐ .

10 If SOME of the taxable FUTA wages you paid were excluded from state unemployment tax, OR you paid ANY state unemployment tax late (after the due date for filing Form 940), fill out the worksheet in the instructions. Enter the amount from line 7 of the worksheet . . . . . **10** ☐ .

11 If credit reduction applies, enter the amount from line 3 of Schedule A (Form 940) . . . . **11** ☐ .

Part 4: Determine your FUTA tax and balance due or overpayment for 2010. If any line does NOT apply, leave it blank.

12 Total FUTA tax after adjustments (lines 8 + 9 + 10 + 11 = line 12) . . . . **12** ☐ .

13 FUTA tax deposited for the year, including any overpayment applied from a prior year . **13** ☐ .

14 Balance due (If line 12 is more than line 13, enter the difference on line 14.)
- If line 14 is more than $500, you must deposit your tax.
- If line 14 is $500 or less, you may pay with this return. For more information on how to pay, see the separate instructions . . . . **14** ☐ .

15 Overpayment (If line 13 is more than line 12, enter the difference on line 15 and check a box below.) . . . . **15** ☐ .

Check one: ☐ Apply to next return.
☐ Send a refund.

▶ You **MUST** fill out both pages of this form and **SIGN** it.

Next ➡

For Privacy Act and Paperwork Reduction Act Notice, see the back of Form 940-V, Payment Voucher.   Cat. No. 11234O   Form **940** (2010)

Department of the Treasury, Internal Revenue Service

PAGE 1 SHOWN

v

FULL FORM
INCLUDED ON
COMPANION
WEBSITE

FIGURE 11.4 FORM 941

Form **941 for 2011:** **Employer's QUARTERLY Federal Tax Return**
(Rev. January 2011)
Department of the Treasury — Internal Revenue Service

950111
OMB No. 1545-0029

(EIN)
Employer identification number

Name (not your trade name)

Trade name (if any)

Address

Number   Street   Suite or room number

City   State   ZIP code

Report for this Quarter of 2011
(Check one.)

☐ 1: January, February, March

☐ 2: April, May, June

☐ 3: July, August, September

☐ 4: October, November, December

Prior-year forms are available at
www.irs.gov/form941.

Read the separate instructions before you complete Form 941. Type or print within the boxes.

Part 1: **Answer these questions for this quarter.**

1 Number of employees who received wages, tips, or other compensation for the pay period
including: Mar. 12 (Quarter 1), June 12 (Quarter 2), Sept. 12 (Quarter 3), or Dec. 12 (Quarter 4) **1**

2 Wages, tips, and other compensation **2**

3 Income tax withheld from wages, tips, and other compensation . . . **3**

4 If no wages, tips, and other compensation are subject to social security or Medicare tax
☐ Check and go to line 6e.

	Column 1		Column 2
5a Taxable social security wages .		× .104 =	
5b Taxable social security tips . .		× .104 =	
5c Taxable Medicare wages & tips.		× .029 =	

For 2011, the employee social security
tax rate is 4.2% and the Medicare tax
rate is 1.45%. The employer social
security tax rate is 6.2% and the
Medicare tax rate is 1.45%.

5d Add Column 2 line 5a, Column 2 line 5b, and Column 2 line 5c **5d**

5e Section 3121(q) Notice and Demand—Tax due on unreported tips (see instructions) . . **5e**

6a Reserved for future use.

6b Reserved for future use.

Do Not Complete Lines 6a-6d

6c Reserved for future use.

6e Total taxes before adjustments (add lines 3, 5d, and 5e) **6e**

7 Current quarter's adjustment for fractions of cents **7**

8 Current quarter's adjustment for sick pay **8**

9 Current quarter's adjustments for tips and group-term life insurance . . . **9**

10 Total taxes after adjustments. Combine lines 6e through 9 . . . . . . **10**

11 Total deposits, including prior quarter overpayments **11**

12a COBRA premium assistance payments (see instructions) **12a**

12b Number of individuals provided COBRA premium assistance . .

13 Add lines 11 and 12a **13**

14 Balance due. If line 10 is more than line 13, enter the difference and see instructions . . . **14**

15 Overpayment. If line 13 is more than line 10, enter the difference _____ Check one: ☐ Apply to next return. ☐ Send a refund.

▶ You MUST complete both pages of Form 941 and SIGN it.

Next ▶

For Privacy Act and Paperwork Reduction Act Notice, see the back of the Payment Voucher. Cat. No. 17001Z Form **941** (Rev. 1-2011)

Department of the Tresury, Internal Revenue Service

FIGURE 11.5 CONTROL SYSTEM

PAYROLL INTERNAL CONTROLS: Small businesses can be seen as defenseless when it comes to fighting payroll fraud. This doesn't have to be true. Just because a veterinary practice might not have the manpower and resources to have an entire department dedicated to accounting and internal controls does not mean that steps cannot be taken to secure the practice's wellbeing by defending against fraud. Don't let your practice be the next victim. Review the following checklist to see if your practice is protected.

✓ Maintain a written policy that provides clarity to each employee in regard to time off work. Include:
  • Definitions of full- and part-time employees, with (1) number of vacation days or hours, (2) number of sick/personal days or hours, and (3) amount of maternity/paternity leave and nonpaid time off.
  • When earned, whether paid time off expires if not used.
  • Paid time-off tracking for each employee. One form of employee theft is using paid time off an employee doesn't have. Periodically review the time-off tracking sheet to ensure its accuracy.

✓ Segregate the duties for updating personnel data from the duties for payroll data accumulation, recording, and reporting. If one person holds all payroll duties, that individual can conceivably manipulate payroll to his or her or other employees' benefit. Without proper segregation of payroll duties, fraud is almost too easy.

✓ Require management approval of any changes made to payroll records and/or personnel information. These records contain sensitive information (e.g., wage rates, benefits, and withholdings) and must be up-to-date and accurate for payroll.

✓ Restrict access to payroll and personnel files to only those employees who work on them.

✓ Securely store blank payroll checks and limit access to them.

✓ Consider eliminating paper checks and mandating direct deposit to employee checking accounts. This avoids the risk of check fraud, especially involving payroll checks.

✓ Process new hires and terminated employees in a timely manner.

✓ Keep a record for each employee that lists (1) anniversary date, (2) paid time off available vs. used, (3) nonpaid time off available vs. used, and (4) tardy incidents by minutes, relative to work start time.

✓ Confirm the number and type of hours worked by each employee before preparing payroll. Do this for each payroll period. Supervisors also can confirm hours worked.

✓ The managing partner should review reports of total payroll at every pay period, including:

paid overtime time, paid time off, and variances between paid time compared with scheduled time.

✓ When using an outside company for payroll services, the payroll manager should compare internal payroll records with those of the payroll company so that any discrepancies are caught immediately.

✓ Periodically review payroll transactions for accuracy:
  • Have transactions been recorded in the correct payroll period?
  • Are there any missing transactions?
  • Are all transactions classified correctly?
  • Do transactions match their source documentation (e.g., pay stubs, payroll register reports)?
  • Verify that all paid employees are valid employees.

✓ Payroll checks and direct deposit pay stubs should be distributed by a nonpayroll manager.

✓ Monitor the time clock to ensure employees are not clocking in or out for one another.
  • Install a biometric or key fob clock, or ensure that there is password control of individual punches to practice management software.
  • Verify when clocked hours have occurred. An easy scam for employees that have after-hours access to the facilities is to clock in and out when the practice is not open. Periodic reviews of hours worked compared with scheduled times and practice hours can reveal abuse.

✓ Track employee advances carefully.
  • The easiest way to prevent abuse is for practice policy to prohibit employee advances.
  • If advances are made, be sure to deduct the amount from the check immediately following the advance. Without strong advance tracking, it can be easy for employees to fail, or forget, to pay back any advance.
  • If an advance is substantial (which is not recommended), obtain a written promissory signed by the employee, stipulating the repayment schedule through regular payroll withholding. Consult the practice attorney prior to implementing such withholding and when using promissory notes.

At the end of year, the bookkeeper will summarize total use. If employees who have received a benefit from the personal use do not reimburse the business for the personal use value they owe, the bookkeeper will include the value in the payroll of the particular employees. Like any regular compensation, such as wages, bonuses, or salaries, the personal use value is subject to usual tax withholdings. The bookkeeper may need to give this information to the accountant or outside payroll service, who makes the correct computations for payroll inclusion. Details must also be correctly reported on tax forms.

REVENUE BOOKKEEPING

The bookkeeper verifies daily income reports and reviews computer audit trails of client transactions in the veterinary practice management software. If the practice is not computerized, receipts and income totals are summarized in the daybook or sales journal and added by hand. The bookkeeper also reconciles the daily bank deposit with the day's total income receipts as reported through computer or manual records.

Sometimes the bookkeeper may be responsible for preparing the daily deposit and making the deposit. As was explained in Chapter 10, it is best that the person preparing and safeguarding records (the bookkeeper) have no access to or control over the related assets (checks and cash to be deposited). However, if the bookkeeper is performing the deposit function, someone else must be reviewing the practice's records of income receipts and deposit slips to mitigate the possibility of embezzlement. (See Chapter 10.)

Refer to Figure 11.5 for a sample procedure to assist in assessing control systems and making improvements to them when you identify weaknesses.

MAINTAINING ACCOUNTS RECEIVABLE

The bookkeeper may be responsible for maintaining the accounts receivable ledger, including individual client ledger cards (if manual), and aging the accounts, assessing financing and billing charges, and preparing and sending monthly invoices. Other duties may include recording payments (but not being in control of such payments), turning accounts over to a collection agency, and writing off accounts receivable that are uncollectible.

Remember that any overlap between record-keeping, authorization, and asset-custody duties can result in significant internal control weakness. If the bookkeeper opens the mail and handles the checks received in payment of accounts, for example, the practice is setting up a potentially risky situation. The risk can be minimized by putting proper procedures in place and following them. In small practices, owners must take adequate steps to ensure sufficient oversight to mitigate possible problems.

Executing decisions related to client account balances is classed as a duty relating to authority. Thus, uncollectible accounts requiring write-off should always be approved by the practice manager or owner. Owner authorization is also required for issuing credits to client accounts as well as refunds to credit cards or by check.

MAINTAINING ACCOUNTS PAYABLE

The bookkeeper receives a variety of documents regarding bills that must be paid, including purchase orders, shipping documents, vendor invoices, and vendor statements. These documents must be compared and reconciled before checks are prepared or a credit card is used to make payment. Each shipping document or service invoice should be signed or initialed by a responsible party. The person signing is verifying that the materials have been received or the service has been completed and that the price has been checked. Many times, the bookkeeper has ultimate responsibility for comparing purchase orders and service contracts with the final invoice to ensure that the vendor did indeed charge the correct price to the hospital.

The bookkeeper also ensures that the invoice is paid accurately and in a timely manner and that it takes advantage of any available vendor discounts for prompt payment. The bookkeeper prepares checks based on the reconciled documents, giving the unsigned check and supporting documentation to a responsible party for review and signing. Usually, a practice owner is the responsible party. For especially large payments, the practice rules may require two authorizing signatures on the check.

All supporting documentation (reconciled purchase orders, shipping documents, vendor invoices, and vendor statements) should be *canceled* at the time the payment is authorized. In this step, all documents are indelibly marked as paid, so that they do not erroneously go through the billing cycle a second time, resulting in duplicate payment. Payment authorization usually occurs before check payment is prepared, but sometimes an experienced bookkeeper knows which bills should be paid and prepares everything ahead of time so that the authorizing party can review the documents, cancel and initial them, and sign the check at the same time.

Because the bookkeeper prepared the checks for signing, signed checks and remittance information should go to someone else for mailing. This person is responsible for stuffing the envelopes with check payment and remittance information and sealing the envelopes for mailing. By segregating duties of record-keeping and custody of the signed checks, the practice reduces the risk of theft.

MONITORING CHECKING, SAVINGS, AND OTHER BANK ACCOUNTS

The bookkeeper records expenditures, deposits, and other transactions that affect any accounts the veterinary practice has at various financial institutions. In addition, the bookkeeper contemporaneously monitors and verifies account balances.

The best practice controls require statements of account from the practice's bank or other financial institution to be mailed to a practice principal (owner or director), who reviews the statement activity, including canceled checks and electronic financial transactions (such as through the *Automated Clearing House* [ACH]). Alternately, the practice principal can review statement activity and check images online. The practice owner then forwards the statements to the bookkeeper, who reconciles them with the practice's ledgers or computer database.

The practice owner, manager, or other party independent of the bookkeeping function should then review the reconciliation report and *source documents* (checking account statement, merchant credit-card summary statements, cleared checks, deposit slips, and so forth) for correctness and correlation with one another. The reconciliation detail is inspected for the number and dates of stale, uncleared checks, as well as deposits that have not cleared, which should be minimal.

A veterinary business can experience a large number of account transactions in the course of a month, including cash and check deposits, electronic fund deposits from credit-card transactions, payroll checks, tax remittances, vendor payments, nonsufficient fund (NSF) checks received from clients, various bank charges, and transfers between accounts.

The time needed to accurately reconcile the hospital's checking accounts can be extensive unless the bookkeeper has developed an organized and methodically maintained system for posting all of the originating data. Yet, the reconciliation process is an essential component of strong internal control systems and should not be deferred. In fact, managers should expect and receive rapid turnaround of account reconciliation documentation from the bookkeeper within a few days of each month's closing, without exception. Business bookkeeping software programs greatly speed the process and increase bookkeeping accuracy.

MAINTAINING JOURNALS AND LEDGERS

Bookkeepers record varying amounts of the data required to keep a current income journal, a disbursements journal, a payroll journal, a fixed asset journal, and a general ledger. Outsourced services, such as for payroll, and internal electronic management of data, such as client invoicing through practice management software, can greatly facilitate the process. Even so, software linkage of the databases and programs in use can be limited. Timely and accurate financial reports rely on a skilled bookkeeper's ability to bring all of the relevant data sources together into a single ledger of all practice financial activity. Usually, this single ledger will be one of the small off-the-shelf business bookkeeping programs that can be used to combine summarized transaction information into a single forum to generate financial reports

For the subsidiary journal that collects all information relevant to current income, most veterinary practices rely on the practice management software. Relevant data includes records of various client payments and amounts, the dates of daily receipts deposits, and details of any receipts not related to fee income, such as insurance proceeds resulting from claims, pharmaceutical rebates, and amounts received for used equipment that was sold.

Disbursement journal data includes all documentation related to purchase orders, inventory receipt, vendor invoices and monthly statements, authorization of service maintenance contracts, dates of insurance contract coverage, and so forth. Any information that provides supporting evidence for the transactions made through disbursements falls under the bookkeeper's supervision.

Payroll journals require the bookkeeper to track and record employee hours worked, hourly rates, employee agreements, and benefit-program payments. Records of tax payments and timely remittance support the payroll journals. With an outside payroll service, detailed journals are availed through the services database. The bookkeeper will use the payroll company's summary reports to create journal entries in the general journal software program, such as QuickBooks or Peachtree.

The fixed-assets journal tracks all of the practice's equipment, furniture, computers, software, and other long-lived personal property. This journal can be maintained through practice property schedules, sometimes referred to as depreciation schedules. Originating with the first equipment purchase on the first day of business, the fixed-assets journal logs every significant item by date of acquisition, name, cost, and useful life expectancy, which usually is defined and recorded pursuant to federal tax regulations. Fixed assets can be tracked through bookkeeping software such as QuickBooks, through standalone software programs, or even through computerized spreadsheet programs. Since equipment can be in use for many years, it is important to keep detailed lists with accurate identification by name and serial numbers. For internal control purposes, these records can be expunged when items are removed from service and sold or disposed of.

PREPARING FINANCIAL REPORTS

In some cases, a bookkeeper may be assigned the task of preparing various financial reports. In past years, the practice accountant routinely prepared the typical business financial reports requested by the practice owner (the *balance sheet* and *profit and loss statement*, discussed in more detail later). However, many practices now rely on bookkeepers to generate management financial reports internally on an interim basis from the bookkeeping software.

With appropriate levels of skepticism, practice directors must be cautious about relying on internally generated financial summaries. They must make sure they are complete and accurate representations of transaction activity and operational results. In most cases, the accountant prepares financial statements at least annually. Any reports that are relied on by outside parties, such as banks or other creditors, will usually be prepared by the practice's accountant, through prearranged agreement about the level of services the accountant will provide.

Outside creditors will usually dictate the timing and the accounting standards required for report preparation. The details of lender requirements will appear in the fine print of loan documentation. A practice manager should be careful to examine the clauses in a loan called the *loan covenants* and make sure the practice reports its financial activity in accordance with them to maintain good credit standing.

The practice's bookkeeping program should include a detailed and well-organized *chart of accounts* (discussed in more detail later in the chapter.) Revenue, expense, asset, and liability accounts should be appropriately established in accord with a veterinary-specific chart of accounts.

Profit and loss statements, also known as income statements or statements of revenues and expenses, should be prepared in such a way as to provide the most valuable information in a single report. For example, if QuickBooks is used, profit and loss statements can include each expense category as a percentage of gross revenues as well as in the form of a monetary total. Expense-to-revenue ratio information is important for benchmarking, budgeting, and controlling costs. Profit and loss statements can also be generated to show the current period results as well as prior period results for the purpose of comparison. Creating statements using the most current twelve months of trailing revenues and expenses is an excellent protocol for minimizing the effects of seasonally related financial fluctuations in the reports and to track practice trends.

Many bookkeeping programs offer export functions allowing report data to be transferred to Microsoft Excel or another spreadsheet format. Exporting reports to computer spreadsheets allows for manipulation of the numbers, as when a planner might want to calculate the effects of hypothesized management actions. As a general rule for the purposes of oversight, all reports should be printed directly from the bookkeeping program or to a PDF format that prevents modification, which can otherwise readily occur in an active spreadsheet version of the exported data.

INITIATED AND ADVANCING PRACTICE BUDGETS

Bookkeepers commonly use historical financial statements to prepare basic budgets for subsequent financial periods. Especially in the case of operating revenues and expenses, it is a relatively easy exercise to project a future period based on a past one. (Revisit Chapter 3 for an introduction to high-level budget concepts, which evolve from strategic, tactical, and operational planning.)

Successful strategy implementation requires a plan of money expenditures to enable tactical and operational actions. Practice owners and managers need to predict, with some semblance of reality, the likely required outlays for equipment, payroll, supplies, and contracted services, and so will use the bookkeeper to both lay a foundation for budget planning and track practice progress against approved budgets. Programs like QuickBooks put reports at your fingertips so that you can compare current results with budgets you have created or with budgets stored within the program database.

The bookkeeper can establish hypothetical budgets for the entire practice or for small segments of the practice. For example, she could formulate budgets for different segments of support staff, including receptionists, technicians, and employee veterinarians, in order to allow practice directors to explore ways of bringing down costs in areas where staffing expenditures have historically been higher than normal.

Through capital budgets, the bookkeeper can help with resource allocation for promotion, marketing, and information-technology investment that supports new communication opportunities with existing clients and potential new clients.

There are two traditional budgeting models that a bookkeeper may use. These are the "top-down" and "bottom-up" approaches. In the top-down approach, the desired gross income of the practice is projected to the desired target amount. In the bottom-up approach, the desired level of profit is established at the outset. Either method will require management consideration and goals for revenues, expenses, and resulting profits; often, both methods are used together to titrate a final budget.

In the top-down approach, expenses are carried forward at the historically experienced percentage of gross income levels. For example, the most recent income statement may indicate that 20 percent of gross income was expended on the total cost of professional services, including laboratory, drugs and professional supplies, and mortuary costs. For the budget, the total cost of professional services is carried forward to the budget at the same ratio.

Other expenses, such as office supplies, salary costs, and so on, are also projected forward at the historically experienced percentage rate. In the course of management discussions, the budgeting team makes decisions as to whether some percentages were too high or too low in prior periods. Concurrently, the means to increase gross revenues may be considered.

In the top-down approach, a bookkeeper may need to know how to budget remaining profits. If profits are inadequate to achieve goals, the bookkeeper may show a high level of competency in forecasting additional increases in certain areas of professional services through volume and fee-adjustment suggestions. The goal of good budgeting is to obtain the necessary profit to allow adequate return on owner investment and to plan reinvestment in the practice.

In the bottom-up approach, where the management team establishes the desired level of profit at the outset, the bookkeeper uses historical trends to adjust projected cash inflow and outflow to meet the profit objective. During this exercise, the bookkeeper will determine how much profit is needed to retire debt or acquire assets. In planning the budget for the next year, the management team would do well to peg the profit target, understanding that taxes will have to be paid in order to acquire the net dollars needed.

PREPARING TAX RETURNS AND INFORMATION RETURNS

Many basic, relatively uncomplicated tax returns may be prepared by the bookkeeper. Typical returns, beyond those for payroll taxes, include returns for remitting sales tax and use tax (see the end of Chapter 9). Information returns reporting miscellaneous payments to outside parties (Form 1099-MISC) are often prepared by the bookkeeper. The bookkeeper might also prepare the corporate annual report for filing with the state's secretary of state. Personal property and local income tax returns may be relatively uncomplicated, depending on the state in question. Otherwise, these may be prepared by the accountant. In fact, when structuring the practice's engagement with the accounting firm for the year, clearly identify whether the bookkeeper or the accountant will be preparing the various requisite tax returns.

RECORD RETENTION

The job of archiving business records often falls to the practice's bookkeeper. Certain hospital records must be maintained permanently: tax returns, annual statements, general ledgers, books of original entry, and certain personnel data. Other records can be kept for periods ranging from one to ten years. Hospital administration should carefully consider its own requirements and consult with a legal professional when adopting or updating a written retention policy.

BOOKKEEPING SERVICES

The bookkeeper's duties are very sensitive since they involve extensive financial transactions and confidential information. Whenever any one person records data entries, maintains records, and also pays bills and manages Internet-based transactions, the risk of embezzlement and fraud increases substantially.

The bookkeeper should be carefully chosen, screened, and bonded, and his work should be monitored. Revisit the internal control principles discussed in Chapter 10 for system design ideas to minimize the risk of embezzlement. The practice's accounting firm is another excellent resource for internal control assessment and recommendations.

Outside bookkeeping services can undertake many of the duties of an in-house bookkeeper. Check references and research the size and experience of the organization. Some bookkeeping services consist of only one or two people, and with such a small organization, you may have more trouble receiving timely reports and financial information. If something happens to the person who has control of all your records, it may be difficult to regroup and carry on with day-to-day bookkeeping tasks. Make sure that contemporaneous back-up data is readily available to expedite a rapid replacement, if necessary.

Many bookkeeping services are quite efficient, whatever their size, with qualified personnel and up-to-date software and bookkeeping systems. A reputable bookkeeping service stays current with changing due dates, reporting requirements, and deadlines for report filings. The service may file some reports on behalf of the practice or can provide an additional reminder about due dates to reduce or eliminate late or missed filings, which would result in penalty and interest assessments.

Some bookkeeping services offer accounting services as well, but these will be less qualified than the services of a certified public accounting (CPA) firm (see the discussion of accountants that follows). For purposes of internal control, it may be advisable to separate the bookkeeping and accounting functions in any case.

As with many other types of services, with bookkeeping services you get what you pay for. Expect to pay a good fee for competent bookkeeping services. Do not weigh the cost of an outside service and reject it out of hand in favor of juggling the work as best as possible with existing employees. The real cost of in-house bookkeeping can easily run as high as or higher than the cost of a bookkeeping service. When considering in-house costs, factor in a reasonable estimate of the time required, the hourly wage amount, payroll taxes, and employee benefit program costs. All of these expenses can match or exceed the fee arranged through outsourcing, even before you consider the cost of errors or fees from late filings or bill payment.

PAYROLL SERVICES
Payroll outsourcing is the one bookkeeping service that should be most seriously considered by any animal hospital employing ten or more workers. Even for smaller practices with as few as five workers, the cost may be very reasonable compared to all of the hassles of in-house payroll bookkeeping. Payroll services use specialized tax and payroll software along with electronic transfers to efficiently process large numbers of client payrolls.

Two well-known, national payroll services are ADP (Automatic Data Processing) and Paychex. Many other companies may provide payroll services in your particular region. When choosing a company, check on its history through the Internet and through customer references and interviews with the company principals, and ask for proof of insurance and bonding.

A payroll service often handles all of the tax deposit and reporting requirements for the clients it serves. To do this, it will draw trust-fund amounts automatically from the clinic checking account and deposit them into its own account prior to making distribution to the various taxing agencies.

One advantage of having a payroll service is that it can handle the practice's tax deposits and reports. Since the payroll company acts as an attorney-in-fact for the veterinary practice, it signs the returns and electronically transmits them to the agencies. If any late notices or other problems occur with payroll, the service is responsible for rectifying all errors. If you have ever had to answer any kind of tax deficiency notice, you know how time consuming and frustrating it can be. Your payroll company will take over this headache if it handles tax deposits and agency reporting on behalf of your veterinary practice.

Keep in mind that if a payroll company transfers a veterinary hospital's trust-fund moneys to its own account and then fails to submit them, the veterinary clinic is still liable to pay the taxes. It is possible for a payroll company to go bankrupt or for its owners to disappear, leaving your clinic to pay the toll. In such a case, the veterinary hospital in effect has to pay the taxes twice, plus probable penalties and interest. To mitigate this risk, it is possible to engage a payroll company to manage all of the data compilation and reporting functions, while the practice personnel manage trust-fund and employee payment transfers internally. In this situation, the practice manager bears crucial responsibility for ensuring that all funds are submitted to tax-collection agencies and employee depository banks before deadlines. Make sure that you choose a reputable, well-established company before entrusting it to handle your business's payroll trust funds. (See textbox, "Payroll Processing Functions.")

The Hospital Accountant

As previously described, accounting services are distinct and different from bookkeeping functions. Accounting firm services are broad and diverse, much like a full-service veterinary hospital. Accountants are not just "bean counters"; they represent a dynamic profession that provides premier business and financial services. Your practice's accounting firm is a valuable resource in these areas of expertise:

- Accounting system design
- Financial report preparation
- Cost studies
- Budget preparation
- Cash flow projections
- Financial forecasts
- Income tax planning
- Estate tax planning
- Forensic accounting (preventing, detecting, and investigating financial fraud)
- Tax preparation and compliance work (assisting the business in reporting requirements for tax purposes and for outside third parties)
- Assurance services (also known as financial audit services), where the accountant attests to the reasonableness of disclosures, freedom from material misstatement, and adherence to generally accepted accounting principles (GAAPs) in financial statements
- Computer application, control, and security implementation in an increasingly electronic business environment

Payroll Processing Functions

A reputable payroll service is a blessing for veterinary practice managers. A full range of employee payroll services are available, from simple calculation of gross pay based on hours worked to assisting in the administration of employer-sponsored retirement plans such as a 401K. Usually the arrangement is as follows:

- The payroll service maintains basic information on the veterinary practice, including all necessary tax identification numbers and applicable tax rates, such as for state unemployment taxes (which are unique by employer).
- The payroll service maintains basic employee information, including full name, Social Security number, number of dependents, hourly rate or periodic salary amount, any voluntary withholdings, hire dates, termination dates, and dates of raises.
- A schedule is set to establish the frequency of pay dates, the day the pay period will end, the day that pay period information will be transferred to the service by the practice, and the day checks will be distributed to employees.
- Pursuant to this schedule, the practice manager or bookkeeper supplies to the service the number of hours worked by each employee in the pay period, along with any special payments or withholding amounts. Phone, fax, or e-mail may be used to relay the information.
- The service prepares paychecks in accord with the information provided by the practice. It calculates taxes and other withholdings. The paychecks are usually direct drafts to the veterinary hospital's checking or payroll checking account, just as if an internal bookkeeper had prepared them at the practice.
- Many practices have moved to electronic paychecks. Employees review paystubs online and the payroll company orchestrates wireless transfers to individual employee bank accounts.
- If paper checks will be issued, they may or may not be signed by the service. Some practice owners like to sign each check personally. Others will choose to supply a sample signature to the payroll company, which then laser prints the signature on each check issued. Each check can then be stuffed and sealed in an envelope by the payroll service to maintain confidentiality of the payments for distribution. In the current environment, paper checks are discouraged because of rising incidences of

CONTINUES >

check fraud. Payroll checks are especially susceptible, since they may be cashed at a variety of risky locations that could present opportunities for perpetuating a check fraud scheme against a veterinary practice.

- The service's payroll software automatically accumulates total wages and taxes paid to date. Summary reports, which can be as detailed as the practice manager desires, are delivered with the paychecks to the veterinary hospital, or by electronic file transfer. The most basic summary reports the total payroll liability, including sum total net of all paychecks transferred to employee depository accounts and payroll tax deposit amounts.

- The payroll service draws from the hospital checking account the required funds to cover all payroll tax liabilities. A lump sum appears on the clinic checking statement.

- In the event the veterinary hospital director prefers to control the tax deposits, the payroll service produces a report that instructs what amounts to pay, to whom, and by when. The in-house bookkeeper is then responsible for making these tax deposits correctly and on time, generally by electronic fund transfer in accord with jurisdictional rules.

- At the end of each quarter, the payroll service prepares and submits tax reports as required by the IRS and by state and local tax authorities. The designated responsible party from the practice receives copies or a link to the payroll company's secured website for download.

- At the end of the year, the payroll service prepares the Forms W-2 for delivery to all employees who worked during the course of the year. Copies are automatically forwarded to the Social Security Administration, as required. Other year-end tax summary reports are filed with the tax agencies, as needed, such as the "Employer's Annual Federal Unemployment (FUTA) Tax Return," Form 940 (see Figure 11.3 earlier in this chapter).

Many other services can be added to this basic scenario. The cost for providing these services is surprisingly low. Because a large payroll company can process huge volumes of payrolls in a very efficient manner, the service can easily beat the cost of a small bookkeeping service, a practice accountant, or an in-house bookkeeper in handling payroll. For more information about using payroll service providers, check out the IRS website at www.IRS.gov. The website includes a list of payroll companies that have passed certain system testing requirements for transmitters of electronic business returns to the IRS.

- Analysis and interpretation of accounting information as an aid in making business decisions
- Corporate governance services
- A wide variety of other business planning and advisory services

Many practice administrators consider the accountant to be their most respected and trusted business adviser.

ACCOUNTING SERVICES

Generally, a veterinary practice maintains an ongoing contracted business service arrangement (or engagement) with an accounting firm. By agreement, the practice's financial data and bookkeeping records are periodically transmitted to the accounting firm. This agreement is generally formalized in writing by means of an engagement letter.

Monthly transmission of records to an accounting firm used to be quite common. However, as practice bookkeeping systems make better and more extensive use of computer technology, inexpensive software programs, and the Internet, information may be transmitted to the accountant as infrequently as once or twice a year.

With the increasing popularity of "cloud computing," more practices are moving their bookkeeping records to an online platform. An online bookkeeping system can be extremely beneficial. Your CPA can have instant access to the books and reports that the practice saves to the system. Practice owners and managers can have access from their homes and other locations. The efficiency of direct connectivity effectively streamlines the transfer of data and enables real-time feedback and communication to take place.

The accounting firm summarizes the income, expense, and other transactional data in the form of uniform reports in accord with professional standards. The accountants will meet with the practice's management team to discuss their observations and any questions they have about specific transactions and business activity. The extent of this clarification and review depends on the nature of the engagement. The accounting firm then creates financial reports and tax returns, as agreed.

Ideally, the practice's directors will then confer with the accountant to review the reports, discuss their meaning, and formalize plans for upcoming financial periods. Facility expansion, employee hiring, expense control, computer improvement, equipment renewal, addition of new owners, business value, and long-range strategic planning are only some of the areas that might be explored in light of financial data analysis. These are all business advisory services that practice owners and managers heavily rely upon when engaging an accounting firm.

Practice managers can make best use of their practice accountants by conferring with them in advance of executing proposed operational plans and business decisions. For example, your accountant will have valuable insight when reading lease and loan covenants, so consult with your CPA prior to finalizing any additional financing arrangements.

The character of the engagement between the veterinary practice and the accounting firm will depend on the size and staff of the hospital. For example, a hospital with a trained book-keeper and few operational changes may not require the services of an accountant more than annually, while another practice might engage an accounting firm that provides bookkeeping services in addition to accounting and management consultation services. Perhaps the best use of an accountant is to talk with her on a regular basis in order to gain the advantage of having expert knowledge that will help grow the practice and mitigate risk.

WHAT CPA CREDENTIALS MEAN

A CPA should be your first choice when deciding on an accountant. To become a CPA, an accountant not only must have extensive on-the-job experience but must also have passed a comprehensive exam that tests knowledge of accounting and tax principles, auditing standards, and business law and ethics. Continuing education requirements to maintain CPA licensure are more strenuous than in any other profession, and CPAs must comply with a strict code of ethics. Accounting firms that are run and owned by CPAs are the only accounting businesses allowed to include the CPA initials in their names.

Be aware that the term "accountant" is much broader and more generic than the designation of "certified public accountant." The title of accountant might be assumed by a bookkeeper as a misleading self-designation. A person who has graduated from a college accounting program might be called an accountant. Some states allow a public accountant designation (PA), which requires much less training and skill and does not require the rigorous CPA examination. One state (Texas) prohibits the designation "accountant" to be used by anyone other than those who are licensed as CPAs. Certain attorneys versed in tax law may provide tax services, but they are not CPAs unless their credentials show otherwise.

CPAs have a duty to clients, colleagues, and the public to perform services competently, objectively, and with integrity. The American Institute of Certified Public Accountants, state boards of accountancy, the SEC, state societies of CPAs, and other regulatory bodies have established strict standards of conduct for CPAs. The purpose of these codes of professional ethics is to instill public confidence in the service quality provided by the CPA profession (Fess and Warren 1987, 15).

LEVELS OF FINANCIAL STATEMENT PREPARATION

A CPA is licensed to prepare three levels of financial reports with corresponding levels of accountant inspection and work, fairness, and reliability. In each type, the accountant subjects the business data accumulated by management to a different level of analysis. When you examine these reports, it is useful to know which level of analysis was used. From least to most detailed and stringent, these service types are compilations, reviews, and audits.

The last two, reviews and audits, are considered *assurance services*. In assurance services, the CPA attests to the reasonableness of disclosures, the freedom from material misstatement, and the adherence to the applicable generally accepted accounting principles in the financial statements.

Compilation

Financial reports *compiled* by a CPA represent the lowest level of service and are the most typical reports included in veterinary practice engagements with CPA firms. Compilation financial statements are a *nonassurance* service. In producing a compiled report, the CPA assesses and makes adjustments to bookkeeping data and supporting documentation provided by the hospital. For compilation reports, *no level of assurance is provided*.

The CPA is required to make inquiries to determine if the information is satisfactory, but no verification procedures are required. However, if the CPA has reason to suspect the fairness of the financial presentation, he is required to obtain additional information. The revised financial data is summarized in a prescribed format and presented in the form of compiled financial statements, signed by the CPA or CPA firm. A sample compilation report is found in Figure 11.6.

Review

Financial reports reviewed by a CPA are subjected to a higher level of analysis than compiled reports. Privately owned veterinary practices may need CPA review engagements when their principals are involved in significant financial transactions, such as when obtaining funds through large bank loans or Small Business Administration (SBA) loans. In a review engagement, the CPA must complete more comprehensive and stringent financial analysis and tests of various accounts and transactions than occurs in a compilation engagement.

Audit

An *audit* engagement represents the uppermost level of assurance and attestation in financial reporting. Audits require independent review of the accounting records in which the CPA examines the records that support the hospital's financial reports. The CPA conducts and analyzes many more tests of transactions and financial activity than in the other reporting levels and attests to the accuracy of the financial statements. For audited financial statements, the CPA gives an opinion of the fairness and reliability of the financial reports. Audit engagements are usually limited to only the largest veterinary business entities, generally those that are publicly owned and traded.

FIGURE 11.6 ACCOUNTANT'S COMPILATION REPORT

Board of Directors
ABC Veterinary Hospital, Inc.

We have compiled the accompanying statements of assets, liabilities, and equity of ABC Veterinary Hospital, Inc. as of December 31, 20XX and 20XY; the related statements of revenues and expenses, retained earnings, and statements of cash flows for the years then ended; and the accompanying supplementary information contained in Schedules I, II and III, which are presented only for supplementary analysis purposes, in accordance with Statements on Standards for Accounting and Review Services issued by the American Institute of Certified Public Accountants. The financial statements have been prepared on the accounting basis used by the Company for income tax purposes, which is a comprehensive basis of accounting other than generally accepted accounting principles.

A compilation is limited to presenting in the form of financial statements information that is the representation of management. We have not audited or reviewed the accompanying financial statements and supplementary information and, accordingly, do not express an opinion or any other form of assurance on them.

Management has elected to omit substantially all of the disclosures ordinarily included in financial statements. If the omitted disclosures were included in the financial statements, they might influence the user's conclusions about the Company's assets, liabilities, equity, revenues and expenses. Accordingly, these financial statements are not designed for those who are not informed about such matters.

Sincerely,

Accountant name and signature

COMPLIANCE ISSUES

While financial reporting is an important function of CPAs, veterinary practices generally rely most heavily on their CPAs to ensure that they are in compliance with the complex laws and regulations of local, state, and federal government. Engaging an accounting firm to prepare financial statements is very different from using a firm's tax-preparation services, although the underlying accountant work for one type of work product can support completion of the other.

Many of the service offerings CPA firms provide are collectively called *compliance work* and involve taxation issues and taxpayer reporting requirements. Besides interpreting regulations and applying taxpayer facts and circumstances to prepare tax returns and legally required disclosures, a CPA may represent the hospital in the event of a tax agency audit of the veterinary practice. For audits by the IRS, only three kinds of tax professional are allowed to represent a taxpayer: a CPA, an attorney, or an enrolled agent (EA).

An EA is an individual who has demonstrated technical competence in the field of taxation. EAs are licensed, or "enrolled," by the federal government, and they are authorized as "agents," that is, they can appear in place of the taxpayer at IRS proceedings about the taxpayer. An enrolled agent can represent taxpayers before all administrative levels of the IRS.

EAs can advise and prepare tax returns for individuals, sole proprietorships, partnerships, corporations, estates, trusts, and any other entity with tax reporting requirements. Unlike CPAs, EAs are required to demonstrate their competence in matters of taxation to the IRS before they may represent a taxpayer in IRS proceedings. They do not have to show competence in other knowledge areas, such as financial reporting and attestation, auditing, basic business-law concepts, and other information that integrates to form expertise in business advisory services. Like CPAs, EAs are bound by strict ethical and procedural requirements, including regular proof of continuing professional education in federal taxation. Accounting firms often have EAs on staff.

USING AN ACCOUNTANT

Every animal hospital should engage the regular services of a reputable accountant. Although the accounting firm you hire may provide bookkeeping services, you do not want to have the CPAs on staff actually doing the bookkeeping. This would be like having your practice's veterinarians performing technician duties. The licensed accountants should be interested in the success of your practice and possess the professional expertise, business wisdom, and technical competencies to help you keep it in good stead. As you can infer from the description of a CPA's credentials, engaging a good accounting firm will entail financial outlay, which should yield favorable return for the investment made.

A good arrangement is to contract with a bookkeeper or bookkeeping service to post transactions and prepare all journals up to and including the *master ledger*, also called the *general ledger*. The general ledger is the principal ledger that contains all of the financial information summarized in the subsidiary ledgers. It is organized chronologically within each of the applicable accounts listed in the practice's chart of accounts. The bookkeeper-prepared general ledger provides the accounting firm with the information it needs to execute its responsibilities to the veterinary practice.

As a manager, you may be serving as bookkeeper or overseeing the work of a bookkeeper and monitoring for internal control functions as well as marking the financial progress of the practice. The bookkeeping data and information you prepare or oversee is transmitted to the accountant on a periodic basis, usually either monthly, quarterly, semiannually, or annually.

For efficiency's sake, coordinate the bookkeeping and accounting software. If both the bookkeeper and the accountant use the same or compatible programs, data transmission, analysis, tax return preparation, and financial reporting can be expedited. Use your accountant to help coordinate and design the practice's bookkeeping system so that this type of compatibility and efficiency will be possible.

The accountant generally prepares the financial statements as often as they are required by the practice owner, in the agreed format outlined in the annual engagement letter for accounting services. A conference to discuss these financial reports and business plans usually occurs at about the same time. At the end of the fiscal year, the accountant prepares the year-end financial statements and the annual tax reports.

The accountant should be able to assist with tax planning, to offer advice on short- and long-term financial strategies, to provide financial reports, to help prepare loan applications, and to customize the internal control procedures. The accountant's primary, overarching function is to help the hospital obtain financial success.

Do not hesitate to ask the practice accountant for advice. Most definitely consult with the practice accountant before embarking on new business ventures, signing loans, or beginning any significant activity that can be anticipated to have a tax or other financial consequence. It is important to recognize that virtually all business and contract decisions that practice managers and owners consider have some related regulation and tax outcome that are best planned through discussion with the CPA before they are executed. Oftentimes, these same sorts of decisions require the expertise of the practice attorney as well. Generally, the CPA will quickly identify issues of business law that in turn require the attorney's expertise to be applied, in order to keep the practice out of harm's way.

Be prepared to articulate your plans and objectives and to clearly explain your expectations. Prudently consider and integrate the accountant's advice into your business planning and operational directives. Investment in accounting fees is expected to yield improved business operations and profitability, assuming the practice director is farsighted enough to ask for more than income tax return preparation.

THE ACCOUNTANT AS A PROFESSIONAL ADVISER

Consider the practice accountant to be a professional adviser, just as an attorney would be. In searching for any type of professional adviser, it pays to take special care to find the right person. Expect to interview several candidates and do your research in order to find a person or firm you can trust. Realize that the trusted advisory relationship with the accountant and the accounting firm will often be life-long, much like the relationships veterinary hospitals have with their clients and patients.

Look for people whose philosophies and personalities are compatible with those of the practice owners, as this is a significant business relationship in which owners must be fully vested. Before hiring an accountant and the related accounting firm, find out about each candidate's commitment to and interest in serving your hospital. Obtain referrals from at least two of their long-standing clients. Do a web search to learn more about selecting an accountant, and do searches of the firms and accountants you are considering to find reviews and background information.

Match the level of service with the need. For example, you would not expect your bookkeeper to be able to do all the things an accountant would do, or an accountant to advise you on legal matters the way an attorney could. Make sure the person's educational background, knowledge, experience, and interests are right for the role you are seeking for her to fulfill.

Whenever choosing an adviser, remember also to look for someone who seems to be dedicated to service. Beware of someone who seems to have a big ego, for example, since ego can get in the way of good service. Good advisers know the limits of their own abilities and will look out for the client's best interest, even if that means referring you to another service for particular needs you may have that they are not qualified to fill.

Choose an adviser who is busy; a busy professional is in demand for a reason. Professionals who have many clients seeking their time are generally highly competent and engaged in their practices. They are loaded with work because they are excellent at what they do.

Investigate how potential accountants and other advisers structure their fees, maintain their level of competence, and choose their staff. Avoid selecting a firm that is too small. You may find that in the event of the sickness or death of the principal, the small firm will not be able to provide continuous services to your veterinary practice. If choosing a larger firm, determine the accessibility of the partners and key personnel who possess the skills your practice requires. Just as your veterinary clients expect excellent communication skills, so should you expect the same from the professionals your practice uses.

Ability to provide instruction is important. Practice advisers must be willing to teach and guide your practice management team to implement effective and efficient systems, to design and generate useful reports, and to summarize accounting functions. Your goal is to obtain a benefit from their consulting services and to manage risk through their compliance services. Make sure your advisers have a constructive approach to service in which the objective is the profitability of the practice.

Check out each candidate's reputation. Your accountant should have a good reputation with other clients and bankers. To make sure they are in good stead with governmental entities such as the IRS and state boards of accountancy, check licensing credentials online. Licensing and professional standing is of increasing importance in the tax-preparation arena, where swelling regulatory scrutiny of preparers is aided by computer database interconnectivity and information sharing among a wide variety of state and federal agencies.

Your accountant should have an excellent understanding of the veterinary profession, and this should be reflected in continuing professional education credits. Ask candidates how they keep current with the veterinary profession specifically. Do they belong to any associations where veterinary management is discussed? Do they subscribe to periodicals on veterinary management issues?

To provide the greatest possible benefit to the practice, the accountant should also be able to work well with your attorney. The practice's law firm is an important resource for addressing many of the day-to-day questions that arise in the course of veterinary practice management that have answers based in points of law. Typically, the attorney will advise on issues regarding employment law, employment and other contracts, buy/sell agreements, real-estate leasing, business entity structure, and negotiation between parties. But most legal issues affect accounting and tax records, so to provide the greatest possible benefit to the practice, the legal firm should collaborate and work well with the accounting firm the practice has engaged, and vice versa.

Ask what services are available from the accountant's firm. Do not assume that the individual accountant will always think to offer every service you may need. Many accountants make the same mistakes veterinarians do, assuming they know what their clients want and what they do not want. The tendency is to offer only that which they predict is needed, so as not to overwhelm you with costs for services in which you may have no interest. Make sure your accountant appreciates your desire to be aware of new ideas and opportunities.

After a candidate has been selected, make sure you are both in agreement about the types of services to be performed, the responsibilities of each party, the personnel assigned to work with your veterinary practice, and the service schedule. The engagement letter should define the exact nature of the work to be completed, and it should be offered without your specific request.

Finally, remember this rule of thumb: No one can know everything. A person who claims knowledge in all areas is a dangerous commodity. When seeking any type of professional adviser, do not preclude other individuals from providing services to your practice. Keep your eyes open to the variety of professionals who can serve on your practice-management and financial team.

Accounting and Bookkeeping by Computer

Bookkeeping and accounting systems through computer and Internet applications are really the only acceptable methods of financial management for veterinary practices strategically positioned for business continuity. Maintaining accounts and ledgers by hand is tedious. Computers can sort and resort data so rapidly that a practice manager relying on a manual system cannot compete with the manager who has access to operational data in virtually unlimited formats. Software has become very user-friendly over years of development, so that personnel can be trained in its use relatively easily. Besides, new generations of employees are highly computer literate and prefer working in electronic environments.

The accounting software used for recording disbursements and performing bank-account reconciliations is often separate from the customized veterinary software program that manages patient records and client invoicing; however, the more sophisticated veterinary practice management software systems allow for some data linking with accounting packages and software.

Off-the-shelf bookkeeping software programs for small business use will generate the various ledgers and journals required for financial control in a nearly transparent manner. Data accumulates to create accounts payable ledgers, payroll ledgers, bank-account and cash-account ledgers, personal property (fixed asset) ledgers, inventory ledgers, and a general ledger.

Bookkeeping software programs also produce daily, monthly, and yearly analyses of income and expenses to compare with past periods. They can also be used to create required payroll reports and prepare checks for accounts payable and payroll. Most programs allow you to generate financial reports as frequently as they are needed internally.

Depending on the extent of bookkeeper training in posting transactions and updating interim journal adjustments, the reports may be quite adequate for internal management purposes. With several years of closely working with the practice's accounting firm and on-the-job training, the bookkeeper may become quite advanced in maintaining highly reliable financial data and producing reports from small business bookkeeping software. For outside users, such as a bank creditor of the practice, reports prepared by the practice's accountant may be necessary and required contractually.

A computerized accounting system rarely eliminates the need for a hospital bookkeeper. Most veterinary practices today seek to employ a practice bookkeeper with advanced training in computerized bookkeeping. Properly used, computerized systems increase bookkeeper efficiency, making that time more productive. Besides staying abreast of bookkeeping software advances, a bookkeeper should be alert to new applications and use other technology that improves practice record-keeping and archiving systems. Efficiency is gained by desktop scanners, well-organized electronic storage of source documents (rather than in file cabinets), and use of two or three flat-screen video monitors. E-mail communications with vendors, electronic transmission of payments, and document receipt via e-mail represent just a small sampling of the ways that computers are changing how bookkeepers perform their jobs.

A computer will never eliminate the need for an accountant but will give the accountant and the hospital management staff much more information, more frequently and more quickly, for use in management decision-making and planning.

Although computerization generates a more identifiable return on the investment in other areas of hospital operations, such as target marketing, reminder processing, and sales invoice standardization, the use of a computer for accounting and bookkeeping serves an essential purpose in veterinary practice management.

Fundamentals of Accounting

Veterinary professionals find that it is easier to communicate with colleagues or employees who have knowledge of medical terminology and basic scientific principles. The same holds true when discussing financial matters. Here we will introduce some fundamental terms and principles of accounting. If this is new material for you, consider following up with a college course or independent study.

ACCOUNTING TERMINOLOGY

With the advent of personal computers, check-writing software, and accounting and spreadsheet software, a greater level of comprehension and interpretation of financial terminology is needed in any successful veterinary practice. Following is an introduction to some basic accounting terms. (See the Glossary for definitions of other commonly used accounting and financial terms.)

What Is the Chart of Accounts?

The backbone of any accounting system is the *chart of accounts* (COA), an organized listing of all of the income, expense, asset, liability, and equity categories used in a business entity for classifying each and every transaction as it occurs. Usually a numeric code is associated with each account name. The account codes allow for daily financial transactions to be coded accurately and consistently, ultimately resulting in reports and financial statements that provide a clear picture of the practice operations.

A suggested chart of accounts that is specifically configured for veterinary practices of all sizes and financial statuses is available from AAHA. Because of the level of detail included and its specialized nature for the veterinary profession, the *AAHA Chart of Accounts* is flexible enough for use in all practices, regardless of size, bookkeeping competency, or the level of accounting detail desired (see List 2002). Another option is the *Equine Veterinary Practice Chart of Accounts* (see Heinke 2006). Both are designed to accommodate a practice's needs with a minimum of difficulty, while at the same time challenging practice managers to obtain better data for financial decision-making and benchmarking.

These COAs promote consistency and accuracy in that they allow your financial data to be compared from year to year and to be compared with the veterinary industry as a whole. With accurate coding and classification using a customized chart of accounts, practice managers come to understand the unique foundations of financial management in their practices, to have a better image of their hospital's real financial status, and to foresee the ramifications of every business decision.

Another reason for using standardized COAs is that doing so results in bookkeeping records that provide virtually all of the information needed for tax reporting purposes. The level of detail accomplished through consistent and correct coding results in well-segregated expense account coding and tax return detail. Increasing the level of detail and disclosure on tax returns may be one way to decrease the probability of undergoing a tax audit and provides good support of a return in the event it is inspected. Veterinary practice appraisers are familiar with the typical veterinary practice accounts organized in accord with the standard chart of accounts and expected benchmarks related to reported data, an advantage when you are seeking an outside analysis of practice value.

Today's accounting software programs are very flexible and can easily accommodate a customized chart of accounts. Once the chart is created, correct implementation is crucial. The chart of accounts should be used with consistent coding of transactions, financial period over financial period. Attention to detail such as posting dates, vendor names, and amounts are other important factors in enhancing the reliability of reports. A chart of accounts that is handled correctly provides the best basis for planning and making prudent business decisions.

What Is the Cost Principle?

The monetary records of properties and services purchased by a veterinary practice are maintained on the *cost principle*, that is, in terms of cost to acquire them (Fess and Warren 1987, 20). For example, if an ultrasound machine is purchased at a cost of $40,000, then $40,000 is the amount recorded in the general ledger and accounting records.

The vendor might have been asking $55,000. The practice owner might have offered $30,000. The machine might be worth only $20,000 if the practice were immediately to resell it to another practice. One month earlier, another hospital might have bought the exact same machine for $45,000. One year later, the machine might only be worth $10,000 because of obsolescence and wear and tear.

But these additional facts have no bearing on the accounting records because they do not originate from an exchange. The cost, or exchange price, of $40,000 determines the monetary amount used in the practice's accounting records until the equipment is exchanged again. This usually occurs when it is resold to another party or is disposed of. Then the historical cost of $40,000 is removed from the practice books and records.

The determination of costs incurred and revenues earned has been fundamental to accounting. In theory, only the exchange price is concrete and objective enough for accounting purposes. Accounting records should not be revised upward and downward on the basis of offers, appraisals, and opinions, under current professional guidelines.

That said, changes to cost-based accounting might occur in the future. Business globalization has resulted in new accounting rule proposals, embodied in ongoing work by accountants to formulate agreed International Financial Reporting Standards (IFRS).

IFRS are a set of accounting standards developed by the International Accounting Standards Board (IASB) (see AICPA, "IFRS FAQs," n.d.). Accounting standards are different in different countries. The purpose of the standards is to codify preparation of public company financial statements so that they are similar around the world. IFRS use is mandatory in the European Union as well as in some other countries around the world. Convergence between IFRSs and the generally accepted accounting principles (GAAPs) required for U.S. public companies is expected to occur, with implementation in 2015 or later. At present, no near-term effect is expected on private companies, such as veterinary practices. Nevertheless, significant changes on a par with other aspects of business operations today can be anticipated.

What Is a Transaction?

A business *transaction* is the occurrence of an event or condition that must be recorded in the financial records of the practice. A loan obtained to purchase an ultrasound machine, a check remitted in payment for a laboratory invoice, or purchase of heartworm preventive on credit are all examples of business transactions that must be recorded.

What Is an Asset?

Any properties or goods owned by a business enterprise are referred to as *assets*. When an ultrasound machine is purchased with cash, this transaction represents the exchange of one asset for another. Cash (an asset of the veterinary practice) was used to purchase the ultrasound machine (a new asset of the veterinary practice). The owners of a practice manage and invest in business assets that are expected to help the practice grow and achieve improving profitability over time. Business assets are acquired based on their planned use to expand client and patient services, and thus revenues.

What Are Equities?

Total financial claims to the properties or assets of the veterinary practice are referred to as *equities*. If the total net practice assets amount to $500,000, then the total financial claims (equities) in these assets must also amount to $500,000. Properties equal the rights in those properties, so that:

$$Assets = Equities$$

There are two principal types of equities: the rights or claims of creditors to the practice's assets, commonly known as *liabilities*, and the rights or claims of the practice owners, called *owner's equity*. Note that an individual or business organization might have both types of equity interests in a practice's assets. A person could be both an owner of the practice, with ownership rights, and also lend money to the practice and thus be a creditor, with a financial claim to the practice's assets.

SUMMARY OF PRIMARY ACCOUNTING ELEMENTS

The primary elements of accounting for any business entity are as follows:

- *Assets* represent all of the economic resources of the practice that can be expressed in monetary terms, meaning anything the practice owns. Examples of assets are: cash, checking and savings account balances, accounts receivable, notes receivable, inventory, land, building and leasehold improvements, tangible property (office equipment and furniture, medical equipment, computers and software, vehicles, etc.), and nonphysical or intangible property of value (software licenses, franchises, copyrights, patents, goodwill, contract rights, covenants not to compete).
- *Liabilities* are legally enforceable obligations resulting from past transactions that require the practice to pay money, provide goods, or perform services in the future. Liabilities can include accounts payable for drugs and professional supplies, maintenance service, and equipment; notes payable (written promises to pay a defined amount at a future date, such as a bank loan); and accrued liabilities (payroll taxes and wages due for hours worked but not yet paid).
- *Owner's equity* represents the interest or claim of the practice owners in the practice assets. Owner's equity is what the practice owes its owners, according to the practice books: the amounts the owners have invested in the business plus the amount of profits that have been retained in the business and that are owed to the owners, less any amounts that have been withdrawn as dividends or draws. It is very important to understand that the amounts recorded on the practice books may very well not be a good approximation of the market value of certain accounts, because of the cost principle discussed previously.

WHAT IS THE ACCOUNTING EQUATION?

The basic accounting equation shows that assets equal liabilities plus owner's equity:

$$Assets = Liabilities + Owner's\ Equity$$

Liabilities are customarily presented before owner's equity because creditors have preferential rights or claims over owners to the assets.

Rearranging the accounting equation emphasizes the residual claim of owners in the veterinary practice:

$$Assets - Liabilities = Owner's\ Equity$$

The accounting equation is always in balance. That is, whenever a transaction is recorded, it will affect at least two accounts at the same time. For example, if the practice bookkeeper pays an outstanding drug bill for $1,000 with a check, the checking account (an asset) will decrease by $1,000 and the accounts payable account (a liability) will also decrease by $1,000. When the current day's receipts are recorded, revenues and thus profits increase, and so does the checking account. Profits affect owner's equity by increasing it.

Let's say that a financial transaction is not recorded. This can skew the accuracy of information present in the financial statement and records. The transaction may be a barter exchange in which no cash is involved. If the value of this transaction is not recorded, revenues from veterinary operations will be understated and so will the cost of operating the practice. Thus, the accounting equation is an important reminder of the importance of keeping consistent and accurate financial records.

EXPLORING FINANCIAL STATEMENTS

Financial statements are important management tools. When correctly prepared and properly interpreted, they contribute to your understanding of the current financial condition of the practice and help you recognize both problems and opportunities. Not only is it important to understand the names of the various components of the financial statements, but you should also understand how the different parts of the statements relate to one another.

Establishing an in-house accounting system, standardized financial-data collection, and internal controls over assets and records are all critical steps in successful organization and planning. You now understand that a standardized veterinary chart of accounts should be in place as your bookkeeper's guide to classifying expenses and income. Appropriate bookkeeper training, with the help of the practice accountant, ensures consistent classification of financial data from period to period.

The level of financial data available to the veterinary practice manager is unlimited when veterinary practice management software and financial software systems are in use. The astute manager must decide what information is the most critical and appropriate for evaluating the success of the practice. The financial statement should be one of those sources of information.

With a computerized system, financial statements can be easily generated in-house within a matter of hours after bank accounts have closed for the month, and statements used to reconcile for the month. Four distinct types of financial statements are used by businesses. Examples of these financial statements are presented in Figures 11.7 through 11.10. The four types are as follows:

1. *Balance sheet:* Also referred to as the statement of financial condition or the statement of assets, liabilities, and owner's equity, the balance sheet summarizes the total assets, liabilities, and owner's equity at a particular date.

2. *Income statement:* Sometimes called the statement of operations, the profit and loss statement, or the statement of revenues and expenses, the income statement reports values that have accumulated between two points in time. This report measures the performance of the practice by comparing the revenue generated with related expenses incurred for a particular period.

3. *Cash flow statement:* This financial statement summates accumulated inflows and outflows of cash between two points in time, depending on sources and uses of cash. This statement differs from an income statement because not all cash inflow results from revenue collection and not all cash outflow is used for paying operating expenses.

4. *Statement of stockholders' equity:* This statement is similar to the statement of owner's equity, the statement of retained earnings, or the statement of partners' capital, depending on the practice's legal and/or tax entity structure, and reconciles beginning and ending owner equity accounts for a given period. Stockholders' equity is increased by net income, stock issuance, and additional capital contributions and is decreased by net losses and shareholder distributions. This statement is sometimes folded into the income statement or the balance sheet, as part of their presentations.

Figure 11.11 ("Financial Statement Timeline") illustrates the basic information presented in the different financial statements. The balance sheet always reports account balances at a specific date. This can be any date, but the most common for formal reporting is at month's end, quarter's end, or year's end. On any given date the balance sheet is prepared, asset, liability, and owner's equity accounts will all be in balance: assets = liabilities + owner's equity.

The statement of revenues and expenses and the statement of cash flows both present account totals that originate from a specific span of time. Usually these reports are generated on a monthly, quarterly, semiannual, or annual basis. For example, a monthly statement of revenues and expenses reports all of the revenues realized and expenditures incurred during the month. The most useful management tool is to prepare these reports on the basis of the most recent twelve months of activity, sometimes referred to as a *rolling twelve-month total.*

These financial statements are prepared and presented using technical accounting terms and rules that are becoming increasingly complex. From the practical standpoint of cost, most practice bookkeepers, managers, and accountants attempt to prepare financial reports in a way that parallels how results will be reported for income tax purposes. Interpretation of statements may be a formidable challenge to managers who are not familiar with the meaning of basic financial terminology.

No matter how technically correct a financial statement is, the statement is not being used to its full benefit unless it is actually used in making sound practice decisions. When the

FIGURE 11.7A   BALANCE SHEET: ASSETS

ABC VETERINARY HOSPITAL, INC.

Statements of Assets, Liabilities and Equity
Income Tax Basis (Unaudited)
See Accountant's Compilation Report
December 31, 20XY and 20XX

ASSETS

	20XY	20XX
Current Assets		
Cash	$22,954	$22,201
Accounts Receivable	12,369	14,460
Drug and Professional Supply Inventory	62,664	64,568
Note Receivable—Other Short-Term	2,274	–
Prepaid Expenses	10,294	7,380
Total Current Assets	110,555	108,609
Property and Equipment		
Medical Equipment	172,885	163,399
Computer Hardware	54,036	46,489
Office Equipment, Furniture, and Fixtures	44,634	42,589
Leasehold Improvements	298,741	274,822
Total Property and Equipment	570,296	527,299
Less Accumulated Depreciation	(180,707)	(145,036)
Total Property and Equipment (Net)	389,589	382,263
Other Assets		
Computer Software Net of Amortization	11,670	12,180
Workers' Compensation Security Premium	990	990
Total Other Assets	12,660	13,170
Total Assets	$512,804	$504,042

FIGURE 11.7B BALANCE SHEET: LIABILITIES AND EQUITY

ABC VETERINARY HOSPITAL, INC.

Statements of Assets, Liabilities and Equity (Cont.)
Income Tax Basis (Unaudited)
See Accountant's Compilation Report
December 31, 20XY and 20XX

LIABILITIES AND SHAREHOLDER'S EQUITY

	20XY	20XX
Current Liabilities		
Accounts Payable	$52,710	$49,852
Credit Card Payable	10,581	9,854
Accrued Wages	20,172	18,779
Accrued Payroll Taxes	1,873	1,285
Sales and Use Tax Payable	1,495	1,126
Federal Income Taxes Payable	–	–
Current Portion of Notes Payable	25,864	24,514
Total Current Liabilities	112,695	105,410
Long-Term Liabilities		
Long-Term Portion of Notes Payable	120,779	203,323
Total Liabilities	233,474	308,733
Shareholder's Equity		
Common Stock—500 Shares Issued and Outstanding	2,000	2,000
Retained Earnings	277,330	193,310
Difference on Rounding	–	(1)
Total Shareholder's Equity	279,330	195,309
Total Liabilities and Shareholder's Equity	$512,804	$504,042

FIGURE 11.8 INCOME STATEMENT

ABC VETERINARY HOSPITAL, INC.

Statements of Revenues and Expenses
Income Tax Basis (Unaudited)
See Accountant's Compilation Report
For the 12 Months Ended December 31, 20XY and 20XX

	20XY	% OF FEES	20XX	% OF FEES
Total Fees—Schedule 1	$1,529,827	100.00%	$1,485,269	100.00%
Total Cost of Professional Services— Schedule II	(316,924)	−20.72%	(311,702)	−20.99%
Gross Profit	1,212,903	79.28%	1,173,567	79.01%
General and Administrative Costs— Schedule III				
Payroll and Employee Costs	742,845	48.56%	687,236	46.27%
Fee Income Collection Costs	33,086	2.16%	28,888	1.94%
Administrative Costs	74,983	4.90%	67,744	4.56%
Facility and Equipment Costs	176,085	11.51%	169,321	11.40%
Depreciation Costs	36,181	2.37%	26,389	1.78%
Total General and Administrative Costs	1,063,180	69.50%	979,578	65.95%
Excess/(Deficiency) of Revenues from Operations Over/(Under) Expenses Paid	149,723	9.79%	193,989	13.06%
Other Revenues and (Expenses)				
Client Finance Charges	4,068	0.27%	4,004	0.27%
Miscellaneous Income	1,851	0.12%	-	0.00%
Dividend Revenue	126	0.01%	100	0.01%
Interest Expense Other	(1,988)	−0.13%	(390)	−0.03%
Gain/(Loss) on Sale of Assets	(1,497)	−0.10%	-	0.00%
Cash Over/(Short)	52	0.00%	(24)	−0.00%
Total Other Revenues and (Expenses)	2,612	0.17%	3,690	0.25%
Excess/(Deficiency) of Revenues Over/(Under) Expenses Paid before Income Taxes	152,335	9.96%	197,679	13.31%
Provisions for Income Taxes				
Federal Income Tax Provisions	53,315	3.49%	69,188	4.66%
Total Income Taxes	53,315	3.49%	69,188	4.66%
Excess/(Deficiency) of Revenues Over/(Under) Expenses Paid	$99,020	6.47%	$128,491	8.65%

FIGURE 11.9 STATEMENT OF CASH FLOWS

ABC VETERINARY HOSPITAL, INC.

Statements of Cash Flows
Income Tax Basis (Unaudited)
See Accountant's Compilation Report
For the 12 Months Ended December 31, 20XY and 20XX

	20XY	20XX
Cash Flows from Operating Activities		
Excess/(Deficiency) of Revenues Over/(Under) Expenses Paid	$99,020	$128,491
Adjustments to Reconcile Net Income to Net Cash		
Provided by Operating Activities:		
Depreciation	35,671	25,879
Amortization	510	510
(Gain)/Loss on Sale of Assets	1,497	-
(Increase)/Decrease in Accounts Receivable	2,091	(1,879)
(Increase)/Decrease in Inventory	1,904	(2,027)
(Increase)/Decrease in Prepaid Expenses	(2,914)	(1,559)
Increase/ (Decrease) in Accounts Payable	2,858	1,101
Increase/ (Decrease) in Credit Cards Payable	727	(111)
Increase/ (Decrease) in Accrued Wages	1,393	925
Increase/ (Decrease) in Accrued Payroll Taxes	588	199
Increase/ (Decrease) in Sales Taxes Payable	369	112
Increase/ (Decrease) in Federal Income Taxes Payable	-	-
Net Cash Provided by Operating Activities	143,714	151,641
Cash Flows from Investing Activities		
Acquisition of Plant, Property, and Equipment	(44,493)	(58,378)
Net Cash (Used) by Investing Activities	(44,493)	(58,378)
Cash Flows from Financing Activities		
Proceeds from/(Retirement of) Loans	(81,194)	(81,062)
Loans and Advances Received/(Made)	(2,274)	-
Purchase of Treasury Stock	-	-
Dividends Paid	(15,000)	(10,000)
Net Cash (Used) by Financing Activities	(98,468)	(91,062)
Net Increase in Cash and Cash Equivalents	753	2,201
Cash and Cash Equivalents at Beginning of Year	22,201	20,000
Cash and Cash Equivalents at End of Year	$22,954	$22,201

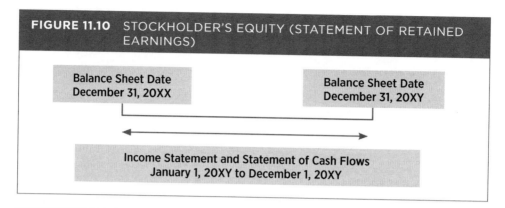

FIGURE 11.10 STOCKHOLDER'S EQUITY (STATEMENT OF RETAINED EARNINGS)

Balance Sheet Date
December 31, 20XX

Balance Sheet Date
December 31, 20XY

Income Statement and Statement of Cash Flows
January 1, 20XY to December 1, 20XY

FIGURE 11.11 FINANCIAL STATEMENT TIMELINE

ABC VETERINARY HOSPITAL, INC.

Statements of Retained Earnings
Income Tax Basis (Unaudited)
See Accountant's Compilation Report
For the 12 Months Ended December 31, 20XY and 20XX

	20XY	20XX
Retained Earnings at Beginning of Year	$193,310	$74,818
Excess/(Deficiency) of Revenues Over/(Under) Expenses Paid	99,020	128,491
Dividends Paid	(15,000)	(10,000)
Difference on Rounding	–	1
Retained Earnings at End of Year	$277,330	$193,310

statements are simply archived without being studied and applied to planning practice goals, managers and owners are missing an opportunity for practice improvement.

ACCOUNTING METHODS: CASH BASIS OR ACCRUAL BASIS?

Another important accounting concept necessary for understanding financial statements is that income and expenses can be reported in two different ways by small, privately owned businesses. The method by which the practice reports income and expenses is usually dictated by how the practice owner has decided to keep the books for federal income tax reporting purposes. The two methods are called *cash-basis* accounting and *accrual-basis* accounting. Here is how these two methods are distinguished:

If *income is measured when cash is received,* and *expenses are measured when cash is spent,* then *the practice is said to be operating on a* cash *basis.*

If *income and expenses are measured when the transactions occur, regardless of physical flow of cash,* then *the practice is said to be operating on an* accrual *basis.*

In the cash basis of accounting, only those fees that have been paid by clients are recognized as revenues for the period in question. When your hospital operates on the cash basis, the balance sheet will not show the level of accounts receivable because they have not yet been paid and, therefore, are not recognized as fee income and not recorded. Likewise, expenses are only recorded when they have been paid.

If your hospital operates on the accrual basis, income is recognized as fees are earned, even when clients have not yet paid their invoices. Fee income that has not yet been collected is recorded as trade accounts receivable. The practice balance sheet will present the total amount of accounts receivable due from clients at the balance-sheet date. The revenue total on the profit and loss statement will include all fees invoiced to clients, regardless of whether they have paid.

In small businesses overall (veterinary or otherwise), the cash basis of accounting is more common than the accrual basis of maintaining records. With cash-based accounting systems, it is somewhat less time consuming and thus less expensive to maintain the books. The time difference from accrual-based bookkeeping is not significantly less, because of the use of computerized bookkeeping systems.

Because cash-basis bookkeeping methods only record revenue when cash is received and only record expenses when cash is paid, this method does not do a particularly good job of matching earned revenues with the expenses incurred to generate those revenues. The comparability of financial statements from one reporting period to the next (e.g., from one month to the next month, or even from one year to the next) will not be as reliable as with the use of accrual-based accounting. Trends will be more difficult to spot and the use of financial statements as a managerial tool can be hampered using the cash method.

Many practice owners prefer the cash basis of accounting because it provides possible tax benefits. Income is deferred as long as it hasn't been received, and expenses are deducted as soon as they are paid, even when they represent the acquisition of supplies, contracted services, and other assets that will not be used until a future financial period in which more patient care occurs. By minimizing revenue and maximizing expenses, taxable profit is reduced. Of course, sooner or later, income will be collected and banked, and the practice will not see the wisdom of accelerating any additional purchases because it is fully stocked. Nevertheless, many business owners try to play out this timing game as long as possible, sometimes without regard to tax rates that may be changing.

Practice managers can implement accounting that has the best of both worlds by using cash-based accounting for tax purposes and accrual-based accounting for managerial purposes. Bookkeeping programs like QuickBooks provide for both reporting options from the same database, contingent on bookkeeper competency. Dual use can occur when the bookkeeper carefully and consistently posts transactions in the correct financial periods using an accurate accrual bookkeeping methodology. This approach also supports better internal control systems, since accrual-based records are complete for all transactions as they occur.

There are other reasons for using the accrual basis rather than the cash basis, especially if merchandise is sold by your hospital. Businesses that provide services (rather than selling products) often use the cash basis of accounting for tax reporting purposes. Veterinary practices generally sell a mix of veterinary services and inventory. For example, sales of dietary products, heartworm preventives, and flea-control products can account for a significant proportion of practice revenues. Veterinary practices are different in this regard compared to other professional businesses like law, accounting, and architecture firms, which do not sell merchandise or maintain inventories.

When the sale of merchandise constitutes an appreciable source of income to a business, the IRS is likely to insist that inventories be accounted for and that the accrual accounting basis be used. In 2005, the IRS updated its *Veterinary Audit Technique Guide* (ATG; see U.S. Dept. of Treasury 2005). The purpose of this second-generation ATG is to guide IRS agents in reviewing veterinary practice activities. The guide discusses merchandise sales by veterinary practices and what constitutes merchandise, inventories, and supplies. It emphasizes that many practices are likely to be deemed ineligible for the cash basis of accounting (for income tax purposes) because of merchandise sales, but they might be eligible for a hybrid methodology. This means that most services can be accounted for on a cash basis, but sales-related merchandise might need to be reported on an accrual basis.

When deciding which method of accounting to use in your animal hospital, discuss these issues with the practice's accountant, since they can be complex. The Internal Revenue Code, or IRC (the U.S. federal tax laws), Section 446, states that "no method of accounting is acceptable unless, in the opinion of the commissioner, it clearly reflects income."

The IRC and the underlying regulations do not themselves define the term "merchandise," but the IRS recognizes that there is a difference between merchandise and supplies, and it relies on how the various courts have defined merchandise. Based on the regulations and the case law, the IRS has determined that "merchandise is property transferred to a customer (including property physically incorporated in that which is transferred to a customer), whereas materials and supplies are property consumed during the production of property or provision of services" (IRS 2005).

The issue becomes confusing because of the difference between the IRS definition of veterinary merchandise and its definition of veterinary supplies. In responding to a request for the definition of inventory and an explanation of the point at which inventory becomes "income producing," the IRS responded, "Items are merchandise if they are transferred to a customer or are physically incorporated in that which is transferred to the customer. Items that are used or consumed during the production of goods or provision of services are materials and supplies. For example, serum is merchandise while the disposable gloves and disposable syringes are materials and supplies." At the same time, the IRS also responded that there is no provision for an exception for "de minimus [sic]" (least, smallest, slightest) amounts of inventory (McCarthy 1998).

As you can see, it is difficult to interpret where merchandise leaves off and supplies pick up. Nearly all veterinary practices dispense pharmaceutical agents at one time or another. Veterinary hospital sales of dietary products, flea-control products, heartworm preventives, antibiotics, and retail items like collars, pet identification tags, and toys are commonplace. Sales of such items definitively constitute merchandise, according to the current IRS view. After ascertaining that your hospital *does have* merchandise, you need to determine whether or not the merchandise is "income producing" to a significant degree. The ATG provides some assistance in determining the issue.

Yet confusion deepens, as years go by and Congress carves out even more exceptions to a complex code and body of regulations. In 2002, Revenue Procedure 2002-28 expanded on a prior exception (Revenue Procedure 2001-10) to provide an exception for businesses with less than $10 million in revenues, on average, from accrual-based accounting and accounting for inventories. What at first glance appears to be simple, however, is not. Ultimately, both of these revenue procedures clarified that the exclusion from accounting for inventories means treating inventory as "materials and supplies that are not incidental." Thus, the cost of such inventory (merchandise) items are deductible only in the year they are used for providing veterinary services and sold to clients, or in the year the practice actually pays for those supplies, *whichever is later*.

It does appear that many practices should evaluate to what extent they have merchandise, whether it is significantly income producing, and how to account for it on tax returns, even when the practice has taken a cash-based position. All of this should be reviewed carefully with your accountant, as should other matters regarding tax preparation. The tax code and its related regulations are constantly changing. Court cases and revised ATG information must also be taken into account. All of these sources should be considered when you are deciding how your hospital will report income on tax returns.

On a positive note, full accrual-based accounting provides better managerial accuracy, as previously discussed. Also, it is less expensive through computerized systems than it was in the past with manual ledgers. For many small animal practices, maintaining all of the books and records and tax reporting on a full accrual methodology may be the simplest and best decision of all.

Be aware that tax laws and regulations are constantly changing. The interpretation and application of the tax laws by the IRS are constantly tested in court. Court decisions affect how a particular law may apply to similar cases.

Your accountant should keep your practice informed of changes that affect how tax reporting is done so that the veterinary business remains in compliance. A particular stance taken in the past may no longer be appropriate today. What is interpreted as correct today may change tomorrow. Pleading ignorance of changes is not a defense in the event of audit or other challenge.

Staying abreast of regulatory changes also saves money. A taxpayer is not obligated to pay more than the minimum legal amount of taxes required. Changes in the law can result in tax savings when they are appropriately applied to the practice's particular situation. A practice that is in compliance also minimizes the risk of penalties and interest for underpayment or late payment of taxes. Since many veterinary practices have federal tax entity structures that result in pass-through of profit and loss to their equity owners, the ramifications of underpayment or overpayment of taxes, penalties, and interest can have very personal ramifications and meaning.

V

MARKETING AND CLIENT RELATIONS

12

The Human–Companion Animal Bond

The human–companion animal bond is the beneficial emotional relationship that forms between a person and an animal companion. The formal definition of this bond is "a continuous, bi-directional relationship between a human and an animal that brings a significant benefit to a central aspect of the lives of each" (Tannenbaum 1989, 125). The relationship is in some sense voluntary. Each party treats the other not just as a living being entitled to respect but also an object of admiration, trust, devotion, or love.

The medical team must understand the human–companion animal bond in order to work and communicate effectively with clients and provide the best possible veterinary care. But the rest of the veterinary team must also understand how this bond works. All team members interact with clients and patients and can help to nurture the bond. Managers must understand the importance of the bond in order to train the team to respect it and support it—and, ultimately, in order to keep clients satisfied and coming back.

Dr. William F. McCulloch, who is known as a pioneer in the study of the relationship between people and their pets, wrote that, "in addition to caring for animal patients, today's veterinarian is responsible, directly or indirectly, for maintaining and improving the physical, mental, and emotional well-being of his or her clients. . . . Society has only recently begun to realize that veterinarians in companion animal practice are more than luxury practitioners serving those who can afford pets. They are increasingly applying their veterinary skills, knowledge, and resources to the protection and improvement of human health" (McCulloch 1985, 423).

When people bring their animal "family" members to the practice, they are placing great trust in the veterinary hospital team. As members of the veterinary profession, hospital team members receive an unmatched reward: the satisfaction of helping people with their beloved companions.

Further, your clients' animal friends cannot talk or complain when they are sick or hurt. Your clients rely on your doctors and team to interpret the signs of disease and recommend both preventive care and medical treatment. Veterinarians and other hospital team members must accept as a responsibility the role that they play in this unique relationship between their clients and their companion animals.

Isn't it an incredible honor and compliment that people seek out your hospital and team to share confidences and their love of animals? Many clients fear that friends, family, and colleagues in their own private lives would not understand how they feel about their animal companions. But they intuitively know the caretakers in a veterinary hospital do understand.

Understanding the Bond

Many studies have shown the human health benefits of owning and living with companion animals.

- Dog walking leads to health benefits, as shown by many studies. A recent one by Cindy Lentino, an exercise scientist at the George Washington University School of Public Health and Health Services in Washington, D.C., measured the general health of 916 middle-aged adults who fell into one of three categories: those who did not own dogs, those who owned dogs but did not walk them, and dog owners who regularly walked their dogs. In her study, regular dog walkers sat less every day, used less tobacco, had more social support, scored lower on body mass index (BMI), and had, overall, fewer chronic conditions and depressive symptoms than non-dog-walking participants (Davis 2010).
- Pets help to lower blood pressure. Several studies have shown that being around dogs, birds, fish, or other animals lowers the blood pressure of people under moderate stress. One of the more recent studies involved a population of individuals with similar characteristics (New York stockbrokers living alone) who suffered from hypertension. Those who adopted a cat or dog registered lower blood pressure readings during stressful situations than those who did not own a pet (Allen et al. 2001).
- Companion animals help people with heart disease. Studies have found more favorable survival rates after heart attack for pet owners as compared to nonowners (Edney 1995).
- Animals help people fight depression. Various studies have shown that interaction with animals delivered a psychological benefit, reducing symptoms of depression. Pet therapy, also known as *animal-assisted therapy*, has been recognized by the National Institute of Mental Health as a type of psychotherapy for treating depression and other mood disorders. Physically being around animals and interacting with them promotes a sense of emotional connectedness and overall wellbeing (Thompson 2011).

The bond that develops between people and their animals is intensely emotional. A survey of pet owners taken by AAHA in 1995 indicated that 55 percent of those surveyed felt like a mom or dad to their pets, and 28 percent felt like a playmate or friend (multiple responses were allowed). In another survey question, 62 percent said that caring for a pet filled a need of parenting (AAHA, "Move Over," 1995). An unpublished 2005 survey conducted by AAHA and Merial found that a critical piece of the bond is the intense sense of responsibility that pet owners feel in caring for their animals. They want their animals to feel taken care of.

A 2011 survey (Milo's Kitchen™ Pet Parent Survey, conducted by Kelton Research, as reported in Goodavage 2011) demonstrated the increasing trend toward people viewing pets as family. The survey said:

- 81 percent of Americans consider their dogs to be equal members of the family
- 77 percent say they talk about dogs as if they were family members
- 71 percent admit they have at least one picture of their pet on their persons to show other people

Truly, the human–companion animal bond is very important; any veterinary hospital that honors and nurtures it will, in turn, create stronger bonds with clients. That process begins at the top, and as practice manager, you set the tone by making it a priority.

Respecting the Bond

Your clients expect more from the veterinary team than excellent medical care and advice. Many people attend veterinary hospitals seeking kind words and empathetic friends in a world that seems increasingly cold and uncaring. In fact, some clients may not even have a significant complaint about their pets but simply enjoy being around other people whom they see as caring, loving, and sharing a common interest.

The human potential for unconditional love of animals is witnessed every day in veterinary hospitals. Contentment, pure joy, anger, and extreme sadness are common extremes of emotion expressed here. Not only do we observe the full spectrum in clients, we see it in our employees and feel it ourselves. This intense, wonderful link between humans and animals makes working in a veterinary hospital simultaneously very rewarding and very demanding. As a manager, you need to recognize the effects this bond has on both the hospital's clients and your team.

As a manager, you must also be aware of another risk that results from the potential intensity of the human–companion animal bond. Veterinary professionals are trained to take care of animals, not people. They should not practice psychology without a license. There is a fine line between empathy and inappropriate advice. Train your team to know when they should wisely, and in the best interest of the animal owner, refer a client to a person competent and licensed to practice psychology or psychiatry.

The "Additional Resources" section at the end of this book includes some selected publications detailing aspects of the human–companion animal bond. Consider adding these and other resources to your hospital's lending library for use by both team members and clients.

ACTIVITIES INFLUENCED BY THE BOND

During normal veterinary hospital activities, a number of circumstances and situations arise in which personnel exercise their understanding of the special relationship between animal and caretaker. Here are a few:

- When giving advice on acquisition of a new pet or companion animal
- When caring for a patient that is in the hospital for treatment or surgery
- During a treatment or handling procedure that might cause pain or fright
- When dealing with animal behavior problems exhibited at the hospital or at home
- When treating conditions and diseases that are potentially contagious to animal owners or family members, or giving advice to owners with family members who are allergic to animals or are immunocompromised
- When advising pet owners who must relocate to places where they are not permitted to take their animals
- When dealing with requests for subsidized-cost or pro-bono veterinary services
- When discussing pet-care needs with young children or in the presence of young children
- When discussing the possible euthanasia of an animal with its owner, whether this is the result of the patient's serious illness or injury or due to financial hardships faced by the owner, behavioral problems in the animal, or other reasons
- When helping a client grieve the death of a companion animal because of an accident, illness, or euthanasia

Anyone who works in the hospital can affect the relationship between any client and companion animal. Each hospital team member can enhance an existing strong bond; nurture a new, tentative bond; or damage an existing relationship irreparably. The client may judge each team-member interaction with the client and animal very critically. Where clients are looking for an especially empathetic, caring veterinary hospital environment, employees who encourage the human–companion animal bond are cherished.

HOW TO SUPPORT THE BOND

Help your team understand the unique bond that people share with their companion animals. Use this understanding to educate, support, and empathize with your clients. Celebrate good times by recognizing pet birthdays, client and pet accomplishments in competitions, or client involvement in animal-related activities such as raising guide- or assistance-dog puppies. Teach your team to help clients through the bad times, too. The sum total of small acts of kindness occurring in your hospital and the generous attitudes of your team will help ensure a rewarding veterinary medical career for your employees and a well-deserved community reputation for caring (Hetts et al. 2004).

There are many ways to help reinforce the bond that are founded in simply taking care of people the way we would want ourselves and our pets to be treated. Develop in your team a habituated perspective about the importance of each client and patient. This perspective says that the client you are dealing with at the moment is the only client in the world, and the most important person in the world, and his companion animal is the most important patient your team will treat. Or, pretend that the animal at hand is your own favorite pet. When you imagine that the client's pet is your own animal "child," it becomes much easier to provide full attention to both client and patient and to give recommendations that meet the standards of care to which the veterinary practice aspires.

Every person on the team must acknowledge the client and patient. Scientific and medical competency is important, but if the connection is not made with the client through rapport with the pet, the scientific and medical competency won't matter. Address both the client and the animal at each fresh interaction. Use eye contact with the client and address the pet in a way that respects its normal boundaries. Be able to read body language and anticipate what you can and cannot do to keep yourself and the animal comfortable relating without looking standoffish to the client. This is a real nuanced art.

Make sure patients are as comfortable as they can be, given that visits can be stressful. Hospitalized patients should be warm, comfortable, and clean. When an animal soils itself or vomits, the team should attend to the patient as quickly as possible.

An extremely important aspect of the bond is that it is reinforced and strengthened by animals with good behavior, and it is strengthened when clients have a good understanding of normal animal behavior. Well-behaved animals are more likely to have long lives in their owners' homes. Animals that have been adopted from shelters may be less likely to be returned to a shelter when the adopting families know what to expect as normal behaviors from their adopted pets. When these new owners have been educated about pets, they can more success-fully integrate a new pet into the family. The veterinary team should be an essential resource in these processes.

Veterinary hospital teams can also help enhance the human-animal bond by embracing and learning to apply concepts of *behavior wellness*. Behavior wellness is more than just the absence of behavior problems, just as good health is more than the absence of a disease. By us-ing behavior wellness concepts and instituting behavior wellness programs in your veterinary practice, you can greatly enhance support of the patient-caregiver-veterinarian bond. (This concept is discussed further below in the section entitled "Extending the Bond.")

Taking these ideas as the bottom line, here are specific ways to strengthen the bond:
- Make the veterinary hospital a behaviorally friendly place for animals and their owners. A veterinary practice that promotes behavioral wellness care and subscribes to the notions

of mental well-being and comfort for their patients must strive to make the hospital itself a behaviorally friendly place.

- The veterinary practice team should apply knowledge of animal behavior to reduce animal stress during visits. This makes visits to the veterinary hospital as pleasant as possible for animals and owners and makes it more likely that owners will bring their pets in for routine wellness and preventive care.

- Encourage behavior wellness, which eases future client and patient interactions. This means taking a real interest in the young patient so as to educate the client about how to improve the odds of having a behaviorally healthy animal that is a great companion. The added benefit is that the animal also becomes a great patient.

- Cats are different from dogs, and your team can enhance the patient-caregiver-veterinarian bond when they learn how to work creatively with the feline species. (A good resource on this issue is the Catalyst Council website at catalystcouncil.org. It describes the cat-friendly practice and showcases techniques that reduce the anxiety that many feline patients experience when visiting the veterinary practice.)

- When handling animals, the veterinary team members should be acutely aware of how they are modeling to owners the practice's philosophy of how pets and companion animals should be treated.

- Behavior wellness enhances a pet's well-being and is based on eliciting and reinforcing desirable behaviors rather than punishing undesirable ones or intimidating a pet into submission. The veterinary team must be educated and trained in how to correctly reinforce wanted behaviors and also in how to pass this knowledge on to clients.

- Make generous use of toys and tidbits whenever possible so that pets will associate pleasant experiences with staff. This reduces their stress and fear about visiting the hospital.

- At the core of a behaviorally friendly practice is a team that can accurately observe and interpret species-specific communication signals and respond in ways that lower animal stress and arousal and promote pet and human safety.

- Establish and adhere to clear guidelines for how animals are handled, using the principles of humane training or guidelines suggested by animal-behavior experts for handling, restraining, and disciplining animals in veterinary hospitals. Additions to these guidelines should include descriptions and examples of alternatives to physical restraint.

- Employees should be trained to identify whether a situation warrants a substantial amount of physical restraint and should know how it can be humanely applied while keeping the animal, the client, and staff safe.

- When difficult-to-handle pets are identified, team members should give owners specific, step-by-step instructions about how to gently and gradually acclimate their pets to handling, mild restraint, and unfamiliar places. Socialization visits to the hospital that only entail food treats and pleasant experiences could be scheduled to help support training and ensure calmer visits in the future.

- Be aware of odors and other hospital conditions that might agitate existing and incoming patients and may be offensive to clients.
- The design of the physical environment is an often overlooked aspect of creating a behaviorally friendly veterinary hospital. Evaluate and enhance reception-area and examination-room aesthetics from the clients' perspective and also from the patient's point of view. Consider what the pet sees and experiences.
- Whenever possible, construction and remodeling should strive to create environments that tend to reduce stress for animals. Separate entrances for dogs and cats in a cubicle layout in the reception area that isolates animals visually can reduce the number of stressful animal interactions that occur.
- Sound-deadening materials that reduce noise, and movement patterns that reduce human traffic in treatment areas, can alleviate stress and fear in animals.
- Towels or sheets can be draped over the front edge of cages of fearful animals to reduce their reactivity.
- Provide timely referrals when owners need expert behavioral counseling. It may not be feasible or desirable for every practice to offer a full range of wellness-care services or behavior-problem resolution services. The practice team must critically assess the client's knowledge, experience, and interest in behavior, and proactively decide when it is in everyone's best interest to refer a patient who needs help.
- Puppy and kitten classes can be a forum to educate owners about animal behavior. Classes can acclimate animals and owners to the veterinary hospital and create fun, interactive experiences that encourage future visits.
- Custom-designed labels for various product lines can include the hospital logo as well as images of client animals. Many software programs now allow patient images to be included as part of the invoice or treatment plan.

Veterinary practice teams want to have clients and patients for life. Consider all of the ways that you can help your clients develop great relationships with adopted pets, especially puppies and kittens. Plenty of resources can help your team structure an ongoing educational environment that helps create a culture of p assion for ever-improving human–companion animal relationships. (For one such resource, see Hetts and Estep 2005.)

HOW THE BOND MIGHT BE DAMAGED

Of course, it is possible for a veterinary hospital team to give correct information to clients or treatment to patients without any consideration of the emotional connection between animal and human. The patients in such a practice may be competently and successfully treated, but to their loving owners, it might seem that team members couldn't care less—about them or their companions. A busy team, possibly suffering from stress or burnout, may miss opportunities to nurture the human–companion animal bond, which in some cases can cause distress to the client and even damage the bond. The relationship between the client and the hospital may be seriously damaged as well, even so damaged that the client seeks services from another provider.

Your team probably cares deeply about both the animal and the client, but keep in mind that this does not matter if the client cannot perceive their concern. Many common daily circumstances can easily lead a client to conclude that the hospital team is less than empathetic. Most often this occurs because of time restrictions—the need to fit as many patient treatments and client visits as possible into a short period of time, leading to a failure to connect because of communication failures.

Do the following scenarios sound familiar?

- A full schedule allows little time for chitchat. The veterinarian and team are hurried, and so they focus only on what is necessary to examine and treat the animals. Little extra time is taken to listen to the client's stories about her companion. The client leaves the hospital believing that the team just doesn't care about her or the animal.

- A hurried doctor doesn't read the record entirely and so calls a cat "it" instead of "he" or "she," or uses the wrong gender entirely. The client looks shocked and says, "Doctor, Tabby is a he, not a she!" To the client, the slip seems to be a sign of carelessness and indifference.

- A busy receptionist doesn't take the time to find out which clients are coming in next. She does not know the names of the clients and pets due for the next appointments of the day, and she looks at them blankly even though one of these clients was in the hospital only a week previously. The client cannot believe that the receptionist still does not know who he is, especially since he just spent such a large sum of money at the clinic so recently.

- An Akita is nervous, and the employees recognize that it might react aggressively during treatment. To keep the pet from hurting itself or others, including the client, they restrain it in a safe but forceful manner in the exam room rather than taking the time to soothe it or to remove it to a separate treatment area. A muzzle is applied while the client watches. These procedures are not adequately explained to the client, who does not see them used every day like the team does, and the client perceives the restraint as abusive and hard-hearted.

- A client overhears a disparaging comment made by a team member about a pet or another client. Although the comment was made in jest to alleviate stress, the client does not understand the context and thinks, "Boy, I wonder what they say about me and my dog?"

- A client brings a stray kitten with a broken leg to the hospital and asks the receptionist if the hospital can just "fix it up" and keep it until it is better. A technician nearing the end of her shift abruptly informs the client, without any explanation, that the kitten cannot be examined without a deposit and release agreement signed by the client. The client, who has brought many pets to the hospital over the years, wonders, "Does Dr. Smith really care about animals?"

All of these examples illustrate that the client cannot know the entire scope of the many stresses and duties your team members face in the course of a day—the constant flow of people and animals, the difficult cases, the emergencies. Clients make judgments solely on the basis of what they hear and see personally. They do not know how full the receptionist's day has been, and they generally do not want to hear excuses.

Clients want to be treated with courtesy, respect, and promptness. They seek reliable and responsive service. They need to see that their four-legged companions are held in caring, professional, and loving regard by veterinary team.

The examples above should spark your thoughts about how policies, procedures, and team training at your practice can promote respect for the human-animal bond and not damage it.

Extending the Bond

The bond that exists between the human and animal also extends to the hospital and its employees. If a healthy bond exists between the hospital team and the client, communication is better and recommendations are more likely to be followed. The patient profits from improved care and is hopefully healthier and better behaved because the team helps the client do a better job as a companion animal owner. Thus, the bond between the animal and the animal's owner is strengthened.

When the client sees how much the team likes the pet, when employees make a big deal about the patient coming to the hospital, and when the animal is treated with patience and kindness, the client learns. The bond between the hospital team and the patient is enhanced, and, by default, the client appreciates both the animal and the hospital team more. Don't you love to hear comments like, "I am always amazed how much Gussy likes to come here!" or "I tell all my friends how much my dog likes the veterinarians here!"?

Each and every team member affects the hospital-client relationship through every interaction with a client or patient. In the veterinary profession, this extended bond is often called the patient-caregiver-veterinarian bond (see Figure 12.1).

Just as each team member can help satisfy the needs of a client and build a stronger relationship between the hospital, patient, and client, each team member can also entirely destroy the relationship. Many times, the relationship simply is not allowed to develop because an employee is insensitive to the feelings of the client, which are built upon the bond between the client and the animal.

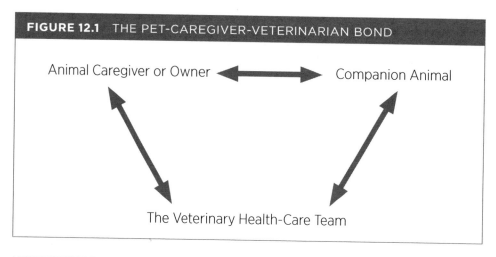

FIGURE 12.1 THE PET-CAREGIVER-VETERINARIAN BOND

Animal Caregiver or Owner ⟷ Companion Animal

The Veterinary Health-Care Team

MONITORING EMPLOYEE ATTITUDES TOWARD PEOPLE AND ANIMALS

We can see how daily hospital routine might easily result in communication breakdown. Every team member has a bad day or a difficult time with a client once in a while. Even people who love working with animals get tired; some days just seem to go on forever, with no break in the number of emergencies or the number of clients seeking undivided attention.

Yet, over the long haul, most veterinarians and team members are able to maintain the excellent bedside manner that results from cherishing the human–companion animal bond. The manner in which individual veterinary professionals and other team members assist clients and treat animals over the course of their veterinary careers will ultimately reflect their own personal beliefs and values. The vast majority of veterinary practice employees started in their careers directly as a result of their own special bond with animals. But this is not universally true in the profession. One veterinarian, for example, might believe that dogs are a disposable commodity and can easily be replaced, and this underlying belief will invade his communications with clients and undermine the trust a dog-lover has in the hospital and in every other team member.

Be aware of your employees' attitudes. Here is another way that being a "walk-around manager" (see Chapter 7) can strengthen your practice. Listen attentively as you monitor conversations between team members and clients. Additionally, open and free discussion celebrating the human–companion animal bond at team meetings and during employee reviews will help build employees' confidence in their own bedside manner. Such training also increases employee awareness of the relationship between client and animal.

Consider ways to honor your employees' bonds with their own animals. For example, throughout the hospital you might display photo portraits of team members with their pets and other companion animals. Employee–companion animal bonds can be celebrated and strengthened in many unique ways, creatively suggested through team brainstorming and ideas from other practices. Facebook is just one example of a venue for sharing favorite images and experiences. Some practices have photo contests or a calendar celebrating the birthdays of employees' pets.

WHEN CLIENT ETHICS CONFLICT WITH PRACTICE ETHICS

Some clients can be extremely demanding or seem to have little respect for animals, even their own. Team members may have a difficult time communicating or working with such clients. Sometimes, ethical considerations and moral values may dictate that the hospital team should not continue to work with such animal owners. And yet, in many situations it may be possible to work with and educate the difficult client. Although the easiest course of action may be to dismiss the difficult client, remember that if the hospital's relationship with the client comes to an end, the animal may lose its best advocate, the veterinary hospital team.

Even so, James F. Wilson, an expert on law and ethics in the veterinary profession, reminds us that veterinary hospitals have no legal duty to see every client who requests care. When team members dislike clients and find their poor treatment of animals impossible to bear, it is best to terminate the relationship. The stress created by the client may not be worth it (Wilson 1988, 356).

Professional veterinary responsibility could even require that your practice report a client to law-enforcement authorities, particularly when the animal shows evidence of abuse. There are excellent materials and guidelines available from different veterinary organizations to help you in responding to suspected animal cruelty, abuse, and neglect (see, for example, AVMA 2010 and AAEP 2009).

When a client is chronically nasty or offensive to team members or when there is evidence that animal abuse may be occurring, you may no longer be able to tip the balance by trying to educate the client. The client has stepped over the line. At this point, discuss the situation with other administrative personnel, the practice owners, and the practice attorney. Determine what documentation needs to be acquired or compiled and how to best proceed with terminating the practice's business relationship with the owner as its client and, in the case of abuse, reporting her to the authorities (see Chapter 7 for more on "firing" clients).

Animal Death and Human Emotion

Perhaps one of the greatest difficulties of working in the veterinary profession is facing animal mortality. Clients whose animal companions die need the support of the veterinary team, because their grief is very real. The team must be trained to understand the grieving process, to engage in active listening, and to communicate empathically with animal owners experiencing grief. As practice manager, it is your role to make sure they get the training they need. This will likely mean organizing extra team training sessions in which you can have team members do role-playing exercises or use other modes of learning.

THE TEAM'S ROLE

The one emotional situation that requires the most team concern and involvement is the death of a companion animal. Whether the death is expected, as with a long illness or advanced age; the result of a humane euthanasia to aid a suffering animal; or abrupt and unexpected, as with poisoning or car accidents, clients will look to the veterinary team for assistance in coping with their grief.

Most often, your practice's veterinarians will be responsible for discussing a patient's serious illness or death with the client. Yet, grieving owners often relate more directly to nonveterinarian team members than to the veterinarians at this time. For some clients, the veterinarian may now be the "bad guy" because the animal was not cured. Anger is a normal phase of the grieving process, and anger can be directed at anyone. The veterinarian becomes an easy target. This is why all team members should understand basic guidelines for delivering bad news to clients and talking empathically with a client who is grieving.

In addition, although nonveterinarian team members usually have no role in the decision-making process, clients often ask them about their own feelings toward euthanasia, seeking validation of their decisions. When a client asks a technician or receptionist, "Am I making the right decision?" or says, "I'm not sure about this choice," the hospital employee must answer very carefully, remembering that the decision has already been made through lengthy discussion and careful consideration by the veterinarian and client. A clear role exists for the team member: to reinforce the client's decision. The employee should assure the client that everything possible has been done for the animal.

If a team member has any personal doubt about the veterinarian's recommendation, that employee should not voice an opinion, either to the client or any other team member. If a team member has questions, those questions should be directed in person and privately to the veterinarian managing the case. Support team members are not usually privy to all of the information that resulted in the euthanasia decision. To suggest to a client that the euthanasia decision is suspect is to invite a malpractice suit. Be very careful.

Whether an animal has died in the hospital or elsewhere, encourage your staff to use good communication skills. This can include methods of consoling clients, handling issues such as client visitation with the body and disposal of the body, writing sympathy letters, and maintaining record management. In Chapter 7, we discussed managing difficult conversations. See "Communicating with Distressed Clients" for information specific to grief communication.

WHY CLIENT SUPPORT IS IMPORTANT

There are good reasons for veterinarians and the veterinary team to be sensitive to a pet owner's emotional needs when a beloved animal must be euthanized. Helping the client resolve the grief of losing a companion animal is an act of kindness that the team can perform for the client. The team members may be the only people with sufficient understanding of the distress the client is feeling to be able to provide this support.

Even other family members may not be experiencing the same emotions and thus may be unable to understand what is happening or how to help. It is common for clients who have been through the bereavement process to later say to the veterinary team, "No one but you understood how dearly I loved that cat."

Some clients are so devastated by the pain of losing a pet that they are reluctant to establish another relationship with an animal. Some former pet owners do not replace lost companions because going through the grieving process was too painful. People who have lost a beloved companion may never own another, unless your team makes the difference.

Skillful delivery of bad news and discussions with clients during critical points of the patient's life can be key to preserving the ongoing bond between the client and the hospital. If you can teach your team how to be supportive to a grieving client, you may be able to increase the probability that the client will adopt a new animal companion.

Even if the client does choose another companion animal, that person may never again attend the veterinary clinic where the patient was euthanized. Many times, owners report that returning to the old veterinary office is too painful a reminder of what happened there.

Increasingly, veterinary practices are incorporating amenities in their buildings that provide a soothing environment at the point a patient's death is imminent and euthanasia will happen. An exam room with comfortable furniture, floor coverings, and indirect lighting that can be lowered can provide a homelike and comforting setting for clients in these situations. In fact, a comfort room like this can be used for private discussions with clients for all sorts of situations, such as the diagnosis of an incurable disease. It can be used during the release of a patient postsurgically or those convalescing from an illness. It can even be used for regular exams of elderly pets.

Another option for a comforting setting is an outdoor walled garden, with a grassy area and seating. In good weather, an outdoor retreat like this is well appreciated by clients for end-of-life rites, including humane euthanasia.

Whatever you and your team can do to improve the likelihood that the client would be willing to engage in another relationship with an animal is important both to the client and to the practice. Certainly, if a grieving client can recall pleasant experiences at the hospital, if he can remember that a bond existed between hospital team, his pet, and himself, then he will be more likely to return with a new animal.

Some clients experience intense anger as part of the grieving process. This is another reason for training your team in client communication. Letting a client leave the hospital with unresolved anger could be hazardous to the reputation of the hospital (Hopkins 1984, 278).

In these days of media frenzy, an unhappy and vindictive client may threaten to go the local newspaper and television reporters. Some may even carry out the threat, expressing their anger to a large audience in the practice's geographic area via the Internet. Such a client tells only one side of the story, and the practice may not even have the chance to defend itself. Litigation can also result from animal deaths, including euthanasia. Good communication and empathetic sensitivity to the client's state of mind can prevent much of the unfortunate aftermath that might otherwise occur subsequent to an animal's death at the veterinary hospital.

COMMUNICATING WITH DISTRESSED CLIENTS

Communication is extremely important at this difficult time, from communicating bad news to offering condolences, but it can also be quite challenging. The good news is that much helpful research exists on this topic. In interviews with experts in the veterinary profession focusing on client communication during patient terminal illness and death, *DVM Newsmagazine* senior editor Lynne Brakeman heard some excellent ideas on communicating bad news skillfully. Included in her synopsis of tips were the following (Brakeman 1998):

Recognize and Cherish the Human–Companion Animal Bond. Every team member is responsible for communication with clients and should respect the special relationship that exists between the client and pet. Clients intuitively pick up on the hospital's belief in the relationship. Clients follow team advice and recommendations because of their trust in the hospital.

Be Realistic. Veterinary health-care providers must guard against being overly optimistic in the face of potentially serious disease or injury. Provide differential diagnoses and relative probabilities of good and bad outcomes. Don't be negative, but don't be overly optimistic or build up client hope unrealistically in a bad situation.

Know the Family Dynamics. Even if only one person is present, others in the family with strong ties to the animal should be included in the decision-making process. Within the medical record, you may wish to identify details about the entire family system, not just the person who is financially responsible.

Deliver Bad News in a Supportive Environment. Avoid using the telephone for this conversation and certainly never use e-mail. If you must use the telephone, think about where the client will be when you call him or her. If it is especially bad news, the client is likely to display some form of grief, so think twice about calling the person at work, where the client may not have the privacy needed to deal with grief and distress. If you can talk to the person directly in the hospital, deliver the news in a quiet, private place. Minimize any barriers to good communication. Laurel Lagoni and Dana Durrance, veterinary grief counselors, suggest a basic framework for communicating with clients in difficult situations. The three-step process includes laying the foundation, conducting the communication, and staying connected through follow-up care. (See textbox, "Three-Step Process for Euthanasia Cases.")

Anticipate Questions. Before you meet with clients, be prepared with answers and treatment options. If you are meeting with the client in the examination room, take a few deep breaths to stay calm and keep your voice modulated and soothing. Have tissues on hand. Brakeman interviewed Dr. Ellen Bogen, who calls the tissue a "symbolic gesture of caring."

Keep paper and pencil handy to write down treatment options and information for the client to refer to later. It is probable that the client will not be able to remember everything you say. You may need to share the information again later with other family members.

Deliver News and Information in Stages. Bad news is best delivered in stages. (See textbox, "Delivering Bad News: A Four-Stage Process.")

Use Proven Communication Techniques. Listen to the clients and validate their feelings. According to Lagoni and Durrance, other communication skills that are helpful in the clinical setting include *normalizing, disclosure, paraphrasing,* and *active listening*. Other team members may become involved and supportive of the veterinarian's recommendations and client's decisions.

Expect Emotion. As Dr. Nan Boss, author of *Educating Clients from A to Z*, commented, be prepared to answer questions, perhaps repetitively. Don't take anger personally, and don't blame yourself. Try to deflect anger by understanding that it is really directed at the disease process that is taking the animal's life. Dr. Kathy Mitchener recommends expressing your own emotion and reminding the client that the hospital employees work with the client as a team to fight the disease or problem. Both the client and the hospital team need to focus on what is best for the animal.

Follow Up. Make sure clients have the information they need before they leave the hospital. If the client must decide among a range of disease treatment options, provide information on each alternative. If the options include euthanasia, then information about the procedure and about the disposal of the body should be provided to the clients so they can discuss preferences with the entire family. Other items that can be given to clients include a list of pet support groups or hotlines available through the various veterinary schools (Brakeman 1998).

Assisting a client with the bereavement process is a very important responsibility for the veterinarians and practice team. After a medical crisis or the loss of a beloved animal, most clients will experience grief. Grief is a normal and healthy process, necessary for healing emotional

Three-Step Process for Euthanasia Cases

The following information may be helpful for any team member who deals with clients before, during, or after euthanasia procedures. As hospital manager, you will need to provide training in this important area.

STEP ONE: LAY THE FOUNDATION

It is important for clients to fully understand the entire process of euthanasia and the protocol that you use. Talk them through the procedure, educating them about what to expect and what drugs you will use. Be very specific and answer any questions they may have.

Encourage clients to stay with their animals during euthanasia procedures. Some clients will want to leave before the euthanasia; many want to stay but might be afraid that they will get emotional in front of you. Reassure clients that it's normal to experience grief and that tears are completely acceptable.

It can be very helpful if you work through the following euthanasia checklist with your clients:

- When and where will it take place?
- How will you take care of your companion's body?
- Consider how you will want to say goodbye to your companion.
- Consider taking a memento of your pet or companion animal.
- How will you take care of yourself in the hours immediately following the euthanasia?

STEP TWO: CONDUCT THE COMMUNICATION

After the pet or companion animal has been euthanized, it is important to let the client cry and hold, touch, and just be with the animal in the presence of its spirit. While uncomfortable, silence is often the most appropriate thing. When you do speak, make sure to continue acknowledging and normalizing the client's grief. Offer the client some private time alone with the pet for a specific time window. For example, "I'm going to step out and let you have a private moment. I will be back in about five minutes to check on you. If you want more time, please just let me know."

STEP THREE: STAY CONNECTED THROUGH FOLLOW-UP CARE

Send a condolence card. Give everyone on the practice team an opportunity to sign it (it should be sent within one week after the animal's death).
Update the client's records.

Schedule a callback if you feel the need. It may also be appropriate to provide outside grief resources and support to your clients after the euthanasia (such as a pet-loss support

CONTINUES >

group, talking to a pet-loss counselor, or visiting a particular website). By educating clients about grief, they will feel more comfortable in seeking out the support that is most helpful to them. You can also create some basic grief materials that describe the normal process of grief and help clients understand what is happening to them.

The most important thing to remember about euthanasia is to realize that while you have been through many of these procedures before, it is often the very first time for the client. Remember the little details that communicate your sensitivity and concern.

Source: Dana Durrance, MA, and Laurel Lagoni, MS, Connecting with Clients: Practical Communication for 10 Common Situations, 2nd ed. (Lakewood, CO: AAHA Press, 2010), 65–67. Used with permission.

Delivering Bad News: A Four-Stage Process

The following information may be helpful for any team member who must deliver bad news to clients about their pets. As hospital manager, you will need to provide training for team members who share this responsibility.

Create a relaxed yet structured environment where you and your client can sit down, touch, and make direct eye contact. Use a soft voice and speak more slowly than usual. Then, deliver bad news in four stages:

- Prepare yourself emotionally for the client's potential responses, keeping in mind that the client may be in shock. Reactions may include sadness, anger, crying, and denial.
- Tell the client that there is bad news that will be difficult to hear. This prepares the client emotionally for what is to come.
- Proceed to offer the client information in brief, step-by-step increments, using clear and concise language. Offer information in slow, deliberate sentences, giving the client the opportunity to process what is being said before continuing to provide information.
- Give the client permission to express himself herself by normalizing his or her feelings and using appropriate self-disclosure. Touch, attend, and paraphrase to deescalate tension and calm the client. Acknowledge your client's emotions, and do not take any comments that he or she makes at this time personally.

Source: Laurel Lagoni, MS, and Dana Durrance, MA, Connecting with Grieving Clients: Supportive Communication for 14 Common Situations, 2nd ed. (Lakewood, CO: AAHA Press, 2011), 34–35. Used with permission.

wounds. By understanding the grieving process, the veterinary team can be more helpful to the bereft client.

In her classic work *On Death and Dying* (1969), Dr. Elisabeth Kübler-Ross described the following stages of the grieving process:

1. Denial and isolation
2. Anger
3. Bargaining
4. Depression
5. Acceptance

Although Kübler-Ross's book was written about the loss of a human loved one, it is generally accepted that owners losing a beloved companion animal will experience most, if not all, of these stages. Each of the stages involves a different emotion, but the stages are not well-defined. Some may be noticed momentarily or not at all. Each blends into the next stage. A grieving person may experience a fluctuation from one emotion to the next and back again. For instance, one might feel anger and then start to cry and then swing back to thoughts of denial ("This can't possibly be happening").

Generally, a person experiencing grief goes through these stages in order, exhibiting different behaviors for which each requires a different response by those assisting and supporting the bereaved person. Veterinary team members are usually much more involved with the client in the early stages of the process, particularly the first three. However, in a lengthy illness where death is the expected outcome, as in cancer and kidney failure cases, the team may have direct contact with the client through all five stages.

Providing the client with information on the grieving process can be helpful. AAHA carries several supportive publications for sharing with clients, including children. So does the AVMA, as well as the American Association of Equine Practitioners (AAEP) for equine patients. These and other helpful resources are listed in the "Additional Resources" section at the end of the book.

Give information to clients early on about the emotions they may experience later. Be supportive and empathetic during their time of need. In most cases, clients deeply appreciate these thoughtful acts.

The Delta Society (www.deltasociety.org) and the Argus Institute at Colorado State University Veterinary Teaching Hospital (www.argusinstitute.colostate.edu) websites include rich resources for animal owners seeking assistance in dealing with pet loss. These sites include helpful information on the decision-making process, resource books, and support guides. The Delta Society website lists telephone hot lines that clients can call to talk about companion animal loss. Most of these are associated with colleges of veterinary medicine and are teamed by veterinary students.

The information contained on these sites and in brochures customized for client use is as helpful to the veterinary team as it is to veterinary clients. Topics include:

- How do I know when it is time?
- What should I do?
- What if the animal is healthy?
- How do I tell my family?
- Will it be painless?
- How can I say goodbye?
- How can I face the loss?
- Should I get another pet?

In cases where the client is experiencing or likely will experience profound grief, recommend that the client seek help from a professional who is trained in grief counseling. Lagoni and Durrance have written a useful practice management resource book entitled *Connecting with Grieving Clients: Supportive Communication for 14 Common Situations*, 2nd ed. (2011, 12). The authors state, "Remember that you are not a psychiatrist, psychologist, social worker, family therapist, member of the clergy, or suicide prevention counselor. Nor do you want to be! These are professional roles that require years of study and experience."

Lagoni and Durrance identified several client support roles that can be provided by veterinary team members, include educating, supporting, facilitating, and providing resource information. They also describe fourteen "common situations" where support of the veterinary team is required. They discuss crises and emergencies, euthanasia decision making, grief responses, and a number of other important issues, such as client viewing of the body, making referrals, and helping children, seniors, and disabled clients with grief.

Team role-playing is a helpful exercise to prepare employees to face discussions about euthanasia and know how to console clients. Employees who interact with clients, especially beginners, should practice dealing with a client who has decided to have a patient euthanized first through role-playing. Experienced team members, especially veterinarians and technicians, can explain to less experienced staff the kinds of suitable responses that can be made. For example: "Mrs. Jones, Tabby is very sick. Every possible treatment has been given to try to help her. You have made the right decision for her. It is a very hard choice for you, but it is the right choice for her sake."

The basis for all these suggestions is the need to understand the unique bond that people share with their companion animals. Use this understanding to educate, support, and empathize with your clients. Keep resource materials on loss and grieving available for your clients. Everything your hospital does to enhance and show appreciation for the human–companion animal bond will help keep clients for life, even as they lose beloved animal friends and find new ones with which to share their life journeys.

Compassion Fatigue

Companion animals will often live their entire lives under the care of a single doctor. Veterinary team members who stay employed at the same hospital will treat many animals from the time they are newborns until they are old, gray, and arthritic. They may know these animals well, and when death comes, they will likely experience it as a personal loss.

Animal death is a very real part of day-to-day animal hospital operations. As a manager, you will need to understand the intense emotional interplay surrounding death, because it affects not only your clients but also you and your employees.

Although the client's emotions are of primary concern during the loss of a companion animal, a patient's death may significantly affect the hospital team. Encourage team members to speak openly with each other about their feelings, whether these are feelings of sympathy for a valued client, self-doubt about treatment decisions, or the helplessness that can arise when veterinarians run out of treatment options and are not able to do anything more for the patient. A wise manager will recognize the signs of stress in the team after an emotional final farewell to a patient. Don't immediately expect a return to "business as usual." It's also important to note that hospital employees can grieve even if they knew the patient only one day or even one hour, because compassion fatigue arises from witnessing critical events repeatedly.

Familiarity with grieving helps hospital team members handle their own emotional discomfort and trauma. Not only do team members become personally attached to patients who die, but they can also become upset when trying to deal with a bereaved client. Once team members are acquainted with the emotional stages of grief, it becomes easier to clearly ascertain what is happening. Knowing what to expect helps ease the trauma of working with upset clients.

Stress of this sort is an inevitable part of practicing veterinary medicine. A workable plan to help veterinarians and team members manage the stress is important. Chapter 5 provides some advice that will help you develop a workable plan for helping your team manage stress, sometimes manifested as what an employee might call "burnout." While burnout "results from stresses that arise from the clinician's interaction in the work environment . . . compassion fatigue evolves specifically from the relationship between the clinician and the patient (Kearney et al 2009). However, some of the tactics that help alleviate burnout will do the same with compassion fatigue.

Be alert to team members who become overly emotionally involved with patients and clients. These individuals may become so burdened by stress whenever an animal requires euthanasia or dies that they cause problems for themselves, other employees, and clients. For instance, an assistant's particularly marked expression of grief may make it very difficult for veterinarians and other employees to assist a client in making a carefully considered decision for euthanasia.

Such individuals may not be suitable employees for an animal hospital, even though their hearts are in the right place. During hiring interviews, be sure to discuss animal death and euthanasia procedures in a limited way and try to gauge the emotional sensitivity of each candidate. Try to avoid hiring individuals who are visibly upset by the idea of animal death.

By understanding the human–companion animal bond and the benefits that it brings to your clients, respecting the bond in the way you manage the practice, and extending the bond so that all team members are building up the patient-caregiver-veterinarian relationships, you will be making a contribution to the lives of clients, patients, and employees alike that is incalculable. You will be making the practice a richly rewarding, deeply satisfying place to visit and to work, and the practice, as a result, will thrive.

13

Marketing Your Veterinary Practice

Ask different people what they think *marketing* is and you will hear a wide variety of definitions. For some, the word evokes television ads for cars or garish newspaper pull-outs and coupons, or even paid advertisements on search-engine results. Some people might describe other forms of *advertising*, particularly attempts to get people to buy things they do not necessarily need.

What these people usually do not realize is that marketing is a much broader term than advertising. Advertising competitively promotes a product or service, typically through paid, public announcements by a business directed to its existing and potential customers. Many doctors are averse to blatant advertising, and, in any case, professional ethical constraints have traditionally prohibited some forms of advertising.

Marketing is something quite different. It is a multifaceted approach to reaching customers and clients. A marketing program may include advertising, but it also includes many other things, such as *public relations*, *publicity*, direct communications, and more.

In veterinary practice, marketing, done well, is all about educating animal owners as to the best ways to keep their pets and other four-legged companions healthy. That education in most cases will help an owner take the veterinarian's guidance and choose the best forms of preventive care.

Most practice managers now realize that increasing clients' knowledge and awareness of appropriate health care is an important aspect of veterinary practice success. As hospital manager, it is essential for you to understand not only what marketing is, but the various aspects of marketing. You will need to be able to plan, organize, direct, and evaluate marketing programs that fit your practice's philosophy of veterinary care and client education.

After defining marketing and marketing concepts, describing the scope and aims of marketing, and outlining marketing techniques and tactics, this chapter provides guidance on how to begin developing and implementing a practice marketing plan.

Marketing Defined

Marketing encompasses all of the activities that you engage in as practice manager to build a *brand*, create awareness of goods and services offered, and fulfill a need. Within marketing, there are many tactics that may be undertaken, including advertising, public relations, *promotion*, sales, a website and other electronic media (for example, pages on social-media sites), and the like. All of these activities build your practice's brand, that is, the overarching concept, image, or perception that people have of the practice.

In the veterinary profession, marketing describes what veterinary hospitals do on a daily basis. Because of the breadth of activities that can help grow a practice, many managers and administrators may not be aware that marketing is a significant effort that integrates seamlessly with many of the daily client communications that already occur.

Veterinary practice marketing has much more to do with educating clients about the availability and scope of services than with announcing cut-rate prices or the deal of the week. Marketing uses knowledge about existing and potential clients to convince them that a particular veterinary hospital is best positioned to ensure their lasting satisfaction with animal health care and related services (Edwards 1983, 35).

In veterinary medicine, successful marketing is geared to education. The goal is to teach people about the personal value of animals. Marketing helps increase awareness of the many ways that clients can help to keep their animal companions healthy. Often, these are things that will involve services provided by the practice that the client needs to know about in order to provide the best possible veterinary care.

The vast array of beneficial animal services provided by veterinarians is relatively unknown to animal owners, who may believe that one visits a veterinary hospital only in case of broken legs, diarrhea, and regulation-mandated rabies inoculations. If you had never worked in a veterinary hospital, it is quite possible that you could not have imagined the level of surgical care provided there. Most people do not realize how important dental cleaning is for their cat or dog, or that nutrition and skin care are areas of veterinary expertise. Nor do they know that pet misbehavior might have a solution through a veterinary hospital, or that older animals can benefit from specialized geriatric care prescribed by a doctor of veterinary medicine. Your marketing program ensures that both the existing client base and potential new clients are familiar with these and other animal-care services and with your hospital as a provider and resource.

Successful marketing depends on a thorough understanding of the market, that is, the clients currently served and the potential clients whom you seek to serve. Understanding existing and potential clients means knowing their needs, wants, and concerns. With this information, a veterinary practice can highlight and showcase where and how it can meet and exceed these needs, wants, and concerns. Furthermore, marketing introduces clients to services they might not have known about before and, therefore, couldn't have wanted. Once clients are educated and understand the benefits, they will want to acquire the services or products. Authors John P. Sheridan and Owen E. McCafferty described this well, explaining that marketing is the task of evaluating the entire veterinary enterprise from the client's point of view (Sheridan and McCafferty 1993, 23).

Brand Management

Perhaps the most important aspect of marketing is the concept of brand and brand management. Throughout this chapter you will learn about a broad array of business marketing concepts that can be applied to the veterinary practice you manage. However there is one important principle that you should remember, and that is to manage your practice's image.

Brand management is a business strategy that started with consumer product marketing in the 1930s (Harvard Business School 2000). In brand management, a team of employees was responsible to work at every level exclusively on the task of distinguishing a specific product sold by a company. The team was tasked to differentiate the product from all the other similar products available to consumers, either through the same company or by competitors.

Product differentiation is a key element of marketing that is applicable to service-based businesses like veterinary practices. Your objective is to differentiate your practice from all the others in your area so that it is easily recognizable to your existing clients as well as to potential ones. Some practices might go so far as to brand-manage their individual service providers (doctors, technicians, groomers, and trainers), and certainly many professionals take special care that their personal "brand image" correlates with the practice with which they are affiliated.

For a doctor of veterinary medicine, a veterinary practice, or any team member, personal or entity reputation is everything. Most people aspire to having a reputation that includes attributes such as being honest, competent, trustworthy, punctual, reliable, courteous, empathetic, and compassionate. Consistently displaying these desirable attributes leads to a solid brand image.

Other attributes might also become part of a person's or a practice's brand image: being cheap or expensive or fairly priced; being well organized and methodical or being disheveled and chaotic; or being plain and durable or high-end and luxurious. You can probably think of many more attributes that might portray brand image. It is also clear that clients may have different ways of perceiving attributes, depending on their own points of reference.

Managing your practice and personal brand means controlling to the extent you can the many perceptions that clients and the community might have. Maintaining reputation should be the first and foremost concern, with physical appearance a close second. If your practice does not yet have a brand image that reflects your core values, refer to the section in Chapter 3 on creating a mission statement and a vision statement and to the section below entitled "Creating a Marketing Plan."

YOUR REPUTATION

The core values discussed in Chapter 3 not only provide a solid foundation for the practice vision or mission statement but also lay the groundwork for expected ethical conduct and goal setting. Stating and living by practice core values is a good starting point for managing the practice reputation, as well as your own, because the practice reputation, ideally, is not just a veneer but a true reflection of the practice and what it stands for.

In his book on ethics, John C. Maxwell wrote, "Companies that are dedicated to doing the right thing, have a written commitment to social responsibility, and act on it consistently are more profitable than those who don't" (Maxwell 2003, 11). Good management requires setting behavioral expectations, being accountable to them, and enforcing them. The leadership capabilities discussed at other points in this book support practice reputation, the first and most important aspect of brand management.

A key aspect of managing professional reputation is to speak directly with and to clients. Doctors often assign team members to make client calls for them, but it is more effective from a relationship standpoint to have many of those conversations personally. On his blog, Dr. Andy Clark stated, "Your Reputation is Your Brand" and then asked, "Who is managing your brand?" Veterinarians work in a world with two outcomes to everything they do: the patient care result and the client perception.

Dialogue happens electronically now, too. Clients are more interconnected than they ever were before. Practices, veterinarians, and managers cannot afford to be unaware of what is being said about them in social-media venues. Being responsive, especially to negative chatter, is an important aspect of brand management.

BRAND MANAGEMENT THROUGH APPEARANCE

After reputation, the image the practice conveys plays an important part in differentiating it from other service providers. Image includes factors such as office decor and overall facility cleanliness, well-landscaped and properly maintained grounds, signs that clearly identify the hospital, and adequate, convenient parking.

As Chapter 3 describes, it is important to decide what message you want to communicate and how you want to be known among your clientele and community. Using the practice vision, determine how your hospital should be designed, decorated, and make people feel in order to accomplish these perception or reputation goals. A logo and all other branding elements should be derived from the brand position, the values the practice represents, what the practice principals want to be known for, and what "space" the practice wants to occupy in the marketplace.

Branding involves creating an image among clients and potential clients so that they see your practice as providing the best and perhaps only solutions to their problems. Brand packaging does not just entail having a logo. Rather, it is an easily identifiable and unified look that becomes linked with the practice reputation and all that the practice stands for.

A key point to remember about managing your practice's brand packaging is to maintain consistency and continuity. Continuity is the strategy and process of coordinating all elements of the practice's overall identity to achieve a consistent, memorable, and overall look and feel for the services it provides (Schakenbach 2007).

Some of the branding or rebranding aspects to consider for a veterinary practice's image continuity include the following:

- *Practice name:* Does it convey an accurate message about what the practice does, and, in applicable circumstances, where it is located?
- *Tagline:* Is it meaningful, concise, actionable, and unique, and does it really say what the practice is and aspires to be?
- *Logo:* Is it up-to-date, unique, and cleanly rendered? Is it memorable? Can it stand the test of time, or is it trendy? Does it accurately reflect the "personality" of the practice? Is it easy to read, and different from others in the same market space?
- *Colors:* Are they consistently reflected throughout the practice's image, including sign, logo, uniforms, facility décor, printed materials, website, ambulatory vehicles, and so forth?
- *Typeface or font:* Are two or three selected and used exclusively everywhere, without exception?

Managing the practice brand through reputation and outward appearances is the foundation of a good marketing strategy. Yet one element is perishable and the other is not. Outward image or packaging can always be completely overhauled when it becomes dated. Reputation is to be guarded pugnaciously as a precious asset. Once lost, it can be very difficult to recover. Again, the brand image should be rooted in the mission and vision statements of the practice (see section below called "Creating a Marketing Plan").

Scope and Aims of Marketing

Seen in its essential elements, marketing involves communications between the marketer (the veterinary practice) and the target audience (the clients and potential clients). This communication should motivate the target audience to seek out and learn more about the services being offered and lead to sales. If the marketer cannot communicate effectively or fails to show the benefits of the services offered, the prospect will quickly get bored and may seek the service elsewhere.

With instantaneous information abounding via smartphones, consumers are demanding and quick to make decisions. Competition for the client's attention and spending money is often steep. A veterinarian's competition often isn't even other veterinarians. It is the other businesses vying for the limited number of dollars the consumer has to spend.

Veterinary clients are typical modern consumers. What are their concerns? Quality, cost, service, reliability, and convenience (Sheridan and McCafferty 1993, 23). Your practice must keep each concern in mind while devising ways of conveying to discerning consumers how you can meet their needs. Client perception is all-important in marketing. Recall, for example, how clients form first impressions (see Chapter 7). These impressions are based on employee phone presence, appearance of the reception area and the receptionist's manner and appearance.

The current veterinary market is consumer driven. Pet and animal owners demand more and more quality veterinary services, efficiently provided at a reasonable cost. The consumer desires good value but may not understand all the factors that lead to good value or the how much it costs the veterinary hospital to make valuable services available for purchase. The practice takes ultimate responsibility for promoting its professional competency, state-of-the-art care, and professional standards so that consumers accept the services and prices as a good value.

Successful practice marketing depends on many little things done right (see textbox, "Marketing: A Multifaceted Approach"). Attracting and retaining clients through marketing spans such a broad range of activities that a practice manager's skills are required to plan the marketing approach and to organize and direct the marketing plan detail. You must also constantly reevaluate and adapt the plan in accord with your observations about which activities give a good return for the investment in time and money.

Often, practice administrators and managers are unaware of the things they do to market their veterinary practices. They may already be promoting practice attributes and performing actions that present an image to the public. However, unless these activities are consciously planned and coordinated, they will not be as effective as they could be, and they could even work in opposition to practice goals. As practice manager, you must design a marketing program in which all of the components of marketing complement each other.

An important concept in marketing veterinary services is realizing that veterinary medicine is a personal service business. The primary goal of most people who have embarked on careers in the veterinary profession is altruistic—working with and helping animals. A surprising revelation occurs in the career education process. Veterinary practice teams do administer medical and surgical services to animals, but only after obtaining the agreement

Marketing: A Multifaceted Approach

Marketing is broad in scope. As the following list of marketing activities shows, marketing is anything that has an impact on the client's impression of the hospital and staff, including many activities that are part of day-to-day hospital operations as well as intentional advertising and promotion efforts:

- Establishing courteous and reliable client relations
- Asking for and listening to clients' opinions and making changes in response to them
- Maintaining a clean, well-lit hospital appearance
- Having a clean, professional, consistent look for printed material and online design
- Offering a convenient practice location
- Providing full-service care
- Sending reminders and making callbacks
- Employing a neat, clean, and well-groomed staff
- Preparing easily deciphered invoices
- Sending digital newsletters
- Sending thank-you notes and condolence cards
- Posting informative articles or hospital updates on your Facebook page
- Providing emergency service
- Giving career talks at high schools
- Providing informational handouts to clients
- Texting clients brief updates about newsworthy issues
- Sponsoring 4-H and dog-show events
- Participating in group advertising about veterinary services

and support of the animals' owners (McCurnin 1988, 116). The goal of working with animals is always attained through concentrated work with and through people.

Marketing is one of the many ways veterinary practice employees can meet their goal of helping animals. The more you can tell animal owners about the amazing care veterinary practices can provide patients, the better the chance to extend the best possible care to the maximum number of animals. Veterinary-practice marketing not only helps people understand how extensive and rewarding the human–companion animal bond is, but also informs and convinces clients that good preventive care from veterinary professionals is an important part of preserving and enhancing that bond.

Marketing Principles

To better plan your practice's marketing strategy, you need grounding in basic marketing concepts, which we will cover in this section. These models include differentiating indirect marketing from direct marketing and distinguishing internal marketing from external marketing.

We will describe a classic model for describing the marketing mix called the "four Ps" and what they mean to veterinary practice managers. The four Ps represent the component parts of a business's offerings to the consumer: product, place, price, and promotion. This section concludes with a summary of other marketing terminology with which you should be acquainted, before moving on to a discussion about specific marketing tactics.

INDIRECT AND DIRECT MARKETING EFFORTS

Two broad types of veterinary practice marketing are indirect marketing and direct marketing. Practically every activity or occurrence in an animal hospital has an indirect marketing component. The way the phone is answered, the smell of the reception area, the cleanliness of the animals in hospital cages, the appearance of the building, and the type of sign—all are a part of the image intentionally or unintentionally conveyed by the hospital itself.

Direct marketing is more deliberate than indirect marketing. With direct marketing, the hospital manager strives to introduce animal owners to specific services and recommendations. For instance, a website might detail the variety of services available and describe the doctors on staff. A special e-mail blast describing an effective new treatment for a common malady might be sent to all practice clients having an animal prone to the problem. The practice digital newsletters or Facebook posts might highlight new products, services, equipment, and staff members. A staff veterinarian might speak at local dog clubs and pass out business cards and client brochures. All these are active forms of direct marketing.

EXTERNAL AND INTERNAL MARKETING

Alongside these two broad types of marketing, indirect and direct marketing, there are two other categories: external marketing and internal marketing. Internal marketing concentrates on existing clients and aims to strengthen their bond with the practice and to increase their demand for veterinary services. Sending letters to existing clients about the benefits of twice annual physical exams for older animals is a good example of internal marketing. Maintaining a relationship with your clients through your business's Facebook page is another example.

External marketing introduces the practice to potential clients, people who have never used the hospital's services, and aims to convince them to use the services. Direct mailings to new people in the area, increasing the practice's Google search engine rank through SEO (search engine optimization), a yellow pages ad, or a newspaper advertisement are examples of external marketing.

Both internal and external marketing can use a combination of direct and indirect techniques. New landscaping, a fresh exterior paint job, or a refurbished sign is an indirect form of marketing that could appeal to and reinforce the patronage of existing clients while convincing drive-by pet owners that this might be a good veterinary practice to visit. A practice open house during National Pet Week is an active form of marketing, but if the open house invites the community at large, both internal marketing and external marketing are accomplished.

In all forms of marketing, effectiveness is founded on one key principle: Practice owners and managers provide serious leadership in planning, organizing, directing, evaluating, and adapting marketing efforts. Like so many aspects of practice administration, marketing is not a static event. The one certainty in today's business environment and consumer-based culture is change. If the veterinary practice isn't constantly responding to consumer demands and expectations, its marketing program will be left behind, with little success in maintaining a healthy practice.

THE FOUR PS OF MARKETING

One way to remember classic marketing concepts is with the memory aid called "the Four Ps": product, place, price, and promotion. Although each of these concepts is integrated to some extent with the others in the way it advances practice services, we will discuss each as a segmented management activity.

Product

The primary *product* of any animal hospital is the veterinary services that are offered, accepted, and provided. In marketing terms, services are identifiable activities that provide buyer satisfaction (AVMA 1988).

The secondary product provided by veterinary hospitals is merchandise. Certain specialized or prescription foods have been sold on the recommendation of veterinarians for many years. Pharmaceutical companies later began to market drugs and other products through veterinarians in a much more direct fashion. In the late 1990s, changes in regulations controlling the advertising of prescription drugs allowed companies to allocate huge budgets to advertise their products. Animal owners sought out veterinary hospitals specifically to purchase the products advertised in these ad campaigns.

These same regulations and the rapidly increasing use of the Internet to sell products have led to massive shifts in consumer purchasing patterns in recent years. The perceived convenience of ordering online and the use of direct shipping, as well as competitive prices, have siphoned pharmacy purchases back away from veterinary practice providers. Keeping practice personnel up-to-date on managing client requests for written prescriptions has become a daily obligation if client satisfaction and perception of service value is to be guarded.

One increasingly popular strategy to retain product sales involves private labeling. In this situation, the practice brands certain popular products, such as shampoos, vitamins, and even certain pharmaceuticals, with its name, logo, and other customized labeling features. Franchises have used this strategy for many years, and it is now catching on in veterinary practices as competitive pressure increases from big-box stores and the Internet.

All veterinary services offered should be within the abilities of the doctors and veterinary practice team, and employees must believe in the value of the services offered. Simply adding new services as they come into vogue can be a mistake, unless they have a good foundation in proper medical care and the professional staff is committed to them.

Even if you want to provide certain services that clients request, the hospital staff may have difficulty recommending them if they themselves do not believe in the value of these services. Examples are chiropractic care, acupuncture, or homeopathy. The doctors on your staff may not have an educational background that allows them to believe these services will give patients the same level of care that traditional Western medicine offers. Even though some clients might be looking for these services for their companion animals, your hospital might make a critical tactical error by adding services that the team is not committed to recommending or even trained to provide.

Place

The *place* is the hospital, clinic, mobile unit, or any other location where the veterinary service is provided. For marketing and other purposes, veterinary operations strive for a convenient and visible location, a location that is centrally located to a population base with animals, money, and a desire to purchase veterinary services. Remember what Realtors say about finding a parcel to build a business: "Location, location, location." This axiom holds true for veterinary practices, too. Location is a key factor in successful business growth.

The convenience of your hospital's location is measured, in part, by how close it is to the client's residence or to main areas of shopping or travel. Convenience also refers to relatively easy entrance to and egress from the parking lot and a lack of physical barricades and obstructions. Making sure the building is accessible to the physically handicapped is another aspect of convenience—one that, in many cases, is required by law.

The physical plant should also market itself through cleanliness and attractiveness, both inside and out. Lack of bad odors is as important as clean floors. You need sufficient equipment, enough exam rooms, and plenty of space. A well-marketed hospital includes staff members who are clean, neat, and personable and who create a climate that the client will want to visit again.

Here's an easy exercise you can perform to evaluate your "place": Mark one reminder on your calendar for each quarter. On the assigned day, take a fresh look at all aspects of your hospital's location and appearance. Carry a digital camera. You will be amazed at what a static image reveals. You may well notice things in the resulting photographs that you did not notice in a personal inspection. Make this kind of physical review a formal event. Note specific maintenance items and improvements that should be addressed. If you do not plan these reviews, easily resolved appearance problems can be all too readily delayed or simply ignored.

Ask yourself, if you were an animal owner driving by for the first time, would you consider visiting your hospital with your companion animal to seek veterinary services? If not, why not? What specific actions could the practice team take to improve the appearance of the hospital and gain attention? Changing the location or the size of the parking lot might be out of the question, but certainly many other proactive changes could be made to enhance the chances of new client acquisition.

If you do not think you can see the practice from a fresh perspective, ask a trusted relative or close friend to help and to give you honest feedback. Have this person visit the practice without you and ask the front-desk staff questions about the services provided. As in so many other crucial matters, it is worth getting a "second opinion."

Price

In a professional service business, *price* should not be as important an issue as it would be if your business were selling furniture or appliances. Even so, price can be factor in areas where clients can choose from a large selection of veterinarians. Clients may be selective about the price of services that are perceived to be either optional or deferrable.

The price that an animal hospital can charge for its services will depend on several factors. Consider how much clients know about proposed services and the hospital. Be aware of the competition in the area for a particular service. Think about the nature of the service being offered: Is it a service that is routinely requested and readily available? For example, a client may be more sensitive to the price of a relatively routine procedure, such as a vaccination, than to the cost of a complex laboratory test.

Services and products that are commonly asked for by name (e.g., pet sterilization procedures, vaccinations, flea-control products) are referred to as "shopped" items. Clients are more likely to compare the fee of one provider's shopped service with another provider's.

Nonshopped services and items are usually related to treatment of medical conditions, nonelective surgical procedures, and diagnostic workups. Clients who already have a relationship with the hospital and the doctor will return there for these services. Although estimates are usually provided, the client will usually not comparison shop the recommended procedures with other veterinary practices, since a level of trust has already been built.

Nonshopped services are viewed as requiring a higher level of expertise and knowledge, whereas shopped services are viewed as more of a commodity that any provider can deliver with the same quality and outcome. Price becomes a more significant decision factor when purchasing a commodity.

Other important factors affect the price charged: the reputation of the hospital and the veterinarians, the quality of the service, and the personal attention given to the client. Many of these factors take years to develop. Reputation is not built overnight, but what took years to acquire can be ruined very quickly, if employees don't abide by the rules. To protect the hospital's ability to charge a fair fee for high-quality medical care and surgical services, carefully guard the reputation of the hospital.

Promotion

You are blessed with a wide array of options for promoting veterinary services. The goals of promotion are to convince your target market of the benefits of your hospital's services, to differentiate the practice from others, and to build a positive practice image. You want to keep the products and services in the minds of the customers in order to stimulate demand.

Promotion involves ongoing advertising and publicity as well as special efforts, such as giveaways at targeted events. The veterinary practice's philosophy about the level of veterinary care it will deliver and about the way clients are informed of potential options will decide which promotional plans will be developed, organized, and directed. Specific promotions can include advertising, public relations, personal selling, and more. The "Marketing Tactics" section below defines these concepts in more depth.

Marketing Tactics

Any veterinary practice has a wide variety of options for maintaining and expanding community awareness of its service offerings. This section describes different vehicles for marketing a practice and the pros and cons of each.

ADVERTISING

Advertising is any paid announcement, especially one that proclaims the qualities or advantages of a product or business so as to increase sales. It is designed primarily to attract new clients to veterinary practice, although it can also inform existing clients about unfamiliar services and new products.

Common conventional advertising media forms include newspapers, magazines, television, radio, direct mail, and the yellow pages. You should be aware of these traditional meth-

Marketing Terminology

Following is a list of marketing terms that you may come across as you read more about marketing in order to develop your practice marketing efforts:

- *Segmentation:* Identification of a specific target group by specific characteristics, such as age, income level, type of animal, or number of pets. It is useful to know how to predict which services the target group might want or what prices they are willing to pay for those services, and to do that you will need to understand the significant characteristics of each group.
- *Target marketing:* An effort to direct promotional efforts toward one or more identifiable segments.
- *Message:* The information you want the prospect to hear, see, or learn.
- *Reach:* The total audience addressed by the message (the target group).
- *Frequency:* The average number of times that the targeted audience is exposed to the message in a given period of time.
- *Media:* The communication channels used to send the message to the potential clients or targeted audience (Engel et al. 1987).

ods, but cutting-edge practices lean toward Internet-based modalities: websites, SEO (search engine optimization), e-mail, social networking, and texting.

When designing a marketing plan, you will weigh choices on the merits of advantages and disadvantages. Because there are so many options, regularly monitor the effectiveness of each method in obtaining your predetermined objectives. You will also need to prioritize the practice's marketing choices in accord with an overall practice budget. When it comes to marketing and advertising, you'll likely find exceeding budget limitations an easy thing to do.

Newspaper Advertising

Newspapers used to be a considered one of the most timely and accessible ways to reach customers, with broad acceptance and wide reach. With newspaper sales dramatically decreasing with the advent of Internet immediacy, smartphone apps, and the like, there may be better ways to attract a potential customer who needs a product or service and is willing to buy it immediately.

Nevertheless, smaller local papers continue to have wide readership because they feature local news stories that may not be covered elsewhere, the results of school athletic competitions, and other family-interest pieces, such as wedding and engagement announcements, graduations, awards, and obituaries. Plenty of clients still enjoy getting and reading newspapers, and local papers still have excellent reach into a practice's potential and existing client base.

Newspaper advertising tends to have several disadvantages: It is readily disposable and can be expensive; newspaper ads are difficult to target to a specific segment; and you may have little control over where your ads are placed in the newspaper, so that your target audience may miss the ad entirely. The advertisements can look dated, since the design may be controlled by the newspaper ad department, but most local papers are very flexible and eager to work with their neighbors, especially small businesses like veterinary practices. Often, the newspaper art department will be very helpful in portraying the brand images practices have worked hard to develop. Remember, keeping your practice's business purchasing local helps to support the economic well-being of the community, and that's good for increasing trust and the amount of veterinary care you can deliver.

Magazine Advertising

Magazines offer superior targeting, have a long life, are well accepted by customers, and are considered by some to be more authoritative than newspapers. The disadvantages to this form of advertising are that magazine ads are expensive and ad placement requires a long lead time. The effectiveness of magazine ads takes a long time to measure. In addition, there may not be a magazine targeted to your local area that would reach prospective clients, unless you are located in a mid-sized or large city. In veterinary medicine, magazine advertising is ideally suited for advertising purchased by groups, such as state and national veterinary associations.

Television Advertising

Although user habits are rapidly changing, television traditionally has had wide appeal, a large reach, and potentially high frequency. It has been considered an effective mass-market advertising format, with 99 percent of all U.S. households having at least one television set (Allbusiness. com 2011). Even if the Internet is rapidly gaining ground, a 2010 study showed that the average adult spent 4.5 hours per day, or 30 hours per week, watching TV (Frederickson 2010).

For small businesses, television advertising is likely cost prohibitive when the full array of advertising options is prioritized. Airtime is very expensive, good commercials are difficult to create, TV offers poor audience segmenting, and influencing consumer behavior usually takes multiple touch points. Television rates can be more affordable in small, local cable markets that can narrow in on your target market, or in off-hour programming time slots, yet the total cost of shooting quality ads that portray a desirable image, and repetitively airing the ads, can still be prohibitive. The bottom line is that veterinary practice managers will probably need to look elsewhere to effectively promote their hospitals in a cost-effective manner.

Radio Advertising

Radio has low cost, easy access, fair segmenting, and high frequency. The disadvantages include audience inattention, as radio broadcasting is often "background noise," and so is tuned out by an audience involved in other activities. Radio ads also have little long-term impact. People may retain relatively low percentages of what they hear unless they perceive it to be important or hear the message many times. Therefore, effectively using radio requires a commitment to regular airing, using consistent messaging that clearly brands the practice. Radio advertising could be useful and more affordable than television advertising for group, association, or institutional advertising.

Yellow Pages

Quickly evaporating as a valued advertising venue, print telephone-directory advertising traditionally ranges from a simple name and number listing to a full-page display ad. These printed book advertisements have limited usage and life today. The immediacy of the Internet provides consumers with much more information about businesses, including powerful testimonials and reviews by others. However, if the demographics of your area indicate that many residents still would look first to the yellow pages (e.g., a high percentage of senior citizens), then the yellow pages are still a valuable place to advertise.

If you do have a yellow pages listing, carefully evaluate your contract and costs each year. Does your contract have an automatic renewal clause? If so, keep the contract renewal date on your management calendar so that you can cancel it, if necessary, in a timely fashion, before a future billing.

To ascertain whether it is worth keeping an ad in the yellow pages, your registration paperwork can include a question about how the new client heard about the practice. When the yellow pages are not being mentioned much, if at all, it may be time to reconsider renewal. (See also section below entitled "Internet Yellow Pages.")

Internet Yellow Pages

As the use of print yellow pages has declined, publishers have created online versions called IYPs, or Internet yellow pages. Most telephone-book publishers are now including IYP listings so as to capture and retain business listings and advertising revenue streams as the transition from print to electronic media rapidly evolves. If you have a print ad in the local yellow pages, you have likely already received an offer of this sort with your annual contract renewal notice. If you have not, this is something to inquire about.

Whether IYP listings are worth the cost compared with those for other ways for clients to find you requires investigation. What is the current status of Internet search results in your geographic area: Specifically, can existing and potential clients find your hospital readily at the top of the results page for any search?

Knowing how most consumers conduct searches is important, too. For example, are consumers going to an IYP site to start their searches (and which one of many IYP options)? Or are they simply using a favorite search engine such as Google, Bing, or Yahoo, and typing in a search request like "vet hospital"? According to various studies, Internet yellow pages still garner only a slim percentage of total Internet searches, with the major search engines being used better than 85 percent of the time. Determining whether IYP advertising makes sense for your practice may require your use of Internet marketing consultants who can provide objective information about consumer usage and preferences.

Ethical Considerations in Advertising

All advertising should comply with the "Principles of Veterinary Medical Ethics" of the American Veterinary Medical Association. Although the U.S. Supreme Court ruled in 1977 that professionals can advertise their services, that ruling was based on the public's right to know and not on the advertiser's right to seek unfair advantage (*Bates v. State Bar of Arizona* 433 U.S. 350). AVMA principles state that "advertising by veterinarians is ethical when there are no false, deceptive, or misleading statements or claims. A false, deceptive, or misleading statement or claim is one which communicates false information or is intended, through a material omission, to leave a false impression" (AVMA 2000, 38). Any animal hospital advertising or contemplating advertising should refer to the AVMA's "Principles of Veterinary Medical Ethics" for more details, and also any rules that are outlined in the state veterinary practice act for the state of practice domicile. (Those in Canada should be aware that the applicable laws and regulations on professional advertising vary from province to province. Research the applicable provincial rules before embarking on an advertising program.)

DIRECT-RESPONSE MARKETING

A textbook definition of *direct-response marketing* is "the use of consumer direct channels to reach and deliver goods and services to customers without using marketing middlemen" (Kotler and Lane 2008, 620). It also "involves sending an offer, announcement, reminder, or other item to a person" (ibid., 622).

Direct Mail

Direct-mail offers are targeted marketing efforts that are geared to client-acquisition goals. They can also be great for promoting a particular service (e.g., "Dental Month"), a new service, or educational efforts (e.g., with a newsletter).

Even so, you can spend quite a bit of money with minimal return: Even good response rates may be only 2 to 4 percent if you are sending mail to a *cold list*, such as potential clients obtained through a purchased mailing list. When direct mailings are sent to current clients, the results should be much better.

There are three basic types of direct mail: postcards, letters, and packages (dimensional mail). Oversized postcards to grab attention may be a good way to alert sales prospects to an upcoming event, but dimensional mail has the highest probability of being read and responded to (5.49 percent, according to the Direct Marketing Association; Gordon 2005).

Direct-mail response rates are readily measurable. If you choose to spend time and money on direct-mail campaigns, try different types of mailings with each effort and keep track of the response rates. Repeat what works, and eliminate whatever does not work. Did you get a good response from a particular mailing list? Did you have a good response when you used a mailing to alert current clients to a special practice offer? What other creative approaches can you try?

Of course, anything done in print can be transitioned to electronic communication, so direct marketing through e-mail may be an alternative to direct mail, if done with the understanding that the readership may be quite a bit different. Some recipients prefer paper and will read and keep a direct-mail offer, but never even see an e-mail version. The opposite may be true for individuals who prefer e-mail. Some clients may follow your comments on Twitter but throw away a piece of direct mail without really looking at it.

Make sure all direct-mail pieces and coupons abide by ethical rules and are professionally acceptable (see also section on "Ethical Considerations in Advertising," below). Before using coupons, also think of the hospital image: Will discount coupons attract the type of clients the hospital wishes to attract and retain? Some clients may perceive coupons negatively as junk mail and, by association, view the hospital in a negative light as well. Direct-mail coupons rely on mailing lists—if you do use them, make sure your database is up to date. Otherwise, you are wasting money on postage.

Patient Care Reminders

One crucial goal of practice management is to make sure each animal receives the ongoing veterinary medical care it needs by reminding the client in a consistently timely fashion of the recommended procedures to be completed. Vaccination and other service reminders have been an integral part of animal hospital procedures for many years. A well-tended reminder system is a proven, essential tool for encouraging repeat client visits and retention, and supporting practice compliance initiatives.

As discussed elsewhere in this book, compliance goals work at closing the gap between the practice's recommended care for any particular species, breed, and preventable or treatable condition and the actual number of patients whose care is in compliance with those recommendation guidelines. Effective reminder systems are an important function supporting compliance goals.

An effective reminder system ensures timely client notification so that clients are aware of necessary care as it comes due. Ideally, the reminders your practice sends are based on a well-planned design of lifelong health-care recommendations. Here are examples of the services and products your practice might include in an effective reminder system:

- Early detection of health problems through annual or biannual physical exams
- Booster vaccinations to prevent various diseases
- Intestinal parasite screens, to evaluate for and treat parasite infestations
- Laboratory tests such as heartworm and leukemia screens
- Dental exams and prophylaxis
- Medical progress exams
- Senior animal medical screens and lab panels
- Weight-management program rechecks
- Therapeutic dietary management and product refills
- Therapeutic-drug organ function screens
- Flea and heartworm preventive product refills

A reminder system can use postcards, letters, magazines, e-mail, phone calls (live and automated), or even text messages. The best practice is to use multiple reminder types, suited to client preference when possible. Regardless of the communication approach, reminders are well-accepted by clients who have come to expect and rely on them for scheduling-required preventive health care. (For example, see the post-visit reminder card in Figure 13.1.) Repeat reminders at set follow-up intervals are necessary to generate as many client returns as possible, since clients do not always answer the first reminder. One estimate is that only 15 to 35 percent of clients will respond to the first vaccination reminder. The second reminder increases overall response to approximately 40 to 65 percent. Third reminders increase compliance to 70 to 85 percent (Remillard 1995, 308).

Traditionally, practices would send reminders once a month for all the patient care coming due the following month, as well as send second or third reminders for clients who had fallen delinquent. The current trend is sending reminders on a continuous basis (weekly). This helps to smooth the workload for reminder preparation as well as for appointment scheduling and handling incoming phone calls or e mail requests for appointments.

Computer databases should be built and continuously reevaluated to maximize automation of reminder generation. This means evaluating every service and product code and the reminders linked to it. Evaluate the messages themselves as well as the timing of the reminders.

FIGURE 13.1 POST-VISIT CARD

How long did you wait in the reception area? _____

Did you consider the waiting time:

❏ Brief ❏ Reasonable ❏ Excessive

Were you treated courteously by all team members?

❏ No ❏ Somewhat ❏ Yes

I saw Dr. _____

Did the doctor listen carefully to all of your concerns?

❏ No ❏ Somewhat ❏ Yes

Was the doctor knowledgeable?

❏ No ❏ Somewhat ❏ Yes

Was the doctor able to explain everything to your satisfaction?

❏ No ❏ Somewhat ❏ Yes

Was the doctor friendly?

❏ No ❏ Somewhat ❏ Yes

Did the doctor spend enough time with you?

❏ No ❏ Somewhat ❏ Yes

Would you recommend this practice to others?

❏ No ❏ Somewhat ❏ Yes

If you answered "No" or "Somewhat" to any question, please tell us how we can improve.

_____

Do you have any other suggestions for improving our practice?

_____

Over time, doctors' ideas about exam frequency may change; make sure the reminder system agrees with what the medical team is telling clients.

Another best practice is to use diagnostic codes with linked reminders. Doctors apply diagnosis codes to the patient records when problems have been diagnosed. The reminders associated with the diagnostic codes cover follow-up services such as progress exams, lab retesting, and therapeutic drug monitoring, including organ function tests.

According to Wendy Myers of Communication Solutions for Veterinarians, the best day to mail reminders via the postal system is Monday, so that clients can contact the practice when it is open and at the midpoint of the week. Appointment schedulers may be less busy at that time than they are the first two days of the week. Send e-mail reminders on Tuesday or Wednesday between 10 a.m. and 3 p.m. for highest readership and effectiveness in appointment generation. Phone calls should be made between 5 and 7 p.m. on weekdays and 9 to 11 a.m. on Saturdays, preferably placed to the client's cell-phone number.

Text messaging is an important means of communicating with clients, especially for reminders. You can remind clients of an appointment, let them know when prescriptions are ready to pick up, or inform them of lab results. An e-mail or text reminder of an appointment should be sent 48 to 72 hours in advance of the appointment time. (See Chapter 2 for more information about e-mail and texting use and etiquette.)

Client retention is improved by repetitive contact. Effective marketing keeps the practice's and doctors' names in the client's mind. The reminder system is one of three classic prongs of client retention. These "3 Rs of client retention" are re-call, reappointment, and reminder. Each client that presents a patient to the hospital should be scheduled for at least one of the three follow-up events so that the hospital automatically contacts each client in the future. With competent use of veterinary practice management software, much of the process should be automated so that the practice is achieving all three contact types for all clients.

A re-call flag on the record results in a follow-up call to see how the animal is doing after the appointment, a surgery, an anesthetic procedure, or any other activity that the practice identifies as important to client feedback. Here is another time that e-mail and texting might be used interchangeably with phone calls, and, of course, with common sense. If the client reports that the patient is having any problems, a new appointment for recheck might be scheduled, or a doctor may be tasked with calling the client to address questions. If the animal is fine, then the caller should make a patient record notation and check the record to assure that all future reminders for routine services, such as vaccine boosters and physical exams, exist as determined by age, breed, and other risk factors for the animal.

BRANDING

Branding was discussed at the beginning of this chapter and is influenced by a company's strategic plan. A key element of branding is product differentiation. A major objective of branding in veterinary medicine is to differentiate your practice from all the other ones in your area so that it is easily recognizable to your existing clients as well as to potential ones.

Hospital Information Brochure

Like the practice website, a well-designed brochure presents essential practice information in an attractive format, projecting an image of professionalism and competency. The purpose of both the website and the general information brochure is to inform existing clients about the practice and to attract new clients to the practice.

Hospital brochures can be concise and simple, with a traditional trifold design and basic information in blocks of text, or more elaborate and colorful, with plenty of images supplementing the text. What you choose will depend on your budget, your competition, your clientele, your marketing focus, and other factors.

When initiating or updating a brochure, consider current practice needs and research your options. Keep in mind that information appearing in the practice brochure can also appear on the practice website, and vice versa. Ideally, both venues work together to create a consistent practice image. A client should be able to see that the brochure and website represent the same practice.

You do not have to start from scratch when creating a brochure. Collect samples from other businesses, including veterinary hospitals. Search online to examine the websites of practices in cities similar to yours. Check out the large selection of veterinary-specific marketing firms that you can engage to help with the appearance and content of your website, brochures, cards, and other materials. If your budget permits, you may wish to consider using their services.

Or, you may want to support your local economy—and the clients who patronize your practice—by using local services. Your local print shop may have samples to show you and can suggest paper, font, and print color ideas, as will local marketing and design consultants. If you choose to go this route, you can credit the local businesses on the printed materials themselves, promoting goodwill among your clients. Is there a local community-college, vocational-school, or even high-school art or web-design class that could help to create your brochure or website as a hands-on learning experience? Perhaps a talented high-school student is looking for a senior project, and working on your materials would be a perfect fit for him or her.

If you decide to create your own materials or assign this job to a talented team member, keep in mind that various document and publication software programs provide a helpful resource for brochure design and format. Many of these programs include options for obtaining more design ideas from the manufacturer's website. Plenty of free templates can also be found from Internet searches.

Whatever layout you choose, you may want to select a font that is large enough for your over-forty clients to read without difficulty. Some font styles are also easier to read than others, so try different looks in mock-up versions and ask team members which ones they think work best. If you include graphics, they should be well composed and interesting. Include the practice logo, recast and modernized, if necessary. Photos should be in focus and professional looking.

Keep the brochure simple. It should not look too cluttered. Remember that the judicious use of white space can make a brochure more attractive. A complex, overly detailed brochure may be more difficult for potential and existing clients to read. They may lose interest before getting to the most important information. In addition, the more complex the design, and the more colors you use, the more expensive the brochure may be to print. If you design a full-color brochure that must be professionally printed on glossy paper, staff may tend to hoard it because of the per-copy expense. It is better to have something that can be distributed liberally without worrying about the cost. Small runs can often be economically handled by an office supply store that offers printing and folding services. If you are considering printing in-house, remember to budget for employee time, color toner replenishment, and wear-and-tear on printer equipment.

Text content is just as important as visual presentation. At the minimum, your brochure should include the following information:

- Hospital name
- Hospital street address (and map, if space allows)
- Web address and e-mail contact information
- Telephone numbers, including emergency phone numbers and area codes (consider listing the main hospital telephone number and web address in several conspicuous areas on the brochure)
- Practice vision statement (see Chapter 3 on strategic planning) and highlights of the practice's strengths.
- Extent or limitations of professional services offered (e.g., "Practice limited to cats" or "Medical and surgical services for all companion animals, including birds, reptiles and amphibians")
- Any nonprofessional or ancillary patient services available, such as pet boarding and grooming
- Appointment hours and procedures for scheduling
- Emergency hours and procedures for reaching emergency coverage
- Patient-care policies, such as ease of obtaining progress reports or visiting hospitalized animals
- Payment policies (e.g., "Check, credit card, or cash deposit required before hospitalization," or "Payment required at time of services, unless prior arrangements have been made with the hospital administrator")
- For some practices, such as emergency, equine, or mixed animal, credit privilege policies, if any (e.g., prequalification requirements, billing charges, interest charges on overdue accounts, and what constitutes an overdue account)

If space allows, you might also consider listing:

- Local community and civic organization membership, such as humane societies, Better Business Bureau, Jaycees, or Rotary Club
- Sponsorships, charity support, and community involvement, such as Future Farmers of America, 4-H, Girl Scouts, Boy Scouts, National Pet Week
- Professional organization membership, such as AAHA, AVMA, state and local veterinary medical associations, and veterinary technician associations

- Marketing copy:
  - » "Please visit and tour our practice at any time. Group tours can be arranged by appointment."
  - » "Our hospital team is available to speak to your group on a variety of animal-care topics."
  - » "Visit our website at [website address] to sign up for newsletters, special offerings, and pet health alerts and to manage your pet's record online."
  - » "Find us on Facebook and be part of our pet parent community with fun contests and prizes."

As you compose the text, watch out for medical and technical jargon. Use language that is easy for the layperson to understand. Many editors recommend writing information at a sixth-grade level. Carefully edit and proofread the final copy before sending it to print. Use a second and third set of eyes or engage the services of a professional copyeditor. Make sure a "spell-check" has been run, but do not rely on the spell-check to catch all errors.

Consider printing only an estimated six-month supply of brochures. This will allow you to update the brochure before ordering a reprint. The cost per brochure may be lower if you print more than you estimate needing during that time, but you do not want to be left with a large supply of brochures that must be thrown away when you decide to change your fees. If you wish to take advantage of bulk printing prices, make sure you do not include the kind of information that may need to be updated soon, such as specific fee information. The mission statement, services offered, strengths of the practice, and contact information are not likely to change and can be included. The practice website is much easier to update and can include the information that changes.

Give brochures to all new clients. Keep copies readily available in the reception area for established clients and visitors. Encourage existing clients to take extras and share them with family members and friends. If you give a presentation to a service club or school classroom, hand them out. If you go to Chamber of Commerce meetings, bring them with you. If you have a specialty practice and receive referrals from more general practices, give brochures to those general practices along with your cards. Practice employees should keep copies in their cars or other handy locations. You never know when someone might need a veterinarian. You will think of other uses over time.

Be sure to review all client handouts, including the brochure, periodically for accuracy, and update as needed. A review once every six months should be sufficient.

While a hospital information brochure can represent a sizable investment, it is a good partner to the practice website, which will include similar information but will link to more detailed pages. The practice brochure and website work together, conveying valuable information to existing and potential hospital clients. They will save the practice time and money by eliminating time-consuming telephone calls and conversations explaining basic hospital guidelines. But the real benefit is in gaining "top-of-mind recognition." With careful planning, your hospital brochure can be a very effective marketing and promotion piece, working in conjunction with the website to build and maintain client awareness of your veterinary practice.

Practice Websites

Once an optional, fun way to market a practice, websites have become a basic business necessity. Potential clients now rely heavily on the information they find on websites to compare service providers and select the ones they will use.

Your practice website should provide basic information about your location and services while maintaining a strong brand image in accord with the attributes described earlier in this chapter. The website can be designed to achieve other practice objectives as well, such as providing reliable information about various health conditions and animal-related topics pertinent to veterinary medicine. Since clients will search for information about diagnosed problems and undiagnosed signs of disease, the practice should consider developing reliable online resources that clients can refer to when questions arise. These resources may be in the form of links to other sites or in the form of blogs and/or an online newsletter created by veterinary team members. This extra touch can cement the trust your clients have in the practice and give them reason to return to the website again and again.

You may wish to subscribe to an Internet-based service that will enable the practice to have a robust Internet presence. These companies usually offer a full array of complementary services, such as the following:

- Domain name registration and management
- Website design, branding, and rebranding
- Website hosting
- Search engine optimization technology, to raise the website to the highest possible level of visibility
- Social-media branding and integration with the website
- E-mail management, including e-mail addresses using the practice domain name
- Statistics about website traffic
- Medical-based content and resources for client education and use
- Online forms for client use, such as new patient registration and boarding registration
- Hosted Internet pharmacy
- Online payment processing
- Secure client log-in to access and self-manage patient information (name, birthdays, images)

Website Design Essentials

Your hospital website should be:
- Visually engaging and attractive
- Easy to navigate, with the desired information easy to find
- Interactive
- Up-to-date
- Helpful, offering the information most users are looking for and solving common problems
- Linked to the practice's selected social-media sites, such as Facebook, and blogs created by practice staff members

- Secure employee log-in to remotely access work schedules, training materials, and other employment resources
- Private social chat rooms for the practice's clients
- Sign-up service for practice electronic newsletters (e-newsletters) and e-mail reminders
- Client survey tools
- Videos that teach and entertain, such as with links to YouTube
- Access to coupons and practice special offers
- Links to helpful information, such as directions for those driving to the practice and maps

Internet users have certain expectations of a web page. You should regularly reassess whether your practice's website reflects an adequate professional image. Website software and code has evolved rapidly. Although the practice website might have been cutting edge a few years ago, its functionality and appearance may now be quite dated.

Keep in mind, too, that the Internet browsers people use are constantly advancing. It is important that the software running the practice website allows the site to function and appear perfectly in whatever browser type and version an Internet surfer might be using.

Consider that many users may be searching the Internet using a smartphone or other small handheld device. A mobile website is a variation of the practice website that is easily viewed in the limited space of a small video display. The typical mobile website information cleanly displayed with a smartphone hit would include practice name, logo, phone number, e-mail link, map link, and Facebook, Twitter, and blog links.

Social Media

In the past, an active Internet presence required ongoing refreshment of the practice's website so that users would keep returning to see what was new. E-mail blasts, e-mailed newsletters, and e-mail reminders helped in pulling clients back to the website if it was seen as the central platform for the practice's Internet interface.

Business use of social media has changed all of that. A foundational premise of social-media use is how it allows an organization to build "social authority" by establishing its expertise (Brauer and Bourhis 2006). A practice cannot completely control its marketing message through social-media platforms, but by participating in the conversation, the practice becomes a significant influencer in client dialogue about veterinary care.

In many regards, social-media platforms are a perfect fit for veterinary practices to reach potential clients. The veterinary profession as a whole is generally put off by direct marketing, and people are for the most part resistant to overt marketing through social media. Social-media marketing strategy relies on building social authority with credibility. In a 2008 report, 58 percent of respondents said they most trusted company or product information coming from "people like me." In 2011, this number dropped to 43 percent, with 70 percent of respondents saying they preferred information from industry experts and academics, as compared to 57 percent in the 2008 report (Edelman 2011).

By using various Internet-based applications such as Facebook and Twitter, practices can focus on creating an interactive dialogue with clients. Information and news, ideas and feedback, opinion and testimony can be easily and passively disseminated through the social networks that each application provides. Social media can provide both benefits and challenges as part of a veterinary practice's integrated marketing strategy, yet most experiences show that the benefits surpass the downsides that can be felt.

In general, a practice's social-media marketing program should center on creating content that attracts the attention of existing clients so that they in turn will share it with their own social networks. People love their companion animals and love to talk about them. Because messages and information flow from user to user and friend to friend, referrals resonate powerfully, just as classic word-of-mouth referrals did in the past. These messages can become an important way of building a practice's client base.

Social media has wide reach while still being very personally targeted to users within the veterinary practice's catchment. Messages posted on social-media sites are also easily accessible through Internet access. Use of social media has a very low cost of implementation.

Social media take many forms. It can be overwhelming to think about using or managing all of them. However, it is not necessary to begin using all of them at once. In fact, payroll and time limitations may make it difficult and expensive for the typical small veterinary practice to do so. Begin small, with one or two platforms, and build from there as your experience with social media increases.

When deciding on a platform to use, consider what you can manage and where clients are most likely to find you. Facebook, for example, is a good place to start. It is probably the platform that is the closest fit for most veterinary practices at this time. Animal owners like to share images and stories, there is a high proportion of women users, and a wide range of ages represented, with many older users.

Facebook's business profiles are also more detailed than Twitter's. A typical veterinary practice profile will be branded, shows images and videos, and features ongoing client and friend interactive dialogue in real time, which leads to word-of-mouth referrals and builds trust. The Facebook platform includes many other tools as well, including the possibility of advertising as well as link placement based on criteria the practice defines.

Some research has shown that consumers with higher-than-average annual incomes have a preference for using Twitter, so this can also be a logical choice. Businesses use Twitter to promote products and services with short messages (tweets) that followers will be likely to read on their home pages. Messages can link to the practice website, to other social-media platforms like Facebook, and to images and more.

Google has launched Google Plus, a social-media site similar to Facebook, which may also soon become a popular option. Google Plus offers innovative opportunities such as organizing contacts into "circles" or groups for sharing across various Google applications and for group video chats.

Practices can use blogs (short for "web logs") to describe service offerings and veterinary medical information at length, personalized by the medical staff. Well-written blogs can result in an increased client following and build the perceived credibility of the practice and its personnel. Blogs can welcome reader input and feedback, and they can link to and from the practice website, Facebook profile, Twitter page, and/or Google Plus page.

Critically assess all of the hospital's marketing efforts on a yearly basis. While branding is important, it is also important keep what's important to your clients center stage: their worries about their animal companions and your practice's expertise in providing health-care solutions that will maximize their well-being and longevity. Do not choose a particular marketing strategy or form of advertisement just because "everyone else is doing it." Ask yourself what the practice truly expects to gain from a marketing technique. Will the practice gain or keep a significant number of clients by using the strategy? Will the use of the strategy help to build trust in its competencies in your community? Measure results by tracking the number of new clients obtained from each type of marketing initiative, and weigh whether the data support the decision to maintain each type.

The Internet has many benefits, but it can have drawbacks as well. When negative feedback about your practice appears on the Internet, it, too, can reach a wide audience, depending on the venue. Sooner or later every practice will experience a bad review by a client who felt he had a poor experience. Sometimes, bad reviews are posted by consumers who are perpetually angry or upset, and seem to cause problems for many of the business from which they purchase goods and services. Nevertheless, it is wise to have a plan of action to deal with these issues quickly and effectively.

First, manage the practice's online reputation by monitoring what is being said. Google Alerts is a free service that will automatically send you messages based on key words you set up. The goal is to understand the conversations going on about your practice, both positive and negative.

Be aware of any complaints or negative chatter that might show up so that you can quickly manage it. You can always choose to ignore negative feedback, and trust that readers will understand that all businesses are going to have bad reviews from time to time. But you can also take the active stance of recognizing such comments and, by doing so, make them an example of your practice's excellent client service.

When you do find an irate client venting about your practice, most advisers state you should respond as quickly as possible in the same forum. Andy Sernovitz, CEO of the Word of Mouth Marketing Association, reported that "most negative conversation is actually a plea for assistance, and the negative stops when you solve the problem" (Griffin 2006). Responding quickly creates a public record of an attempt at a quick resolution. For example, you might post a response that says, "We are very sorry you had a bad experience, and would like to talk with you as soon as possible so that we can correct the situation. Please contact me at _____." Your goal is to get the conversation taken off line, so that you can talk with the person directly and not through the Internet. You can then resolve the problem in a professional manner. Do not get into a dialogue with the person online, even though she may try to continue it there. Other people will see your professional response of offering help and understand that the practice takes complaints seriously.

Your practice should view negative comments posted on the Internet as an opportunity. A client has alerted you to a potential problem, and now you have the ability to publicly help that client. If you are able to successfully resolve the issue and please the customer in such a public avenue as Facebook or another website, potential clients will see your strong efforts at customer service. Your response turns this possibly harmful situation into a positive incident to boost your practice's public image.

A proactive method of dealing with customer issues in the Internet age is to post updates to your company's website or to Facebook, Twitter, your blog, or another form of social media. If a sizable number of customers are sharing complaints on the same issue, you may want to address this common concern in a post so that clients know that you are working to resolve the issue (Nolan 2010).

Newsletters

Newsletters can be prepared in house or purchased from companies that specialize in creating veterinary newsletters. Increasingly, electronic versions are used as a cost-effective way to reach clients. You can also archive the information through the practice website, use newsletter-like content in blogs, and post excerpts from your newsletter in the practice's social-media profiles. Over time, you can create a large electronic library of credible information related to veterinary care.

Electronic media also allows you to link and cross-reference information to other parts of the practice's array of integrated marketing and communication resources. An electronic newsletter featuring an article on ear care could include a YouTube video link showing how to correctly clean and medicate a dog's ear canal. Explanatory audio narration can supplement the video clip.

Purchased newsletters can incorporate customized articles and announcements specific to your practice. Use of computers makes it easy to modify newsletter content so that it uniquely reflects the practice and current information. For example, the newsletter service you subscribe to might send you generic pieces addressing animal health-care issues; to customize them, you might rewrite the articles slightly to incorporate information supplied by veterinarians at your practice and personal accounts of their experiences in dealing with the issues covered (using pseudonyms for client and animal names, of course). Make sure you understand what your agreement is with the organization or company producing these newsletter items, especially in terms of making modifications and citing the source.

Keep the newsletters attractive, fun, easy to read, and interesting. The articles should be simple and short. Do not try to educate the client about every aspect of a disease or condition. The goal is to show your expertise, but not overwhelm the reader with technical information. Use pictures, quizzes, and fun facts about animals. Biographies of employees can add human interest. Briefly introduce new service offerings and products that provide effective solutions that your clients will want for their companion animals.

Preparing, printing, and mailing newsletters can be costly, especially if they are published frequently, and the newsletter's effectiveness in reaching clients and promoting services may be difficult to determine. The best use of newsletters may be as an internal marketing tool aimed at the needs of existing clients. Newsletters can be a part of your client-education program, support retention of clients, and encourage repeat visits. Blogs and other forms of communication, however, can in many ways replace the traditional newsletter. Consider the demographics of your area when deciding how to best reach and inform your new and existing clients.

Sympathy Letters

Expressing condolences to an owner about the loss of a beloved companion animal creates goodwill. Direct mailing of team-signed sympathy letters or cards to clients and donations in the name of patients that have died usually result in deeply felt client appreciation. As noted in Chapter 12, these actions have a very positive effect on your relationship with current clients and can increase the probability of retaining the client, even after the death of a companion animal.

PUBLIC RELATIONS

Public relations is any activity initiated by your animal hospital that is designed to create a positive image while communicating with present and potential clients. It is marketing through any unpaid communication conveyed through the media, be that newspaper, radio, television, or the Internet. It can be initiated by the practice (for example, through press releases), or it can be initiated by a third party (such as a newspaper reporter investigating a piece about animals, a blogger, or, unfortunately, a dissatisfied client). Public relations allows for excellent segmenting and target marketing with limited reach and frequency. Several of these public relations tools are described below.

Press Releases

Press releases are specialized documents that convey news about your veterinary hospital to the media. If you create press releases, make sure they are well written and to the point. They may be used in whole or in part by the media outlet. A reporter may call you for more information and revise the piece, but more often, it will only be used if it is in good shape to begin with.

Use press releases to inform the community about positive practice developments, such as the opening of new facilities, the addition of specialized equipment, or new doctors joining the staff. Using a third party, the media, to tell your story will give it more legitimacy and credibility than will direct mail or advertising.

Consider developing good relations with local newspaper reporters and radio reps so they will respect you as a reliable source of accurate news about animal-related issues. You then have contacts for e-mailing press releases on local animal-health issues and your own hospital news. Properly written press releases can be the basis for news stories while also positioning you as a news resource. Supplement your faxes and e-mails containing press releases with phone calls.

News releases present information presumed to be of interest to the readers of the publications in which they will appear. The content should avoid sounding like an advertisement, as the editor will likely not run such copy.

Keep copies or obtain reprints of any newspaper articles or news releases about your veterinary hospital. If the feature is also carried on the newspaper website, you can link to it from Facebook or the practice website, but be aware that the linked article may eventually disappear. Scanning or saving an image file of the article is a good idea, using media like Adobe Acrobat, and it can be added to the website or a Facebook profile for sharing with current and prospective clients.

Whenever a special article is published about the hospital or its staff, consider having a copy professionally mounted and framed for permanent display in the reception area. Prominently display the logo of the publication along the top of the page, but remove the date so the article always seems current.

If you live in a small community, the local paper may be open to having a veterinarian write a regular column about animal-health issues. This may be time consuming, as you will want to make sure each column is well written and contains accurate information. However, if a veterinarian has a talent for writing, this effort can provide a means of keeping the hospital name prominently front and center while educating potential clients about services they may not have been aware of previously.

Public Appearances

Public appearances, such as talks before a service club, kennel club, school class, scout group, or other similar groups, are a useful means to educate the public about veterinary care and the range of services available at your animal hospital. Presentations may be made by veterinarians or any other knowledgeable staff member. Speaking before groups can be a bit intimidating at first, but personal relationships developed through live presentations are very valuable. You will gain new clients while giving the practice a more visible presence in the community.

Presentations are an excellent opportunity to educate the public about the human-animal bond and the veterinary practice's important role in promoting it. The presenter can go to other sites (such as schools and service club meetings) to make presentations, or the practice can invite groups in for a tour. Presentations at the hospital allow you to introduce your facility, equipment, and abilities. Potential clients can learn that veterinarians are interesting and approachable people (Bower et al. 1994, 48). However, making presentations at other places in the community allow you to reach larger audiences. Consider incorporating both types of presentations into your marketing plan.

Your state veterinary medical association may have presentation kits to help your staff prepare for speaking engagements and open houses. A wide selection of PowerPoint presentations from various professional organizations should give you lots of easily accessible material through the Internet, or you can create your own. Children at events represent your practice's potential future clients, and they also may encourage their parents to seek veterinary services for the family pets. Your efforts may also attract faculty members, scout parents and other parent volunteers, and the like, who will know some of your hospital's staff personally because of the presentation.

Service club meetings are a great place for presentations. Because they often have presentations monthly, and need to fill their calendar, you may well be able to come up with a presentation idea that will interest them. For example, the presenter could focus on work with therapy animals or service dogs. Service clubs often have members that are leaders in the community, and they may tell many other people about the good work that you are doing at the practice.

Special Events

Special events such as hospital open houses, National Pet Week celebrations, and other creative venues offer opportunities to communicate with and educate the public about veterinary services.

Open houses can be quite simple or elaborate. An open house can celebrate a hospital anniversary, a new associate hire, or a hospital renovation. For National Pet Week, check with the American Veterinary Medical Association for marketing ideas and resources.

Other special events sponsored by the hospital might include pet fun shows, pet walks, and pet talks. Talk about these sorts of live social events on Facebook and send invites from the practice Facebook page. Scheduling events like this is one of the many ways that you can increase the number of fans of the practice Facebook business page.

A pet fun show is a hospital- or community-sponsored event for pet owners and pets. Usually participants compete for prizes, but the criteria are different from breed-fancier-club show guidelines. Competition may be based on silly categories, such as "the pet that looks most like its human companion," "the pet with the best tricks," or "the pet with the longest (or shortest) tail." Better yet, the competition can be a test of practical caregiver knowledge, such as being able to explain the origin and purpose of the animal's breed or knowing facts about proper nutrition and animal husbandry.

Veterinarians might also volunteer to be on call for dog, cat, and horse shows or to officiate at pet parades. This may sound at first like a big time commitment; however, the contacts made at such events can be very valuable.

PERSONAL SELLING

Another powerful marketing tool is simply personal selling, the effort made by every hospital staff member to use direct personal communication to inform and persuade a client, either in person or on the telephone. Personal selling includes both verbal and nonverbal techniques.

Examples of personal selling attributes are personal appearance, telephone manners, and listening skills. Effective personal selling activities include taking adequate time to explain procedures, advising clients of additional services needed for their pets, and informing clients about additional services and products available at the hospital.

Team training is essential to successful personal selling. The information and recommendations employees give clients must be correct and consistent with practice guidelines of animal care. (See Chapter 7 for more information on how to train employees to convey a clear and consistent message to clients.) An important axiom states that no client should be left with unanswered questions, and every client should leave with unquestioned answers.

Business cards are a personal selling tool that helps to promote the hospital image and services. They are inexpensive to print, so each veterinarian should have personalized business cards to give to acquaintances. In some practices, each employee has personal business cards. If the practice goes to this expense, the employees must keep their cards available and hand them out.

Take time to teach employees how to use their cards effectively: Have cards readily available in your pocket, hand the card to the client or prospective client, and say, "Please permit me to give you my business card. Please ask for me when you visit or if you have questions. It would be my pleasure to help you." Personalizing the card with a handwritten note on it helps improve client retention of a card.

From time to time, evaluate the cards to see if they need to be modernized or updated with current clinic information. Keep them available at the reception area so that clients can take a few to pass on to referrals. Business cards may never go out of style, even in an age when smartphones have replaced wristwatches and maps.

In established veterinary practices, the main sources of continued business revenue are current clients and referrals directed to the hospital by those clients. Clients who are sold on what your practice does and how it does it will refer other clients to you. The best way to transform clients into practice ambassadors is through personal selling. Clearly, social-media sites also help to advance personal selling. When multiple employees help manage the practice Facebook page, their personal messages and dialogue with clients effectively reinforce relationships. The contacts are more frequent than in physical, face-to-face meetings, thus bringing the practice to the client's attention more often.

Many attributes of favorable client interactions have been previously described throughout this book, as well as what to avoid. When training employees in how to manage client communication in social-media sites, it is a good time to remind them to avoid poor personal selling techniques—such as using high-pressured sales talks that come off as pushy, or making clients feel guilty about the care they decide not to purchase for their animals. Lack of empathy, being argumentative, appearing apathetic or disengaged, and being too soft-spoken or indecisive are also to be avoided.

Clients who are pleased with patient care, thoughtful advice, and prompt, courteous service will wholeheartedly promote the practice to others. By the same token, the easiest way to turn a client away from the hospital (and possibly create a negative voice in your community) is with poor personal selling.

Creating a Marketing Plan

An effective marketing plan requires many decisions that can only be made by the owners of a business. Leadership beliefs and attitudes about the practice's history, reputation, and image and about how that image should be publicly displayed will affect the ultimate plan. Marketing can require significant financial commitment that only owners are able to authorize.

Nevertheless, as practice manager you can play an important role in the success of any marketing plan. A good starting point is to discuss and clarify practice leadership opinions and beliefs and what the owners would like to accomplish through the marketing plan. How do they see the practice, as compared with other practices in the surrounding market?

The practice may be undergoing changes that call for a marketing plan. The practice might be opening a new satellite facility; moving to a new location; acquiring new hospital owners, new doctors, or other staff; adding specialty services; changing hours of operation; or responding to changes in client base demographics. These and similar developments may indicate that it is time to consider a formal marketing plan.

The practice manager has a significant role to play in assisting in the plan design and ensuring the implementation and adaptation of ideas. The manager will monitor the response to and the success of the various marketing endeavors, give feedback to the owners, and suggest improvements as the plan develops.

The steps in designing, creating, and implementing a marketing plan are discussed below. In each step, queries are posed to help you channel your efforts. The steps and questions relevant to your practice will depend on the stage of growth or decline that the hospital is experiencing.

GOALS

First, meet with the practice owners and directors to recall the mission, scope of activities, and goals of the practice. If your practice has not already determined its mission, vision, values, and strengths and weakness, or if these need to be revised or improved, refer back to Chapter 3. Without a clear understanding of the practice's current culture and future direction, the marketing plan will be a hit-and-miss endeavor.

Keep in mind that no single practice is able to satisfy the requirements of all the people all the time. In fact, a major objective of your marketing plan is to show how and where your practice is different from others competing in the same area. A practice that is perceived to be the same as all the rest has no image (Sheridan and McCafferty 1993, 24).

When formulating your marketing plan, you will need to set goals so that you will be able to measure your level of success. These goals usually come directly from your SWOT analysis and ongoing analysis of key performance indicators and the market (described in detail in Chapter 3). Here are some questions to consider when thinking about the goals you will establish:

- What is your goal to increase or sustain the number of visits per year from present clients?
- Do you want to attract new clients? If so, what types of clients do you want to attract?
- Where will the new clients come from?
- What are the financial goals of the practice?
- What are the goals for team career development, performance improvement, and education and training?

You will need to compare your unique selling points to the perceived needs and desires of people in your surrounding area and your clientele. Though some of these questions are discussed in Chapter 3 on strategic planning, they are important enough to revisit when beginning to create coordinated marketing plan.

ANALYSIS

As you determine your brand image and your marketing plan, you'll need to be aware of your strengths, weaknesses, opportunities, and threats. Here are some questions to answer that will help to bring hospital's strengths into focus:

- Are you open twenty-four hours a day? Or only eight hours? Perhaps twelve hours? What days of the week is the hospital open?
- Do the veterinarians have any special skills or offer any unique services?
- What are the internal strengths of practice veterinary staff, technical staff, and office staff?
- Does your practice board, groom, or train animals?
- Does the practice sell pet supplies or increase therapeutic food sales through nutritional counseling?
- At what price-point do you offer your services? Are you a competitively priced practice or do you offer high-end services and excellent customer service commanding premium prices?
- Is your practice conveniently located? Does it have ample parking? What are the facilities like?

Next, turn to opportunities and threats in the market area. Evaluate the practice's general area to assess its current condition and to identify projected or proposed changes. These changes may be out of the control of the practice (e.g., municipal decisions for new road construction or impending development of new residential communities).

Assess the impact that such changes may have on your practice. Try to read the crystal ball and make predictions. These predictions will help to shape the goals you establish:

- Who are the potential new clients the practice can attract?
- What kinds of animals do your clients and potential clients own?
- How many animals are owned in the area?
- How many animal owners are in the area?
- What is the proportion of current clients to potential clients in the area?
- Where are the potential clients whom the practice may be able to attract? Are there any new opportunities, such as new companies about to begin hiring that will attract new people to the area?
- What are the demographics of the area from which you draw clients? What is the percentage of elderly residents? What is the percentage of families with young children?
- Is there a marketing technique that will allow you to reach demographic groups that you are not yet reaching? To draw more clients from the groups that are already attracted to the practice?
- What are your current clients' needs, wants, and concerns?
- What can you do to meet those needs?
- Who in the average family unit takes care of the pet and determines the purchase of services? Is there a way to target these family members more effectively?
- Who and where is your competition?
- Can you differentiate your services from the competition by providing services that the competition does not provide, or by providing a veterinary staff with board certification or specialty training?
- Will other competition be moving in? Can you buy up the competition, or combine forces?
- How many veterinarians are in the area? What is the full-time equivalency number of veterinarians?
- What is the proportion of animal owners to full-time veterinarians in your area? How has this changed from the last time you measured?
- Who are the major employers in the area? What is the economic base of the community or metropolitan area?
- Are there any external threats, such as downturns in major industries, or other changes that should be considered?
- In an economic recession, are there particular industries, companies, or demographic groups that are faring better than others? Would it be feasible to try to reach these groups through your marketing program?

The primary sources for this information will be the hospital files, local news media, local chamber of commerce information, client satisfaction surveys, and massively increasing data available through Internet search and investigation, using tools like Google and Google maps.

Client Surveys

Client surveys can yield a wealth of information to help improve client satisfaction, evaluate current offerings, test client interest in new offerings, and determine client needs, wants, and concerns. They can be done in-house, mailed to every client, or completed with online survey tools, which are inexpensive and easy to use. You could choose to survey all clients or only a random selection of clients (see Figures 13.2A and 13.2B).

Client questionnaires should be easy to read and complete. If you ask too many questions, the client is less likely to complete the survey. Before investing the time and money needed to send it to your entire mailing list, test it first with a small sampling of clients. If you conduct the survey by regular postal service, enclose a self-addressed, stamped envelope for the highest probability of return. Otherwise, consider using an online service.

One way to use an online survey is to have the client complete it at the time of service. A laptop or touch pad computer with an Internet connection is an easy way to interview clients while they are waiting for whatever reason. Exit surveys completed before the client leaves the practice can provide an accurate assessment of client opinion, since the client's thoughts and feelings are contemporaneous with hospital contact.

Some practices hand clients a card with a link at the conclusion of an appointment and ask them to visit the website and complete the survey. Others include survey links on the practice website. Facebook provides a survey option that is easy to construct on a practice profile page. You can tweet single-question surveys through Twitter. All of these methods allow you to keep in touch with what your clients think and what they want from the practice.

If you survey clients who have not visited your hospital in a while, they may not be able to answer specific questions, since memory and accurate assessment have a way of fading with the passage of time. Choose questions that can help you find out why they have not been back. This is very valuable information to know. Some consultants advocate conducting surveys through third-party providers. If the hospital can afford it, a survey that is written, distributed, and analyzed by a trained professional will give a more reliable picture of the hospital's performance and will provide more useful decision-making criteria. It might also provide a means for contemporaneous benchmarking against other practices participating in the same survey.

Client Interviews

You may decide to have face-to-face conversations with key clients. A meeting over coffee with a top-referring client or someone who has spent a good deal of money with the veterinary practice can be revealing. A significant advantage of personal interviews is that you can clarify responses with additional questions. Personal interviews can bond the client even more to the practice. Asking for a person's opinion is flattering and shows respect. The client feels important and valued.

PAGE 1 SHOWN

˅

FULL FORM
INCLUDED ON
COMPANION
WEBSITE

FIGURE 13.2A   AAHA CLIENT SATISFACTION SURVEY

As an accredited member of the American Animal Hospital Association, we are dedicated to providing excellence in small animal care. Our hospital is evaluated by AAHA to ensure that we meet or exceed the association's standards of excellence. AAHA standards are recognized around the world as the benchmark for quality care in veterinary medicine.

Thank you for taking time out of your busy day to let us know how we are doing. Your feedback is very important to help us continue to grow and enhance your experience at our practice.

1. How long have you been bringing your pet to our hospital?
a. Less than 6 months
b. 6 months – 2 years
c. More than 2 years

2. Are you aware that we're an AAHA-accredited hospital?
a. Yes
b. No

3. Please rank the top five attributes you value in a veterinary hospital (1st most valuable through 5th most valuable).
a. The location and parking are convenient. _____
b. The hours of operation meet my needs. _____
c. The appointment begins promptly at the scheduled time. _____
d. The hospital staff is friendly and courteous. _____
e. The hospital staff really care about my pet. _____
f. The veterinarian listens to what I have to say. _____
g. The veterinarian explains any problems and treatments clearly. _____
h. The veterinary hospital provides good value for my money. _____

4. When scheduling an appointment, I (yes, sometimes, no):

a. Encounter a busy signal	❏ Yes	❏ Sometimes	❏ No
b. Obtain put on hold	❏ Yes	❏ Sometimes	❏ No
c. Obtain an appointment that fits my schedule	❏ Yes	❏ Sometimes	❏ No
d. Am contacted to confirm my appointment	❏ Yes	❏ Sometimes	❏ No

5. The front desk staff (yes, sometimes, no):

a. Greets me and my pet by name	❏ Yes	❏ Sometimes	❏ No
b. Are welcoming and courteous	❏ Yes	❏ Sometimes	❏ No
c. Are helpful and concerned about my pet	❏ Yes	❏ Sometimes	❏ No
d. Are knowledgeable about hospital services and policies	❏ Yes	❏ Sometimes	❏ No
e. Are able to answer my questions	❏ Yes	❏ Sometimes	❏ No

6. The veterinary technicians/assistants are (agree, disagree):
a. Friendly and outgoing
   ❏ Agree strongly   ❏ Agree somewhat ❏ Disagree somewhat   ❏ Disagree strongly
b. Knowledgeable
   ❏ Agree strongly   ❏ Agree somewhat ❏ Disagree somewhat   ❏ Disagree strongly
c. Able to answer my questions
   ❏ Agree strongly   ❏ Agree somewhat ❏ Disagree somewhat   ❏ Disagree strongly
d. Kind and careful with my pet
   ❏ Agree strongly   ❏ Agree somewhat ❏ Disagree somewhat   ❏ Disagree strongly

PAGE 1 SHOWN

˅

FULL FORM
INCLUDED ON
COMPANION
WEBSITE

FIGURE 13.2B CLIENT SATISFACTION SURVEY

In a continuing effort to improve the quality of care that we provide, we are asking a number of our clients to respond to the enclosed questionnaire. By taking a few minutes to fill out this form and return it to us in the enclosed envelope, you can help us determine how best to serve your veterinary care needs.

Please circle one letter for each question.	Always	Usually	Sometimes	Seldom	Almost Never	Never
1. When Calling for an Appointment:						
Is the reception staff polite and helpful?	A	B	C	D	E	F
Do you encounter a busy signal?	A	B	C	D	E	F
Are you put on hold?	A	B	C	D	E	F
Are you able to get an appointment as promptly as you would like?	A	B	C	D	E	F
Are your questions answered to your satisfaction?	A	B	C	D	E	F
If you leave a message, does someone return your call within the same day?	A	B	C	D	E	F
2. When You Arrive for Your Appointment:						
Is the parking lot clean?	A	B	C	D	E	F
Is the parking adequate?	A	B	C	D	E	F
Are you greeted warmly by our receptionist?	A	B	C	D	E	F
Is your appointment acknowledged?	A	B	C	D	E	F
Is there adequate seating in the waiting room?	A	B	C	D	E	F
Is the waiting room clean and neat?	A	B	C	D	E	F
Do you have to wait longer than 15 minutes to see the veterinarian?	A	B	C	D	E	F
3. When You See the Veterinarian:						
Do the veterinary technician and other staff treat you courteously?	A	B	C	D	E	F
Is the veterinarian courteous and helpful?	A	B	C	D	E	F
Is the veterinarian professional in manner and appearance?	A	B	C	D	E	F
Do the veterinarian and staff seem interested in your pet?	A	B	C	D	E	F
Does the veterinarian take time to answer your questions?	A	B	C	D	E	F
Did the veterinarian fully explain your pet's condition and the prognosis for your pet's illness or accident?	A	B	C	D	E	F
Were you satisfied with the treatment received?	A	B	C	D	E	F
4. Our Staff:						
Are they neat in appearances?	A	B	C	D	E	F
Do they have a thorough knowledge of our products and procedures?	A	B	C	D	E	F
Are they able to answer your questions to your satisfaction?	A	B	C	D	E	F
Are they professional in manner and appearance?	A	B	C	D	E	F

Adapted from VHMA materials

The disadvantage to this approach is that it takes a lot of time to complete individual interviews. You may also obtain skewed results compared to a survey of the entire client base, because the sampling size will be much smaller than with a written survey questionnaire. Interviewing the top clients of the practice may in itself skew the results because these clients already have shown that they like what you do. You might not acquire the kind of feedback that you can use to improve overall services. To counter this tendency, be sure to interview clients who will give you valuable, constructive input rather than simply complimenting you on the practice's positive attributes.

Focus Groups

Focus groups are used by large companies to find out which products are of interest to the consumer and how they should be marketed to effectively achieve a high sales volume. Veterinary businesses can implement focus groups in the same manner. A neutral facilitator can work with a small group of six to twenty participants. There might be a major topic of discussion or a series of ideas that are bounced off the focus group members. Videotaping or audiotaping (of course, with everyone's permission) helps memorialize the comments and conclusions. The interplay between the interviewer and the focus group provides a synergy of its own. Ideas or topics that may not have been posed through a questionnaire can be developed and pursued within the freedom of a focus group (McCafferty 1995).

You might even consider conducting a focus-group discussion or client interviews by electronic means. For example, you could arrange a chat-room conference. If your practice has a website, questionnaires could be routinely posted to gain information from clients and anyone else visiting the site.

Each survey method has its own pros and cons. The most important task is to collect data that will be useful in monitoring and assessing the objectives of the practice. Objectives may change as a result of the surveys. The assessment should be part of an ongoing, methodical process. Gathering information is important, but it is only helpful if subsequent compilation and analysis occurs.

OBJECTIVES

Now you are ready to set the practice's marketing objectives. Once you have recalled your mission and goals, completed a market analysis, and gathered information from surveys and interviews, the next step will be to set definite objectives for the marketing plan. Ultimately, you will establish a budget to implement the objectives.

Your objectives might be to increase total numbers of patients seen, to see the same number of clients or more, or to increase the number of services provided and the average transaction charge (ATC) per client visit. Some objectives could be directed toward improving client relations, especially if the client survey identified client relations as a problem. For example, if client feedback included complaints about unexpectedly high invoices, providing prompt and accurate estimates might be a practice objective. If clients have appeared to be confused about how to follow up with home care after hospitalization, and your investigation showed that illegible doctor handwriting on the instruction sheets are part of the problem, you might decide to develop printed instructions incorporating the practice brand image for many routine issues.

Your objectives should be specific. For example, you might say, "We will increase the number of feline patient visits by 25 percent," or, "We will increase the per patient transaction charge by 12 percent." Or, your objectives could be more general, such as, "Our goal is to perform more prophylactic dental procedures on feline patients than we did last year."

Keep in mind that stated targets should be attainable and realistic, with goals based on improving past performance. For example, the foregoing general objective could be restated more specifically to: "Last year, we completed dental care on 42 percent of our feline patients for which it was recommended. Our goal for this year is 55 percent."

Work with doctors, and especially owners, to establish agreed-upon goals for patient care and client compliance. At the end of the day, all objectives must be carefully considered in light of the owner's willingness to provide the time and resources necessary to implement them.

STRATEGIES
Now you can select the marketing strategy to implement these objectives. The following questions will help you define your marketing strategy:
- Will advertising be used?
- If so, what media will be used?
- Will a digital newsletter or targeted marketing letters be used?
- Will a new approach to personal selling be used, for instance, hospital renovations or new staff uniforms?
- Will the practice subscribe to an e-mail reminder system?
- How will the reminder system be systematically maintained?
- Will texting be used? If so, by whom?
- Will social media be used? If so, with what platform?
- Who will speak in the coming year, and at what organizations and events?
- Will open houses be scheduled?
- If new services are to be added, how will present and prospective clients be informed about them?

Since you will likely come up with a variety of strategies, consider ranking the list. Prioritize each strategy according to potential monetary benefit, most probable success for the amount of required resources (money and time), and ease of completion. Prioritizing will help you to concentrate on the most worthwhile projects first. Also, try to include a few tasks that can be finished quickly, so that the successes will produce a feeling of accomplishment and encourage further work on more complicated tasks.

ACTION PLAN

Take time to develop the practice's marketing action plan carefully. The action plan will list the specific marketing strategies you will use one by one and provide a timeline for accomplishment. A budget can then be estimated detailing the cost of each segment of the strategy: labor, printing costs, postage, ad rates, equipment or software requirements, and so on.

If a newsletter, a new reminder system, or targeted letters are part of the strategy, does the budget include subscribing to outsourced services and incorporating design software? If the strategy includes website updating or Facebook or Google ads, who will write, proofread, streamline, brand, and upload the message? Is the budget sufficient to cover the expense, including labor cost?

If new services, such as advanced dental surgery or ultrasound imaging, are to be provided, does the budget include the purchase of the equipment, the continuing education and training for the veterinarians and technicians, and the allocation of hospital space, as well as the promotion of the service to potential clients? If one strategy is to improve personal selling, the allocated time and related payroll budget must include the funds required for team member product and service training and coaching.

When large equipment acquisitions will be made, you might want to calculate a break-even analysis. The break-even analysis is most helpful when the equipment is medically or surgically based. Since the equipment will be used over a long period of time to generate fees from added or improved services, the actual fee structure needed to cover its acquisition and ancillary costs can be estimated from the projected number of transactions produced.

An important step in creating the action plan, and often the most difficult, is to design some system to measure the results of the marketing strategy. If an objective sets a specific, measurable goal, then monitoring the practice's activity in dollars or transaction numbers can give you the answer. For example, if you decide to send a targeted mailing about senior pet exams, the goal might be to increase the number of exams in sixty days to 20 percent over what was achieved in the entire twelve-month period prior to the mailing. You would then count senior exams completed in the prior twelve months and compare this with the exams conducted in the sixty days following the target mailing.

Reminder systems and target letters can be measured by comparing the number of reminders or letters sent with client return rates. It is more difficult to measure the success of newsletters, hospital brochures, advertising, or other promotions, such as open houses. Many times, the only measure will be the level of satisfaction felt by owners and staff, or a rough gauge of success from client feedback.

PLAN EXECUTION

By the time you reach this point, you and the practice owners and other stakeholders have already carried out a number of complex tasks. You have carefully considered and identified the practice mission and goals. You have analyzed the market and set the practice objectives. You have selected marketing strategies and developed an action plan, and you have identified the evaluation methods. You are now ready to execute the plan.

If implementing the plan will require equipment purchases for new services that will be provided, now is the time to purchase them. Negotiation for such purchases may require the oversight of practice owners. You will also need to schedule time for the relevant staff members to learn how to use the equipment and to train the team about how to succinctly explain the new services to clients with a common voice in order to accomplish the plan directives.

If the practice will use consultants, website designers, and the like, you will need to interview providers, and, with practice owners, determine who these people will be. Establish a schedule for each promotional activity, and be sure to keep track of the allocated budget and the results of your efforts from the start.

Hiring a marketing agency may be right for your practice if you feel you need more guidance. Marketing agencies can also execute the plan on your behalf, write copy, design mailings, and so on. Engaging the agency early in the process will increase your success. They can even do the analysis and create the plan.

However, a marketing plan does not have to be a long, time-consuming process to be effective. The following questions can serve as reminders of the essential elements of a marketing plan:

- What are the strengths and weaknesses of the practice now?
- What does the practice want to be?
- What are the opportunities and threats in the surrounding market?
- What do you have to do to move the practice from where it is now to where you envision it being in the future?
- How will you reach your objectives?
- By when will these objectives be accomplished, and who will be involved?
- How will you measure the results?

As you implement the plan, keep the owners and directors updated with periodic reports of progress and outcomes. Adapt the plan as necessary as you learn from experience. Don't keep plowing the same ground if a particular strategy is not yielding results. The market is continually changing, and marketing plans need to be flexible to new ideas and consumer quirks.

Marketing and Data Segmentation

Your computer system should be able to sort clients and patients by a variety of criteria so that you can use targeting marketing to specific groups. As your staff collects more detail, your computer's sorting capacity will increase—that is, it will be able to identify more specific segments and generate more sophisticated target lists from your database. You will know more about your client base and will be able to better identify opportunities and understand client wants, needs, and concerns.

A well-maintained database, with thorough and accurate data collection and input and regular software upgrades, will become the foundation of many of your marketing strategies and implementation. (See also defined database in Glossary.)

Marketing the practice will be an ongoing effort. Your first step should be to make sure your team is united in the mission of the practice. Employees must be well educated and trained to clearly communicate important issues of animal care to existing and potential clients. Personal relationships are probably one of the most important factors leading to referral of the types of clients who best fit with your practice's philosophy of veterinary service delivery.

Nearly as important is practice appearance. Because clients will judge professional aptitude on the basis of what is easily observed, an attractive hospital building, visible signage, a clean reception area, and neatly appointed personnel will indirectly market your practice.

Finally, regular contact with the practice's existing client base is a crucial marketing tool and results in ongoing income generation. Gaining new clients requires great effort and expense. Your existing clients already know the reputation, convenience, and people of your practice. Be attentive to the reminder system, and treat your existing clients with a level of courtesy and respect that will ensure their continued patronage. One way to show this respect is by making sure your clients are fully aware of all the veterinary services your hospital can provide to protect their animals as fully as possible from preventable health problems, with a life-long plan for each.

Glossary

ABC analysis A process for prioritizing or ranking inventory items based on annual usage value, so that inventory management systems can be structured to selectively control prioritized categories of items based on that value.

accounting The process of identifying, measuring, and communicating economic information, often in the form of professionally prescribed and standardized reports, to permit informed judgments and decisions by users of the information, such as practice owners and managers.

accounts payable Bills and vendor liabilities due for payment by the practice as part of the normal course of practice activity; money the practice owes to regular business creditors and practice vendors, and generally accruing from the previous month of supply and service purchases. These accounts may be aged over longer periods depending on vendor contracts and practice ability to meet its debts as they come due. Under international accounting standards, accounts payable are called "creditors."

accounts receivable Debts owed to the veterinary practice, usually from client sales on credit. Accounts receivable are called "debtors" under international accounting standards. Client amounts owed are generally due within thirty days of the invoice date. With each passing day, accounts are said to age. See also aging accounts receivable report.

accrual An expense incurred during an accounting period for which payment is postponed to a later period, or revenue earned during an accounting period for which cash is received in a later period.

accrual basis accounting The accounting method based on recognition of a transaction's occurrence. The method recognizes revenue as income in the period in which it is earned because a transaction occurred (provision of service), regardless of when the client pays. Accrual-based accounting recognizes expenditures in the period in which the liability for paying them is incurred, regardless of when payment is made. See also cash basis accounting; revenue recognition principle; transaction.

accrue To increase gradually, to accumulate, to have due after a period of time.

advertising The paid, public announcement of a persuasive message by a veterinary practice directed to its existing and potential clients.

aging accounts payable report A report that segregates amounts owed to vendors into increments of 30-day periods, based on the number of days from the inception of the practice debt to the date of the report. An aging report can be sorted by individual vendor or by total amount owed to all vendors. Current accounts are less than 30 days old. Accounts payable greater than 30 days old will generally result in finance charges assessed by the vendor to the practice. See also accounts payable.

aging accounts receivable report A report that segregates amounts owed from clients into increments of 30-day periods, based on the number of days from the inception of the client debt to the date of the report. An aging report can be sorted by individual client, by a group of clients, or by practice totals. Current accounts are less than 30 days old. See also accounts receivable.

ambulatory services Veterinary services that are provided at the client's home, farm, or other location where the animals being treated are housed. May also be referred to as a house call or farm call.

annual usage value Annual demand (volume) multiplied by cost.

assets Things of value owned by a business enterprise, such as cash, accounts receivable, and equipment.

attorney (or attorney-at-law) A lawyer (a person who is learned in law) who is licensed to practice law (has passed the bar examination) and is thereby legally empowered to represent or act on behalf of another person within a given jurisdiction. This is somewhat similar to a veterinarian who is empowered to practice veterinary medicine in a specific state by means of licensure in that state. Some lawyers earn a law degree, but do not take and/or pass the bar exam to be licensed to provide legal services. Generally, unlicensed lawyers should not be used for writing a practice's legal documentation (Salzieder 2007, 438).

attorney-in-fact An organization or person formally identified by a taxpayer as his legally authorized representative. For example, the taxpayer may hire a payroll company to prepare all payroll-related tax returns and sign the returns as the taxpayer's legally authorized agent for that specific purpose. See also power of attorney.

at-will employment Terms of employment whereby employees may quit and employers may terminate as a matter of their own preference unless a specific provision in an employment agreement states an agreed-upon duration of employment. There are many exceptions (see Chapter 5).

audit An examination or verification of financial records or accounts by a qualified professional.

audit trail A record of financial transactions from which an accountant can reconstruct the sequence of events.

authoritarian leadership A style of leadership whereby the manager primarily directs the worker, setting goals and objectives; plans and organizes the work to be done; and constantly shows the worker how to do the job. This style is also known as autocratic, directive, or task-oriented leadership. See also participative leadership and democratic leadership.

Automated Clearing House (ACH) An electronic network for processing financial transactions, such as direct deposit payroll and vendor payments. Increasingly, practices are opting to use ACH business-to-business payments for many reasons, including reducing risk of loss from check-fraud schemes.

average transaction charge See client transaction charge.

balance sheet Also referred to as the statement of financial condition, the balance sheet summarizes the assets, liabilities, and owner's equity at a particular date.

balanced scorecard A powerful strategic planning tool that helps managers focus on four vitally important pillars of effective practice management and that supports identification of objectives, goals, and measurements in each of the four areas. The balanced scorecard concept was advanced and popularized by Harvard Business School's Dr. Robert Kaplan and Dr. David Norton in the early 1990s.

behavior wellness The condition or state of normal and acceptable pet conduct that enhances the human-animal bond and the pet's quality of life.

behavior wellness care The planned attention to a pet's conduct and active integration of behavior wellness programs into the delivery of pet-related services, including routine veterinary medical care.

behavior wellness programs Protocols, procedures, services, and systems to educate pet owners and professionals about factors that constitute a behaviorally healthy pet; promote behavior wellness through positive proaction, behavior assessments, early intervention, and timely referrals; and decrease unrealistic human expectations and interpretations of pet behavior that can lead to neglect, euthanasia, or relinquishment (Hetts et al. 2004).

billing charge A charge added to a bill sent to a client to compensate the veterinary practice for the costs of billing when the usual practice policy requires payment at time of services. Full, advance disclosure of billing charges is generally legally required.

biologics A wide range of medicinal products, such as vaccines, blood and blood components, allergenics, gene therapies, and tissues, that are created by biological processes, as distinguished from chemistry.

body condition score (BCS) A method of evaluating fatness and giving a grade on a point scale. The BCS is a tool for managing body weight and one aspect of monitoring an animal's health and overall condition.

bookkeeping The systematic recording of a practice's financial transactions, including sales, purchases, deposits, and payments. See also transaction.

brand The overarching concept, image, and perception of a veterinary practice.

breach of contract A violation of any of the terms of a contract, intentional or not.

business organization The legally prescribed and recognized organizational structure of a business, often called "entity structure" or referred to as "business entity type." Specific federal and state laws regarding the type of business all have bearing in determining the available choice of organizational structures. See also corporation; partnership; sole proprietorship.

buy-sell agreement A legal document describing and defining the events causing a shareholder or partner to sell her interest in a business (a corporation or partnership), and the conditions and terms for resolving those interests with the business entity and other individuals having ownership in it.

cancel In regard to bookkeeping and internal control processes, the act of indelibly marking or otherwise defacing documentation so that is invalidated for reuse. For example, marking a vendor invoice with a "paid" rubber stamp shows that the invoice should not be paid again.

card swipe terminal Electronic equipment used to read the magnetic strips on credit and debit cards and transmit the transaction information to the financial institution for credit authorization and approval. See also point of sale; POS terminal.

CareCredit A company that provides a dedicated health-care credit card to be used specifically for veterinary services; recommended by AAHA.

cash basis accounting An accounting method that measures income when cash is received and expenses when cash is spent. See also accrual basis accounting.

certified veterinary practice manager (CVPM) A designation awarded by the Veterinary Hospital Managers Association for individuals who have proven education and competence in a wide range of veterinary hospital operations and management skills. Proof of experience as well as successful completion of rigorous tests and interviews are required for certification as a CVPM.

chart of accounts A list of the names of the financial accounts a practice uses to record, organize, sort, and report transactions, usually including numeric coding. The list organizes accounts in order of their permanence and appearance in the financial statements: asset accounts, liability accounts, equity accounts, operating revenue accounts, operating expense accounts, nonoperating revenues and gains, and nonoperating expenses and losses.

check verification service A company that helps manage the risk of accepting client payment by check by validating checks presented to the practice and/or using extensive data analytic predictions to statistically assess the level of risk associated with checks, and sometimes including check guarantee protection.

circle sheet See tracking sheet.

client satisfaction survey Survey designed to determine the level of satisfaction provided to the client by the hospital. By offering clients a way to express their opinions, the surveys also serve to indicate that the hospital values client input.

client transaction charge (or average client transaction charge) The average amount of money charged to a client for a single invoice. Compared to the average patient dollar transaction, which refers to the average amount charged per invoice attributable to single patient, average client dollar transactions are often higher because several animals may be invoiced through a single client bill.

cold list A mailing list not previously used by the practice, usually consisting of the names of people who are not currently clients.

compassion fatigue Progressive loss of empathy experienced by caregivers through oversaturation of the senses by disturbing and/or stressful situations, who may describe symptoms of emotional exhaustion, depression, feelings of hopelessness, and constant stress. Compassion fatigue has been described in various aspects of working in the medical professions and in veterinary medicine may be associated with shelter work and with extensive euthanasia of animals without homes and with economic euthanasia.

compilation A standardized, CPA-prepared financial report that presents transactional information provided by management in a prescribed format. A compilation is the representation of management, not of the CPA, and is the most common type of financial statement presentation prepared by CPAs for veterinary businesses. Accounting profession guidelines and rules dictate protocols and presentation requirements for CPA-prepared compilations.

corporation An organization or business formed and authorized by law to act as a single legal person (even though it may be constituted by more than one person) and legally endowed with the various rights and duties of individuals, including the capacity of succession, the right to enter into contracts, and the right to buy and sell property.

cost of professional services (COPS) The direct patient costs associated with producing veterinary service and related revenues. In benchmarking veterinary practices, COPS does not include employee labor costs. It does include drugs, professional supplies, laboratory expenditures, hospital supplies, mortuary costs, and similar expenses that can be traced to a specific patient.

covenant not-to-compete An agreement (generally, a written agreement) in which one party promises not to compete with another party within a prescribed geographical area around the practice and for a given period of time after employment or ownership ends. The second party gives something in return, called consideration. Commonly, veterinarian employment agreements and sales agreements contain covenants not-to-compete. Their purpose is to protect the value of the practice for a period of time by prohibiting competition by a person who has intimate knowledge of the practice's client base and business practices. Covenants not-to-compete must be reasonable as to time and distance and are not enforceable in some states.

curriculum vitae A written overview of a person's life accomplishments and qualifications that elaborates on education to a more comprehensive extent than does a résumé, and is meant to be refreshed regularly for special training, academic credentials, publications, professional contributions, and professional interests. A Latin expression loosely translated as *the course of my life*.

customer vs. client In the context of a veterinary hospital, these are usually synonymous terms, but, as in any profession, "client" is the preferred term to describe the person who has engaged the veterinary practice to provide veterinary services to the client's animal.

defined database An organized collection of specified details that pertain to a particular subject or area of interest, resulting in a database that can be sorted by any of the defined details. A good example is a client database, which would typically require the same information fields to be completed for each client added: first name, middle initial, last name, address, town, state, Zip Code, home telephone number, work telephone number, e-mail address. An electronic address book is another example, with details including first name, last name, company name, address, city, state, country, zip code, phone, fax, and e-mail address.

Defined databases allow data to be sorted and subsorted according to the user's specifications, but the search capacity is only as powerful as the completeness and accuracy of the data.

democratic leadership A style of leadership that encourages workers to participate in the decision-making process by sharing ideas and opinions, while the leader retains power over final decisions. See also authoritarian leadership; participative leadership.

details-person (or drug detail-person) A representative of a company that provides supplies to a veterinary practice, often called "sales representatives" or "sales reps" for short. Pharmacy companies, medical equipment companies, and pet nutrition companies educate their representatives about all aspects of the products offered, so that details-people have a full understanding of each product: how the product works, when to use it, current pricing, available discounts, and so on. These trained employees visit practices and are present at veterinary conferences to explain these important details of product use so that the practice's buying agent can make more educated decisions about acquisition.

diagnostic code In health care, a method for classifying diseases, disorders, clinical signs, and other medical conditions through the use of standardized naming conventions otherwise called "nomenclatures." The purpose of diagnostic codes is to enable computer systems to automate retrieval and categorization of various health issues, leading to better care, such as by evaluating the relative success of one therapy over another for the treatment of a specific disease or condition. In veterinary medicine, AAHA has refined diagnostic code nomenclature to approximately 5,600 clinical signs and diagnostic terms commonly used in companion animal practices. Also see SNOMED.

DICOM (Digital Imaging and Communications in Medicine) A technology standard established to ensure that medical image data files would include patient information that could not accidently be separated from the patient image, and that would allow images to be universally shared easily among devices that create, transmit, and view them. See also PACS.

differential diagnosis One of several possible etiologies or causes of observed health conditions identified by signs, symptoms, examination, and laboratory findings. Listing possible differential diagnoses helps in the process of choosing tests to narrow possibilities to a definitive cause, or definitive diagnosis.

digital image technology Computer technology that allows images to be made, stored, transmitted between computers, and re-created for viewing. In veterinary medicine, digital image technology is an effective and efficient means of documenting case progression, obtaining diagnostic information (radiographs, ultrasound, endoscopic, and laparoscopic images), and rapidly transmitting this data over long distances. It also makes possible compact storage of what would otherwise be voluminous printed documentation.

direct costing A cost accounting method in which cost of a product or service is determined by allocating to it the variable (direct) costs attributed to it. Direct costing treats practice fixed costs as overhead and does not apply them to sales units.

directive behavior See authoritarian leadership.

disability As defined under the Americans with Disabilities Act (ADA), a physical or mental impairment that substantially limits one or more of the major life activities of an individual.

disbursement journal A bookkeeping record that chronologically records expenditures made. In modern electronic veterinary bookkeeping, the disbursement journals are integrated through software with other aspects of the practice's accounting for receipts, investment in equipment, payroll, debts, and other transactions.

discrimination As defined by the Civil Rights Act of 1964, discrimination is the failure or refusal to hire, the discharge, or the prejudicial treatment of any individual with respect to compensation, terms, conditions, or privileges of employment because of such individual's color, religion, sex, or national origin. Under federal law, the definition has been extended to include disability, pregnancy, and age, and state law may include additional conditions, such as sexual orientation.

display ad A purchased advertisement designed to attract new business to the hospital, generally including artwork or graphic information. May be found in the yellow pages or in a newspaper or magazine.

doctor medical notes Notations made by the veterinarian in the patient record describing physical examination findings, patient assessment, treatment plans, surgical procedures, and other aspects of patient care.

economic euthanasia Generally, the euthanasia of a healthy animal that an owner cannot or will not support financially or of an animal with a medical condition that the client chooses not to treat. Economic euthanasia is emotionally and mentally challenging to veterinarians and employees and can contribute to compassion fatigue and burnout.

economic order quantity (EOQ) formula A mathematical formula that allows calculation of optimal order quantities. The EOQ formula recognizes three specific costs incurred in ordering and holding drug and professional supply inventory: (1) the unit cost, (2) the ordering cost, and (3) the holding cost.

The economic order quantity formula determines the optimum quantity of any one item to be ordered each time an order is placed, when the demand for the item is constant. This formula is:

$$EOQ = Economic\ ordering\ quantity$$

where:

$$A = Annual\ demand\ in\ units$$
$$F = Fixed\ ordering\ costs\ incurred\ per\ order$$
$$H = Holding\ costs\ expressed\ on\ an\ annual\ basis\ as\ a\ percentage\ of\ unit\ cost$$
$$UC = Unit\ cost\ to\ purchase\ item\ from\ vendor\ or\ supplier$$

economies of scale A business consolidation concept that suggests that increased profits can be realized through better use of underutilized assets, such as equipment or skilled employees, by combining disparate economic units (e.g., separately owned but similar types of veterinary practices) to create more transactional volume over a given period of time. Increased profits occur by reducing the fixed cost per transaction.

emotional intelligence (EI) A variety of psychological theories that describe the capabilities and/or developed skills people use to identify, assess, understand, and control emotions, of oneself, of others, and of groups of people.

employee A person engaged by another or by an organization to provide labor and services, usually in exchange for wages or salary. Under the rules of the Internal Revenue Service, an individual is an employee if the person or organization for whom the individual performs the service has the right to control and direct that individual as to the results to be accomplished by the work and as to the details and means by which the result is accomplished. See also independent contractor.

employee stock ownership plan Plan that provides employees with an opportunity to own stock in the company where they are employed. The company would generally be organized as a corporation, and the plan would require that contributions be invested into securities of the sponsoring corporation as an employee benefit.

employment agreement or employment contract The legal relationship between an employer and an employee, which may or may not be in writing. Under contract law principles, three elements underlie the formal relationship between employee and employer: offer, acceptance, and consideration.

employment practices liability insurance (EPLI) A type of insurance that provides coverage for claims arising out of employment practices—any type of employment process that involves selection in hiring, promoting, terminating, or related functions. The types of claims against which EPLI provides coverage include wrongful termination, discrimination, and sexual harassment.

environmental scan A strategic planning activity that involves analysis of the practice in relation to its external environment and how various factors such as competition and regulations might develop in the future to affect the practice. Also known as situational analysis.

equity Rights or claims to the properties or assets of the veterinary practice. Owner's equity is what the practice owes its owners: the amounts the owners have invested in the business plus the profits that have been retained in the business and that are owed to the owners. Also called capital.

ergonomics The study of the physical aspects of work. In the context of the Occupational Safety and Health Administration, ergonomics focuses on how the work is performed to determine whether workers are at risk of developing cumulative trauma or musculoskeletal disorders.

essential functions A complete list of the duties expected to be performed by an employee. The list should include not only skilled or specialized duties but also physical duties, including the amount of time and stress involved.

exam-room report cards A written summary report, usually in checklist format, of the veterinarian's findings during patient physical examination. The report findings are usually grouped according to bodily systems or areas examined (such as oral cavity, eyes, skin, musculoskeletal system, skin and hair, etc.). The exam-room report card is given to the client as a source of useful, easy-to-understand information about the patient, but it can also be included in the permanent patient record maintained by the hospital. When problems are noted during the physical examination, specific recommendations can be noted on the report card to reinforce verbally communicated information.

exit interview Interview between an employer and a departing employee, conducted in part to determine why the employee is leaving the employment, regardless of the circumstances, and to gather other information that may be helpful in the ongoing effort to improve the veterinary practice and the employment experience.

experiential knowledge "Hands-on" experience, skills, and knowledge gained by employees in the performance of their jobs.

external marketing Marketing that introduces the practice to potential clients and aims to convince them to use the veterinary practice's services. Direct mailings to new people in the area, a yellow pages ad, or a newspaper ad are examples of external marketing.

financial control Systems and protocols for ensuring the management and protection of monetary and investment aspects of the veterinary practice. These controls are framed by the protocols, policies, and activities that ensure that the practice's accounting system is strong and intact. Good systems provide safeguards against loss and theft and ensure that records are accurate, with transactional information collected and recorded in a consistent manner in each accounting period. See also internal controls.

financial statement A type of business report that presents financial information about the economic impact on the entity of completed transactions and other events. General-purpose financial statements for external use report financial information relevant to (1) investors, (2) creditors, and (3) public policy decision makers. The most commonly used financial statements include the statement of financial position (also know as the balance sheet or the statement of assets, liabilities, and equity), the statement of income (also known as the statement of revenues and expenses or the profit and loss statement), and the statement of cash flows. Terminology can be confusing because common vernacular use often differs from the nomenclature prescribed by accounting profession standards, which has very specific application and meaning.

five-force analysis A strategic planning activity described by Michael Porter of Harvard Business School that organizes the practice's evaluation of the external environment and its opportunities and threats.

fixed asset Tangible assets of a durable nature, which are expected to help generate revenue over a period of a year or longer. Property and equipment are examples of fixed assets that would not normally be intended for sale and that are used repetitively for the production of veterinary service revenues.

fixed cost (or fixed expense) An expense that tends to remain constant in monetary amount, regardless of variations in the volume of activity. For example, the amount of electricity used (purchased) is approximately the same on any two days of business operations even if ten patients are seen on one day and twenty are seen on the other. See also variable cost.

flat fee A fixed fee for services rendered, as opposed to charging by the hour or based on a percentage of the service.

formulary A veterinary formulary is a list of medicines used for animal treatment, generally including clinical information such as dosages, side effects, and contraindications. From a practice management perspective, a practice specific formulary helps streamline the practice's in-house inventory of stocked supplies and defines which will be kept on hand as compared to scripted by the veterinarians for preparation by an outside pharmacy.

freight on board (FOB) Describes typical points in transfer of ownership title from a vendor to the purchaser. FOB shipping point means that title transfers as supplies are loaded to the shipping carrier at the vendor location, while FOB destination means that ownership title to the shipment occurs when the carrier unloads it at the purchaser's location.

401K plan A retirement savings plan based on employer and employee contributions and investment earnings. The employer may promise a defined contribution for each employee, but no exact benefit is promised at retirement. The employee must meet certain requirements to be eligible for inclusion in the plan.

full absorption analysis or costing A cost analysis that not only considers the directly assignable costs of the product or service, but also matches other overhead costs of operation (e.g., utilities, rent, administrative and personnel costs) with the units of product or service. This method is intended to ensure that all incurred costs are recovered from the selling price of a service or product. See also direct costing.

full-time equivalency (FTE) A term describing the hours worked by one person working full time to fulfill the requirements of a particular job position for one year. FTEs are a useful measurement when at least some employees in a practice work part time. For example, we can figure the number of FTEs for a practice that employs five veterinarians, some on a part-time basis. Let's assume that full-time is defined as 45 hours per week, or 2,340 hours per year. The total number of work hours required to fulfill the duties and responsibilities of all veterinary activities in this practice is 7,956. To find the number of FTEs for this practice, divide the total hour requirement (7,956) by the defined number of full-time hours that constitute an FTE (in this case, 2,340). The practice has 2.4 veterinarian FTEs.

Note that there is no specific number of hours that established or accepted as industry standard for an FTE for doctors of veterinary medicine or for practice managers. Many consultants and managers hold that a professional should expect to devote 45 to 50 hours per week on average. For support staff, full-time is usually based on a 40-hour workweek, or 2,080 hours per year. Therefore, if the practice budgets for 6,000 hours of technician time, 2.88 veterinary nurse FTEs are needed.

general ledger The complete and permanent chronological record of all of a practice's transactions, organized by financial accounts, that summarizes other supporting journals, such as those listing details of sales, cash receipts, and cash disbursements.

gross profit For a specific item, the difference between revenue realized by and the cost of selling a product (like dog food or a drug). In veterinary practice, gross profit reflects the mix of services and product sales and appears on the income statement, as the difference of revenues (fee income) and cost of professional services. See also cost of professional services.

gross revenue The veterinary practice's total operating income, before any deductions for discounts, account write-offs, or operating expenses, and without adding other sources of cash, such as consumer sales tax collections and nonoperating income. See also operating income.

Hazardous Communication Standard A standard adopted by the Occupational Safety and Health Administration that requires all employers to develop prescribed programs to ensure that all employees are aware of the existence of hazardous materials in their workplace and are trained in their use.

holding cost The cumulative costs of owning and keeping inventory on the premises in anticipation of its future use during service provision or its sale to clients.

human resources Collectively, the employees of a business who provide the services for which they were employed.

imprest An adjective describing a fund or cash reserve that is maintained at a constant level for lengthy periods of time. A petty cash fund and cashier's drawers are examples of imprest funds that are regularly restored to their original cash balances.

inbound processes Part of the value chain framework for strategic and tactical planning, these are the operational activities related to the mechanics of establishing appointments and admitting clients and patents to the hospital. Identification and memorialization of all aspects of the inbound process allows a manager to establish concrete goals, train to those goals, and assess performance of team members.

incentive program Compensation arrangement by which employees who successfully convince the client to purchase services or products receive a bonus or percentage of revenue earned.

income A gain or recurrent benefit, usually measured in money, that derives from capital or labor. Veterinary hospital income results from services and products purchased by clients. See also accrual basis accounting; cash basis accounting; revenue.

income journal A bookkeeping record that chronologically records transactions related to sales and other sources of revenues, such as rent and interest. Like disbursement and payroll journals, income or receipt journals may be integrated within the electronic bookkeeping programs now used by the majority of veterinary practices.

income statement A type of financial report that presents the total income earned and expenditures made for a specific period of time. When income for the period exceeds expenses, a profit occurs. When expenses exceed income for the period measured, a loss occurs. The period of time can span one day, one month, one calendar or fiscal quarter, a full year, or another time frame that gives management the information it wishes to examine. The terms "profit and loss report," "P & L," and "statement of revenues and expenses" all have similar meanings, but very specific meanings and nuanced differences to accountants and the financial industry, which are beyond the scope of this book.

independent contractor An individual who is contracted to perform a service but who, based on the unique set of facts and circumstances, does not meet the criteria that define an employee as described by the Internal Revenue Service. Payments made to an independent contractor are generally not subject to payroll tax withholding, as is the case with an employee, but the independent contractor is required to attest to exemption from backup tax withholding by the veterinary practice on a Form W-9, and total payments to the contractor are reported annually on a Form 1099. See also employee.

informed consent A person's agreement to allow something to happen, such as a medical diagnostic or surgical procedure, that is based on full disclosure of the facts necessary to make an intelligent decision (Scott 2007, 442). Although this is a common doctrine of human medicine, the preferred veterinary terminology for informing the client and obtaining consent to proceed with care is called owner consent.

inpatient A patient receiving medical care within the hospital.

internal controls All measures, systems, and protocols used by a business to prevent errors, waste, and fraud; to ensure the reliability of accounting data; and to promote compliance with all company policies. See also financial control.

internal marketing Marketing that concentrates on existing clients, aiming to strengthen their bond with the practice and to increase their demand for veterinary services. Sending letters to existing clients about the benefits of twice annual physical exams for older pets is a good example of internal marketing.

Internal Revenue Code (IRC) Law passed by the U.S. Congress and subsequent regulations created under that law and through which the Internal Revenue Service functions with regard to taxation of individuals and businesses.

interstate commerce "Commercial trade, business, movement of goods or money, or transportation from one state to another, regulated by the federal government according to powers spelled out in Article I of the Constitution," and, "theoretically . . . by the Interstate Commerce Commission (ICC), under authority granted by the Interstate Commerce Act, first enacted by Congress in 1887" (The Free Dictionary by Farlex, http://legal-dictionary.thefreedictionary.com/interstate+commerce).

inventory All goods owned and held for sale or use in the regular course of business. See also perpetual inventory; physical inventory.

job description An outline of the definition of a job, listing the special skills required, the essential duties and responsibilities involved, and the relevant bounds of authority in the veterinary hospital.

jurisdiction The geographical area over which a court or government body has the power and right to exercise authority in accord with laws and regulations.

just-in-time pricing A method of pricing that adjusts the sales price of an item as contemporaneously as possible to the sale, based on its most current replacement acquisition cost and regardless of how much was originally paid for that item.

key performance indicator (KPI) Also called key success indicator, an industry jargon term for any metric or measurement that is deemed important to monitor for evaluation of the practice's success in meeting objectives and goals.

key person loss The loss of a practice employee or owner whose role in the practice unit is so important that the loss causes prolonged financial detriment to the practice. Loss can occur through death, retirement, resignation, disability, divorce, or another reason. The more sudden the loss, the more devastating the financial impact.

laid off Temporarily suspended or permanently terminated from employment due to business causes, such as seasonal business demand fluctuation or economic downturn and financial decline. Termination of employment through lay-off implies there is no fault of the employee, while termination by firing occurs due to cause, such as employee performance failure or gross misconduct.

lead time The time between ordering and receiving a particular inventory SKU, also known as delivery time. The longer the lead time, the greater the quantity of items that must be on hand when the order is placed with the vendor (reorder point).

liabilities Present obligations resulting from past transactions that require the practice to pay money, provide goods, or perform services in the future.

loan covenant Clauses in a written document of borrowing that requires the borrower to do, or refrain from doing, certain things. Protective covenants define terms and conditions the borrower must fulfill in order to satisfy the lender's concerns about the risks it has taken in lending. The higher the lender's perceived risk, the more restrictive the covenant requirements, which generally define several areas: the minimum level of practice working capital, amounts of insurance coverage, adherence to repayment schedules, and periodic financial reporting requirements to the lender. In the event a borrower does not comply with the loan covenants, the lender can call the loan, requiring it to be immediately paid in full.

lunch and learn A training or light educational event, usually held over the lunch hour for about forty-five minutes, where food is brought in to feed attendees. They can be volunteer events and are generally not meetings that must be documented to the employee, such as workplace safety training. In veterinary practices, the meetings are most often led by a vendor representative (pharmaceutical company, supplier, or equipment vendor) who provides pizza or other fun food and gives the presentation. Lunch and learns are usually focused on jazzing up employees about something interesting in patient care and/or client service.

macroeconomics A branch of economics that examines aggregate market perspectives (regional, national, and global) of production, distribution, and consumption of goods and services, and upon which models and forecasts are developed to assist in policy and business strategy formation and evaluation.

malpractice A dereliction of professional duty or a failure to exercise an accepted degree of professional skill or learning by someone (e.g., a veterinarian) rendering professional services that results in injury, loss, or damage.

malpractice suit A legal complaint against a veterinarian or veterinary hospital based on actions that allegedly resulted in patient injury or death or based on indications that the professionals involved did not exercise the care and diligence ordinarily exercised by skilled veterinarians.

marketing Techniques and activities used for finding and keeping clients, increasing public awareness of a need for veterinary services, advertising products and services available, and enhancing the image and reputation of the practice in community.

medical history Past and current information about a patient that is useful in formulating a diagnosis and in planning and providing medical care, both from a preventive standpoint and from the perspective of treating diagnosed abnormal conditions. Medical history can be collected by forms and interviews with the patient's owner and by observations recorded from previous interactions with the patient.

metadata Called "data about data," the term has two different meanings that are both applicable to veterinary practices. The first is related to descriptive information about what is in an electronic file, such as the client and patient information that links to an image file and identifies it. The second kind of metadata is information related not to the specifics of what is in the file but to important facts about the file, such as when it was created and the computer language it was written in and the last time it was modified, such as for an electronic medical record. The first kind of metadata is like the label on a manila folder that explains what the file is used for and what is in it, and the second kind of metadata is analogous to information about the weight and type of paper stock, the size of the folder, its color, and when it was manufactured.

mission statement An inspiring description of the practice's purpose and primary objectives that defines key measures of the practice's success, directed primarily to guide the practice's leadership in the decisions they make in their service to shareholders, employees, and clients. See vision statement.

Modified Accelerated Cost Recovery System (MACRS) The current mandatory depreciation method required by U.S. federal regulation for most tangible depreciable property (equipment, furniture, signs, computer hardware, buildings, and improvements) placed in service after December 31, 1986. MACRS depreciation does not accurately reflect the actual useful lives of assets purchased and placed in service in a veterinary hospital.

negligence Neglectful or heedless behavior; doing something that a person of ordinary prudence would not have done under similar circumstances. Negligence in the context of a veterinary hospital primarily relates to business and medical practices that can result in injury to clients, patients, and/or others on the premises.

negotiable instrument A paper document that can move freely in financial transactions as a substitute for money, such as a check.

on-boarding The planned and executed process of welcoming, orienting, and training a new employee.

one-write system A bookkeeping system that utilizes overlapping carbonless papers to record the same transaction to several records simultaneously. For example, a one-write check recording system results in a permanent record of the payee, amount, check number, and other information within a ledger at the same time the check is prepared for remittance to the payee. A one-write receipting system results in a ledger entry of specific information about a specific sale at the same time a receipt is completed to give to the client.

operating income Revenues or income resulting from veterinary activities and veterinary-related sales, such as pharmacy sales. Operating income does not include income from sources other than veterinary-related, such as interest income, income from selling used practice equipment, subleasing retail space, and the like. See also gross revenue.

ordering cost The cumulative costs of negotiating for and obtaining inventories of various supplies required for practice operations, not including the actual cost of the supplies themselves. Ordering costs do not include sales tax or freight charges incurred when a purchase transaction occurs.

out-of-line expenditure Practice expenses are grouped into general categories, such as postage, office supplies, advertising, and laboratory supplies. An out-of-line expenditure is an expense category amount that exceeds or falls short of the projected amount based on comparison to other practices or national or regional benchmarks.

outpatient A patient being treated at home or at a farm or stable after examination and diagnosis is made by the doctor, generally in the hospital.

owner consent A client's agreement to allow veterinary care to be given to his animal that is based on full disclosure of the facts necessary to make an intelligent decision and involves a process of providing medical findings and treatment recommendations to the client, including disclosure of possible adverse outcomes and reasonable estimated cost of care. See also informed consent.

PACS (picture archiving and communication system) PACS is a medical imaging technology which provides economical storage of, and access to, digital images from different sources and machine types, such as digital radiography, ultrasonography, and magnetic resonance imaging. PACS appliances for local integration with the veterinary practice information management system (VPIMS) or remote application use and storage (through a "cloud"-based application service provider) use the universal format for electronic storage and transfer called DICOM (Digital Imaging and Communications in Medicine).

participative leadership A style of leadership whereby the manager listens to the problems of the worker; praises and encourages the worker; and asks for suggestions. This style is also known as supportive or relationship oriented. See also authoritarian leadership and democratic leadership.

partnership A legally recognized association of two or more persons who are co-owners and joint principals in a for-profit business. Ownership may be divided equally or unequally. Partnership can be classified as general or limited, depending on the relationships agreed to by the partners, both to each other and to the partnership, and on state statute (limited partnerships must be allowed by state law and require state filing). Most typically, veterinary partnerships are general partnerships, wherein each partner shares in management and has unlimited personal liability.

patient-health pocket records A type of commercially available pet health record that is given to the client to keep track of the animal's vaccination history, parasite-control medications, surgery dates and events, and so forth. Usually these records are imprinted with the practice name, address, telephone number, and other practice information.

patient record A record of all information pertaining to the medical history, diagnostic processes, and treatment provided to a single animal. It may or may not include financial data. There are various forms of patient records (see Chapter 8).

patient tracking sheet (or patient service tracker [PST]) See tracking sheet.

payroll journal A bookkeeping record that chronologically records transactions related to payment of employees, employee taxes, employer payroll taxes, and various amounts withheld from employee pay, such as employee copayment of health insurance premiums, garnishments, and voluntary retirement contributions.

performance evaluation An employee evaluation that provides the hospital manager with the information necessary for measuring the employee's job performance and giving constructive feedback for improvement.

perpetual inventory Inventory system that can provide accurate, up-to-date detail at any time because items are added to inventory records as soon as they are received and are subtracted from inventory records as soon as they are sold or used.

petty cash Imprest cash fund maintained for minor expenditures. Petty cash improves the practice's internal controls by providing a system for tracing cash expenditures and eliminating such cash disbursements from the daily receipts. Major expenditures should always be made by means other than cash (check, credit card, electronic fund transfer).

physical inventory The accounting for all items of inventory on hand at a given time, accomplished by performing an actual count of each item.

point of sale (POS) In the context of veterinary practice, the location a sales transaction is completed, such as the receptionist-cashier's checkout desk. Increasingly, technology is used to process transactions at the point of sale, such as with credit/debit card terminals and check-swiping equipment. See also POS terminal.

POS terminal An electronic device that provides an interface between the practice cashier and the Internet for processing client payments. See also card swipe terminal.

power of attorney A legal instrument authorizing someone to act as the attorney or agent of the grantor, and generally authorizing the actions to a specific purpose.

practice act A state's or commonwealth's law, codified into regulations, describing what licensed and nonlicensed employees can and cannot do as such activities pertain to the practice of veterinary medicine.

pretax benefits Employee benefits paid by the employer, such as health insurance premiums, that are identified by law and not subject to employment taxes. Qualified pretax benefits provide a valid and legal deduction to the employer and provide a specified, nontaxable benefit to the employee. If the benefit were not provided by the employer, the employee might have to buy that benefit personally with net wages available after various employment taxes were deducted.

privity of contract The mutual and unique legal relationship of each party to an agreement, recognizing their individual rights and duties to the agreement. It does not generally confer rights to or impose obligations on anyone other than the contracting parties.

problem list A part of the medical record that summarizes each patient abnormality identified by professional staff (e.g., not eating; diarrhea; weight loss; discharge, right eye; overgrown toenails). The problems noted might be related as part of a single disease process or not related at all. Each problem indicates a need for further assessment and a treatment plan for resolution.

problem-oriented medical records (POMR) A record that is chronologically ordered according to each identified health problem. The POMR links all record information to various patient health problems as they arise, are identified, and are resolved or managed.

procurement The planned acquisition of appropriate goods and/or services at the optimum total cost of ownership to meet the needs of the practice in terms of quality, quantity, time, and location.

profit and loss statement See income statement.

promotion The act of demonstrating to a client the quality and benefits of a certain service or product in order to differentiate your practice from others and to build a positive practice image.

publicity Information about a practice or other entity conveyed through the media, be that newspaper, radio, or television. Unlike public relations, publicity is initiated by a third party and can be positive or negative. See also public relations.

public relations Marketing tools initiated by a practice to reach current or prospective clients. The public relations tools most commonly used by veterinary practices are news releases or press releases, which are specialized documents that convey news about a veterinary hospital to the media. Other public relations tools include practice newsletters, the practice website, a brochure, and hospital tours or speaking engagements in the community. See also publicity.

purchase order The form issued by the purchasing department to document and order inventory items from a supplier, including supplies, merchandise, equipment, or any other purchased item. Purchase orders can also be generated when the hospital purchases services, such as routine copier maintenance. The form indicates the date of order, desired items, quantity, and quoted price.

qualified fringe benefit A form of pay in exchange for the performance of service that is explicitly excluded from taxation through federal tax law as written in the Internal Revenue Code and related tax regulations. Unless the law specifically excludes a fringe benefit from taxation , it must be included in the recipient's pay subject to tax withholding.

qualified person with a disability As defined by the Americans with Disabilities Act, this is an individual who satisfies the skill, experience, education, and other job-related requirements of the position such individual holds or desires, and who, with or without the assistance of a reasonable accommodation, can perform the essential functions of such position. See also reasonable accommodation.

quality assurance A program for the systematic monitoring and evaluation of the various aspects of a project, service, or facility to ensure that preestablished standards of quality are being met.

quality control An aggregate of activities (such as design and system analysis and inspection for defects) designed to ensure adequate quality of services offered and provided to clients and patients.

realized revenues Revenues that are or will be collected because all events have occurred that establish the practice's legal right of receipt from the client.

reasonable accommodation As defined by the Americans with Disabilities Act, a modification or adjustment to a job or to the work environment that enables a qualified applicant or employee with a disability to participate in the application process or to perform the job. See also qualified person with a disability.

remittance information Information accompanying payment that informs the vendor which invoices are being paid, including the customer account number, invoice number(s), and so on.

reorder point (ROP) The time at which the purchasing manager places a restock order with the vendor. Reorder point is determined by the SKU quantity that will meet predicted normal operating needs until the restocking supplies arrive on premises (also called lead time) plus the selected emergency stock quantity (safety stock) . Reorder point quantity equals safety-stock plus lead-time quantity.

requisition order The form used by employees for requesting purchase of a supply, pharmacologic agent, equipment item, or service, such as maintenance or repair.

résumé A written record of the goals, education, work history, other accomplishments, activities, and references presented by an individual applying for an employment position.

revenue The income from goods sold and services rendered during a given period of time, equal to the inflow of cash and receivables from sales made during that period. See also realized revenues.

revenue recognition principle An accounting concept wherein a revenue transaction is marked at the moment the revenue is earned, regardless of when cash is ultimately received for services or products provided. See also accrual basis accounting.

review The second level of CPA financial statement presentation, which involves more analytic review and cross-checking of account balances than does the compilation report, and unlike the compilation report, provides a minimum level of assurance to the reader. CPA-reviewed financial statements are commonly required by lending institutions as part of the terms for loaning money to a veterinary practice. This higher level of CPA attestation requires more in-depth transactional analysis and work by the CPA. See also compilation.

RFID Radio-frequency identification is tracking and identification technology using radio waves. In veterinary practice, RFID is the underlying technology for animal identification microchipping. It is also used for controlling access and securing areas (for example, in key fobs and key-fob readers that activate door-locking mechanisms). It may also supplant bar-reading technology for inventory management in the future.

running charge An up-to-date, cumulative tally of services provided to and supplies consumed by a hospitalized patient. Given this convenient record of current charges, the client is better able to make informed decisions about electing additional procedures and care. Eventually, the running charge will be completely tallied when an invoice is closed. New charges then begin to accumulate that will be totaled in the next completed invoice.

safety stock The minimum quantity of an inventory SKU that is held as a protection against shortages due to higher than expected use between placing an order and receiving it. Safety-stock quantity plus delivery-time quantity equals the reorder-point quantity.

salary and wage pool An amount of money budgeted for a certain period of future time to cover salary and wages for a group of employees. The salary and wage pool is valuable for planning hourly wage rates, employee work schedules, and new employee acquisition.

script out Abbreviated practice jargon to describe the writing of a prescription for a drug or medication that the client will purchase elsewhere. Many drugs and medications require a licensed veterinarian's authorization and directions for use, but the veterinary practice may not maintain stocks of those items. In these cases, a prescription is prepared by the veterinarian, and the client uses this written authorization to purchase the item from a pharmacy or other supply outlet.

search engine optimization (SEO) The process of improving a website's visibility using unpaid algorithmic search results.

seasonal marketing program A program that increases client knowledge about practice services that are more frequently required during specific times of the year. For example, heartworm testing and prevention and flea prevention medications are usually marketed before mosquito and flea season, and seasonal marketing programs are often planned for National Pet Dental Month in February of each calendar year.

seed capital The initial money investment necessary to start up a practice that allows it to cover initial operating expenses as well as equipment, technology, and organizational cost.

selective inventory control A materials management system that methodically ranks the importance and value of items used by business processes to enable application of different levels of control (time and money). See also ABC analysis.

service industry The segment of all industry primarily involved in providing services rather than products to clients.

service write-off See write-off.

sexual harassment Unwelcome verbal or physical conduct of a sexual nature on the job. Quid pro quo sexual harassment is defined as unwelcome sexual conduct in which submission to or rejection of such conduct by an individual is used as the basis of employment decisions affecting the individual. Environmental sexual harassment includes unwelcome sexual conduct that unreasonably interferes with the individual's job performance or creates an intimidating, hostile, or offensive working environment.

shipping document Vendor document included with ordered items shipped to the veterinary practice. The shipping document presents details of the size, strength, and quantity of the shipped items in addition to other important information.

shrinkage Inventory loss, usually unexplained or difficult to isolate. Sales records and original purchase quantities are compared with the current physical inventory to determine the amount of shrinkage; when the physical counts are less than the documented amounts, inventory shrinkage has occurred.

situational analysis A strategic planning step. See also environmental scan.

slotted safe A safe with a deposit slot. When the safe is locked, items can be deposited through the slot, but they cannot be removed. Usually locked with a key, combination, or pass card.

SMART goals A useful acronym to remember when establishing inspirational objectives for the practice team. Such target goals are defined using five parameters that must be included in their description: Specific, Measurable, Attainable, Relevant, and Time-limited.

SNOMED (Systematized Nomenclature of Medicine) In health care, a comprehensive system for classifying diseases, disorders, clinical signs, and other medical conditions through the use of standardized naming conventions otherwise called nomenclatures. SNOMED CT is a nomenclature of clinical terms (CT) that allows computer processing of clinical data groups such as diseases and signs. It can be used to record as codes the clinical details of individual patients in electronic medical records. If consistently applied to every patient encounter and recorded, it should reduce variability in how data is encoded and used for clinical care of patients and in research. Also see diagnostic code.

sole proprietorship A form of business organization in which only one owner has any financial or legal interest. The owner has unlimited personal liability.

source document An accounting term that describes the originating record of details supporting and substantiating a transaction. Some examples include canceled checks, voided checks, cash register slips, deposit slips, invoices, packing slips, loan documents, financial reports, and tax returns.

specialization (or specialty) Certification in advanced veterinary medical knowledge. A doctor of veterinary medicine who has completed advanced scientific education and rigorous training in recognized bodies of knowledge may obtain certification as specializing in the specific tested area of study. Pursuant to American Veterinary Medical Association (AVMA) ethical guidelines, only specialty organizations that are members of the AVMA American Board of Veterinary Specialties (ABVS) may award certification in a specialty to a qualified veterinarian. Such certified doctors are allowed to call themselves "specialists." Otherwise, veterinarians who have concentrated their careers in specific areas of focus, such as a particular species, may only say that they have "special interests in" the described areas. See AVMA website for more information about board specialties and ethical considerations.

statement of cash flow Financial statement detailing inflows and outflows of cash between two points in time.

statement of revenues and expenses See income statement.

stock-keeping unit (SKU) An item of inventory or stock that is completely specified as to function, style, size, color, and usually location and assigned a unique code or number for purposes of inventory tracking and management. For pharmacy items, the stock keeping unit might be a single capsule or tablet at a given strength, for example, or one milliliter of injectable solution, that an inventory system can accurately track as to resupply and depletion with each and every related transaction. The SKU code or number is assigned by the individual hospital through its inventory management system. For a perpetual inventory management system to accurately track all stock, every variation of a given product must have a unique SKU code or number assigned to it so that even very similar items are distinguished from one another.

stock-out The event of running out of a supply item before the next order arrives.

strategic planning The formalized process of defining a practice's vision, mission, and future course of action and aligning resources such as money, equipment, and people to achieve these purposes and objectives.

supportive behavior See participative leadership.

SWOT analysis A strategic planning technique that analyzes the practice's internal strengths and weaknesses and external opportunities and threats.

tangible property Physical assets, such as buildings, inventory, and equipment.

ten key An adding machine used by cashiers, bookkeepers, and accountants to quickly tally long lists of numbers, and providing an option for printing to a narrow roll of paper to create a printed tape used as a proofing mechanism for bank deposit totals, among other number lists.

Theory X A management theory popularized by Douglas McGregor that assumes that people prefer to be directed, are not interested in assuming responsibility, and are motivated primarily by financial incentives and the threat of punishment. See also Theory Y.

Theory Y A management theory popularized by Douglas McGregor that assumes that people can be self-directed and creative at work, if properly supported and motivated. Motivation can come from individual desire for recognition, from a sense of self-worth and pride, and from an interest in work well done. See also Theory X.

tickler system An electronic or manual method of keeping dates that cues a practice manager when tasks should be completed; a reminder methodology facilitating follow-through on specific parts of a project.

tracking sheet A printed list of coded services and products that provides a way of identifying completed services and dispensed items when preparing the invoice. Typically a user will highlight or circle codes on the list to identify the services or medications provided to a particular patient. Also called a patient service tracker (PST) or circle sheet, the tracking sheet is a valuable source of information about the recommended services and completed procedures that should be paid for by the client.

trade account payable Amount owed to a vendor. See accounts payable.

trade account receivable Amount owed from a client. See accounts receivable.

transaction 1. (usual practice management usage) The process of providing a service or product and receiving revenue in return. 2. (accounting definition) Any exchange of or binding promise to exchange goods, services, or money at a sum certain (that can be measured in monetary units).

undue hardship As defined by the Americans with Disabilities Act, significant difficulty, disruption of business, or expense that would be incurred by a business entity if it were to provide a reasonable accommodation. See also reasonable accommodation.

unit cost The amount paid to a vendor for an item of inventory, including applicable sales taxes and shipping costs, divided by the quantity of the item ordered. See also stock-keeping unit.

value chain A powerful analysis tool for strategic planning and goal setting, originating as a management concept developed and advanced by Michael Porter, that describes the series of activities an organization conducts, with each stage adding value to the final product or service outcome.

value proposition Part of a business strategy involving a practice promise to the client that gives convincing reasons for purchasing services and/or products, and serving to differentiate the practice's offerings from those of the competition, through two primary attributes: price and quality. A service or product must be superior in price and/or quality in order to sustain sales in the face of competition.

variable cost (or variable expense) An expense that directly and proportionately fluctuates in amount in relation to the volume of activity. For example, for each canine distemper vaccination procedure, one dose of vaccine must be used. The cost of total vaccine doses used increases proportionately with each vaccination sale. See also fixed cost.

variance A difference between the physical count of an item and the count as calculated from the records maintained for that item. A positive variance indicates that there is more of the physically counted item than a perpetually maintained record indicates there should be. A negative variance indicates that the physical count is less than the recorded count. Any variance suggests a system weakness or problem.

vendor invoice A document sent by a supplying vendor to the practice describing the products or services provided and listing the cost per item, quantity, and other information. In general, a vendor invoice is sent separately from the product shipment or service provision directly to the practice's bookkeeping department.

vendor statement A document sent once a month by a vendor to the practice that lists all of the invoices that have been completed during that month.

veterinary hospital vs. veterinary clinic Generally speaking, a facility with overnight hospitalization provisions is a hospital; one without these provisions is a clinic.

veterinary practice information management system (VPIMS) The network of computer hardware, human interface devices, operating systems, and software written specifically for running the veterinary practice operations, including client invoicing, patient reminder notifications, and medical records functions. To centralize and organize data for optimal efficiency, veterinary management software increasingly integrates with other practice technology, such as digital imaging equipment of all sorts, laboratory equipment, bar code scanners, point-of-sales terminals, electronic signature capture, flat panel whiteboard displays, and time-keeping applications. VPIMS also include various programs that assist in education and communication with clients.

veterinary practice scorecard (VPS) A management processes tool adapted by Marsha L Heinke, CPA, Inc., based on concepts entailed in the balance scorecard methods widely published starting in the early 1990s. The VPS concept assists managers in identifying and targeting measurable performance goals in four operational quadrants: client perspective, patient perspective, employee perspective, and owner perspective. The VPS is intended to supplement and dovetail with other strategic planning systems and tools and to assist in the implementation, management, and outcome measurement of strategy.

vision statement An inspiring description of the underlying human values of the practice's mission that serves to guide beliefs and energize behaviors about how the practice team goes about its day-to-day activities. When shared publicly, the vision statement emotionally shapes client understanding about why they want to use the veterinary organization. See mission statement.

voice recognition software Computer software that allows a computer to recognize speech and convert it into a written format or perform specific actions in response to speech commands. The user of voice recognition software with a headset and microphone does not have to use the keyboard or mouse.

wait time The amount of time between the prearranged appointment time and the time the appointment actually begins; the amount of time the client has to wait to see the veterinarian or other veterinary professional.

wastage Loss of supplies and other purchased inventory items through waste or misuse. A form of inventory shrink. See also shrinkage.

wellness plan An insurance or prepaid service plan that pays for veterinary care provided to an animal for those services generally considered to be necessary to prevent disease and/or promote a healthy life. Most plans include vaccinations, periodic examinations, neutering, parasite management, and possibly dentistry.

wellness visit A patient appointment that centers on preventive health care and early detection of impending health problems, usually through complete physical examination and laboratory testing. As prevention is a hallmark, vaccination boosters and parasite management protocols may be part of the overall wellness visit. Practice plans can be devised to organize recommendations for frequency and timing of lifelong wellness visits, based on species and breed, as well as the services that should be generally included in the wellness visit at each stage of life.

workweek As defined by the Fair Labor Standards Act with reference to determining compliance with minimum wage laws, a workweek is 7 consecutive, regularly recurring, 24-hour periods totaling 168 hours.

write-off An amount charged to a client that is later removed from the financial records and deemed unrecoverable because of nonpayment.

References

Allbusiness.com. 2011. "Television Advertising Pros and Cons," May 17, www.allbusiness.com/small-business-tv-advertising/15583543-1.html.

Allen, Karen, Barbara E. Shykoff, and Joseph L. Izzo Jr. 2001. "Scientific Contributions: Pet Ownership, but not ACE Inhibitor Therapy, Blunts Home Blood Pressure Responses to Mental Stress." *Hypertension* 38: 815–820, http://hyper.ahajournals.org/content/38/4/815.full.

Allison, Thomas H. n.d. Lecture notes, course in medical records and documentation, Cleveland, Ohio.

American Animal Hospital Association (AAHA). n.d. *Medical Records Manual.* Lakewood, CO: AAHA Press.

———. 1995. *The 1995 AAHA Report: A Study of the Companion Animal Veterinary Services Market.* Lakewood, CO: AAHA Press.

———. 1995. "Move Over Cindy Crawford: Fido Has More Clout." Cyberpet.com, www.cyberpet.com/dogs/articles/general/crawford.htm.

———. 1997. "The Cost of Compassion." Lakewood, CO: AAHA Press.

———. 2000. *Hospital Standards and Accreditation Manual.* Lakewood, CO: AAHA Press.

———. 2003. *The Path to High-Quality Care.* Lakewood, CO: AAHA Press.

———. 2009. *AAHA Guide to Creating an Employee Handbook,* 3rd ed. Lakewood, CO: AAHA Press.

———. 2010. *Standard Abbreviations for Veterinary Medical Records.* Lakewood, CO: AAHA Press.

———. 2011. *Financial and Productivity Pulsepoints,* 6th ed. Lakewood, CO: AAHA Press.

American Association of Equine Practitioners (AAEP). 2009. "Equine Welfare: Unwanted Horse." AAEP, February, www.aaep.org/health_articles_view.php?id=334.

American Institute of Certified Public Accountants (AICPA). n.d. "IFRS FAQs: International Financial Reporting Standards." AICPA, www.ifrs.com/ifrs_faqs.html#q1.

———. 2005. *Management of an Accounting Practice Handbook,* rev. New York: AICPA.

American Veterinary Dental College. n.d. "Dental Charts," www.avdc.org/dental-charts.pdf.

American Veterinary Medical Association (AVMA). n.d. "AVMA Policy: Principles of Veterinary Medical Ethics of the AVMA," www.avma.org/issues/policy/ethics.asp.

———. *Marketing and Practice Strategies.* 1988. Schaumburg, IL: AVMA.

———. "Principles of Veterinary Medical Ethics." 2000. In *2000 AVMA Directory.* Schaumburg, IL: AVMA.

———. 2007. "AVMA Guidelines on Euthanasia." June, www.avma.org/issues/animal_welfare/euthanasia.pdf.

———. 2007. "Owner Consent in Veterinary Medicine." November, www.avma.org/issues/policy/owner_consent.asp.

———. 2007. Public Perceptions Survey. Schaumburg, IL: AVMA.

———. 2010. "Practical Guidance for the Effective Response by Veterinarians to Suspected Animal Cruelty, Abuse and Neglect." Schaumburg, IL: AVMA.

Ancom Business Products. 1999. Records Management catalog.

Association of Electrical and Medical Imaging Equipment Manufacturers. n.d. Digital Imaging and Communications in Medicine (DICOM) brochure. National Electrical Manufacturers Association, http://medical.nema.org/dicom/geninfo/brochure.pdf.

Beaulieu, Ken, ed. 2009. "The Key to Speaking Clearly: Know Your WPM to Deliver More Effective Sales Pitches." In "Effective Sales Techniques," Step by Step Marketing, Pohly Company, August 14, www.stepbystepmarketing.com/daily/effective_sales_techniques/the-key-to-speaking-clearly/.

Be Safe: Veterinary Safety Training for Medical and Technical Staff. 2007. DVD. Lakewood, CO: AAHA Press.

Be Safe: Veterinary Safety Training for the Whole Practice Team. 2007. DVD. Lakewood, CO: AAHA Press.

Boss, Nan. 2011. *Educating Your Clients from A to Z: What to Say and How to Say It*, 2nd ed. Lakewood, CO: AAHA Press.

Bower, John S.M., John N. Gripper, and S. Dixon Gunn. 1994. *Veterinary Practice Management*. Oxford, U.K.: Blackwell Scientific Publications.

Brakeman, Lynne. 1998. "Experts Share Techniques on Breaking Bad News Skillfully." In "Career Builder: A Business Primer for Veterinary Students," special supplement of *DVM Newsmagazine*, December.

Brauer, Markus, and Richard Y. Bourhis. 2006. "Social Power." *European Journal of Social Psychology* 35, no. 4.

Bregman, Peter. 2009. "When to Confront Someone: The Rule of Three." *Harvard Business Review* (HBR Blog Network), November 30.

Burns, Katie. 2011. "Solo Practitioners See a Place for Themselves." *JAVMA News*, December 15, www.avma.org/onlnews/javma/dec11/111215c.asp.

Carlson Learning Company. n.d. *Understanding Personal Listening Approaches: Introducing the Personal Listening Profile*. Minneapolis: Carlson Learning Company.

———. 1994. *Personal Profile System Facilitator's Manual*. Minneapolis: Carlson Learning Company.

Catanzaro, Tom. Veterinary Consulting International, Queensland. Interview with author.

———. 2009. *Zoned Systems and Schedules in Multi-Doctor Practices*. VCI Signature Series Monographs. Morrison, CO: Veterinary Consulting International.

Center for Educational Development and Assessment. n.d. "Communication Styles." The CEDA Meta-Profession Project, www.ceda.net.com/meta/communication_styles.htm.

Civil Rights Act (PL 88-352, 78 Stat. 241, enacted July 2, 1964). Title VII, 42 U.S.C., 2000e[2]. Available at Equal Employment Opportunity Commission website, www.eeoc.gov/laws/statutes/titlevii.cfm.

Clark, Andrew. 2011, "Your Reputation Is Your Brand . . . Who Is Managing Your Brand?" Blog, July 13, www.dvmmba.com/blog/2011/07/13/your-reputation-is-your-brand-who-is-managing-your-brand/.

Clinical Informatics n.d. Wiki. "Problem-Oriented Medical Information System," http://clinfowiki.org/wiki/index.php/Problem-Oriented_Medical_Information_System_(PROMIS).

Cohen, Mark. 2009. "Text-Message Marketing." *New York Times*, September 23, www.nytimes.com/2009/09/24/business/smallbusiness/24texting.html?pagewanted=all.

Collins, James C., and Jerry I. Porras. 1996. "Building Your Company's Vision." *Harvard Business Review*, September.

Collins, Jim. 2001. *Good to Great: Why Some Companies Make the Leap . . . And Others Don't*. New York: HarperBusiness.

Corley, Robert N., and Peter J. Shedd. 1990. *Fundamentals of Business Law*, 5th ed. Englewood Cliffs, NJ: Prentice Hall.

Cottle, David W. 2011. "Billing Myths." In American Institute of Certified Public Accountants (AICPA), *Management of an Accounting Practice Handbook*, rev. New York: AICPA, chap. 203.

Crook, D. Scott. n.d. "Best Practices for Employee Recordkeeping." Smith Hartvigsen PLLC, Salt Lake City, Utah, www.smithlawonline.com.

Crossen, Cynthia. 1997. "The Crucial Question for These Noisy Times May Just Be: 'Huh?'" *Wall Street Journal*, July 10.

Davis, Jennifer. 2010. "Dog Walking May Lead to Big Health Benefits." *Arthritis Today*, June 11.

Drucker, Peter F. 1954 [1993, 2006]. *The Practice of Management*. New York: Harper and Row.

Dun & Bradstreet Credibility Corp. n.d. "Why Do Many Small Businesses Fail?" http://smallbusiness.dnb.com/business-planning-structures/business-plans/1440-1.html.

Durrance, Dana, and Laurel Lagoni. 2010. *Connecting with Clients: Practical Communication for 10 Common Situations*. Lakewood, CO: AAHA Press.

Edelman. 2011. "Edelman Trust Barometer Executive Summary." Edelman.com, www.edelman.com/trust/2011/uploads/Trust%20Executive%20Summmary.PDF.

Edney, Andrew T.B. 1995. "Companion Animals and Human Health: An Overview." *Journal of the Royal Society of Medicine* 88: 704P–708P.

Edwards, Francis G. 1983. *Marketing of Professional Services.* Tulsa, OK: Pennwell Publishing.

Engel, James F., Martin R. Warshaw, and Thomas C. Kinnear. 1987. *Promotional Strategy: Managing the Marketing Communications Process.* Homewood, IL: Irwin.

Eppinger, Catharine T. 1997. *Creating Job Descriptions for Your Veterinary Support Staff.* Lakewood, CO: AAHA Press.

Equal Employment Opportunity Commission (EEOC). 2002. "Facts about Sexual Harassment." June 27, www.eeoc.gov/facts/fs-sex.html.

Federal Trade Commission (FTC). 2011. *Protecting Personal Information: A Guide for Business.* November, http://business.ftc.gov/sites/default/files/pdf/bus69-Protecting-Personal-Information-guide-business_0.pdf.

Fess, Philip E., and Carl S. Warren. 1987. *Accounting Principles*, 15th ed. Cincinnati: South-Western Publishing.

Finch, Lloyd. 1997. *Telephone Courtesy and Client Service.* Los Altos, CA: Crisp Publications.

Fisher, B. Aubrey, and Leonard C. Hawes. 1972. "An Interaction System Model of Small Group Decision Making." Unpublished mimeographed manuscript, University of Minnesota.

Frederickson, Clark. 2010. "Time Spent Watching TV Still Tops Internet." EMarketer.com, December 15, www.emarketer.com/blog/index.php/time-spent-watching-tv-tops-internet/.

Friedman, Nancy. 1987. "Five Forbidden Phrases." DVD no. 5, *Telephone Doctor Complete DVD Library.* St. Louis: Telephone Doctor.

———. 2011. Webinar sponsored by the Veterinary Hospital Medical Association, September 7.

Fritz, Kathy. 2008. "Managing Your Inventory Investment." Paper presented at Illinois State Veterinary 126th Annual Convention, Lombard, Illinois, November.

Froehlich, Robert E. 1987. *Successful Financial Management for the Veterinary Practice.* Lakewood, CO: AAHA Press.

Fulghum, Robert. 1988. *All I Really Need to Know I Learned in Kindergarten: Uncommon Thoughts on Common Things.* New York: Ballantine.

Gaedeke, Ralph M., and Dennis H. Tootelian. 1985. *Small Business Management*, 2nd ed. Glenview, IL: Scott Foresman.

Garbarino, John B. 1984. "Management of the Enterprise." Management 101, Lecture Notes. Fall.

Gawande, Atul. 2009. *The Checklist Manifesto: How to Get Things Right.* New York: Metropolitan Books.

Gerber, Michael. 1995. *The E-Myth Revisited: Why Most Small Businesses Don't Work and What to Do About It.* New York: HarperBusiness.

Gill, Brian. 1997. "Cross-Training Can Be a Win-Win Plan." *American Printer*, October.

Gillum, Bryan. 2011. "The Role of a Manager." Webinar sponsored by Ohio Society of CPAs, August 31, Columbus, Ohio.

Goldhaber, Gerald M. 1974 [1993]. *Organizational Communication*, 6th ed. Dubuque, IA: Wm. C. Brown.

Goleman, Daniel. 1995. *Emotional Intelligence: Why It Can Matter More Than IQ.* New York: Bantam.

Goodavage, Maria. 2011. "Survey: Dogs Really Are the New Kids." Dogster for the Love of Dog Blog, June 20, dogblog.dogster.com/2011/06/20/survey-dogs-really-are-the-new-kids/.

Gordon, Kim T. 2005. "Get in Front of Customers with Direct Mail." *Entrepreneur*, June, www.entrepreneur.com/magazine/entrepreneur/2005/june/77868.html.

Griffin, Matt. 2006. "Word of Mouth: Five Steps to Deal with Negative Customer Feedback." Retail Online Integration, November 28, www.allaboutroimag.com/article/word-mouth-five-steps-deal-with-negative-customer-feedback-41355_1.html.

Hannah, Harold W. 1996. "Veterinary Medical Records—Some Legal Issues." *Journal of the American Veterinary Medical Association* 209, no. 3.

Hansen, Heather E., and Jeffrey P. Brien. 2011. "Legal Concerns of EMR and PACS." Advance for Imaging & Radiation Oncology, February 7, http://imaging-radiation-oncology.advanceweb.com/Features /Articles/Legal-Concerns-of-EMR-and-PACS.aspx.

Harvard Business School. 2000. "American Business, 1920-2000: How It Worked—P&G: Changing the Face of Consumer Marketing." Working Knowledge for Business Leaders Archive, May 2, http://hbswk.hbs .edu/archive/1476.html.

Heagle, Chris, and Robb Heagle. 2005. Edited by Jim Stowe. *Receptionist Training Manual*. Guelph, Ontario: Lifelearn.

Heath, Chip, and Dan Heath. 2010. *Switch: How to Change Things When Change Is Hard*. New York: Random House.

Heathfield, Susan M. n.d. "How to Welcome a New Employee: Welcome Is More Than an Announcement." About.com, http://humanresources.about.com/od/orientation/a/welcome_letter.htm.

Heinke, Marsha L. 1998. "Don't Lose Out on a Great Profit Relationship." *Columbus Serum Company Journal*, Fall.

———. 1999. "The New Communication: E-Mail Etiquette Planner." *DVM Newsmagazine*, February. Adapted from Bill Howard, "Avoiding Clueless E-Mail," *PC Magazine*, May 26, 1998.

———. 1999. "Using Breakeven Analysis as a Starting Point for Product Pricing." *Columbus Serum Company Journal*, October-December.

———. 2006. "Ethics and Professional Laws Affect Strategic Planning." Paper presented at the AVMA Convention, Honolulu.

Hersey, Paul, and Kenneth Blanchard. 1982. *Management of Organizational Behavior*, 4th ed. Englewood Cliffs, NJ: Prentice Hall; 9th ed., 2007.

Hetts, Suzanne, and Daniel Q. Estep. 2005. *Raising a Behaviorally Healthy Puppy: A Pet Parenting Guide*. Littleton, CO: Island Dog Press.

Hetts, Suzanne, Marsha L. Heinke, and Daniel Q. Estep. 2004. "Commentary: Behavior Wellness Concepts for General Veterinary Practice." *Journal of the American Veterinary Medical Association* 225, no. 4: 506–513.

Hopkins, Alton F. 1984. "Pet Death: Effects on the Client and the Veterinarian." *In the Pet Connection: Proceedings of Conferences on the Human–Companion Animal Bond, June 13–14, 1983*. Minneapolis: University of Minnesota.

IBM. 2010 "Our Values at Work on Being an IBMer," www.ibm.com/ibm/values/us/.

Isadore, Chris. 2011. "Fed Gloomier about the Economy." CNN Money, June 22, http://money.cnn .com/2011/06/22/news/economy/federal_reserve_meeting/index.htm.

Johnson, Paul 2004. "The Top Five Reasons Why Strategic Plans Fail." Panache and Systems, August 20, http://archive.webpronews.com/ebusiness/management/wpn-36-20040820TheTopFiveReasonsWhy StrategicPlansFail.html.

Johnson, Spencer. 1998. *Who Moved My Cheese? An Amazing Way to Deal with Change in Your Work and in Your Life*. New York: G. P. Putnam's Sons.

Kahn, Steven C., Barbara Berish Brown, and Michael Lanzarone. 1999. *Legal Guide to Human Resources*. Boston: Warren, Gorham and Lamont.

Katz, Daniel, and Robert Kahn. 1966. *The Social Psychology of Organizations*. New York: John Wiley and Sons.

Kotler, Philip, and Kevin Lane Keller. 2008. *Marketing Management*, 13th ed. Upper Saddle River, NJ: Prentice Hall.

Kübler-Ross, Elisabeth. 1969. *On Death and Dying*. New York: Collier Books/MacMillan.

Lagoni, Laurel. 2011. *Connecting with Grieving Clients: Supportive Communication for Fourteen Common Situations*, 2nd ed. Lakewood, CO: AAHA Press.

Lawrence, P., and J. W. Lorsch. 1967. *Organization and Environment: Managing Differentiation and Integration*. Boston: Harvard University Graduate School of Business Administration.

List, Lorraine Monheiser. 2002. *AAHA Chart of Accounts*, 2nd ed. Lakewood, CO: AAHA Press.

London, Sheldon. 1998. *How to Comply with Federal Employee Laws: A Complete Guide for Employers Written in Plain English*, rev. ed. Rochester, NY: Vizia.

Love, Thomas. 1998. "Keeping the Business Going When an Executive Is Absent." *Nation's Business*, March.

Maxwell, John C. 2003. *Ethics 101: What Every Leader Needs to Know*. New York: Time Warner.

McCafferty, Owen E. 1989. "Computers: Luxury or Necessity?" *Veterinary Economics*, March.

———. 1990. "Selecting Professionals to Work with Your Veterinary Practice." *DVM Newsmagazine*.

———. 1995. "Improve Outcomes: Ask Clients for Their Opinions." Unpublished paper.

———. 1998. "Associate Burnout: Do You Know the Signs?" *DVM Newsmagazine*, May.

———. 1999. "Associate Burnout: Know Strategies and Signs," Parts 1 and 2. *DVM Newsmagazine*, January and March.

McCarthy, John B. 1998. "IRS Publishes Audit Technique Guide for Veterinary Medicine." *Journal of the American Veterinary Medical Association* 212, no. 11.

McCulloch, William F. 1985. "The Veterinarian's Education about the Human-Animal Bond and Animal Facilitated Therapy." *Veterinary Clinics of North America* 15, no. 2.

McCurnin, Dennis M. 1988. *Veterinary Practice Management*. Philadelphia: J. B. Lippincott.

McIntyre, Marie G. n.d. "Ten Steps to an Exceptional Coaching Discussion." Your Office Coach, www.yourofficecoach.com/Topics/conducting_coaching.htm.

Meigs, Walter B., and Robert F. Meigs. 1986. *Financial Accounting*, 4th ed. New York: McGraw-Hill.

Meyer, John L., and Carolyn C. Shadle. 1994. *The Changing Outplacement Process: New Methods and Opportunities for Transition Management*. New York: Praeger.

Miller, George W., III. 1998. Notes from the Annual Meeting of the Veterinary Hospital Managers Association, Atlanta.

Murray-Hicks, Margo. 1988. "Marketing Basics for Small Entrepreneurs." Lecture presented at Training 88 Conference, Margo Murray-Hicks and Associates, Oakland, California, December 14.

Myers, Wendy. n.d. Communication Solutions for Veterinarians. Website, www.csvets.com.

National Association of Veterinary Technicians in America (NAVTA). 1998. "Bits & Pieces." March.

Nolan, Monica. 2010. "Turning Negative Customer Feedback into a Positive." Ezine Articles, February 15, http://ezinearticles.com/?Turning-Negative-Customer-Feedback-Into-a-Positive&id=3139145.

Nyland, Heidi, with Marsha L. Heinke. 2006. "At the Core: Incorporate Your Values into Your Practice." *Equine Veterinary Management*, Spring, 24–28.

Osborne, Jayne, ed. 1995. *CPA's Human Resource Administration Handbook*. San Diego: Harcourt, Brace.

Pear, Robert. 2011. "As Health Costs Soar, G.O.P. and Insurers Differ on Cause." *New York Times*, March 3, www.nytimes.com/2011/03/05/health/policy/05cost.html.

Pogue, David. 2010. "Talk to the Machine: Progress in Speech-Recognition Software." *Scientific American*, December 20, www.scientificamerican.com/article.cfm?id=talk-to-the-machine.

Porter, Michael E. 1980. *Competitive Strategy: Techniques for Analyzing Industries and Competitors*. New York: The Free Press.

———. 1985. *Competitive Advantage: Creating and Sustaining Superior Performance*. New York: The Free Press.

"Presentation Tips: Porter 5 Forces Analysis." n.d. Presentation Help Desk, www.presentationhelpdesk.com/porter-5-force-html.

Princeton Insurance. 2008. "Electronic Medical Records: Patient Safety & Risk Management Guide," www.pinsco.com/downloads/EMRUsersGuide_final.pdf.

Pritchett, Price, and Ron Pound. 2008. *The Employee Handbook for Organizational Change*. Dallas: Pritchett and Associates.

QuickMBA. n.d. "The Strategic Planning Process." Internet Center for Management and Business Administration, http://quickmba.com/strategy/strategic-planning/.

Raps, Andreas. 2004. "Implementing Strategy: Tap into the Power of Four Key Factors to Deliver Success." *Strategic Finance*, June.

Reference for Business. n.d. "Cross Training," www.referenceforbusiness.com/small/Co-Di/Cross-Training.html.

Reh, F. John. n.d. "Cross Training Employees Saves You Money, Makes Them Happy." About.com, http://management.about.com/cs/people/a/crosstrain.htm.

Remillard, James. 1995. "Essentials of Internal Practice Promotion." *In Business Management for the Veterinary Practitioner*, ed. David Chubb. Denver: Chubb Communications.

Rezendes, Allison, and Susan C. Kahler. 2007. "Executive Board Coverage." *JAVMA News*, December 15, www.avma.org/onlnews/javma/dec07/071215d.asp.

Rogerson, Lynda. 1993. "Cover Your Bases." *Small Business Reports*, July.

Russell, Ray. 1996. *The Miracle of Personal Leadership*. Dubuque, IA: Kendall/Hunt.

Salmon, Peter, Ann Rappaport, Mike Bainbridge, Glyn Hayes, and John Williams. 1996. "Taking the POMR Forward." Proceedings of the American Medical Informatics Association (AMIA) Annual Fall Symposium, http://www.ncbi.nlm.nih.gov/pmc/articles/PMC2233232/pdf/procamiaafs00002-0500.pdf.

Salzieder, Karl R. 2007. *The 5-Minute Veterinary Practice Management Consult*. Ames, IA: Blackwell.

Schakenbach, Jim. 2007. "Continuity: Creating an Image Greater Than the Parts." About.com, http://marketing.about.com/od/brandstrategy/a/mktgcontinuity.htm.

Schultz, Jan R. 1988. "A History of the PROMIS Technology: An Effective Human Interface." In *A History of Personal Workstations*, Adele Goldberg, ed. Reading, MA: Addison-Wesley.

Scott, John F. 2007. *The 5-Minute Veterinary Practice Management Consult*. Ames, IA: Blackwell.

Seibert, Philip J. 2007. *Be Safe! Manager's Guide to Veterinary Workplace Safety*, AAHA Press.

"Selective Inventory Control." n.d. National Institute of Calicut, http://124.124.70.22/nitc/bulletin/files/opt_25422_2146861206.pdf.

Sheridan, John P., and Owen E. McCafferty. 1993. *The Business of Veterinary Practice*. Terrytown, NY: Pergamon Press.

Slater, Bruce. 2007. "Online Health Records." Session in online course, "Electronic Commerce and Online Market for Health Services." George Mason University, Online Market for Health Services, http://gunston.gmu.edu/722/OnlineMedicalRecord.asp.

Smith, Carin A. 2009. *Client Satisfaction Pays: Quality Service for Practice Success*, 2nd ed. Lakewood, CO: AAHA Press.

Starch, Daniel. 1988. In *Harvard Business Review* 1, no. 1 (1922). Quoted in *Harvard Business Review* 66, no. 3.

Stevenson, William J. 2009. *Operations Management*. New York: McGraw-Hill.

Stockner, Priscilla K. 1983. *A Practice Management Manual for Veterinarians*. Lake San Marcos, CA: Stockner and Associates.

———. 1995. "What to Do with 'Old Records.'" In *Business Management for the Veterinary Practitioner*, ed. David Chubb. Denver: Chubb Communications.

———. "Inventory Control Equals Hidden Profits." *Trends* 111, no. 2.

Stone, Kathlyn. 2011. "Drug Shortages." About.com, February 15 (rev. November 22), http://pharma.about.com/od/Manufacturing-and-Technology/i/Drug-Shortages.htm.

Tannenbaum, Jerrold. 1989 [1995]. *Veterinary Ethics: Animal Welfare, Client Relations, Competition and Collegiality*, 2nd ed. St. Louis: Mosby.

Tapper, Ron. n.d. Practice Orientation Notes. Emerald Hills Animal Veterinary Hospital, Florida.

Thill, John V., and Courtland L. Bovee. 1993 [1996]. *Excellence in Business Communication*, 2nd ed. New York: McGraw Hill.

Thompson, Dennis, Jr. 2011. "Pet Therapy and Depression." Medically reviewed by Niya Jones, MD, MPH. Everyday Health, October 26, www.everydayhealth.com/depression/pet-therapy-and-depression.aspx.

Tootelian, Dennis H., and Ralph M. Gaedke. 1984. *Small Business Management*. Boston: Scott, Foresman.

Trupanion. n.d. "European Influence and Market Share," http://trupanion.com/pet-insurance/european-influence-and-market-share.

U.S. Citizenship and Immigration Services (USCIS). n.d. Website, www.uscis.gov/portal/site/uscis.

U.S. Department of Justice, Drug Enforcement Agency. 1990. *Physicians Manual: An Informational Outline of the Controlled Substances Act of 1970*, rev. ed. Washington, DC: Government Printing Office.

U.S. Department of Labor. n.d. "ELaws: Fair Labor Standards Act Advisor. Exemptions," www.dol.gov/elaws/esa/flsa/screen75.asp.

U.S. Department of Labor, Employee Benefits Security Administration. n.d. "Health Care Reform and COBRA: Frequently Asked Questions," www.dol.gov/ebsa/faqs/faq-healthcarereform.html.

U.S. Department of Labor, Wage and Hour Division. n.d. *Fair Labor Standards Act*. PowerPoint presentation, produced in conjunction with the Employment Standards Administration, www.dol.gov/whd/flsa/comprehensive.ppt.

———. 1993. "Family and Medical Leave Act," www.dol.gov/whd/fmla/.

———. 2008. "Fact Sheet #21: Recordkeeping Requirements under the Fair Labor Standards Act (FLSA)." July (revision), www.dol.gov/whd/regs/compliance/whdfs21.pdf.

———. 2008. "Fact Sheet #170: Technologists and Technicians and the Part 541 Exemptions under the Fair Labor Standards Act (FLSA)." July (revision), www.dol.gov/whd/regs/compliance/fairpay/fs17o_technicians.htm.

———. 2010. "Fact Sheet #28A: The Family and Medical Leave Act Military Family Leave Entitlements." February (revision), www.dol.gov/whd/regs/compliance/whdfs28a.pdf.

U.S. Department of the Treasury, Internal Revenue Service. n.d. Website, www.irs.gov.

———. 1998. *Audit Technique Guide—Veterinary Medicine*. Market Segment Specialization Program. Washington, DC: Government Printing Office.

———. 2005. *Veterinary Audit Technique Guide (ATG)*. April, www.irs.gov/businesses/small/article/0,,id=141316,00.html.

———. 2008. "Independent Contractor or Employee . . . " Publication 1779, August (revision), Catalog no. 16134L, www.irs.gov/pub/irs-pdf/p1779.pdf.

———. 2009. "Proper Worker Classification." Video. June 17. Available with transcript at www.irsvideos.gov/ProperWorkerClassification.

———. 2011. "Barter Exchanges." Updated July 11, www.irs.gov/businesses/small/article/0,,id=113437,00.html.

U.S. Food and Drug Administration. n.d. "What Is MedWatch?" www.fda.gov/medwatch.

U.S. Small Business Administration. n.d. "FAQs: Frequently Asked Questions: Advocacy Small Business Statistics and Research," http://web.sba.gov/faqs/faqIndexAll.cfm?areaid=24.

Usry, Milton F., and Lawrence H. Hammer. 1991. *Cost Accounting: Planning and Control*, 10th ed. Mason, OH: South-Western Publishing.

Veterinary Hospital Managers Association (VHMA). n.d. "Certified Veterinary Practice Manager: A Professional's Recognition in Veterinary Practice Management," http://vhma.org/displaycommon.cfm?an=1&subarticlenbr=214.

———. n.d. "Code of Ethics," www.vhma.org/displaycommon.cfm?an=1.

Veterinary Pharmacy Reference (VPR). n.d. Website, www.vpronline.com.

Veterinary Study Groups, Inc. n.d. Website, www.veterinarystudygroups.inc.

Weed, L. L. 1968. "Medical Records That Guide and Teach." *New England Journal of Medicine* 278, no. 11: 593–599, and 278, no. 12: 652–657.

Welsch, Glenn A., and Charles T. Zlatkovich. 1989. *Intermediate Accounting*, 8th ed. Homewood, IL: Richard D. Irwin.

Wiio, Osmo. 1978. *Wiio's Laws—and Some Others*. Expoo, Finland: Welin-Goos.

Wilson, James F. 1988. *Law and Ethics of the Veterinary Profession*. Yardley, PA: Priority Press.

———. 1995. "Managing Your Credit Policy." In *Business Management for the Veterinary Practitioner*, ed. David Chubb. Denver: Chubb Communications.

———. 2006. *Legal Consent Forms for Veterinary Practices*. Lakewood, CO: AAHA Press.

Wilson, James F., and Karen Gendron. 2005. *Job Descriptions and Training Schedules for the Veterinary Team*. Lakewood, CO: AAHA Press.

Wilson, James F., and Carol McConnell. 2002. *The Veterinary Receptionist's Training Manual*. Lakewood, CO: AAHA Press.

Additional Resources

Accounting and Bookkeeping Management

BOOKS

Cavanaugh, David C. Lorraine Monheiser List, and Byron G. Porter. *AAHA Chart of Accounts*, 2nd ed. Lakewood, CO: AAHA Press.

Chamblee, Justin, and Max Reiboldt. 2010. *Financial Management of the Veterinary Practice*. Lakewood, CO: AAHA Press.

Heinke, Marsha L. 2006. *The Equine Veterinary Practice Chart of Accounts*. Published courtesy of Pfizer Animal Health, Webster Veterinary Supply, and Milburn Equine.

Heinke, Marsha L., and Rachel A. Forthofer, et, al. 2014. *VMG Companion Animal Chart of Accounts and Financial Management*. Las Vegas, NV: Veterinary Study Groups, Inc.

OTHER RESOURCES

American Institute of Professional Bookkeepers. Bookkeeping Tips (e-newsletter subscription). www.aipb.org

North American Business Association (NABA). www.aahanet.org/Membership/NABA.aspx.

Computer Systems

BOOKS

Oberst, Byron B., and John M. Long. 2011. *Computers in Private Practice Management*. New York: Springer-Verlag.

ARTICLES

Hardesty, Constance. 2013. "Management Case Study: Electronic Medical Records Planning." *Trends*, June.

Williams, Ben. 2013. "Virtual Software Roundtable: Experts and Vendors Opine on Top Software Questions." *Trends*, Sept. and Oct.

PERIODICALS

PC Magazine

Financial Management

BOOKS

Cavanaugh, David C. Lorraine Monheiser List, and Byron G. Porter. 2002. *AAHA Chart of Accounts*, 2nd Ed. Lakewood, CO: AAHA Press.

American Animal Hospital Association (AAHA). Publishes biennially. *Financial and Productivity Pulsepoints*. Lakewood, CO: AAHA Press.

American Animal Hospital Association (AAHA). Publishes biennially. *The Veterinary Fee Reference*. Lakewood, CO: AAHA Press.

CCH Inc. *The U.S. Master Tax Guide*. Published annually. Chicago: CCH.

Chamblee, Justin, and Max Reiboldt. 2010. *Financial Management of the Veterinary Practice*. Lakewood, CO: AAHA Press.

Hammer, Lawrence H. 2005. *Cost Accounting*, 14th ed. Boston, MA: Cengage Learning.

Internal Revenue Service. 2011. Internal Revenue Code. www.irs.gov.

North American Business Association (NABA). www.aahanet.org/Membership/NABA.aspx.

TRAINING PROGRAMS

American Animal Hospital Association. Veterinary Management School. www.aahanet.org/Education.

American Animal Hospital Association. Veterinary Management Institute. www.aahanet.org/Education.

OTHER RESOURCES

American Institute of Certified Public Accountants (AICPA). www.aicpa.org.

General Management

BOOKS

Ackerman, Lowell. 2013. *Blackwell's Five-Minute Practice Management Consult*. New York: Wiley-Blackwell.

American Animal Hospital Association (AAHA). *Hospital Standards and Accreditation Manual*. Lakewood, CO: AAHA Press.

Blanchard, Ken, Susan Fowler, and Laurence Hawkins. 2005. *Self Leadership and the One-Minute Manger: Increasing Effectiveness Through Situational Self Leadership*. New York: HarperCollins.

Cottrell, David. 2005. *Twelve Choices That Lead to Your Success*. Cornerstone Leadership Institute.

Drucker, Peter F. 1954. *The Practice of Management*. Reprint, New York: Harper and Row, 1993.

Gaedeke, Ralph M., and Dennis H. Tootelian. 1985. *Small Business Management*. Glenview, IL: Scott Foresman.

Gerber, Michael E. 2004. *The E-Myth Revisited: Why Most Small Businesses Don't Work and What To Do About It*. New York: HarperCollins.

Heath, Chip, and Dan Heath. 2010. *Switch: How to Change Things When Change Is Hard*. New York: Crown Business/Random House.

Maxwell, John C. 2005. *Ethics 101: What Every Leader Needs to Know*. New York: Center Street.

ARTICLES

Blaney Flietner, Maureen. 2013. "Making the Grade: Using Benchmarking to Improve Your Practice's Performance." *Trends*, Dec.

PERIODICALS

DVM Newsmagazine. Published by Advanstar Communications, Inc.

Harvard Business Review

Inc. Magazine

Trends Magazine. Published by the American Animal Hospital Association (AAHA), Lakewood, Colorado.

Veterinary Economics. Published by the Veterinary Medicine Publishing Company, Lenexa, Kansas.

Veterinary Forum. Published by Forum Publications, Fairway, Kansas.

Veterinary Practice News. Published by Fancy Publications, Irvine, California.

Wall Street Journal

TRAINING PROGRAMS

American Animal Hospital Association. Annual Meeting. www.aahanet.org/Education.

American Veterinary Medical Association (AVMA). Annual Meeting. www.avmaconvention.org.

American Animal Hospital Association. Veterinary Management School. www.aahanet.org/Education.

American Animal Hospital Association. Veterinary Management Institute. www.aahanet.org/Education.

OTHER RESOURCES

American Animal Hospital Association (AAHA). www.aahanet.org.

American Veterinary Medical Association (AVMA). www.avma.org.

DVM Newsmagazine. http://veterinarynews.dvm360.com/.

Food and Drug Administration. www.fda.gov.

North American Veterinary Technicians Association (NAVTA). www.avma.org/navta/default.htm.

Veterinary Hospital Managers Association (VHMA). www.vhma.org.

Veterinary Information Network (VIN). www.vin.com.

Veterinary Hospital Managers Association (VHMA). www.vhma.org. Forms bank.

Veterinary Hospital Managers Association (VHMA). www.vhma.org. Guidelines for Applying for Veterinary Practice Manager Certification.

Veterinary Practitioners' Reporting Program (VPRP). www.usp.org/prn/vprp.htm, or call 800-487-7776.

Human–Companion Animal Bond Management

BOOKS

Ayl, Kathleen. 2013. *When Helping Hurts: Compassion Fatigue in the Veterinary Industry.* Lakewood, CO: AAHA Press.

Durrance, Dana, and Laurel Lagoni. 2010. *Connecting with Clients: Practical Communication for 10 Common Situations* (2d ed.). Lakewood, CO: AAHA Press.

Figley, Charles R., and Robert G. Roop. 2006. *Compassion Fatigue in the Animal Care Community.* Humane Society Press.

Hetts, Suzanne, and Daniel Q. Estep. 2005. *Raising a Behaviorally Healthy Puppy: A Pet Parenting Guide.* Littleton, CO: Island Dog Press.

Montgomery, Mary, and Herb Montgomery. 1991. *Good-bye My Friend: Grieving the Loss of a Pet.* Minneapolis: Montgomery Press.

Montgomery, Mary, and Herb Montgomery. 1993. *A Final Act of Caring: Ending the Life of an Animal Friend.* Minneapolis: Montgomery Press.

Smith, Patricia. 2009. *Healthy Caregiving: A Guide to Recognizing and Managing Compassion Fatigue.* CreateSpace.

ARTICLES

Shadle, Carolyn, and John Meyer. 2013. "Empathy in the Veterinary Clinic." *Trends,* Feb.

OTHER RESOURCES

American Veterinary Medical Association (AVMA). www.avma.org/PersonalDevelopment.

Argus Institute, Colorado State University Veterinary Teaching Hospital. csu-cvmbs.colostate.edu/vth/diagnostic-and-support/argus.

Pet Partners. www.petpartners.org.

Inventory Control and Management

BOOKS

Guenther, James E. 2010. *101 Veterinary Inventory Questions Answered.* Lakewood, CO: AAHA Press.

Marketing Management

BOOKS

Brogdon, Robin. 2011. *101 Veterinary Marketing Questions Answered*. Lakewood, CO: AAHA Press.

Schultz, Mike, and John E. Doerr. 2013. *Professional Services Marketing: How the Best Firms Build Premier Brands, Thriving Lead Generation Engines, and Cultures of Business Development Success*. New York: Wiley.

Scott, David Meerman. 2011. *The New Rules of Marketing and PR: How to Use Social Media, Online Video, Mobile Applications, Blogs, News Releases, and Viral Marketing to Reach Buyers*. John Wiley & Sons.

ARTICLES

Fernandez, Kim. 2013. "Leap Ahead: SIVA Marketing Goes Beyond Ads and Postcards." *Trends*, Dec.

Medical Records Management

BOOKS

American Animal Hospital Association (AAHA). 2000. *Standard Abbreviations for Medical Records*, 3rd ed. Lakewood, CO: AAHA Press.

American Animal Hospital Association (AAHA), and Pfizer Animal Health. 2009. *Six Steps to Higher-Quality Patient Care*. Lakewood, CO: AAHA Press.

Gawande, Atul. 2011. *The Checklist Manifesto: How to Get Things Right*. Picador.

Wilson, James F. 2006. *Legal Consent Forms for Veterinary Practices*, 4th ed. Yardley, PA: Priority Press, Ltd.

OTHER RESOURCES

American Animal Hospital Association (AAHA). Forms and Logs. Lakewood, CO: AAHA Press.

American Animal Hospital Association (AAHA). Progress Notes stickers. Lakewood, CO: AAHA Press.

Ancom Business Products, www.ancom-filing.com. Comprehensive filing systems, alpha and numeric; color coding; office filing systems; furniture.

Personnel Management

BOOKS

ADA Handbook (Title I). 2010. Washington, DC: U.S. Department of Justice and Equal Employment Opportunity Commission (EEOC). www.ada.gov.

American Animal Hospital Association (AAHA). 2009. *AAHA Guide to Creating an Employee Handbook*, 3rd ed. Lakewood, CO: AAHA Press.

American Animal Hospital Association (AAHA). Publishes periodically. *Compensation and Benefits*. Lakewood, CO: AAHA Press.

Americans with Disabilities Act Compliance Manual for [your state]. Available for some states.

Blanchard, Ken, and Spencer Johnson. 2003. *The One Minute Manager* (10th anniv. ed.). Berkeley Trade.

Boss, Nan. 2011. *Educating Your Clients from A to Z: What to Say and How to Say It*. Lakewood, CO: AAHA Press.

Pittampalli, Al. 2011. *Read This Before Our Next Meeting: The Modern Meeting Standard for Successful Organizations*. Do You Zoom.

Seibert, Philip J. 2014. *Manager's Guide to Veterinary Workplace Safety*, 2nd ed. Lakewood, CO: AAHA Press.

Wilson, James F., Jeffrey D. Nemoy, and Alan J. Fishman. 2009. *Contracts, Benefits, and Practice Management for the Veterinary Profession*. Yardley, PA: Priority Press.

Wilson, James F. 2006. *Legal Consents for Veterinary Practices*, 4th ed. Yardley, PA: Priority Press.

Wilson, James F., and Karen Gendron. *Job Descriptions and Training Schedules for Veterinary Hospital Staff*. Yardley, PA: Priority Press.

PERIODICALS
Veterinary Safety & Health Digest. Write to Philip Seibert, RR 1 Box 313, Calhoun, TN 37309-9608.

TRAINING PROGRAMS
American Animal Hospital Association. Veterinary Management School. www.aahanet.org/Education.

American Animal Hospital Association. Veterinary Management Institute. www.aahanet.org/Education.

WEBSITES
Occupational Safety and Health Administration, www.osha.gov.

U.S. Department of Health and Human Services, www.hhs.gov.

U.S. Department of Labor, www.dol.gov.

OTHER RESOURCES
American Animal Hospital Association (AAHA). Employment Application. Lakewood, CO: AAHA Press.

Compliance Poster Company. www.complianceposter.com/. Employee law posters.

Equal Employment Opportunities Commission (EEOC). *ADA: Your Employment Rights as an Individual*. Washington, DC: EEOC.

Equal Employment Opportunity Commission (EEOC). *ADA: Your Responsibilities as an Employer*. Washington, DC: EEOC.

Equal Employment Opportunity Commission (EEOC). *Questions and Answers on the ADA*. Washington, DC: EEOC.

G. Neil. www.gneil.com. Forms, software, labor law resources, greeting cards, employee screening resources.

Lab Safety Supply. www.labsafety.com/. Safety posters and workplace safety supplies.

Reception and Front-Desk Procedures and Management

BOOKS
Durrance, Dana, and Laurel Lagoni. 2010. *Connecting with Clients: Practical Communication for Ten Common Situations*, 2nd ed. Lakewood, CO: AAHA Press.

Lagoni, Laurel, and Dana Durrance. 2011. *Connecting with Grieving Clients: Supportive Communication for Fourteen Common Situations*. Lakewood, CO: AAHA Press.

Lee, Fred. 2004. *If Disney Ran Your Hospital: 9½ Things You Would Do Differently*. Second River Healthcare.

McClister, M.T., and Amy Midgley. 2014. *The Veterinary Receptionist's Handbook*, 3rd ed. Lenexa: KS: Veterinary Medicine Publishing Group.

Renfrew, Jill. 2013. *AAHA's Complete Guide for the Client Service Representative*. Lakewood, CO: AAHA Press.

Smith, Carin. 2009. *Client Satisfaction Pays*, 2nd ed. Lakewood, CO: AAHA Press.

Strategic Planning

BOOKS
Catanzaro, Thoman E. 1997–1998. *Building the Successful Veterinary Practice* (three-book series). Wiley-Blackwell.

Collins, Jim. 2001. *From Good to Great: Why Some Companies Make the Leap … and Others Don't*. New York: HarperBusiness.

Collins, Jim, and Morten T. Hansen. 2011. *Great by Choice: Uncertainty, Chaos, and Luck—Why Some Thrive Despite Them All*. New York: HarperBusiness.

Index

About the Author

MARSHA L. HEINKE, DVM, EA, CPA, CVPM, earned her Doctor of Veterinary Medicine degree in 1979 and followed that with Enrolled Agent, Certified Public Accountant, and Certified Veterinary Practice Manager certifications. Most recently, Dr. Heinke has dedicated herself to the veterinary profession through her accounting and consulting practice, Marsha L. Heinke, CPA, Inc. In addition to speaking at veterinary conferences and facilitating study groups, she shares knowledge and advice through her writing, having written numerous articles and authored and coauthored books for the veterinary profession.